Neuropsychology

A CLINICAL APPROACH

To Francis Patrick Bowler

For Churchill Livingstone:

Commissioning editor: Michael Parkinson
Project editor: Barbara Simmons
Production controller: Frances Affleck
Design direction: Erik Bigland

Neuropsychology

A CLINICAL APPROACH

Kevin Walsh AO
BA MB BS MSc FBPsS
Senior Associate, University of Melbourne

David Darby
MB BS PhD FRACP
Associate (Behavioural Neurology), University of Melbourne

FOURTH EDITION

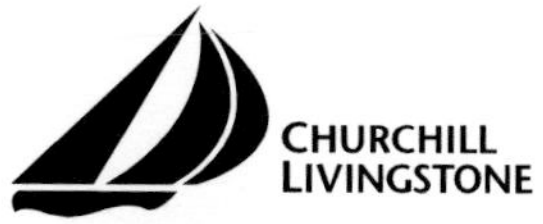

EDINBURGH LONDON NEW YORK PHILADELPHIA SYDNEY
TORONTO 1999

CHURCHILL LIVINGSTONE
An imprint of Harcourt Brace and Company Limited

Churchill Livingstone, 1–3 Baxter's Place, Leith Walk,
Edinburgh EH1 3AF

ISBN 0443 060517

British Library of Cataloguing in Publication Data
A catalogue record for this book is available from the British Library.

Library of Congress Cataloging in Publication Data
A catalog record for this book is available from the Library of Congress.

Medical knowledge is constantly changing. As information becomes available, changes in treatment, procedures, equipment and the use of drugs become necessary. The author and publisher have, as far as it is possible, taken care to ensure that the information given in the text is accurate and up-to-date. However, readers are strongly advised to confirm that the information, especially with regard to drug usage, complies with current legislation and standard of practice.

The publisher's policy is to use **paper manufactured from sustainable forests**

Printed in China

Preface

The expansion of neuropsychology continues and the growth of such subspecialities as cognitive neuropsychology and experimental neuropsychology means that even in a general introductory text like our own there must be restrictions. To cope with this expansion there has been a light pruning of some previous sections to allow for treatment of clinical issues in line with our major orientation. This pruning has been in the areas of such topics as sensory disturbances, experimental neuropsychology and some of the more detailed neuroanatomy. Major parts of the outline of neuroanatomy have been retained so that those without formal training in the subject will have a ready source with which to read the appropriate medical journals in which many of the clinical conditions of interest to neuropsychologists are described. This is more important than ever as the dissection of psychological functions by cognitive neuropsychologists proceeds and is related in an increasingly specific and detailed way to the structure of the brain.

The growth of cross-fertilization between the psychological and neurological disciplines, which is a heartening sign of the present times, is being greatly aided by the presence of specialists in different areas who take the effort to 'learn two (or more) languages'. The coming together of the major disciplines is treated in the final chapter.

A final new section on forensic neuropsychology has been added to introduce some of the special issues to be considered when neuropsychologists are requested to assist the courts.

As in the previous edition, an attempt has been made to make up for the limited treatment of some subject matter by providing in the body of the text reference to more specialized sources of information.

Melbourne
1999

K.W.
D.D.

Acknowledgements

We would like to express our thanks to the Medical Librarians, in particular the Senior Librarian Ann McLean, and Philippa McEniry who were the backbone of the enterprise. We would also like to acknowledge the assistance of all those colleagues who regularly contributed to case presentations and discussions in meetings.

Contents

1

History of neuropsychology

ANCIENT CIVILIZATION

The earliest written information we possess on localization of function in the brain is contained in the Edwin Smith Surgical Papyrus. The copy acquired by Smith in Luxor in 1862 is thought to date from the 17th century BC, while orthographic and other evidence would place its origin some thousand years earlier, somewhere between 2500 and 3000 BC. It contains the earliest known anatomical, physiological and pathological descriptions and has been described as the earliest known scientific document.

The papyrus contains reports of some 48 cases of observations and description of treatment of actual cases, many of them suffering from traumatic lesions of various parts of the body including many injuries to the head and neck. Translation of the papyrus was undertaken in 1920 and the detailed examination of the text and commentary was published by Breasted in 1930. It is in this papyrus that a word for brain appears for the first time. The papyrus 'opens the door on cortical localization of function with its description of injuries to the brain' (Gibson 1962).

The material of the papyrus may be divided into two parts, namely, the original text and the explanatory comments which have been added at a later date to expand and clarify the text. That these glosses which appear on the back (verso) of the manuscript are of a much later date is witnessed by their explanation of terms in the texts which had, by the time of our extant copy, apparently become obsolete.

Of the 48 cases the first eight deal directly with injuries to the head and brain. Though some of the injuries may have been sustained in civilian occupations, it is more than likely that many of them, as well as wounds described in other parts of the body, were sustained in war. If so, this would be the earliest recording of the contribution of the study of war wounds to the study of brain–behaviour relationships, a source which has been of paramount importance in more recent times.

The following cases serve to illustrate the careful observations made by the ancient medical practitioner. The direct quotations are from Breasted (1930). Thirteen cases of most interest to the neurological scientist have been reprinted in Wilkins (1965).

1. The examination of case four reads in part:

> If thou examinest a man having a gaping wound in his head, penetrating to the bone, (and) splitting his skull, thou shouldst palpate his wound. Shouldst thou find something disturbing therein under thy fingers, (and) he shudders exceedingly…

The shuddering which occurred upon the surgeon's palpation may refer to convulsive movements produced by pressure upon the exposed brain. It is reminiscent of the extraordinary case described by Gibson (1962).

2. Case six described a skull fracture with rupture of the coverings of the brain.

> If thou examinest a man having a gaping wound in his head, penetrating to the bone, smashing his skull, (and) rendering open the brain of his skull, thou shouldst palpate his wound. Shouldst thou find that smash which is in his skull (like) those corrugations which form in molten copper, (and) something therein throbbing (and) fluttering under thy fingers, like the weak place of an infant's crown before it becomes whole - when it has happened there is no throbbing (and) fluttering under thy fingers until the brain of his (the patient's) skull is rent open – (and) he discharges blood from his nostrils, (and) he suffers with stiffness in his neck, (conclusion in diagnosis).
>
> The commentator has written two glosses in clarification:
>
> *Gloss A*
> As for: 'Smashing his skull, (and) rendering open the brain of his skull,' (it means) the smash is large, opening to the interior of his skull, (to) the membrane enveloping his brain, so that it breaks open his fluid in the interior of his head.
>
> *Gloss B*
> As for: 'Those corrugations which form on molten copper,' it means copper which the coppersmith pours off (rejects) before it is forced into the mould, because of something foreign upon it like wrinkle.

Here is a clear description of the meninges and an awareness of the cerebrospinal fluid which bathes the brain, together with a picturesque but apt description of the appearance of the brain's convolutions.

3. In a further example (case eight) we are introduced to statements which obviously relate brain injury to disordered function, that is, the earliest recorded findings in neurophysiology or functional neurology.

> If thou examinest a man having a smash of his skull, under the skin of his head, while there is nothing at all upon it, thou shouldst palpate his wound. Shouldst thou find that there is a swelling protruding on the outside of that smash which is in his skull, while his eye is askew because of it, on the side of him having that injury which is in his skull; (and) he walks shuffling with his sole, on the side of him having the injury which is in his skull…

The ancient Egyptian has noted that injury to the brain may affect other parts of the body, here the eye and the lower limb. The shuffling of the foot presumably refers to the weakness of one side of the body produced by damage to the motor pathways from their origin in the cortex of the brain, what would now be termed hemiparesis. The manuscript had been written so long before that the commentator had to explain the obsolete word for shuffle. The physician who wrote the manuscript also appears to have been aware that the effects of brain injury varied according to the side of the brain receiving the injury.

Breasted notes that the physician has reported weakness of the limb on the same side as the head injury and suggests that the physician may have been misled by a *contre-coup* effect. If so, this could be the first of innumerable occasions in the history of neurology where an incorrect inference has been made on the basis of accurate observation through lack of sufficient information. The contre-coup effect refers to the fact that trauma to the head may produce injury to the brain either beneath the site of external injury (*coup*), or to an area of brain opposite to the external injury (*contre-coup*). Examples are depicted in Figure 3.8. Since damage to the motor region of the brain produces weakness or paralysis of the opposite side of the body, a contre-coup injury may give the appearance of weakness on the same side as the scalp or skull wound.

Apart from these examples of effects resulting from brain injury, the papyrus also describes several effects of spinal injury, e.g. seminal emission, urinary incontinence and quadriplegia as a result of injury to the cervical portion of the spine. There appears to be no evidence, however, that the author considered the brain and spinal cord to be part of a single system.

While the Edwin Smith Surgical Papyrus described head injury there was no reference to common behavioural manifestations such as post-traumatic amnesia. Another work, the Papyrus Ebers (Ebell 1937), contains a general recognition of organic causes of forgetfulness.

Turning from Egypt to the other ancient cradle of civilization in the Tigris and Euphrates valleys we find evidence that medical and surgical practice was well organized and legally regulated in this region in the latter part of the third millennium BC. Information from this civilization was however recorded on fragile clay tablets which have largely perished and even the few surviving fragments from a much later period provide us with no evidence of knowledge of brain–behaviour relationships possessed by these great peoples. It is unfortunate that no surgical treatise, if such existed, has survived from ancient Assyria and Babylon to compare with the Egyptian papyri.

Craniotomy

No history of the brain and behaviour, no matter how brief, would be complete without reference to the neurosurgical procedure of craniotomy or surgical opening of the skull. This serious and difficult surgical intervention was carried out with extraordinary frequency from late Palaeolithic and Neolithic times and has continued without interruption to the present century. Whether such procedures also included operation upon the brain itself is open to conjecture. Some of the interventions show associated skull fractures but many do not. It is likely that only a relatively small proportion of operations was undertaken for traumatic injury.

The widespread use of craniotomy is evidenced by the discovery of prehistoric trepanned skulls from Europe (Italy, France, Austria, Germany, The Netherlands, England), Africa (Algeria, Zimbabwe), South America (Peru, Bolivia, Colombia), North America and numerous islands of the South Pacific region. In some places such operations continued in their primitive form into the 20th century. Apparently no skulls showing prehistoric trepanation have been reported from China, Vietnam or India (Gurdjian 1973).

Early instruments were made of obsidian or stone while, with the development of later civilizations, metallic instruments of iron and bronze were employed. Hundreds of examples of trepanation have been reported from the Peruvian civilizations, beginning with the Paracas culture around 3000 BC and extending up to the end of the Inca civilization in the 16th century AD. In their examination of these pre-Columbian craniotomies Graña, Rocca and Graña (1954) have provided us with illustrations of: (i) operations in every part of the human skull; (ii) operative openings of different shapes – circular, oval, rectangular, triangular and irregular; (iii) sets of craniotomy instruments from different eras which include chisels, osteotomes, scalpels and retractors as well as bandages and tourniquets.

That many patients successfully survived such major cranial surgery is amply attested by skull specimens which show more than one surgical opening and having evidence (such as the bony changes around the opening) of different dates of operation in the same individual's lifetime. As many as five separate craniotomies have been discovered in a single specimen. The illustrator Froeschner has provided two more detailed drawings from Inca skulls studied at the Smithsonian Institution (1992).

In 1953 Graña and his colleagues successfully employed a set of these ancient instruments for the relief of a subdural haematoma (a large clot of blood pressing on the brain) in a patient who had suffered a head injury resulting in aphasia and right hemiplegia.

An elegant example from the Peruvian collection of instruments is shown in Figure 1.1. Known as a tumi, it depicts on its handle an operation on a patient where the surgeon is employing a similar instrument.

One can only speculate about the reasons for many of these early operations. Gurdjian lists as possible indications for operation headaches, the releasing of demons from the cranial space, certain religious and mystical exercises and also 'the fact that some of the openings in the skull have been repaired with silver alloy suggests surgical treatment for the possible skull wound caused in battle' (Gurdjian 1973, p. 3).

How much evidence regarding brain functions was brought to light by these ancient operations is lost to us because of the absence of a written language among these various early peoples.

CLASSICAL GREECE

The writer from this period most frequently referred to is Hippocrates. As Clarke and O'Malley (1968) point out, the Hippocratic writings were clearly the product of a group of physicians between the latter part of the 5th century BC and the middle of the 4th century BC. These physicians probably had little

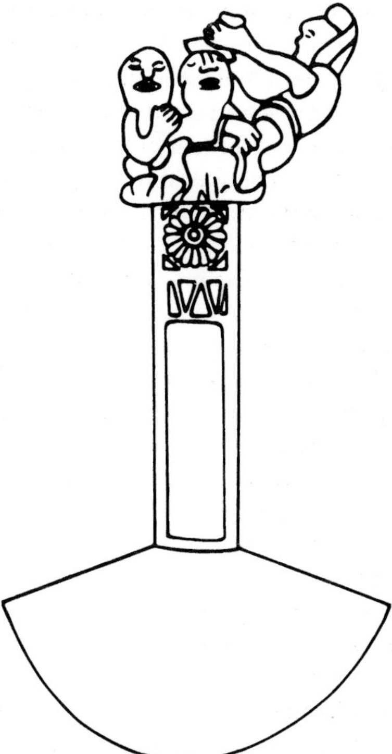

Fig. 1.1 Ancient Peruvian tumi.

familiarity with the human brain because of the aversion for dissection of the human body which existed in Greece at that time, but they did open the skulls of certain animals. Despite this lack of anatomical knowledge they considered that the brain was the seat of the soul or of mental functions and offered comments which showed that they had made very careful observation of their patients. Many would agree with McHenry (1969) that the Hippocratic tract *On The Sacred Disease* contains antiquity's best discussion of the brain and demonstrates the care with which a number of epileptic patients were studied. Another of the Hippocratic writers observed that damage to one hemisphere of the brain produced spasms or convulsions on the other side of the body though little was made of this observation and it appears to have been forgotten in the period which followed.

Hippocrates also 'warned against prodding blindly at a wound of the temporal area of the skull lest paralysis of the contralateral side should ensue' (Gibson 1969, p. 5).

THE VENTRICULAR LOCALIZATION HYPOTHESIS

This theory of localization of function postulated that the mental processes or faculties of the mind were located in the ventricular chambers of the brain. The cavities were conceived of as cells, the lateral ventricles forming the first cell and the third ventricle the second cell, while the fourth ventricle made up the third cell. Hence this doctrine is often termed the Cell Doctrine of brain function.

In its almost developed form the ventricular doctrine was first put forward by the Church Fathers Nemesius and Saint Augustine around the turn of the 4th century AD and it was to remain very much the same for well over 1000 years, that is, well into the beginning of the Renaissance. Outlines of the doctrine together with excellent pictorial representations are given in Magoun (1958) and Clarke and Dewhurst (1972).

The ventricular theory had its roots in a number of earlier ideas, particularly those of Aristotle and Galen. Aristotle had discussed the separate sense modalities and their contribution to perception. To account for the unity of sense experience he proposed a mechanism of integration which he called the common sense or *sensus communis*. Aristotelian psychology divided mental activity into a number of faculties of thought and judgment, e.g. imagination, fantasy, cogitation, estimation, attention and memory. These faculties were to become allotted to the ventricular chambers in the Cell Doctrine. Even as early as 300 BC Herophilus of Alexandria had localized the soul in the fourth ventricle.

Galen, in the 2nd century AD, contributed his theory of the psychic pneuma or gas and, though he himself did not propound the ventricular theory, he contributed to it in no small way. The reverence in which the writings of the 'prince of physicians' were held in the centuries which followed helped to set the doctrine in a form which was to remain unchanged for the next millenium. Unfortunately, Galen's followers were to copy his ideas slavishly without developing further his knowledge of the brain's anatomy and his careful and detailed observations of behavioural change.

As Gibson (1969) has it, Galen's 'brand of orthodoxy overcame medical science for a thousand years so that it required a Leonardo and a Vesalius to overcome it'.

With the intellectual ascendancy of the Arabic speaking peoples around the 8th century all the important Greek medical works were translated into Arabic and preserved in this way for some 500 years until retranslated, this time into Latin, where they formed the basis of medical science at the beginning of the Renaissance and, indeed, long after. The anatomy of the great Arabian medical writers, Avicenna, Hali Abbas, and Rhazes around the 10th century depended to a great extent on translations of Galen.

Galen had incorporated into his system the knowledge of the anatomy of the ventricles already present in Alexandrian medicine. He described the ventricles in detail and, though he laid the foundation for the final form which the Cell Doctrine was to take, did not himself do more than hint at the association of the ventricles with intellectual functions, preferring to locate the faculties in the brain substance itself.

Magoun (1958) gives the following concise account of Galen's theory of the 'psychic gas'.

> Nutritive material passed from the alimentary canal through the portal vein to the liver, where natural spirits were formed. These ebbed and flowed in the veins, taking origin from the liver, to convey nutriment to all parts of the body. A portion of these natural spirits passed across the septum, from the right to the left side of the heart, and joined with material drawn from the

> lungs to form the vital spirits. These ebbed and flowed to all parts of the body through the arteries, taking origin from the heart, to provide heat and other vital requirements. A part of these vital spirits passed to the base of the brain, to be distilled there in a marvellous vascular net, the rete mirabile, and to mix with air inspired into the cerebral ventricles through the porous cranial base, for, at this time, the pulsing of the brain in the opened cranium was conceived as an active process, much like that of thoracic respiration. As a consequence, animal spirits were formed, and 'animal', in this use, was derived from the Latin 'anima' and Greek 'psyche', meaning soulful, and was not animal in any lowly sense. This psychic pneuma, stored in the brain ventricles, passed by the pores of the nerves to the peripheral organs of sense and to the muscles, to subserve sensory and motor functions. Its equivalently important role in managing central functions of the brain was affected either within the ventricles themselves or in the immediately bordering substance of their walls.

Sherrington pointed out how the movement of the brain, which is a passive or transmitted pulsation, misled Galen and his followers by apparently supporting their notion of the ventricular system as pumping the fluid to the different parts of the body. Sherrington supposed that Galen had not only seen it in the scalp of the young child before the vault closes but had also observed that 'war and the gladiatorial games were the greatest school of surgery' (Sherrington 1951).

It was as cells to contain the animal spirits that the ventricular chambers took on their great significance. A number of writers have pointed out that, of course, the ventricular cavities are the most striking features on gross dissection of the untreated brain.

Sherrington comments: 'It is interesting to speculate how much this concentration on meninges and ventricular cavities, an obsession that was to dominate thought about the brain for nearly two thousand years, was due to the simple fact that, unless fixed and hardened, the brain resembles an amorphous gruel, of which one of the few distinguishing features is that it possesses cavities'.

After Galen there was no significant development of anatomical knowledge for many centuries and Galen's influence can be most clearly seen in the slavish copying by those who followed of the *rete mirabile.* This network which appears in ungulates such as the pig and the ox is not found in man, and those who followed Galen's findings for so long were apparently unaware that, although the master had knowledge of the human brain and that of the Barbary ape, his neuroanatomical descriptions were mainly derived from the ox. This also explains how his descriptions of the ventricles seem erroneous for man while they are highly accurate for the ox.

Two early 16th-century woodcuts serve to illustrate the Cell Doctrine. Because of its clarity, Figure 1.2 has been reproduced very frequently. It is from an encyclopedia produced by the Carthusian monk, Gregor Reisch, about 1504.

It shows the senses of smell, taste, sight, and hearing connected to the *sensus communis* at the front of the first chamber. This chamber is the seat of fantasy and imagination, the second that of cogitation and estimation, and in the third

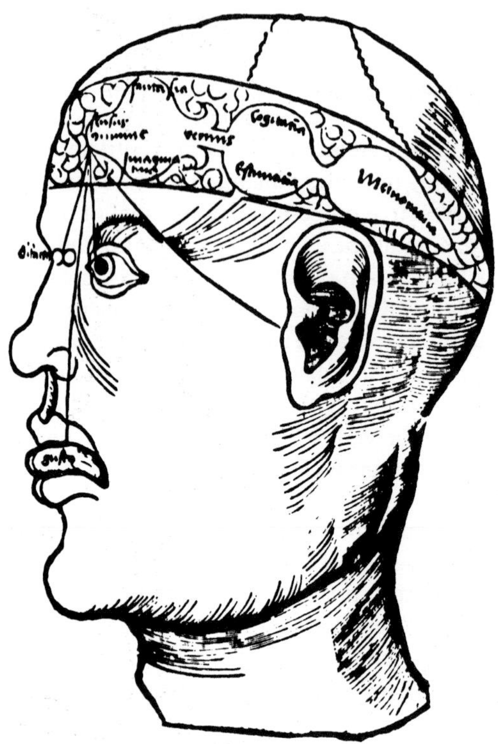

Fig. 1.2 Cell doctrine. Gregor Reisch (1504).

resides memory. There is also a possible depiction of part of the cerebral convolutions. The label 'vermis' or worm would seem to refer to the choroid plexus which passes through the opening connecting the lateral ventricle (first cell) with the third ventricle (second cell) (see Fig. 1.3).

The second illustration (Fig. 1.4) is noteworthy for its reproduction of the rete mirabile at this late date. It is taken from Magnus Hundt, 1501, and illustrates not only the Cell Doctrine but also the cranial nerves according to Galen's classification together with the skull sutures and the different layers of the scalp. Magoun (1958) gives us a liberal interpretation of the Cell Doctrine.

> On passing to the brighter functional aspects of these early views, they first proposed that incoming information from a peripheral receptor was conveyed to a sensory portion of the brain, where it could be interrelated with other afferent data. Activity was thence transmitted to a more central integrative region, equivalently accessible to internal impressions related to sense and to general memory. Last, activity was capable of involving a motor portion of the brain, so as to initiate movement or behaviour. The sequential ordering of these Aristotelian faculties from the front to the back of the brain conveyed an implication that central neural function normally proceeded through such successive stages. Such conceptualization is not excessively different from that reached by Sherrington in his founding studies of modern neurophysiology nor from that which confronts us continually today.

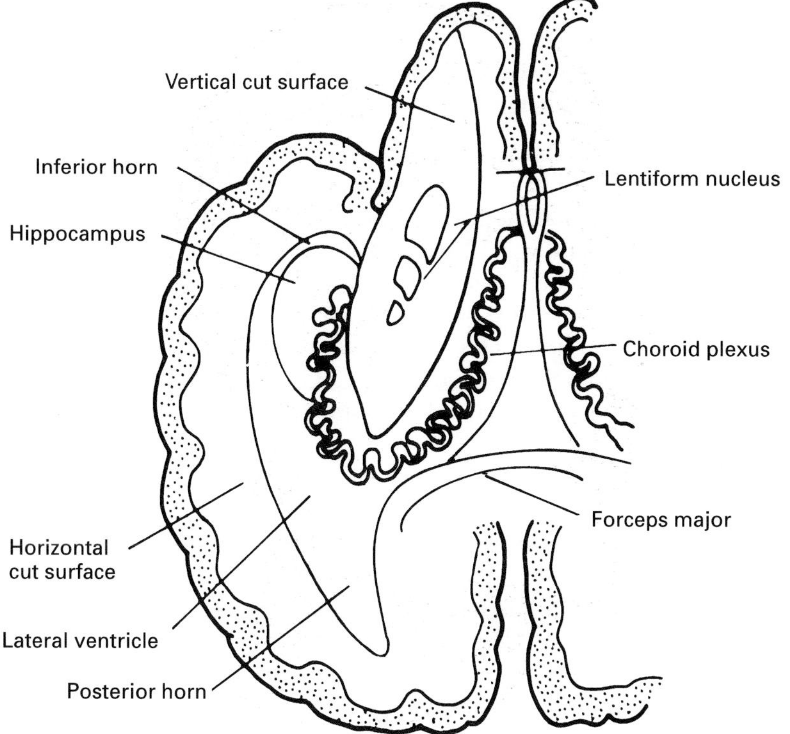

Fig. 1.3 Worm like appearance of the choroid plexus.

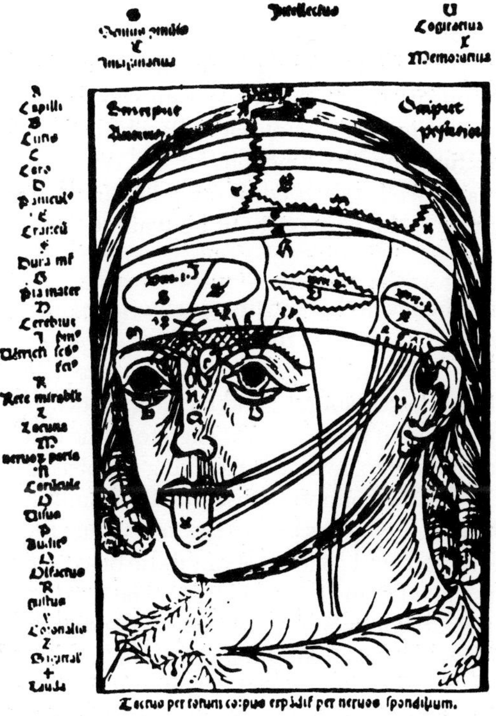

Fig. 1.4 Cell doctrine. Magnus Hundt (1501).

This interpretation may be overgenerous but the crudity of depiction should not be taken as the only measure of the state of development of ideas. In reviewing such ideas from antiquity Woollam (1958) warns of the danger of imputing too much knowledge to our predecessors.

> The great scientific names of the ancient world, Aristotle, Democritus, Galen and Hippocrates have received so much tribute, that it is easy to fall into the belief that all our modern scientific belief already existed in embryo as it were in the ancient world…Hippocrates described how a blow on the head could produce paralysis on the opposite side of the body. It is not too difficult to fall into the trap of reading backwards from our knowledge of the anatomy of the brain and see in this statement the first reference to the crossing of the pyramidal tracts. The study of the knowledge of the anatomy of the brain displayed in the Hippocratic Corpus proves a salutary corrective to this view.

Vesalius

With Andreas Vesalius (1514–1564) came the era in which careful scientific observations began to triumph over the dogmatic statements which had been handed down from the time of Galen.

His anatomical masterpiece, the *De humani corporis fabrica*, and its companion volume the *Epitome* were published at Basle in 1543. This work has been called the embodiment of the spirit of the Renaissance and many have considered it the most influential factor in establishing the modern era of observation and research.

Vesalius was a pupil of Sylvius (1478–1555) who was known as a great follower of Galen. Vesalius was instructed in the ventricular hypothesis and recounts how he and his fellow students were shown the illustration from Gregor Reisch's *Margarita Philosophica* (Fig. 1.2) which they had to copy as an adjunct to their lectures on the functions of the ventricular chambers. The teaching of the time is well preserved in the following extract which records what Vesalius learned at the University of Louvain (Clarke & O'Malley 1968, p. 468).

> Indeed, those men believed that the first or anterior, which was said to look towards the forehead, was called the ventricle of the sensus communis because the nerves of five senses are carried from it to their instruments, and odours, colours, tastes, sounds, and tactile qualities are brought into this ventricle by the aid of those nerves. Therefore, the chief use of this ventricle was considered to be that of receiving the objects of the five senses, which we usually call the common senses, and transmitting them to the second ventricle, joined by a passage to the first so that the second might be able to imagine, reason, and cogitate about those objects: hence cogitation or reasoning was assigned to the latter ventricle. The third ventricle (our fourth) was consecrated to memory, into which the second desired that all things sufficiently reasoned about those objects be sent and suitably deposited.

The detail of Vesalius' anatomy (Figs 1.5 and 1.6) is in sharp contrast to the

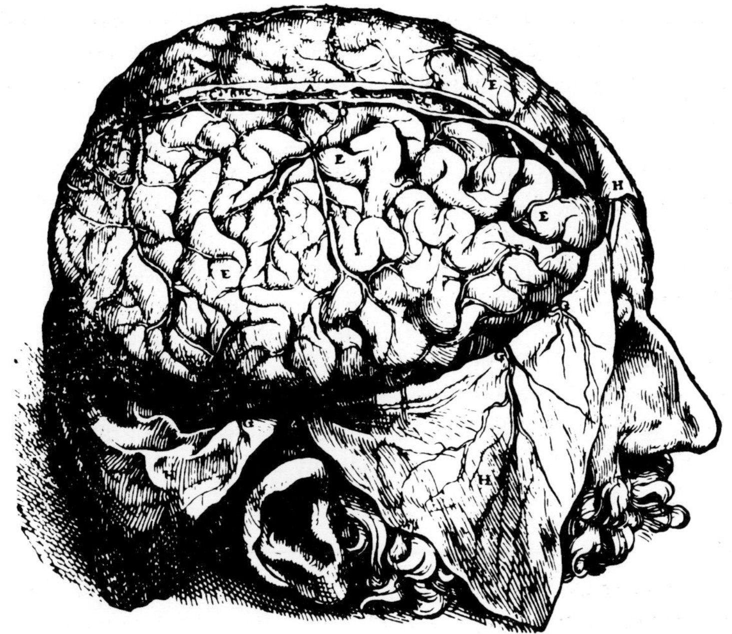

Fig. 1.5 Brain anatomy. Vesalius.

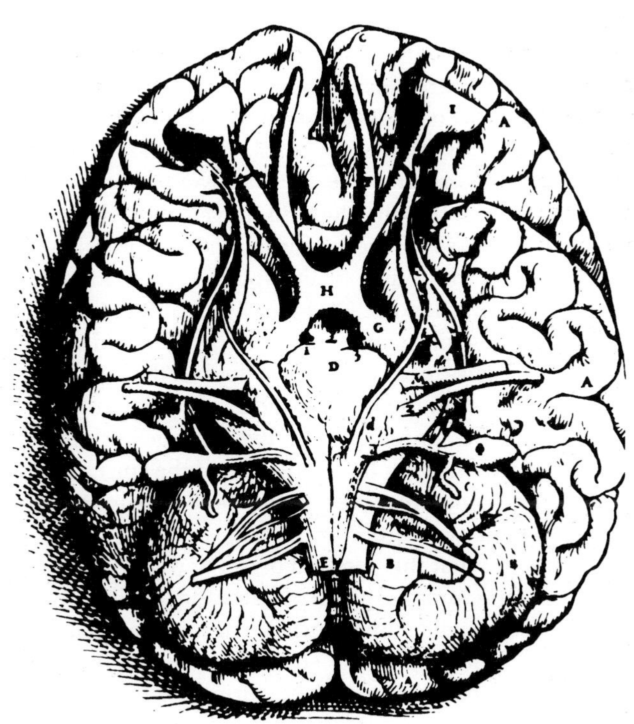

Fig. 1.6 Brain anatomy. Vesalius.

crudity of the earlier 16th-century woodcuts, yet, despite the artistic excellence of the drawings and their dependence upon actual observation of anatomical specimens, the influence of the early Galenical teaching can be seen in the perpetuation of errors which cannot have been present in dissections. Though later commentators have stressed his anti-Galenism and though he was attacked by his contemporaries for his departure from their slavish following of the Galenical teachings, Vesalius himself was at pains to point out his respect for the greatness of the 'prince of physicians and preceptor of all'. What he would not condone was an indiscriminate acceptance of every one of Galen's teachings. His greatness lay in using the observational method to confirm earlier postulations and to note whether the observations were at variance with the accepted dogma.

Unfortunately, this sudden increase in knowledge of structural neuroanatomy was not paralleled by an increase in knowledge of the brain's functions and this discrepancy between anatomy and physiology continued well into the 20th century.

SEARCH FOR THE CEREBRAL ORGAN

During the second half of the 17th century and the early part of the 18th, a number of separate investigators attempted to find the one part of the brain that was the seat of the mind or soul. The essential feature of these attempts is the fact that they were based on speculation, not on clinical observation or experimentation.

The most well-known of the theories was that of Descartes, who in selecting the pineal gland as the seat of the soul argued that it was so strategically situated with regard to the ventricular chambers that it could influence and be influenced by the flow of the spirits between them: 'a certain very small gland situated in the middle of its (the brain's) substance and so suspended above the channel by which the spirits in its anterior cavities have communication with those of the posterior, that the slightest movements which take place in it can greatly alter the course of these spirits; and reciprocally that the least changes which occur to the course of the spirits can greatly alter the movements of this gland' (from Clarke & O'Malley 1968, p. 471).

Descartes reasoned that since our experience of the world is unitary despite the multiple organs of sense, each of which is double, there must be some place where these separate sense impressions could come together 'before they reach the soul'. 'It can easily be conceived how these images or other impressions could unite in this gland through the mediation of the spirits that fill the cavities of the brain. There is no other place in the body where they could be thus united unless it be in this gland' (op. cit., p. 472).

Other writers thought that this cerebral organ or organ of the soul might be represented by such structures as the corpus striatum (Willis), the white matter (Vieussens), or the corpus callosum (Lancisi). The fact that many were preoccupied with the search for a single vital structure does not mean that excellent observations and inferences were not made during the 17th and 18th centuries. They were greatly overshadowed by the search, however, and the clues to the nature of brain organization found in such fine examples as those cited by

Gibson (1962) seem to have been overlooked when interest in the problem of localization blossomed some two centuries later.

FACULTY PSYCHOLOGY AND DISCRETE LOCALIZATION

In the period which followed, the notion of the unity of conscious experience gave way to the 'faculty psychology' which divided mental processes into a number of separate, specialized abilities and this was to precipitate the search for the neural substrate of such faculties or powers of the mind. In founding the system which came to be known as phrenology, Gall leaned heavily on the lists of faculties provided by the Scottish philosophers Thomas Reid (1710–1796) and Dugald Stewart (1753–1828). Gall's was not the only attempt to relate separate mental functions to discrete parts of the brain but it was certainly the most influential, its influence persisting for a century. For all its drawbacks phrenology proved a more fertile notion than the earlier search for 'the single organ'.

Gall taught his doctrine in Vienna from 1796 onwards, and was soon joined by Spurzheim who in fact coined the term 'phrenology' and was to develop a moralizing version of Gall's ideas which was to become as keenly supported as it was contested. The essence of this movement is simply stated. The brain is composed of a number of separate organs each of which controls a separate innate faculty, i.e. there are as many cerebral organs for mental processes as there are faculties. The location of the faculties according to Spurzheim is shown in Figure 1.7.

The development of the cerebral organs led to prominences in the individual's skull so that, by the process of 'cranioscopy' or palpation of the prominences, the practitioner of phrenology could divine the nature of the person's propensities.

Gall stressed the role of the cortex in which he located his faculty organs. This was an advance since the cortex had been considered relatively unimportant up to this stage. Gall made a number of important discoveries in neuroanatomy but these have been greatly overshadowed by his speculative physiology.

When one reads the original work one is struck by the extraordinary lack of evidence given in support of what seem today to be strange and sweeping claims. Nevertheless, it certainly stimulated the scientific thought of the period. Boring (1929) called it 'an instance of a theory which, while essentially wrong, was just enough right to further scientific thought'. Although not providing proof it established the belief in many minds that the localizationist position was a tenable one.

Critchley (1979) considered that phrenology stimulated the careful recording and correlation of anatomo-clinical data which formed the beginnings of our ideas on brain localization. At the time there were those who espoused the notion of silent areas of the brain and pointed to such cases as Phineas Gage (see Ch. 4) where major damage did not appear to lead to any obvious loss of mental capacity. The phrenologists highlighted the gross personality changes in this patient and 'rightly asserted that proper testing and enquiry would always uncover considerable modifications in character and comportment

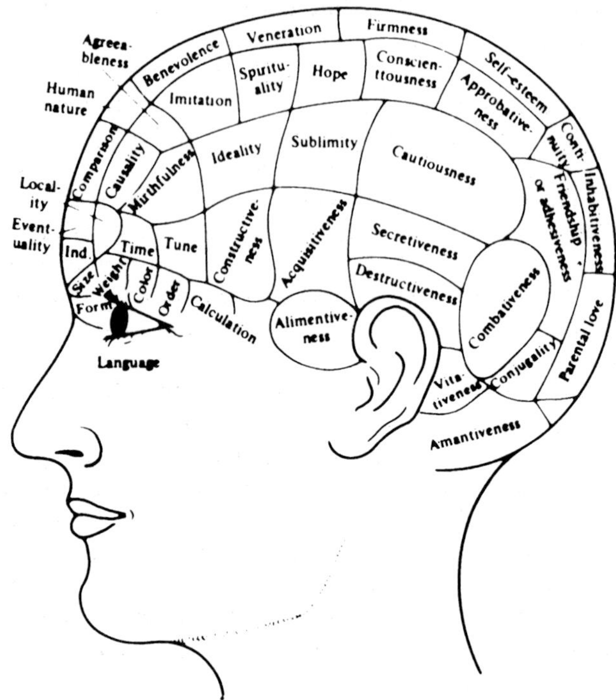

Fig. 1.7 A phrenological map (from Miller G A & Buckout R: Psychology: The science of mental life, courtesy Harper and Row).

...the so-called silent areas of the brain are eloquent to those who know how to listen' (p. 251). The modern neuropsychologist would also add subtle but incapacitating changes in cognitive function.

The most powerful and influential opponent of phrenology was Flourens (1794–1867). He is commonly credited with beginning the movement that resulted in the holistic theory of brain function which held that mental functions are not dependent upon particular parts of the brain but, rather, that it functions as a whole.

Flourens experimented mainly with birds; he demonstrated that animals may recover after ablations of part of their central nervous systems and that the same recovery takes place irrespective of the site of the ablation. This work anticipated the notion of equipotentiality, the ability of other parts of the brain to take over the functions of damaged neural tissue. Flourens stated quite clearly that he did not believe that the nervous system was a homogeneous mass but he did believe that it operated in a concerted, integrated fashion, unlike the theory of discrete localization.

LESION STUDIES OF THE 19TH CENTURY

During the long controversy between the supporters of Gall on the one hand and those of Flourens on the other, what one writer refers to as the controversy between the skull palpators and the bird brain ablators, numerous clinicians were making valuable observations on brain–behaviour relationships. In fact, clinical observations of language disturbance with brain trauma had been recorded for at least two centuries before aphasia become a major focus of attention. Many examples are provided in the fine historical paper of Benton and Joynt (1960). Unfortunately, even the more important of these were not seen in their true light because of their association in people's minds with one or other side of the controversy, e.g. Bouillaud in 1825 pointed out the frequent association of loss of language with lesions of the anterior or frontal lobes but clouded the contribution by stating that this could be taken to support Gall's contention that the faculty of language lay in this region.

It was quite some time later that Broca was to publish his well known dictum. Even when Dax read a paper in 1836, clearly relating the left half of the brain with aphasia, it remained unpublished until his son brought it forward 25 years later. A number of factors may have conspired to bring about this delay, not the least of which may have been Dax's political unpopularity in the region at the time he delivered his paper. Details surrounding these events are given in a recent paper (Finger & Roe 1996). It is clear that Dax understood the specific role of the left hemisphere in the production of aphasia since he searched for cases of right-handed aphasics with right hemisphere lesions but was unable to find one such case.

Broca and the localization of speech

Broca's role in this history of functional localization is a particularly complex one which has been discussed in many places. Joynt's (1964) paper provides a brief but clear outline of the main contentions. Broca himself made no claim for priority in the discovery of the relation between the frontal region and language disturbance. He acknowledged more than once the contributions of Bouillaud. His sustained and systematic observations did, however, greatly advance the cause of the localization of function in the brain.

In 1861 Broca exhibited the brain of his patient 'Tan' who had died only the day before and who had in life lost the power of speech so that the only word which he was able to utter was 'Tan'. The lesion lay in the posterior part of the left frontal lobe. Later in 1861 Broca exhibited a similar case which confirmed his notion that the lesion in cases of aphasia was situated in the frontal lobes of the brain. At this stage, like the cautious observer he was, Broca posed the question of whether a more exact localization was possible, leaving the question open for further investigation.

> It is a much more doubtful question to know if the faculty of articulate speech is dependent upon the whole anterior lobe or particularly upon one of its convolutions; in other words, to know if the localization of cerebral faculties happens by faculty and by convolution, or only by groups of faculties or by groups of convolutions. Further observations must be collected with the object of solving this question. It is necessary for this purpose to indicate exactly the name and place of the diseased convolutions and, if the lesion is very extensive, to seek, wherever possible by anatomical

> examination, the place or rather the convolution where the disease appears to have begun. (Clarke & O'Malley 1968, pp. 496-497)

However, he did consider that even his first observations were more consistent with the system of localization by brain convolutions than the phrenological notion that he termed the 'system of bumps'. Even with the further accumulation of cases over the next two years he was still restrained in his statements. 'Here are 8 cases where the lesion is situated in the posterior portion of the third frontal convolution...and, a most remarkable thing, in all of these patients the lesion is on the left side. I do not dare to make a conclusion and I await new findings' (Benton 1965). At this time Broca also speculated on the possibility of localizing functions other than speech. Finally, in 1885, Broca published his famous dictum which was to become such a landmark in the history of brain function: 'Nous parlons avec l'hémisphère gauche'.

Broca's work stimulated a good deal of clinical research into the anatomical basis of language; numerous workers published findings in his support and soon others began to report observations which supported the view of localization in other areas of functioning.

Broca himself noted, with other workers, that exceptions to the location of language in the left hemisphere appeared to occur in left-handed individuals and from such observations began the notion that a crossed relationship existed between hand preference and hemispheric dominance for language, a notion that has bedevilled us ever since and one that is only now beginning to be clarified (see Ch. 8).

Wernicke and the beginning of modern neuropsychology

In 1874, several years after Broca's demonstration of the importance of the left posterior frontal region for spoken language, Wernicke described a case where a lesion of the left superior temporal gyrus caused difficulty in the comprehension of speech. The addition of this finding to that of Broca meant that at least two separate functions could be affected by lesions in two separate locations. This could not fail to reinforce the ideas of those leaning towards a theory of localization, and the search for similar 'centres' for other mental functions was greatly stimulated.

Wernicke's place in the history of brain function has been overlooked by most writers. Even the comprehensive and thoroughly documented work of Clarke and O'Malley does not mention him while other writers see him as merely subscribing to the notion that the 'discovery of a lesion in a particular area of the brain in an individual with a concomitant definite type of disturbance (signifies) that the area containing the lesion is the 'centre' for the function that had been impaired' (Luria 1966, p. 12).

Geschwind (1966, 1967) considers that Wernicke's contribution was very much greater, pointing out that his paper on receptive aphasia provided a potentially productive theoretical approach which made possible scientific method in the study of aphasia.

> On the basis of this theory it was possible to predict the existence of syndromes not previously seen and to devise experimental means of testing hypotheses. Wernicke's reasoning was simple. He applied Meynert's

> teaching on the fiber tracts of the brain to the problem of aphasia. The phrenologists, he argued, had been wrong in their attempt to localize such complex mental attributes as magnanimity or filial love; what was actually localizable were much simpler perceptual and motor functions. All the complex array of human intellectual attributes must somehow be woven from these threads of different texture. The cortex could at its simplest provide two means of achieving this higher integration, it could store sensory traces in cells for long periods of time and, by means of association fiber tracts, it could link together different parts of the system. (Geschwind 1966, pp. 4, 5)

Subsequent workers such as Lichtheim (1885) and Déjerine (1892) used this method both to predict and explain specific defects of psychological processes with localized brain lesions. Geschwind summarizes Wernicke's position in the following way.

> Wernicke was one of the first to see clearly the importance of the connections between different parts of the brain in the building up of complex activities. He rejected both of the approaches to the nervous system which even today are often presented as the only possible ones. On the one hand, he opposed the doctrine of the equipotentiality of the brain; on the other, he rejected the phrenological view which regarded the brain as a mosaic of innumerable distinct centers. He asserted that complex activities were learned by means of the connections between a small number of functional regions which dealt with the primary motor and sensory activities. Although this third view dominated research on the neurological basis of behavior for a period of nearly 50 years, it has been omitted almost entirely from the discussions of the higher functions in recent times. (Geschwind 1967, p. 103)

Wernicke's point of view has been fully developed in Geschwind's logical analysis and development of the notion of 'the disconnexion syndrome' described later in this chapter (Geschwind 1965a–c). In a very real sense Wernicke could be considered the father of neuropsychology.

Memory disorder and the brain

In a series of reports from 1887 to 1891, Korsakoff reported the association of various mental disorders with polyneuritis. Sometimes the patient retained clear consciousness but was agitated while in others the agitation was part of a confusional state. In most of the patients an amnesic disorder was a prominent feature. Soon after these observations Korsakoff, along with others, noted that the amnesic syndrome could be seen without the polyneuritis. The most common factor in the overwhelming number of cases was heavy indulgence in alcohol. It was some decades before the neuropathological basis began to be established (see Victor et al 1971) and even today the necessary and sufficient lesions are still not settled.

A recent review (Levin et al 1983) reminds us that, even before the classical papers of Korsakoff, Ribot (1839–1916) was the first to develop a systematic theory of memory and its derangement, and a classification which incorporated important distinctions still in use, e.g. amnesia with forward extension (anterograde amnesia) and extension into the past (retrograde amnesia).

In modern times clinical and experimental studies have revealed that lesions in widely separated collections of cells and tracts can affect discrete subfunctions of the complex set of functions which are included under the rubric of memory and learning. Many of these are considered in subsequent chapters.

THE CORTICAL MAP MAKERS

From the era of Broca and Wernicke until well into the 20th century there were numerous reports of the discovery of similar localized centres in the cortex, so that maps of the brain surface with functional labels attached to different areas appeared frequently in the literature. The cortical cartographers were aided by the widespread acceptance of associationism in the new science of psychology which was beginning to assert its independence. They were also in tune with the discoveries on the finer anatomical detail of the cortex and its physiology. The diagrams of the cortical map makers began to relate these latter findings, such as the location of primary sensory and motor functions (mainly derived from ablation and stimulation experiments in animals), to the human brain and to add possible sites for higher mental processes, many of which were as speculative as the assignment of functions to particular areas by the phrenologists.

Cytoarchitecture and myeloarchitecture

Cytoarchitectonics refers to the study of the architecture of cells or the disposition of cells and their type and density in the layers of the cortex. This study was dependent on the discovery of methods for fixing and staining the nerve tissues so that adequate examination of cell populations could be made. Soon after the early development of these techniques of neurohistology by Ramon y Cajal and others, it became apparent that the composition of the cortex was not everywhere the same, and the discovery that the cortex could be subdivided into differently composed areas invited the possible inference that differences in structure might mean differences in function. Again the relationship between morphology and function could be demonstrated for the sensory and motor areas of the cortex which left the tantalizing possibility that the same might hold for higher functions. Though few such relationships have been found to date, this story is not yet concluded.

The corresponding study of the fibre structure of the brain is known as myeloarchitectonics, and quite early on Flechsig (1849–1929) had related the time of development of the myelin covering of fibres to the development of different areas of the cortex. This suggested that the neural bases of higher functions might lie in cortical–subcortical systems rather than being restricted largely or wholly to the cerebral cortex.

The first major work in this new field by Campbell (1905) *Histological Studies on the Localization of Cerebral Function* shows in its title the avowed aim of the author to correlate function with histological structure. His map divided the cortex into some 20 regions. Shortly after, Brodmann (1909) produced his map with the separate zones now numbering around 50. This map has been widely reproduced and referred to ever since (see Fig. 7.3). Still other workers increased the number of subdivisions until 200 or more separate areas were differentiated in some systems. Milner comments: 'The difference between many adjacent regions in these later maps were so small as to be imperceptible to all but the anatomists who first described them. This problem was pointed out by Lashley and Clark (1946), who found only a few regions of the cortex that they could recognize from anatomical sections alone *if they did not know beforehand what part of the cortex the sections had come from*' (Milner 1970, p. 109).

The earliest subdivision of the cortex related large areas of the brain's surface to the name of the overlying bones, and this division into frontal, temporal, parietal and occipital lobes remains with us today. It has been stressed very often that these are artificial abstractions. However, 'as far as the psychologist is concerned the acid test of (any) such subdivisions is whether or not they can be shown to mean anything behaviourally. Does a lesion of an anatomically or physiologically defined area produce a more isolated and clear cut behavioural disturbance than a lesion that ignores such boundaries?' (Milner 1970, p. 112). A century of lesion studies has demonstrated that these abstractions, the 'lobes' of the brain, are still more useful at this stage in discussing brain–behaviour relationships than those based on the finer subdivisions of cytoarchitecture.

MODERN NEUROPSYCHOLOGY

The past four decades have seen an accelerated growth in the new or reawakened science called neuropsychology as lines of evidence converge from the parent disciplines of neurological medicine and psychology and as the special methods of each are modified for use in the new field. As with other areas where scientific endeavours overlap, new conceptions and formulations arise which not only advance the new science but also provide useful stimulation for the progenitors. The two principal aspects of clinical neuropsychology are clearly outlined by Luria, one of its ablest practitioners and developer of an influential theory whose principal features are outlined below:

> The study has two objectives. First by pinpointing the brain lesions responsible for specific behavior disorders we hope to develop a means of early diagnosis and precise location of brain injuries…Second, neuropsychological investigation should provide us with a factor analysis that will lead to better understanding of the components of complex psychological functions for which the operations of the different parts of the brain are responsible. (Luria 1970, p. 66)

This twofold nature of neuropsychology means that by utilizing appropriate tools and concepts to examine brain–behaviour relationships we may be in a position to further our knowledge of the nature of the psychological processes themselves. Neuropsychology has already given us greater insight into some of the processes of perception, memory, learning, problem solving and adaptation, a branch of study much expanded in recent years and termed cognitive neuropsychology. The sophisticated techniques and methodology of modern psychology have also allowed a more detailed analysis of higher nervous disorders than was previously possible.

Leaving aside the psychological measures themselves, since they are dealt with later, there seem to be a number of concepts developed only in recent years which are proving very fruitful. Among these the following four are chosen as they provide a basis for what follows: (i) the adoption of the syndrome concept as against the unproductive 'unitary' concept of brain damage; (ii) a re-evaluation of the concept of 'function' and the development of the concept of functional systems as the neural substrates of psychological processes; (iii) the use of 'double dissociation' of function to strengthen the certainty with which statements may be made concerning the relation between anatomical lesion and behavioural disturbance; and (iv) the development of the notion of the 'disconnection syndrome' to explain neuropsychological findings and to predict others.

Though these notions are interrelated with each other and with other ideas in the field they will be outlined separately.

Neuropsychological syndromes

The general failure of psychological tests to provide suitable measures of 'brain damage' was one of the key factors in moving neuropsychologists in the direction of describing the effects of cerebral malfunction in terms of syndromes. Those with a background in medicine and neurology are already familiar with the utility of the syndrome as a conceptual tool in everyday practice. More and more psychologists have moved in the direction of syndrome analysis, at least in clinical diagnostic practice. Piercy (1959) and McFie (1960) favoured this approach – 'a patient's performance should be described not so much in terms of extent of deviation from statistical normality as in terms of extent of approximation to an established syndrome or abnormality' (McFie 1960). The use of psychological test methods in the appraisal of the patient's preserved abilities as well as deficits has helped to clarify the definition of some syndromes and is already beginning to describe new ones. The syndrome concept has allowed the more realistic use of psychological test procedures aimed at gauging patterns of impairment on appropriately selected measures. In discussing the objections to the syndrome method in clinical research as opposed to practice, Kinsbourne (1971) reminded us that the association between the constellation of signs and symptoms which we term a syndrome and the presence of a disease is a probabilistic not an invariant one. 'Partial syndromes abound, and it is often not clear how many ingredients have to be present to justify the diagnosis. This is particularly true since not all ingredients of a syndrome are of equal importance, their relative valuation being an unformulated outcome of the interaction of medical instruction and clinical experience, and thus a somewhat individual process' (Kinsbourne 1971, p. 290). On the research front he points out that correlative studies between lesion and syndrome need to employ valid experimental designs and that appropriate statistical procedures such as cluster analysis should prove useful in the validation of clinical syndromes. 'Pending validation by appropriate testing, the clinically observed 'syndrome' represents an educated guess at a relationship which has value in generating hypotheses and experimentation' (op. cit., p. 291). One of the major tasks of present day neuropsychology is to increase the degree of confidence with which such probabilistic statements can be made.

Strub and Geschwind (1983), in their discussion of the Gerstmann syndrome (see Ch. 6), have pointed out that some neuropsychologists have a basic misunderstanding of the medical use of the term syndrome. All would agree that a syndrome may be considered as a constellation of signs and/or symptoms which indicates the presence of a disease or lesion. It is not necessary for there to be a high correlation between the elements, though this would strengthen the diagnosis were it to occur. What should be characteristic is the uniqueness conveyed by the total *Gestalt*, and statistical techniques such as cluster analysis might be relevant in distinguishing syndromes from pseudosyndromes.

Closely related to the interpretation of signs and symptoms as a syndrome is the medical concept of differential diagnosis. This means the awareness that similar constellations may be seen in several different diseases or disorders. Ignorance of some of the possibilities will result in a proportion of incorrect diagnoses. This may occur in two directions. Either the pattern of signs and symptoms may be ascribed to the wrong cause or the pattern may not be recognized as a result of a particular disease, or both. The seriousness of the error will depend on the implications for prognosis and treatment.

One of the principal advantages of the differential diagnostic approach is that it allows hypotheses to be set up both to confirm the presence of one disorder and to disconfirm the possibility of others. This approach using psychological tests is exemplified with clinical case examinations in the final chapter. Unfortunately, in neuropsychology there are fewer pathognomonic signs than there are in medicine. The term pathognomonic refers to a sign or symptom which is specifically characteristic of a particular disease. Most symptoms and signs in neuropsychology have multiple significance.

The syndrome approach is close to the distinction between monothetic and polythetic classification in biological taxonomy. 'The ruling idea of monothetic groups is that they are formed by rigid and successive logical divisions so that the possession of a unique set of features is both sufficient and necessary for membership in the group thus defined' (Sokal & Sneath 1963, p. 13). With regard to the description and classification of brain damage such a system is not applicable in the light of present knowledge. On the other hand the notion of 'polytypic' (Beckner 1959) or polythetic groups is very much of value since no single attribute or set of signs and symptoms defines the group. A polythetic classification would place together in one group or syndrome all those cases which share a sufficient number of common characteristics. However, 'no single feature is either essential to group membership or is sufficient to make an organism a member of the group' (Sokal & Sneath 1963, p. 14). The first major attempt to apply a taxonomic key approach to the problem of assessment of brain lesions was that of Russell, Neuringer and Goldstein (1970).

The description of syndromes in neuropsychology is of the polythetic type and is of undoubted value in the preliminary allotment of a patient to a diagnostic category which may then be checked further in the process of differential diagnosis.

Functional systems

The idea of a functional system as the neurological underpinning of a complex psychological function was developed over a long period by Luria and is clearly outlined in his textbook (Luria 1973). At the outset he draws attention to the fact that the term 'function' may be used in at least two principal ways. Firstly one may describe the function of particular cells or organs, e.g. one of the functions of the liver is to produce bile, the function of the islet cells of Langerhans is to produce insulin. This usage is readily understood. On the other hand, the term function is widely used to describe more complex processes involving the integrated participation of a number of tissues and organs in a functional process, e.g. the function of digestion, circulation, and respiration. Such organizations are termed systems and though the final result, such as the absorption of nourishment or the provision of oxygen to the tissues, remains constant, the way in which the system performs the function varies considerably according to a wide variety of factors. 'The presence of a constant (invariant) task, performed by variable (variative) mechanisms, bringing the process to a constant (invariant) result, is one of the basic features distinguishing the work of every functional system' (Luria 1973, p. 28).

The systemic approach has a second advantage which proves useful in topical diagnosis. While it is true that damage in any part of a functional system may lead to disruption of a psychological process it is also true that damage to different parts of a system will impress a different character on the complex of symptoms and signs which result from the damage. Thus it is of paramount importance to establish not only that there is an alteration in a particular psychological function following a brain lesion but also what qualitative features this loss of function has. It was principally for this reason that psychological tests, particularly some of the more widely used psychometric measures, proved of such limited value in diagnosis since they did not allow this difference in the quality of performance to be brought out or psychologists were too impressed with the scores or level of performance to see the significance of qualitative changes. Indeed, workers like Goldstein were roundly attacked because of their lack of norms, standardization and other features of the epitome of psychological assessment, the intelligence test. This overgeneralization is easy to make with hindsight and it is true, particularly of the British clinical psychologists, that they quite early realized the shortcomings of dependence upon test scores alone. Shapiro (1951) expressed it pithily when he commented 'the test scores do not communicate the responses in full'.

The notion of functional systems is a marked advance on the notion of strict localization of function in discrete areas of the cortex. The functional system has as its anatomical basis a number of cortical and subcortical areas working in concert through the action of fibre pathways and it is for this reason that a fairly detailed knowledge of the anatomy of the brain should be indispensable for the neuropsychologist. This becomes apparent in the understanding provided by the disconnection model discussed below.

Double dissociation of function

This concept was put forward by Teuber (1955, 1959) and has been widely accepted and quoted by other workers. In discussing whether certain visual discrimination difficulties described after temporal lobe ablations in animals were specific to those particular areas Teuber commented:

> To demonstrate specificity of the deficit for visual discrimination we need to do more than show that discrimination in some other modality, e.g. somesthesis, is unimpaired. Such simple dissociation might indicate merely that visual discrimination is more vulnerable to temporal lesions than tactile discrimination. This would be a case of hierarchy of function rather than separate localization. What is needed for conclusive proof is 'double dissociation', i.e. evidence that tactile discrimination can be disturbed by some other lesion without loss on visual tasks and to a degree comparable in severity to the supposedly visual deficit after temporal lesions (Teuber 1955, p. 283).

A more general statement appeared a few years later in discussion of Teuber's findings in his extensive studies of human subjects with wounds to the brain: '…double dissociation requires that symptom A appear in lesions in one structure but not with those in another, and the symptom B appear with lesions of the other but not of the one. Whenever such dissociation is lacking, specificity in the effects of lesions has not been demonstrated' (Teuber 1959, p. 187).

Numerous examples of double dissociation of function appear in the later chapters. The concept has proved extremely useful but care must be exercised in transposing the word 'symptom' in the above quotation to mean the patient's performance on a psychological test. Kinsbourne has discussed the application of the concept to groups of individuals with damage in different parts of the brain.

> If a patient group with damage centered at location A is superior to one damaged at B in respect to task P, but inferior in task Q, a double dissociation obtains between these groups. This permits the inference of at least one difference between the two groups specific to location of damage, for P may be a nonspecific task, relating, say, to general intelligence or some other variable in which the groups are imperfectly matched. But then it must be admitted that function Q must have been selectively impaired by a lesion at location A; since the inferiority in performing Q cannot be accounted for by failure of matching on the other task. The search for double dissociation is a valid means towards progress in neuropsychology. (Kinsbourne 1971, p. 295)

This author warns that the converse situation, namely the failure to find dissociations, should not lead us to conclude that specific relationships do not exist between performance on specific tasks and particular anatomical sites or structures since performance on a particular task may be affected by a number of factors. The recognition of the multiple determinants of the performance on many psychological tests should lead to the design of more 'discrete' tasks which are tied to single factors which might then be studied for their association with or dissociation from particular brain structures.

With the double dissociation paradigm Weiskrantz (1968) points out that

> ...the maximum information is conveyed when two treatments are alike in all but one critical aspect (e.g. for brain lesions – same mass, same damage to meninges, but different in locus) and that the two tasks similarly are alike in all but one critical aspect (e.g. same training procedure, same cue-response contingencies, but difference in sensory modality). This is simply to restate the essence of analytical control procedures, and the double dissociation paradigm is simply a way of combining two control procedures into a single pattern. But there are also great risks of reifying a dissociation between tests into a dissociation between functions and arguing that the affected function has been isolated by a single instance of dissociation.

Finally, the principle of double dissociation is proposed by Luria and others. 'The initial hypothesis in this line of work is the assumption that in the presence of a given local lesion which directly causes the loss of some factor, *all functional systems which include this factor suffer, while, at the same time, all functional systems which do not include the disturbed factor are preserved*' (Luria 1973, pp. 13–14). As one of numerous examples he points to the different effects of damage in the left temporal region in man as opposed to the effects of damage in the parieto-occipital region. Temporal damage leads to disturbance of acoustic analysis of that class of acoustic stimulation which we term phonemes and this leads to disturbance of any function which depends to any marked extent on this analysis; the greater the dependence of any function on the analysis of phonemes the greater will be the secondary disturbance of the function, e.g. repeating what another person has said or writing to dictation will be markedly affected. On the other hand functions such as spatial perception which do not depend to any extent on phonemic analysis will be unaffected. Conversely, parieto-occipital damage will spare all those functions dependent upon phonemic analysis but disrupt all functions which have a dependence on spatial orientation. Recent studies such as that of Papagno et al (1993) on apraxia versus aphasia continue to strengthen the usefulness of the concept.

Congruent dissociations

Since naturally occurring lesions are liable on most occasions to affect portions of functional systems which are geographically adjacent, the establishment of two or more 'double dissociations' will render the location of the causative lesion more and more certain. In other words the establishment of one dissociation may suggest application of an appropriate test in the form of a 'crucial experiment' in single cases. We might term such situations congruent dissociations. Table 1.1 depicts one such possible situation based on data given in Chapter 5.

Jones (1983) points out that the paradigm of double dissociation is essentially a type of crossover interaction and, viewed as such, it is not absolutely essential for each group to perform at a normal level as in the example cited above on one of the two tasks in each dissociation. The performance on the tasks may be lowered by non-specific factors as well as by the specific factors involved in the dissociation. This opinion is shared by Shallice (1979) in his analysis. The representation of the relative performances of the two groups on the tasks is shown in Figure 1.8.

Table 1.1 An example of congruent dissociation

Tests	Lesion site		
	Left temporal	**Right temporal**	**Non-temporal**
Verbal memory	Poor	Normal	Normal
Meaningful sounds	Poor	Normal	Normal
Non-verbal memory	Normal	Poor	Normal
Meaningless sounds	Normal	Poor	Normal

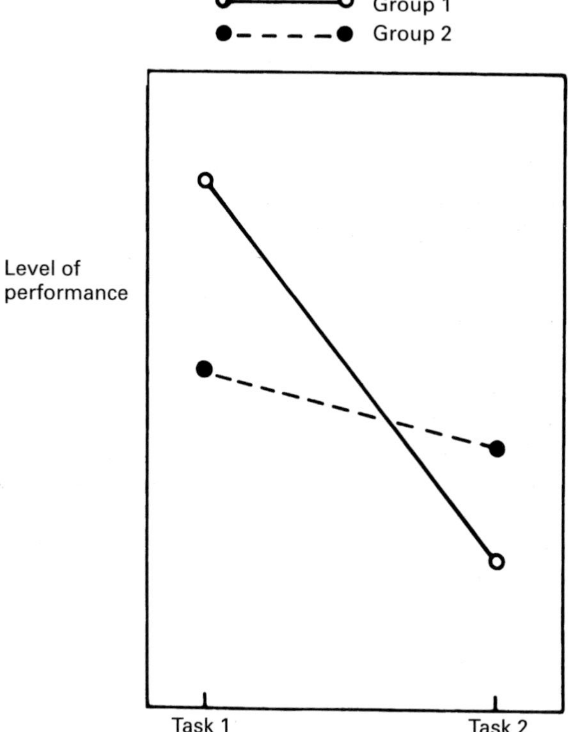

Fig. 1.8 Double dissociation as a form of crossover interaction (after Jones 1983).

The disconnection syndrome

The notion of the disconnection syndrome dates back to the classical neurologists of the latter half of the 19th century. With their conception of specialized sets of cells disposed over the cerebral cortex and the emerging knowledge of the fibre pathways connecting the various parts of the cortex with nearby and distant structures, a distinction arose between 'cortical' and 'conduction' syndromes. Wernicke, for example, knowing the effects of damage to the motor speech area and the quite different effects of damage to the sensory speech area which he himself described, was able to predict what would result if these areas were disconnected or isolated from each other. Though his anatomical assumptions about the pathways involved were not correct, the value of the concept of disconnection was validated by the discovery of the so-called 'conduction aphasia' (see Ch. 3).

The late 19th century and the early years of the present century produced a number of findings consistent with the disconnection theory, particularly those of Liepmann whose analysis of apraxia was in terms of disruption of connections. He was also aware that 'disconnection' symptoms or syndromes could be brought about by interrupting connections between the hemispheres, interhemispheric or callosal disconnection (Liepmann & Maas 1907), as well as by interrupting connections between different parts of the same hemisphere.

However, the disconnection theory for all its factual support gradually lost ground in the first three decades of the present century under the impact of holistic theories espoused by such neurologists as Head, Marie and von Monakow. When Akelaitis and his group published their findings on sectioning of the corpus callosum for the relief of epilepsy in the early 1940s the apparent absence of any of the predicted interhemispheric disconnection effects in their patients seemed to sound the death knell of the disconnection theory (Akelaitis 1940, 1941a–c, 1942a, b, 1943, Akelaitis et al 1941, 1942, 1943, Smith & Akelaitis 1942). It was only much later that it became obvious that the negative findings resulted from lack of appropriate techniques for eliciting disconnection signs. Another 10 years was to pass before the elegant experimentation of Myers and Sperry (1953) in animals demonstrated convincingly that such callosal effects do in fact occur, and the 'split-brain' techniques which they developed were soon applied to the small number of commissurotomy operations being performed on human subjects for the relief of epilepsy. The detailed findings of these hemisphere disconnection operations and their contribution to our understanding of the asymmetry of function in the two halves of the human brain are discussed in Chapter 8.

The split-brain work in animals also stimulated Geschwind and his colleagues both to re-examine the older clinical literature and to reassess their patients with disturbances of the higher functions. They were soon to find excellent examples (Geschwind 1962, Geschwind & Kaplan 1962, Howes 1962).

The following brief summary is condensed from the extensive treatment by Geschwind (1965b, c).

1. Disconnection syndromes are those produced by lesions of association pathways (see Ch. 2).

2. These pathways may be within the same hemisphere (intrahemispheric) or between the two hemispheres (interhemispheric or commissural).

3. Following 'Flechsig's principle' primary receptor areas of the cortex have neocortical connections only with adjacent 'association' areas.

4. The association areas on the other hand receive information, i.e. have connections with several other cortical areas, and send their outgoing connections to other areas at a distance.

5. Flechsig's principle also applies to linkages between the two hemispheres. There are no direct connections between the primary receptor areas of one side and the primary receptor areas of the other, only commissural connections between 'association' cortex. The effects of such an anatomical arrangement are summarized by Geschwind.

These anatomical facts imply that a large lesion of the association areas

> around a primary sensory area will act to disconnect it from other parts of the neocortex. Thus, a 'disconnexion lesion' will be a large lesion either of association cortex or of the white matter leading from this association cortex. The specification of the association areas as way-stations between different parts of neocortex is certainly too narrow, but it is at least not incorrect. This view, as we shall see, simplifies considerably the analysis of effects of lesions of these regions. Since a primary sensory region has no callosal connections, a lesion of association cortex may serve both to disconnect such an area from other regions in the same hemisphere and also to act in effect as a lesion of the callosal pathway from this primary sensory area (Geschwind 1965b, pp. 244–245).

This notion of a disconnection syndrome has been expressed in several ways in recent years, depending upon the theoretical background of the author, and is closely related to the notion of a functional system, a concept which is widely used in electronics and other sciences where 'the systems approach' has proved useful in pinpointing the site of lesions or faults in the system.

> The brain may be considered as a communication network, incorporating multiple information transmitting channels which lead to and from decision points. A limitation of function, namely the impairment or abolition of the ability to make particular decisions, may result from damage to the decision point and from interruption of input to or output from that point. Those points of the system which are most closely aggregated in cerebral space will be most vulnerable to selective inactivation by focal cerebral injury. The extreme example is the corpus callosum, division of which reliably induces a pure disconnection syndrome (Geschwind & Kaplan 1962, Myers 1956) without damage to decision points in either hemisphere...*The neurons that constitute a decision point are widely diffused over the cerebral cortex. But their distinctive function depends on their mode of linkage rather than on physical features of individual neurons, and this is not necessarily reflected in morphological differentiation.* (Kinsbourne 1971, p. 287) (emphasis added)

Midline surgical commissurotomy forms such a clear and dramatic example of disconnection that many students fail to appreciate that many naturally occurring lateral lesions must, of necessity, produce disconnection effects. If one considers the hypothetical case shown in Figure 1.9 it becomes apparent that for the purposes served by the functional link A–B, disconnection is essentially the same whether the interruption takes place laterally in the left hemisphere (1), the right hemisphere (2) as shown, or by surgical division in the midline (3).

Gazzaniga reminded us that cortical lesions also have the same effect: 'Hemisphere disconnection can also result, of course, from the degeneration of the callosal fibers normally innervating a region of extirpated or damaged cortex. Such lesions produce a partial commissurotomy much like those produced surgically – and they result in the same behavioural characteristics' (Gazzaniga 1970, p. 146).

We might summarize by observing that there are two major sets of connecting fibres, viz. those which link areas within the hemisphere (intrahemispheric, often termed association fibres) and those which link the two hemispheres

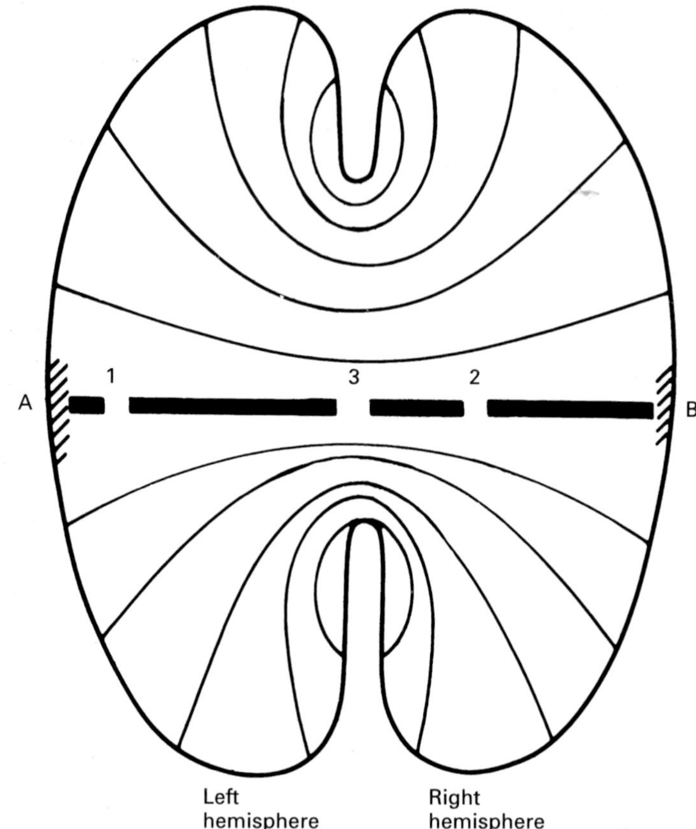

Fig. 1.9 Disconnection produced by a lateral lesion. Horizontal section through the corpus callosum.

(interhemispheric or commissural fibres). This allows for three basic forms of disconnection: (i) intrahemispheric disconnection (see conduction aphasia, Ch. 3); (ii) interhemispheric disconnection (see callosal or left-sided apraxia, Ch. 3, and commissurotomy, Ch. 8); and (iii) compound disconnection where both types of connection are conjointly interrupted (see Alexia without agraphia, Ch. 7).

References

Akelaitis A J 1940 A study of gnosis, praxis and language following partial and complete section of the corpus callosum. Transactions of the American Neurological Association 66: 182–185

Akelaitis A J 1941a Psychobiological studies following section of the corpus callosum. American Journal of Psychiatry 97: 1147–1157

Akelaitis A J 1941b Studies on the corpus callosum. VIII. American Journal of Psychiatry 98: 409–414

Akelaitis A J 1941c Studies on the corpus callosum. II. Archives of Neurology and Psychiatry 45: 788

Akelaitis A J 1942a Studies on the corpus callosum. V. Archives of Neurology and Psychiatry 47: 971–1008

Akelaitis A J 1942b Studies on the corpus callosum. VI. Archives of Neurology and Psychiatry 48: 914–937
Akelaitis A J 1943 Studies on the corpus callosum. VII. Journal of Neuropathology and Experimental Neurology 2: 226–262
Akelaitis A J, Risteen W A, Van Wagenen W P 1941 A contribution to the study of dyspraxia following partial and complete section of the corpus callosum. Transactions of the American Neurological Association 67: 75–78
Akelaitis A J, Risteen W A, Van Wagenen W P 1942 Studies on the corpus callosum. III. Archives of Neurology and Psychiatry 48: 914–937
Akelaitis A J, Risteen W A, Van Wagenen W P 1943 Studies on the corpus callosum. IX. Archives of Neurology and Psychiatry 49: 820–825
Beckner M 1959 The biological way of thought. University Press, New York
Benton A L 1965 The problem of cerebral dominance. Canadian Psychologist 6: 332–348
Benton A L, Joynt R J 1960 Early descriptions of aphasia. Archives of Neurology 3: 205–221
Boring E G 1929 A history of experimental psychology. Appleton Century Crofts, New York
Breasted J H 1930 The Edwin Smith surgical papyrus. University of Chicago Press, Chicago
Brodmann K 1909 Vergleichende Lokalisationslehre der Grosshirnrinde. Barth, Leipzig
Campbell A W 1905 Histological studies on the localisation of cerebral function. Cambridge University Press, Cambridge
Clarke E, Dewhurst K 1972 An illustrated history of brain function. Sandford, Oxford
Clarke E, O'Malley C D 1968 The human brain and spinal cord. University of California Press, Berkeley
Critchley M 1979 The divine banquet of the brain and other essays. Raven Press, New York
Déjerine J 1892 Contribution a l'étude anatomo-pathologique et clinique des différents variétés de cécité verbale. Comptes Rendus, Société de Biologie 4: 61–90
Ebell B 1937 The papyrus Ebers. Levin and Munksgaard, Copenhagen
Finger S, Roe D 1996 Gustave Dax and the early history of cerebral dominance. Archives of Neurology 53: 806–813
Froeschner E H 1992 Two examples of ancient skull surgery. Journal of Neurosurgery 76: 550–552
Gazzaniga M S 1970 The bisected brain. Appleton Century Crofts, New York
Geschwind N 1962 The anatomy of acquired disorders of reading. In: Money J (ed) Reading disability. Johns Hopkins Press, Baltimore
Geschwind N 1965a Alexia and colour-naming disturbance. In: Ettlinger G (ed) Functions of the corpus callosum. Churchill, London, pp 95–101
Geschwind N 1965b Disconnection syndromes in animals and man. Part I. Brain 88: 237–294
Geschwind N 1965c Disconnection syndromes in animals and man. Part II. Brain 88: 585–644
Geschwind N 1966 Carl Wernicke, the Breslau School, and the history of aphasia. In: Carterette E C (ed) Language and communication. University of California Press, Berkeley
Geschwind N 1967 Brain mechanisms suggested by studies of hemispheric connections. In: Darley F L (ed) Brain mechanisms underlying speech and language. Grune and Stratton, New York
Geschwind N, Kaplan E 1962 A human cerebral deconnection syndrome. Neurology 12: 675–685
Gibson W C 1962 Pioneers of localization in the brain. JAMA 180: 944–951
Gibson W C 1969 The early history of localization in the nervous system. In: Vinken P J, Bruyn G W (eds) Handbook of clinical neurology. North-Holland, Amsterdam, vol 2, ch 2
Graña F, Rocca E D, Graña L 1954 Los trepanaciones craneanas en el Peru en la época pre-Hispanica. Santa Maria, Lima, Peru
Gurdjian E S 1973 Head injury from antiquity to the present with special reference to penetrating head wounds. Thomas, Springfield, Illinois
Howes D 1962 An approach to the quantitative analysis of word blindness. In: Money J (ed) Reading disability: progress and research in dyslexia. Johns Hopkins Press, Baltimore
Jones G V 1983 On double dissociation of function. Neuropsychologia 1983: 397–400
Joynt R J 1964 Paul Pierre Broca: His contribution to the knowledge of aphasia. Cortex 1: 206–213
Kinsbourne M 1971 Cognitive deficit: experimental analysis. In McGaugh J L (ed) Psychiobiology. Academic Press, New York, ch 7

Lashley K S, Clark G 1946 The cytoarchitecture of the cerebral cortex of Ateles. Journal of Comparative Neurology 82: 233–306
Levin H S, Peters B H, Hulkonen D A 1983 The early concepts of anterograde and retrograde amnesia. Cortex 19: 427–440
Lichtheim L 1885 On aphasia. Brain 7: 433–484
Liepmann H, Maas O 1907 Fall von linksseifigen Agraphie und Apraxie bei rechtsseifigen Lahmung. Journal für Psychologie und Neurologie 10: 214–227
Luria A R 1966 Higher cortical functions in man. Basic Books, New York
Luria A R 1970 The functional organization of the brain. Scientific American 222: 66–78
Luria A R 1973 The working brain. Allen Lane, The Penguin Press, London
Magoun H W 1958 Early development of ideas relating the mind with the brain. In: Wolstenholme G E W, O'Connor C M (eds) The neurological basis of behaviour. Churchill, London
McFie J 1960 Psychological testing in clinical neurology. Journal of Nervous and Mental Disease 131: 383–393
McHenry L C 1969 Garrison's history of neurology. Thomas, Springfield, Illinois
Milner P 1970 Physiological psychology. Holt, Rinehart and Winston, New York
Myers R E 1956 Functions of corpus callosum in interocular transfer. Brain 79: 358–363
Myers R E, Sperry R W 1953 Interocular transfer of a visual form discrimination habit in cats after section of the optic chiasma and corpus callosum. Anatomical Record 115: 351–352
Papagno C, Della Sella S, Basso A 1993 Ideomotor apraxia without aphasia and aphasia without apraxia: the anatomical support for a double dissociation. Journal of Neurology, Neurosurgery and Psychiatry 56: 286–289
Piercy M F 1959 Testing for intellectual impairment – some comments on tests and testers. Journal of Mental Science 105: 489–495
Russell E W, Neuringer C, Goldstein G 1970 Assessment of brain damage: a neuropsychological key approach. Wiley, New York
Shallice T 1979 Case study approach in neuropsychological research. Journal of Clinical Neuropsychology 1: 183–211
Shapiro M B 1951 Experimental studies of a perceptual anomaly. 1: Initial experiments. Journal of Mental Science 97: 90–100
Sherrington C S 1951 Man on his nature, 2nd edn. Cambridge University Press, Cambridge
Smith K U, Akelaitis A J 1942 Studies of the corpus callosum. 1. Laterality in behavior and bilateral motor organization in man before and after section of the corpus callosum. Archives of Neurology and Psychiatry 47: 519–543
Sokal R R, Sneath P H 1963 Principles of numerical taxonomy. Freeman, San Francisco
Strub R L, Geschwind N 1983 Localization in Gerstmann syndrome. In: Kertesz A (ed) Localization in neuropsychology. Academic Press, New York, pp 295–321
Teuber H L 1955 Physiological psychology. Annual Review of Psychology 6: 267–296
Teuber H L 1959 Some alterations in behavior after cerebral lesions in man. In: Bass A D (ed) Evolution of nervous control from primitive organisms to man. American Association for the Advancement of Science, Washington
Victor M, Adams R D, Collins G F 1971 The Wernicke-Korsakoff syndrome. Davis, Philadelphia
Weiskrantz L 1968 Some traps and pontifications. In: Weiskrantz L (ed) The analysis of behavioral change. Harper and Row, New York, ch 15
Wilkins R H 1965 Neurosurgical classics. Johnson Reprint Corporation, New York
Woollam D H M 1958 Concepts of the brain and its functions in classical antiquity. In: Pointer F N L (ed) The history and philosophy of knowledge of the brain and its functions. Blackwell, Oxford

2

Basic anatomy of the brain

ANATOMICAL TERMS OF RELATIONSHIP

Because some readers may be unfamiliar with anatomy while still wishing to gain a basic knowledge of the structure of the nervous system, it will be worthwhile to explain a few commonly used terms. Some appreciation of the basic structure of the brain is essential for (a) an understanding of the literature which is becoming more detailed with regard to anatomical localization of lesions, (b) understanding relevant details communicated in patients' hospital files, and (c) the development of the neuropsychologist's thinking about brain-behaviour relationships in the understanding of individual cases.

Firstly, the six principal terms are illustrated in Figure 2.1. The alternative terms in brackets may still be found occasionally. Secondly, an appreciation of the relative position of structures within the nervous system can be gained from studying series of sections. There are three principal planes of reference:

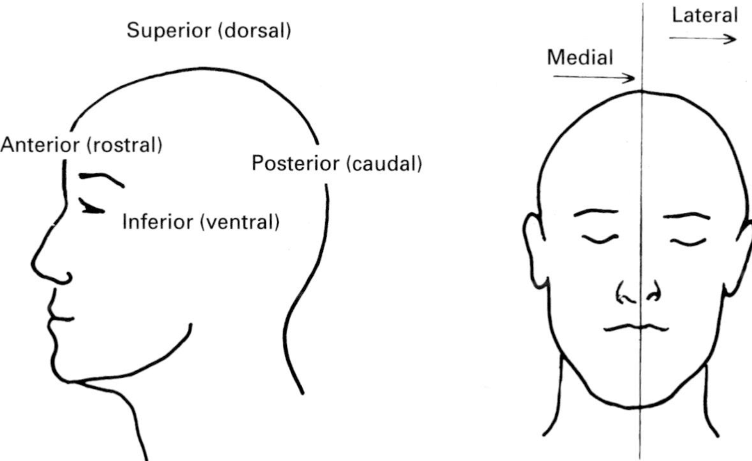

Fig. 2.1 Terms of relationship in neuroanatomy.

(i) *Coronal* or frontal sections are parallel to a vertical plane through both ears.

(ii) *Sagittal* or longitudinal sections are at right angles to the coronal plane in a vertical direction. A median or midline sagittal section would divide the brain into its two hemispheres.

(iii) *Horizontal* sections are at right angles to the other two (Fig. 2.2).

Multiple sections in one or more of these planes are shown in imaging techniques (see Ch. 3).

THE COVERINGS OF THE BRAIN (MENINGES)

Dura mater

The tough outermost layer, called the *dura mater*, is closely attached to the inner surface of the skull and also provides several partitions which divide the skull cavity into relatively separate compartments. Since these partitions are anchored to the skull, they help to prevent the very soft and fragile brain tissue from excessive movement which would result in tearing of the brain substance whenever the head was suddenly accelerated, decelerated, or rapidly rotated. Even this protection breaks down when such movements are very violent.

The two major partitions of the dura mater are the *falx cerebri* and the *tentorium cerebelli* (Fig. 2.3).

The falx cerebri provides a vertical partition between the major divisions of the cerebrum, the left and right cerebral hemispheres. Its narrow end is attached to the skull anteriorly. Its upper edge is attached to the vault of the skull in the midline while its lower edge arches over the upper edge of the *corpus callosum* to join on to the other major partition, the *tentorium cerebelli* which separates the base of the posterior parts of the cerebral hemispheres

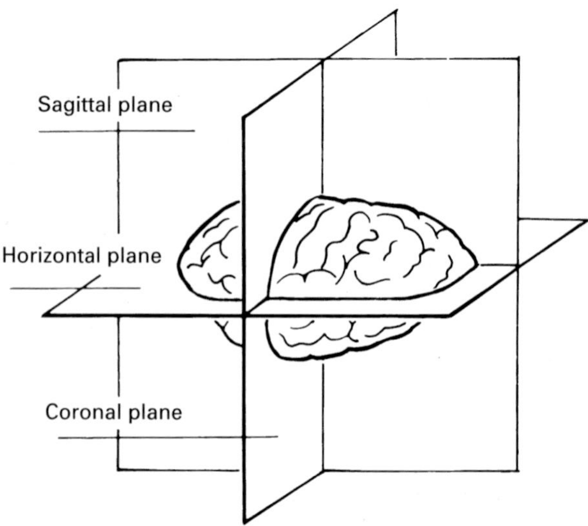

Fig. 2.2 Planes of reference.

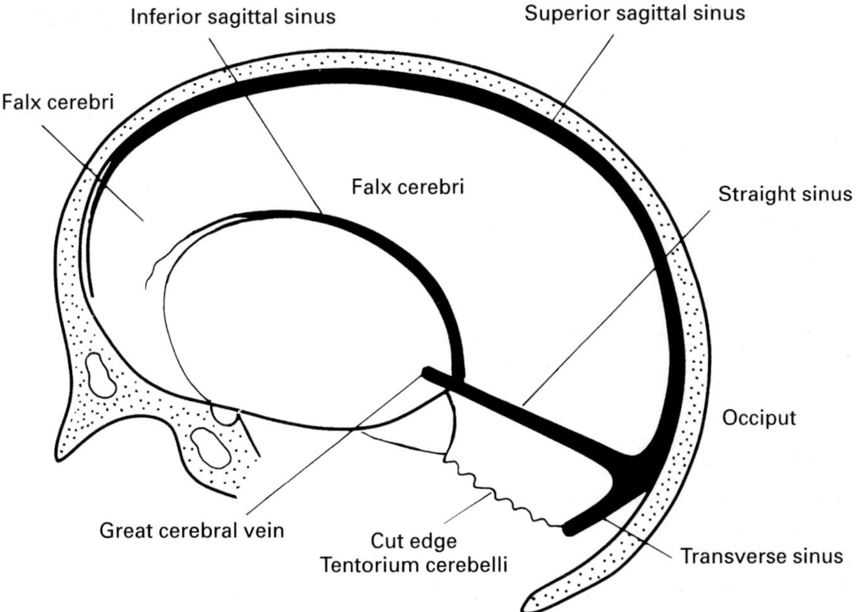

Fig. 2.3 Partitions of the dura mater.

from the cerebellum below. The tentorium and falx cerebri are stretched taut.

In the outer layer of the dura mater are embedded arteries which are termed meningeal arteries though their main purpose is to provide blood supply for the bones of the skull as well as the relatively avascular dura mater. The dura also forms the walls of the large channels or sinuses which drain the venous blood from the brain. The narrow space between the dura and arachnoid mater is termed the *subdural space*.

Arachnoid mater

The second meningeal membrane is also avascular but, unlike the dura, it is very thin and delicate. It is separated from the dura only by a very thin layer of fluid and is attached by cobweb-like strands of tissue to the third membrane which closely follows the conformation of the outer layer of the brain and spinal cord. This latter layer is known as the *pia mater*, and the fluid-filled space which separates the arachnoid from the pia mater is termed the *subarachnoid space*. The blood vessels of the brain are distributed in the *arachnoid mater* and send branches through the pia mater to supply the outer layer of the cerebral hemispheres known as the *cerebral cortex*.

Pia mater

The inner membrane, the pia mater, closely follows the convolutions or *gyri* of the cerebral hemispheres and dips down into the fissures or *sulci* which separate them.

THE CEREBROSPINAL FLUID SYSTEM

The subarachnoid space

The subarachnoid space is filled with cerebrospinal fluid (CSF) which is a crystal clear, colourless fluid composed largely of water. The subarachnoid space is narrow over the cerebral hemispheres but is expanded around the base of the brain, particularly around the brain stem where the subarachnoid space communicates with the ventricular cavities within the brain. The cerebrospinal fluid acts as a buffer to protect the brain and spinal cord. It also helps to provide a constant pressure within the bony cavity under normal conditions. The numerous other functions of the cerebrospinal fluid are beyond the scope of the present outline.

Ventricular cavities

There are four ventricular cavities within the brain. These are continuous with each other and the central canal at the upper end of the spinal cord. Each cerebral hemisphere contains a *lateral ventricle*. Each of these communicates with the midline *third ventricle* which in turn communicates with the *fourth ventricle*. The named parts of the system are shown in Figure 2.4.

GROSS TOPOGRAPHY OF THE BRAIN

The brain has three major divisions, the cerebral hemispheres, the brain stem,

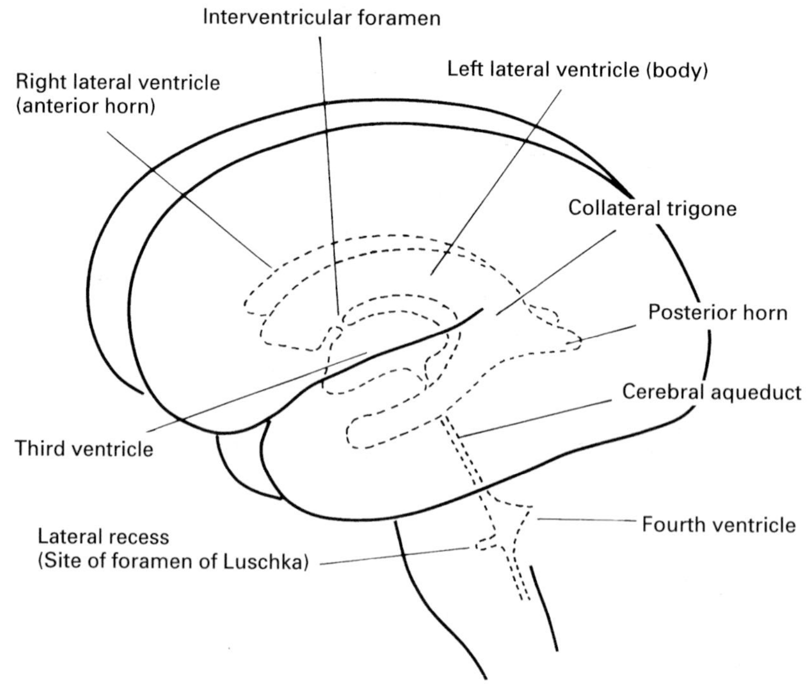

Fig. 2.4 Outline of the ventricle projected onto a lateral view of the brain.

and the cerebellum. Our main concern will be with the cerebral hemispheres and, to a lesser extent, with the midbrain. Description of the cerebellum will be omitted since it is little concerned with man's higher functions. The cerebellum is concerned primarily with motor co-ordination and the control of muscle tone and equilibrium.

The cerebral hemispheres

The paired hemispheres appear to be mirror images of each other. They are covered by a convoluted layer of grey matter, the *cerebral cortex* (Fig. 2.5), which covers the internal white matter and deeply placed collections of grey matter or neuronal masses collectively known as the *basal ganglia*. The grey matter represents nerve cell collections while the white matter represents cell fibres which unite the various regions of the brain with each other (Fig. 2.6).

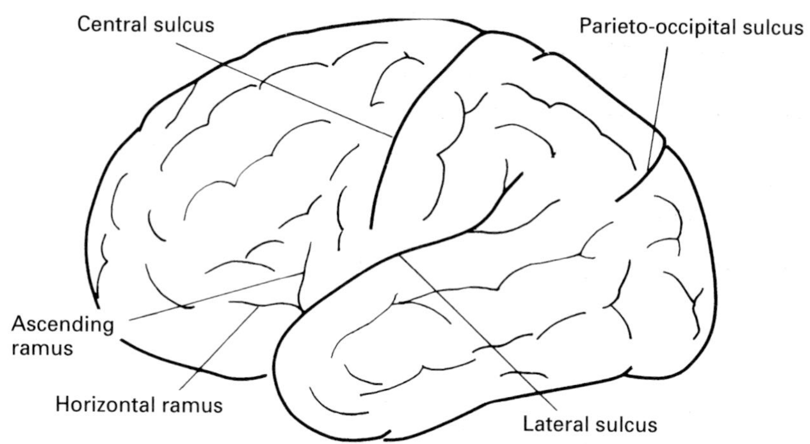

Fig. 2.5 Lateral view of the left cerebral hemisphere.

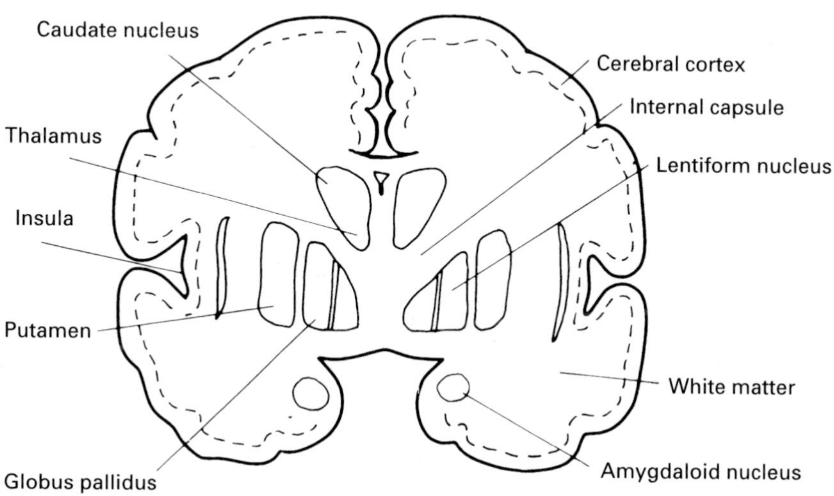

Fig. 2.6 Coronal section of the hemispheres.

The two hemispheres are separated by the *longitudinal fissure* which completely separates them in the anterior (frontal) and posterior (occipital) regions (Fig. 2.7). The falx cerebri forms a partition between the two sides. In the central region the two hemispheres are united by a thick band of white matter, the *corpus callosum* (so called because of its firm consistency), which is the chief functional link between them.

Superolateral surface

Each cerebral hemisphere has three surfaces, the large convex superolateral surface, the flattened medial surface in contact with the falx cerebri, and the inferior surface which lies on the floor of the anterior and middle cranial depressions (fossae) in front and on the tentorium cerebelli behind.

The convoluted portions of the cerebral cortex are known as gyri. They are separated from each other by fissures or sulci. Some of these sulci and gyri are relatively constant features of most human brains and form the basis for describing the general external topography of the brain. On the lateral surface three prominent sulci are used as a basis for dividing each hemisphere into four major areas or lobes. A fifth 'lobe', the limbic lobe, will be described separately. The three sulci are (1) the lateral sulcus, (2) the central sulcus, and (3) the parieto-occipital sulcus.

The *lateral sulcus* is a very deep division between the frontal and temporal lobes anteriorly and portions of the parietal and temporal lobes posteriorly.

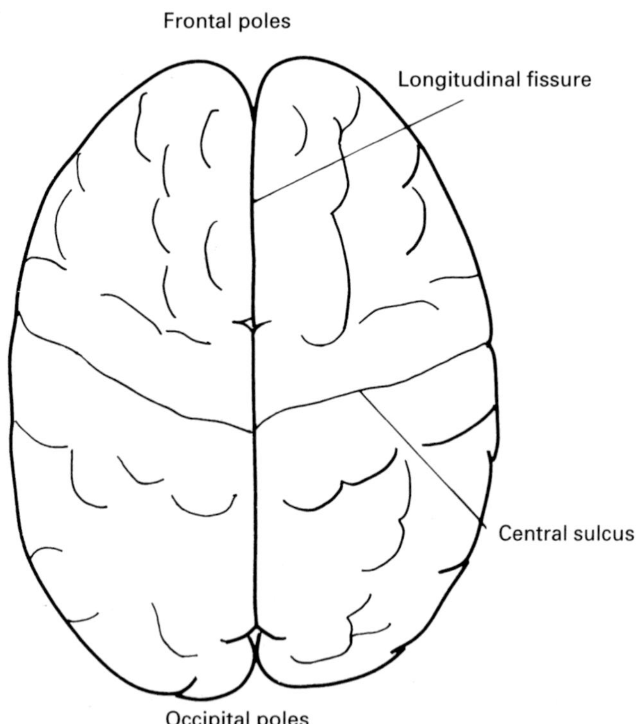

Fig. 2.7 Superior view of the hemispheres.

Towards the anterior end two small branches (rami), the *anterior horizontal ramus* and the *anterior ascending ramus,* run for about 2 cm into the lower part of the frontal lobe while the terminal ascending ramus extends into the inferior part of the parietal lobe. Buried within the lateral sulcus is a cortical area known as the *insula*. This can only be seen when the lips of the fissure are drawn apart (Fig. 2.8).

The areas of cortex overlying the insula are called the opercula (lids). The superior surface consists of the *frontal operculum* which lies between the anterior horizontal and ascending rami, and the *frontoparietal operculum*. The *temporal operculum* is below the posterior ramus and is made up of the superior temporal gyrus and the transverse temporal gyri.

The *central sulcus* is less easy to find. It runs from the superior margin of the hemisphere downward and forward towards the lateral sulcus separating the frontal from the parietal lobe. The central sulcus is variable in form and runs only a little way over the superior border of the hemisphere to the medial surface.

The *parieto-occipital sulcus* is a fairly constant deep sulcus which cuts into the superior border of the hemisphere some 5 cm anterior to the occipital pole and runs on the medial surface in an anterior and inferior direction to intersect the well marked *calcarine sulcus* about midway along its length.

Lobar divisions

The arbitrary boundaries of the lobar divisions are shown with respect to the major sulci in Figure 2.9.

The *frontal lobe* is that part of the hemisphere above the lateral sulcus and in front of the central sulcus.

The *parietal lobe* is bounded in front by the central sulcus and below by the lateral sulcus before it turns upwards to the line which forms the posterior boundary of the lobe. This line runs from the point where the parieto-occipital

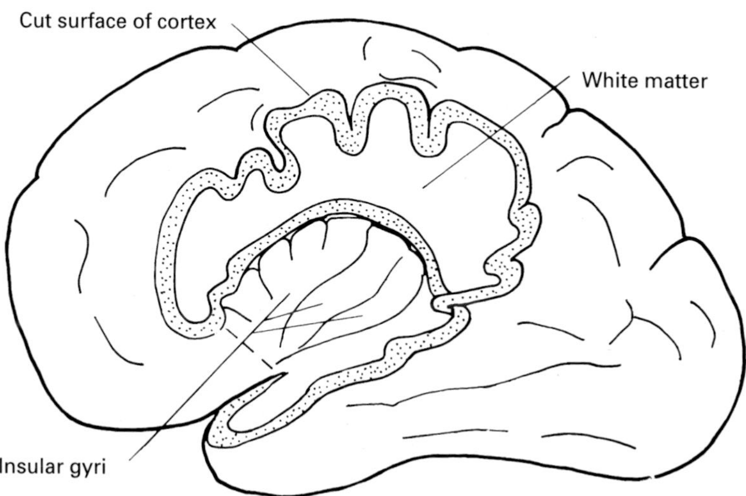

Fig. 2.8 The insular gyri with overlying cortex removed.

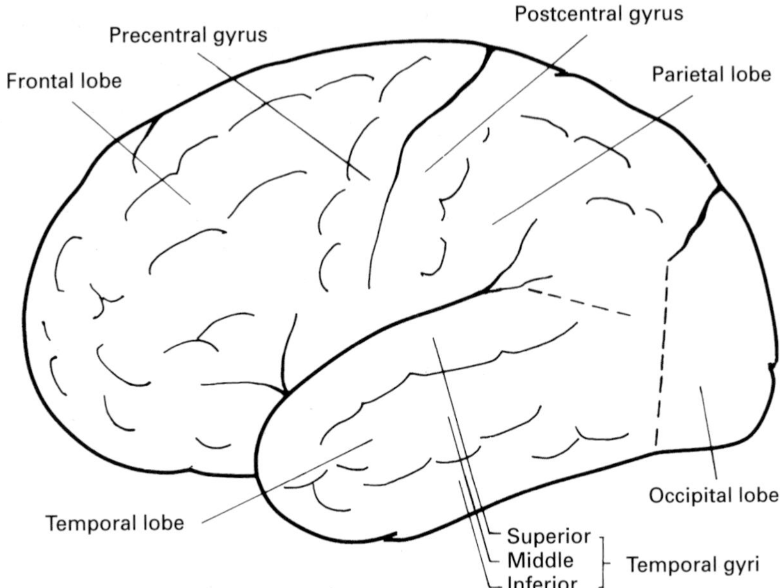

Fig. 2.9 Lobar divisions of the hemisphere.

sulcus crosses the superior border of the hemisphere to a small notch (pre-occipital notch) some 4 cm in front of the occipital pole.

The *occipital lobe* lies posterior to the vertical boundary line on the convex surface and, on the medial aspect, to the parieto-occipital sulcus and a line joining the junction of the parieto-occipital sulcus with the pre-occipital notch.

The *temporal lobe* is bounded by the lateral sulcus and the artificial line of demarcation described above.

Further details of the frontal, temporal, parietal and occipital lobes are described in the separate chapters devoted to each lobe.

Apart from the major divisions into lobes, certain gross features of the external topography of the brain may be described on the three surfaces of the hemispheres, the superolateral, medial, and inferior surfaces.

The superolateral surface is divided into more or less constant gyri as depicted in Figure 2.9.

Medial surface

The medial surfaces of the hemispheres are seen after cutting through the corpus callosum which joins them (Fig. 2.10). The corpus callosum is some 8 cm in length. The anterior curved portion is known as the genu of the corpus callosum and this tapers inferiorly and posteriorly as the *rostrum*. The corpus callosum ends posteriorly in a blunt enlargement termed the *splenium* which lies over the pineal body and the midbrain. The corpus callosum is separated on its upper surface from the *cingulate gyrus* by the callosal sulcus. Posteriorly this gyrus curves around the splenium of the corpus callosum to enter the temporal lobe as the *parahippocampal gyrus*.

Above the cingulate gyrus is a well marked fissure which runs from a position just below the genu (the *subcallosal area*) to a point just in front of and vertically above the splenium where it turns upwards as the *marginal sulcus*

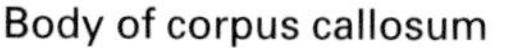
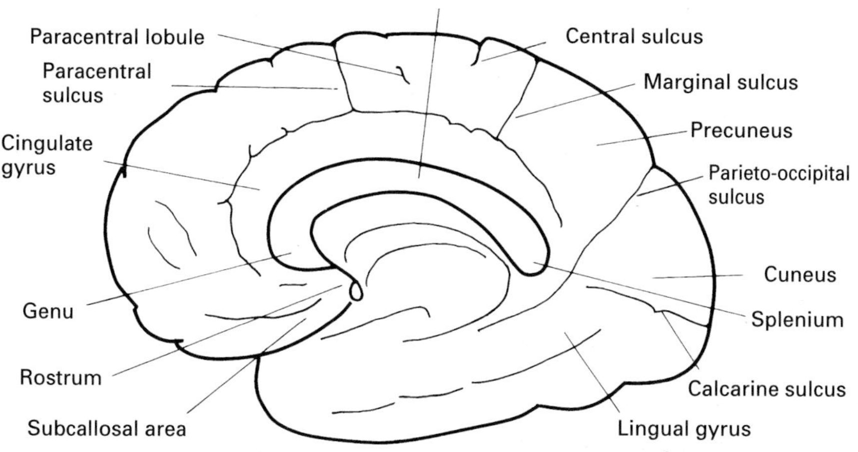

Fig. 2.10 Medial view of the right hemisphere.

(or marginal branch of the cingulate sulcus), above the splenium. Usually the cingulate sulcus gives off a prominent branch, the *paracentral sulcus,* which crosses the upper medial border of the hemisphere vertically above the middle part of the body of the corpus callosum. The area between the paracentral sulcus and the marginal sulcus is the *paracentral lobule.* The lobule is divided by the small part of the central fissure which just reaches the upper medial surface of the hemisphere so that the *paracentral lobule* contains the extension over on to the medial surface of the *precentral* and *postcentral gyri.* The area between the marginal sulcus and the parieto-occipital sulcus is the *precuneus.* This is the extension medially of the *superior parietal lobule.* The *calcarine sulcus* runs forward from the occipital pole to divide the occipital lobe into the cuneus above and the lingual gyrus below.

Inferior surface

The inferior surface of the hemisphere consists of two parts (Fig. 2.11). The smaller anterior portion is the inferior or orbital surface of the frontal lobe while the larger posterior portion represents the inferior surfaces of the temporal and occipital lobes.

The orbital surface of the frontal lobe has a deep straight sulcus, the *olfactory sulcus,* with the *olfactory bulb* and *tract* lying on it. Medial to this sulcus lies the gyrus rectus while lateral to it lie the *orbital gyri.*

The inferior surface of the occipital lobe and the posterior part of the temporal lobe lie on the tentorium cerebelli while the anterior portion of the temporal lobe lies in a depression in the skull, the *middle cranial fossa.* The gyri in this posterior portion are the *lingual gyrus* medially, the *parahippocampal gyrus* and *uncus,* and the *occipitotemporal gyri* laterally.

The limbic lobe and limbic system

On the medial surface of each cerebral hemisphere there is a ring of structures which surrounds the anterior (rostral) part of the brain stem and the commissures uniting the hemispheres. The major portion of the limbic lobe is made up

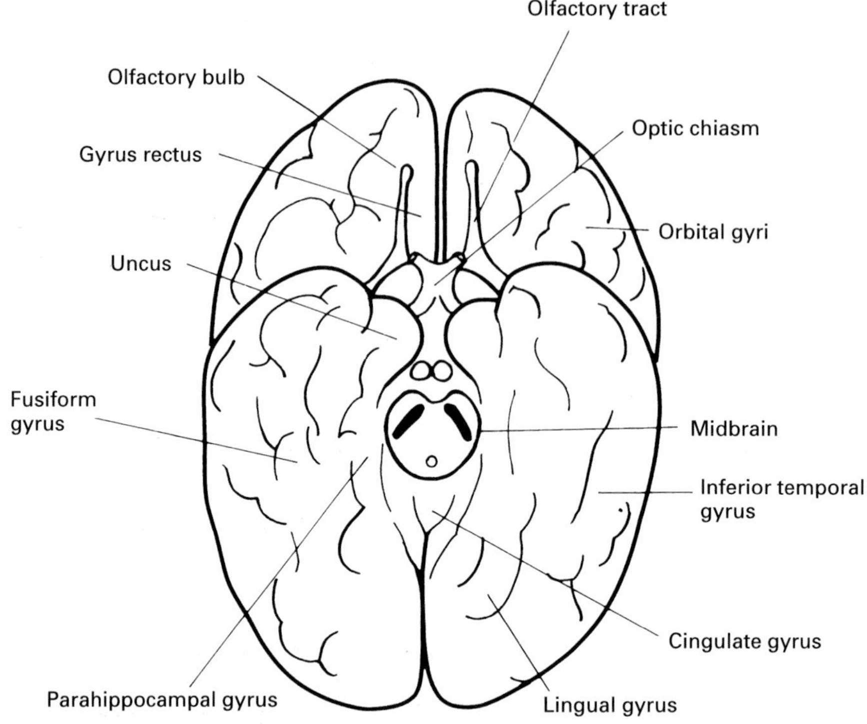

Fig. 2.11 Inferior surface of the hemispheres.

of the *cingulate gyrus* above and the *parahippocampal gyrus* below (Fig. 2.12). It also includes the smaller *subcallosal gyrus* and the *hippocampal formation* and *dentate gyrus*.

The term 'limbic system' refers to a much more extensive complex of structures which includes not only the structures of the limbic lobe but also the temporal pole, anterior portion of the insula, posterior orbital surface of the frontal lobe, and a number of subcortical nuclei. These subcortical nuclei include thalamic, hypothalamic, septal and amygdaloid nuclei, and there is also evidence of a close relationship with the midbrain reticular formation and the reticular nucleus of the thalamus.

The term 'limbic system' includes so many structures and pathways that the general usefulness of the concept of a unified system is open to question. Certainly it is a region where a large number of circuits relating to different functions come together. Since they lie generally towards the middle axis of the brain mass we will later refer to them as axial or medial structures (Fig. 2.13).

As early as 1937 Papez defined a recurrent or 'closed' part of the system, now known as the 'circuit of Papez', as the substratum for controlling emotions and emotional expressions. The Papez circuit forms the following linkage: hippocampus–fornix–mamillary bodies–thalamus–cingulate cortex–hippocampus. A good deal of evidence has also accumulated in recent years to associate lesions of the hippocampal–fornix–mamillary body connections with a disorder of memory of the type known as the Korsakoff or general amnesic syndrome. The importance of the limbic system in emotional experi-

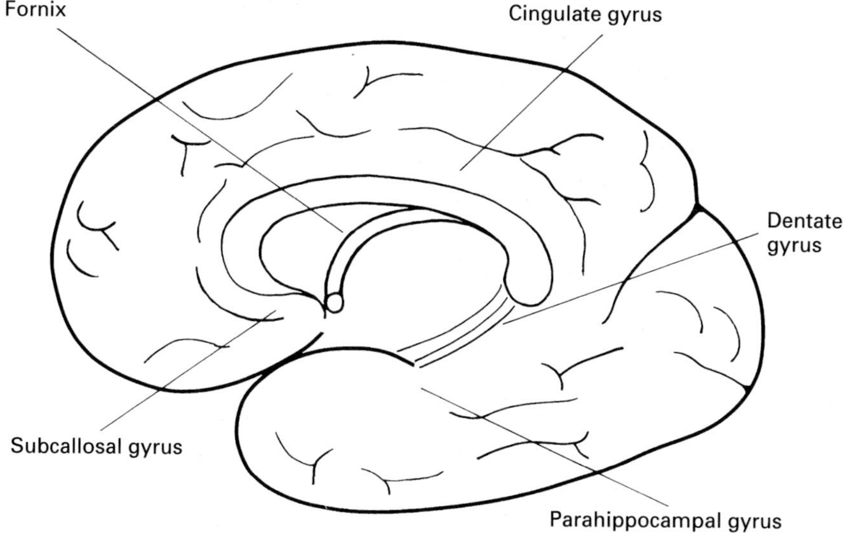

Fig. 2.12 The limbic lobe.

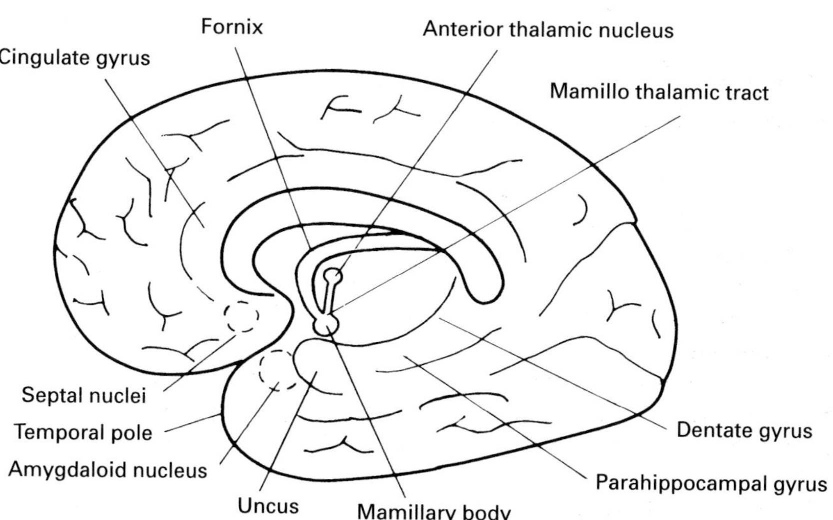

Fig. 2.13 The limbic system.

ence and expression has also been demonstrated by bilateral removal of the limbic structures in the temporal lobe, amygdaloid nucleus, hippocampus, and parahippocampal gyrus as well as the temporal neocortex overlying these structures.

Despite the general use of the terms *limbic lobe* and *limbic system* there are those who see dangers in grouping structures under such headings: 'It is difficult to see that the lumping together of these different regions under one anatomical heading, "the limbic lobe" serves any useful purpose…It is even less justifiable to speak of a "limbic system"…the "limbic system" appears to be on its way to including all brain functions' (Brodal 1980, pp. 537–538).

The hippocampal system

The *hippocampal system* (Fig. 2.14) is one of the more primitive parts of the cerebrum and has an extremely simple three-layered cortex, the *archipallium*. The hippocampal system is made up of the *parahippocampal gyrus* and *uncus*, the *hippocampal formation, dentate gyrus, gyrus fasciolus, indusium griseum, fimbria* and *fornix*. These structures form a pair of arches extending from the region of the interventricular foramina to the tip of the inferior horn of the lateral ventricle (Figs 2.13, 2.14).

The *parahippocampal gyrus* and *uncus* have been seen on the inferior surface of the brain towards the midline. The *hippocampus* is a slightly curved elevation in the floor of the inferior (temporal) horn of the ventricle. Its broader anterior end is just posterolateral to the uncus and the hippocampus diminishes rapidly as it moves posteriorly. The structure of the hippocampus and its relation to neighbouring structures can be further appreciated in a transverse or coronal section through the temporal lobe (Fig. 2.15).

Fibres on the medial surface of the upper convexity of the hippocampus form a flattened band, the *fimbria*, which increases posteriorly as the hippocampus diminishes and, as the pair of fimbria curve dorsomedially the fibres become the *crura of the fornix* which then pass forward beneath the corpus callosum. Figure 2.16 shows the corpus callosum cut away to reveal these structures.

Ventral (inferior) to the fimbria there is a narrow notched band, the *dentate gyrus*. It lessens posteriorly accompanying the hippocampus, curves around the splenium of the corpus callosum having separated from the fimbria and passes on to the superior surface of the corpus callosum in the form of the delicate *fasciolar gyrus*. It then spreads out into a thin grey sheet termed the *indusium griseum* or *supracallosal gyrus*.

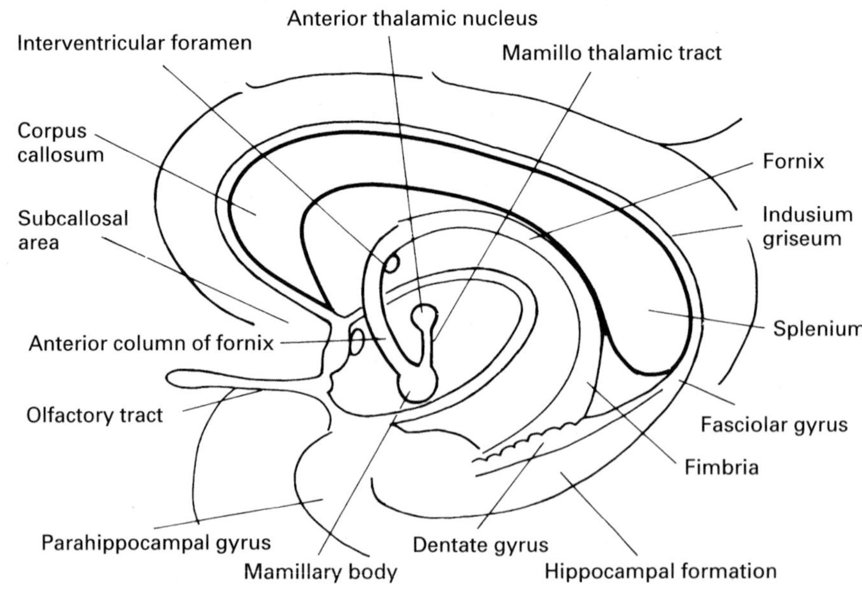

Fig. 2.14 The hippocampal system.

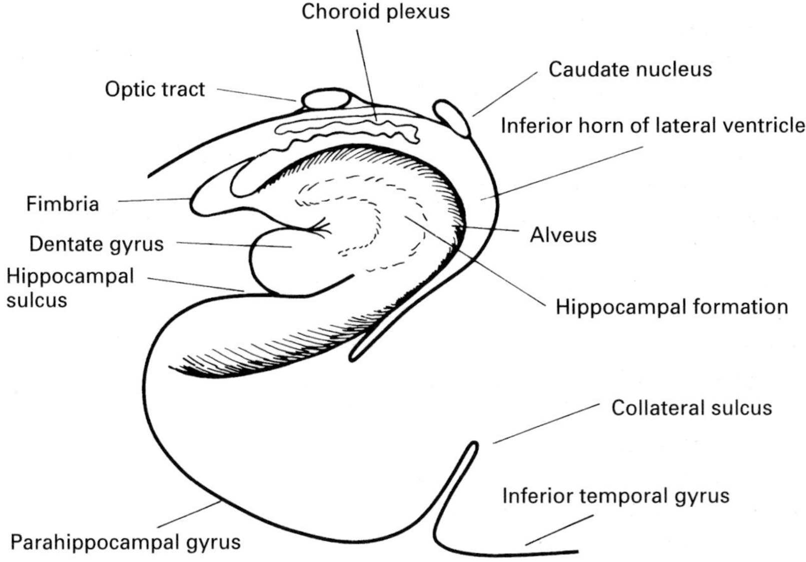

Fig. 2.15 Coronal section through the hippocampus.

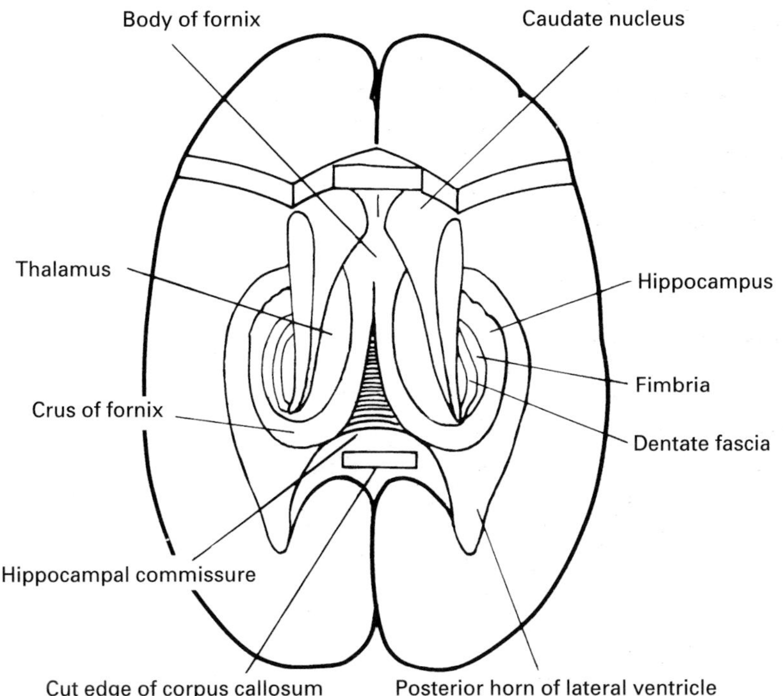

Fig. 2.16 Overlying tissue removed to show the hippocampus and fornix.

The fornix forms the principal efferent fibre system of the hippocampal formation. It has both projection and commissural fibres. The commissural fibres of the fornix (*hippocampal commissure*) are described below. As the crura of the fornix come together under the ventral surface of the corpus callosum they form the *body of the fornix* which travels forward to the rostral margin of the thalamus where they separate again into bundles forming the *anterior columns of the fornix*. The bundles again diverge from each other, arch in front of the *interventricular foramina* and posterior to the anterior commissure and incline slightly posteriorly to terminate in the mamillary bodies.

Further detail about the anatomical connections and functional contributions of the hippocampus and related structures can be found in the extensive reviews in the books edited by Isaacson and Pribram (1976) and Seifert (1983).

THE CEREBRAL CORTEX

The cerebral cortex is the most recently elaborated structure in the central nervous system. It is only in the mammal that it takes on special significance, and it reaches its greatest size relative to other structures in man.

The notion of architectonics was mentioned in Chapter 1. Though the cellular arrangement of the cortex varies in different areas of the brain, it is customary to describe a sample of 'modal' or 'typical' cortex made up of six layers. This six-layered pattern distinguishes the *neocortex* or new cortex from the *paleocortex* which predominates in lower animals and is largely concerned in them with olfaction. Though a certain amount of more primitively structured cortex has been preserved in man, it has become displaced to deeper parts of the brain where it is almost completely covered by the neocortex which comprises the major part of the cerebral cortex in man. The paleocortical structures, because of their earlier association with smell, are sometimes termed collectively the *rhinencephalon* or nose brain. In man, as in other higher mammals, the functions of these structures have little to do with olfaction. They might best be described as being made up of (1) olfactory components and (2) the limbic components described elsewhere.

Functional areas of the cortex

Functional areas of the cortex have been defined in a number of ways including the study of electrical potentials evoked in the cortex on the presentation of different stimuli, the stimulation of the exposed cortex in conscious human subjects undergoing neurosurgery, and more recently with newer neuroimaging techniques (Ch. 5). The *motor area* is situated in the precentral gyrus and the *sensory area* in the post-central gyrus, both having somatotopic representation. The *visual area* is situated in the cortex of the occipital lobe on either side of the calcarine sulcus, mainly on the medial and partly on the superolateral aspect of the hemisphere. The *auditory area* is situated in the *transverse gyri of Heschl* and is largely concealed in the depth of the temporal cortex in the lateral fissure just extending on to the lateral surface of the hemisphere (Fig. 5.4). The remainder of the post-central cortex of the parietal, temporal, and occipital lobes is concerned with the integration and elaboration of incoming sensory information.

Cortical zones

Luria (1973) has divided the whole area of the brain behind the central sulcus into three types of cortical region. He describes how disruption of these different functional types of cortex, known as cortical zones, may confer characteristic properties on the deficits observed. The following brief description scarcely does credit to the elegance of the conception nor the great value which this system has for the understanding of the individual case and for its usefulness in gaining a deeper appreciation of the psychological processes themselves. The principal features of Luria's system have been sketched in Chapter 1. Here a brief relation will be made to the cortical structure itself.

The *primary zones* of Luria are what are commonly termed primary projection areas. They possess high modal specificity, i.e. each particular area responds to highly differentiated properties of visual, auditory, or bodily sense information. They are also topologically arranged so that specific aspects of the stimulus are located systematically in order in the cortex, e.g. sense information from different parts of the body projects to particular sensory cortical areas, specific tones project to specific areas of the auditory cortex, and specific parts of the visual field to specific areas of the visual cortex. These primary zones consist 'mainly of neurons of afferent layer IV' of the cortex and their specificity and topological organization may be of considerable help in neurological diagnosis.

Each primary zone is made up largely of cells which respond only to a specific sense modality but also possesses a few cells which respond to other modes of stimulation and may be concerned with the property of maintaining an optimal state of arousal or alertness in the cortex, or what Luria terms 'cortical tone'. Cortical tone is regulated by the reticular formation of the brain stem. Information on cortical arousal may be found in textbooks of physiology and physiological psychology.

The *secondary zones* are the areas adjacent to the primary projection areas where the modality specific information becomes integrated into meaningful wholes. In a general sense the primary zones may be said to be concerned with sensation while the secondary zones are concerned with perception or gnosis. In the secondary zones 'afferent layer IV yields its dominant position to layers II and III of cells, whose degree of modal specificity is lower and whose composition includes many more associative neurons with short axons, enabling incoming excitation to be combined into the necessary functional patterns, and they thus subserve a synthetic function' (Luria 1973, pp. 68–69). Disruptions of these secondary zones will give rise to gnostic or perceptual disorders restricted to a perceptual modality, e.g. auditory or visual or tactile agnosia.

The *tertiary zones* serve to integrate information across sense modalities. They lie at the borders of the parietal (somato-sensory), temporal (auditory), and occipital (visual) secondary zones. In these *zones of overlapping* of the parieto–temporo–occipital association area, modal specificity disappears. The tertiary cortex is typified by a predominance of cells from the upper cortical layers, and this type of cortex is seen only in man. These are the last portions of the brain to mature in ontogenetic development, not reaching full development until around 7 years of age. Disruption of the tertiary zones gives rise to disorders which transcend any single modality and hence may be thought of as *supramodal* in character (see Ch. 6).

Luria's concept of the post-central cortical territory (or retrofrontal cortex) is thus a hierarchical one which moves from regions of high modal specificity to those which are supramodal in nature. The nature and connections of the frontal cortex are dealt with in Chapter 4.

THE BRAIN STEM

The brain stem is divided into four parts – the medulla oblongata, pons, mesencephalon or midbrain, and the diencephalon; but only the uppermost portion is of major interest to neuropsychology. It is surrounded by the hemispheres on all sides except for a small region between the mamillary bodies and optic chiasma and is one of the most complex regions of the central nervous system. It extends from the region of the interventricular foramen to the posterior commissure above and is continuous with the midbrain (mesencephalon) below (Fig. 2.17).

The superior surface of the diencephalon forms part of the floor of the body of the lateral ventricle. The diencephalon encloses the third ventricle and has a number of named components, the one of principal interest being the thalamus. Consideration is given to the higher functions of the diencephalon in Chapter 9.

The *thalamus* is an oblique mass of grey matter on either side of the midline. The two lateral halves have been divided into a number of nuclei whose classification and nomenclature varies somewhat from one authority to another. Some classifications include more than 20 nuclei but a simpler division is used here (Fig. 2.18). This is related below to the projection of fibres to the cortex (Figs 2.19 and 2.20).

Bowsher (1970) points out that 'with the exception of certain areas in the temporal lobe, the whole neocortex and the corpus striatum receive specific fibres from the thalamus' (p. 125).

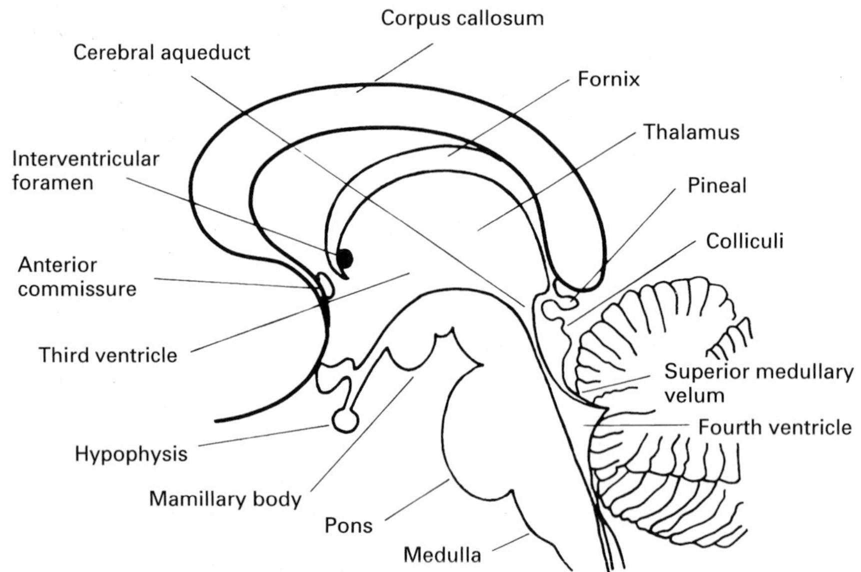

Fig. 2.17 Mid-sagittal section of the brain stem.

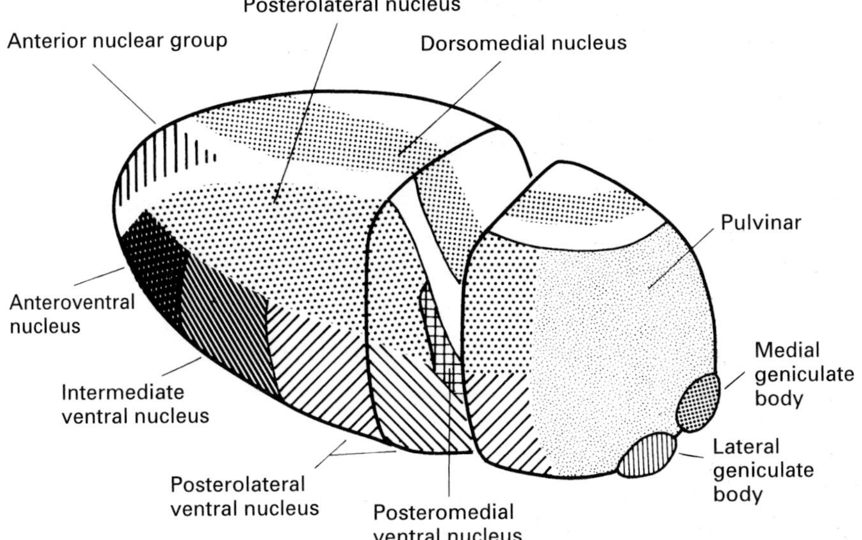

Fig. 2.18 Nuclei of the left thalamus.

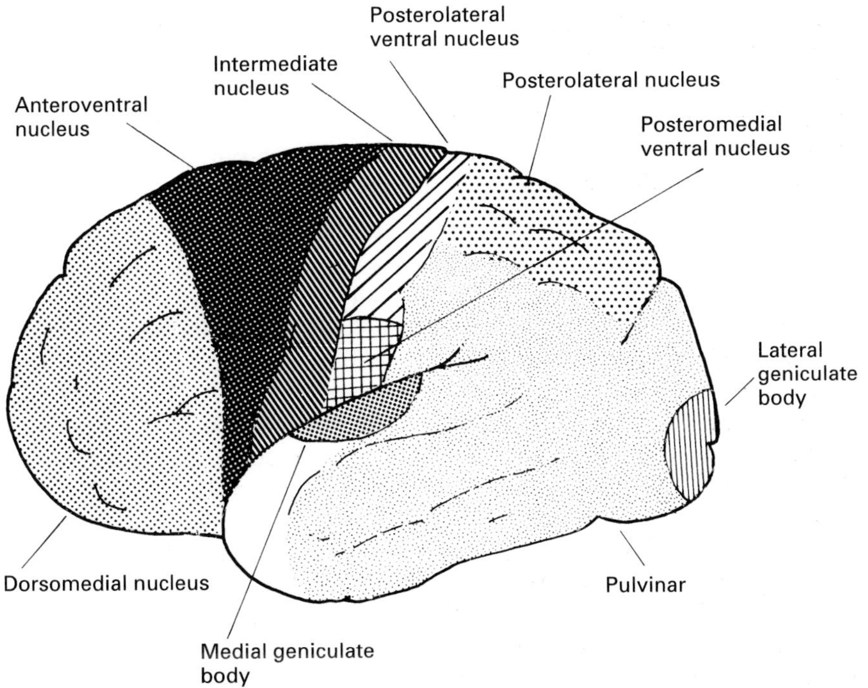

Fig. 2.19 Cortical projections of the thalamus (lateral).

Thus the whole telencephalon (cerebral hemisphere) except some of the neocortex of the temporal lobe, can be regarded as an umbrella cover, whose hub is the thalamus and the spokes of which are the specific thalamo-telencephalic projections . . . It can be seen from this that the true

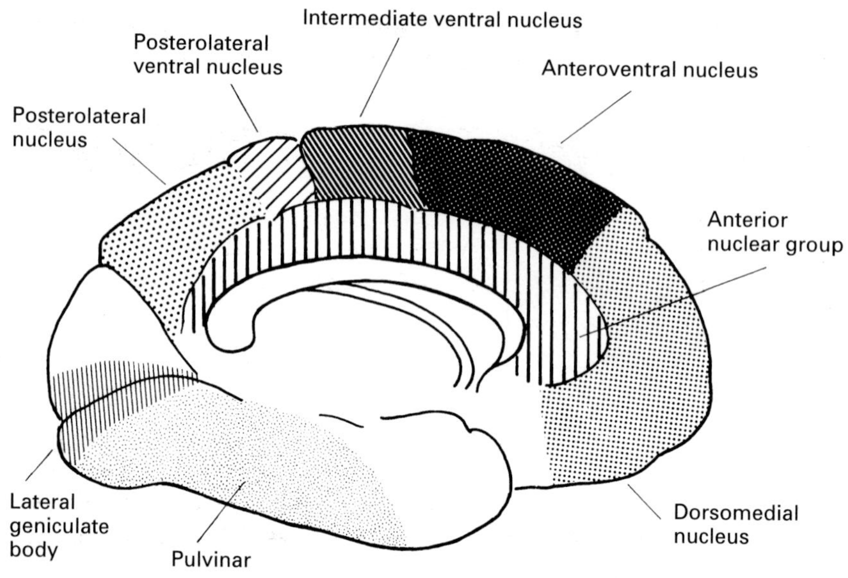

Fig. 2.20 Cortical projections of the thalamus (medial).

> definition of a functional cortical area depends not upon the fortuitous folding of its surface into sulci and gyri, nor upon its cytoarchitecture (though this is related), but upon its specific projection from a particular thalamic nucleus. For example, the primary somatosensory cortex (roughly defined as the post-central gyrus) is, in precise terms, only and entirely that area of cortex which receives its specific projections from the ventroposterior nucleus of the thalamus. (Bowsher 1970, p. 125)

The thalamic nuclear complex lies between the interventricular foramen and the posterior commissure and extends laterally from the third ventricle to the posterior limb of the internal capsule. Sometimes the medial surfaces of the thalami are joined across the midline of the third ventricle by a mass of grey matter termed the *interthalamic adhesion* or *massa intermedia*. Though it crosses the midline it is certainly not to be considered as a commissure.

Apart from its role in projecting sensory information, the thalamus also plays a part in controlling the electrical activity of the cortex and helps in the integration of motor functions by providing relays through which the cerebellum and parts of the basal ganglia can influence the motor cortex.

The *metathalamus* is the collective name for the medial and lateral geniculate bodies which lie underneath the pulvinar (Fig. 2.18). From the *medial geniculate body* fibres of the acoustic radiation pass to the auditory area in the temporal lobe, while the *lateral geniculate body* gives rise to the optic radiation.

The *hypothalamus* forms the inferior and lateral walls of the third ventricle. The hypothalamus is divided into medial and lateral groups of nuclei by fibres of the fornix which terminate in the mamillary bodies. These nuclei are concerned with a wide range of functions, e.g. emotion, sleep, temperature regulation, hunger, and thirst.

The *subthalamus* is a small transitional region lateral to the hypothalamus and ventral to the thalamus. It contains a large lens-shaped discrete nucleus (subthalamic nucleus) on the inner aspect of the internal capsule.

THE INTERNAL STRUCTURE OF THE HEMISPHERES

The principal structures within the hemispheres are (i) the white matter, (ii) the basal ganglia, and (iii) the lateral ventricles. Only the first of these will be dealt with. For details of the basal ganglia readers should consult standard neuroanatomy texts.

The white matter

The white matter or medullary substance is made up of millions of fibre processes or axons of nerve cells. The white colour is conferred by the myelin sheaths which coat the fibres and act as an insulating layer around the fibre as it transmits nerve impulses from one spot to another. The fibres may be divided into three categories:

1. The *association* or intracerebral fibres connect various regions within one hemisphere. These may join areas which are close together or the fibres may be very long.
2. Intercerebral or *commissural* fibres unite homologous or equivalent areas or structures in the two hemispheres.
3. *Projection* fibres convey impulses from deeper structures to the cortex or from the cortex to deeper structures. These deeper structures include the thalamus, hypothalamus, brain stem, cerebellum, and spinal cord.

An understanding of the pathways linking the various parts of the brain is of paramount importance in understanding one of the central concepts in neuropsychology, that of the disconnection syndrome, i.e. many symptoms and signs can best be understood as the result of a break in the normal connections between brain areas or systems. It is possible only to outline the major sets of connections here. Those interested in a more thoroughgoing treatment may consult references such as Krieg (1963) and Wright (1959).

Association fibres. Association fibres may be divided into short fibre groups and long association groups. The short fibres lie beneath the cortex and arch around the bottom of the sulci to join adjacent convolutions or gyri. The long fibres lie more deeply and may be gathered into rather indefinite bundles or tracts which connect the different lobes. A number of the tracts are sufficiently circumscribed to warrant description (Figs 2.21–2.24).

The *superior longitudinal fasciculus* courses backward from the frontal lobe to the occipital lobe and this tract sends some fibres to the posterior part of the temporal lobe. Fibres at the bottom of this fasciculus sweep around the region of the insula connecting the superior and middle frontal gyri with parts of the temporal lobe. These fibres, known as the *arcuate fasciculus,* are important for an anatomical understanding of the aphasias.

The *inferior longitudinal fasciculus* runs from the occipital to the temporal poles.

The *uncinate fasciculus* connects the anterior and inferior parts of the frontal lobe with parts of the temporal lobe by a bundle which is fan shaped at either

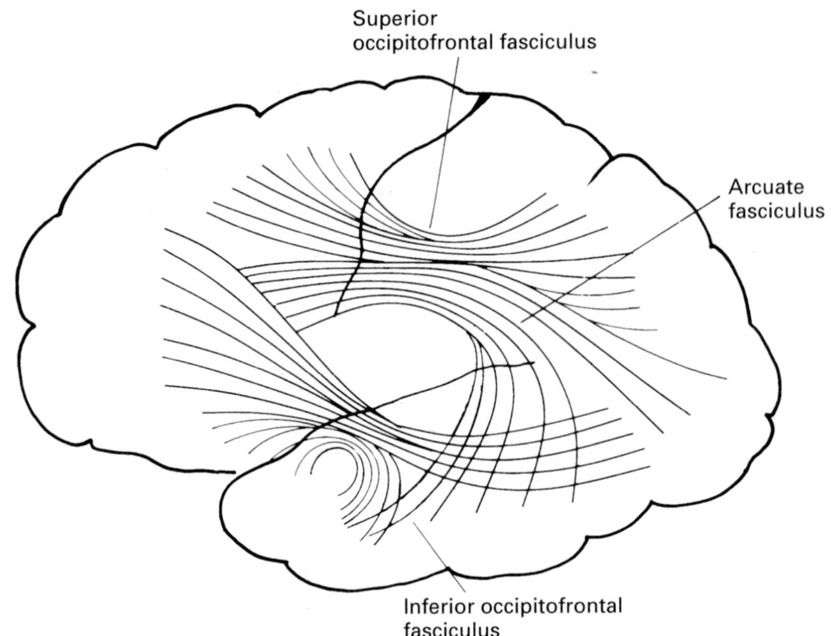

Fig. 2.21 Long association tracts. Lateral view.

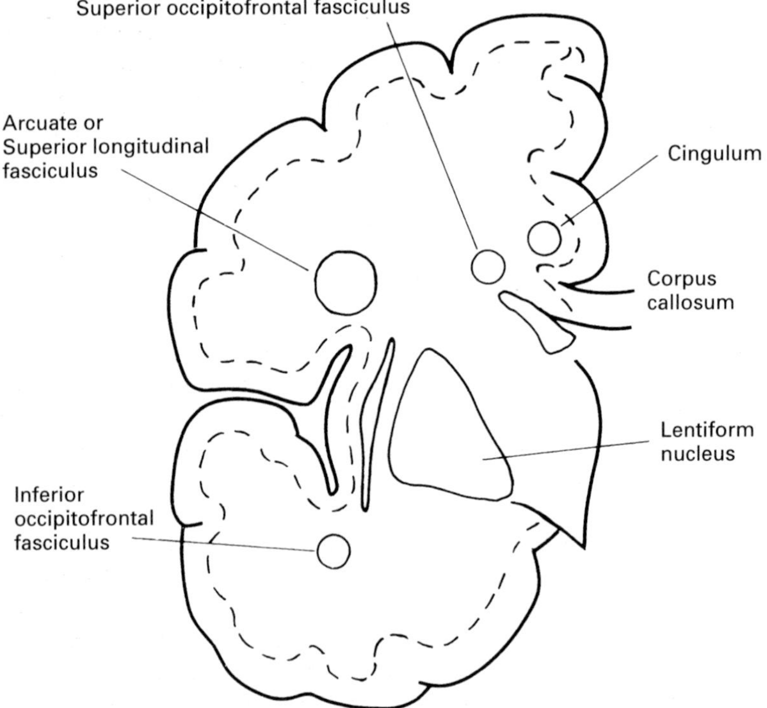

Fig. 2.22 Long association tracts. Coronal view.

end and drawn together in a compact bundle as it arches sharply around the stem of the lateral sulcus.

On the medial aspect the principal association tract is the *cingulum* which

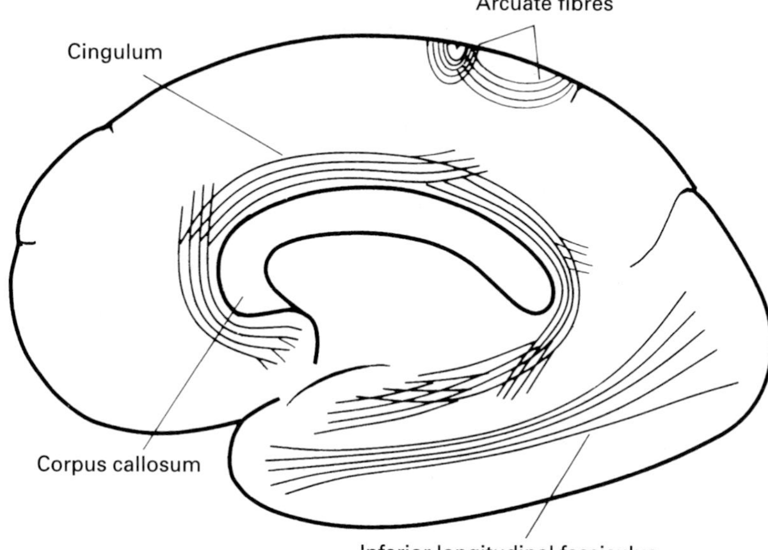

Fig. 2.23 Medial view with association tracts superimposed.

lies within the cingulate gyrus (Fig. 2.23). Like the cingulate gyrus, the cingulum runs an arched course over the corpus callosum beginning below the rostrum and terminating in the uncus. The cingulum contains fibres of different length and it connects regions of the frontal and parietal lobes with parahippocampal and adjacent temporal regions. The tract is much reduced in the parahippocampal gyrus and uncus.

A coronal section through the hemisphere shows that in certain locations certain of the long association bundles are gathered together discretely, so that a relatively small lesion could produce a major disconnection (Fig. 2.24).

Commissural fibres. Interhemispheric fibre systems have three well marked commissures, namely the corpus callosum, the anterior commissure, and the hippocampal commissure or commissure of the fornix.

The *corpus callosum* is the largest mass of connecting fibres in the nervous system. It joins corresponding areas in the neocortex in the two hemispheres. Fibres enter it from practically every part of the cortex (Fig. 2.24). The degree of development of the corpus callosum in animal species is proportional to the degree of development of the neocortex itself, hence its prominence in the human brain. The major named portions of the corpus callosum, i.e. the rostrum, genu, body and splenium, have already been mentioned (Fig. 2.10).

Sunderland (1940) described the distribution of the fibres in the corpus callosum of the macaque. The distribution can be considered to be essentially similar in man. Fibres from the frontal lobes occupy the genu and the anterior third of the body. Other frontal fibres, together with fibres from the parietal and temporal area, occupy the middle third of the body. The posterior third of the body contains fibres from the parietal, temporal, and occipital lobes, those from the parietal regions being more numerous. The splenium is given over to fibres from the occipital regions.

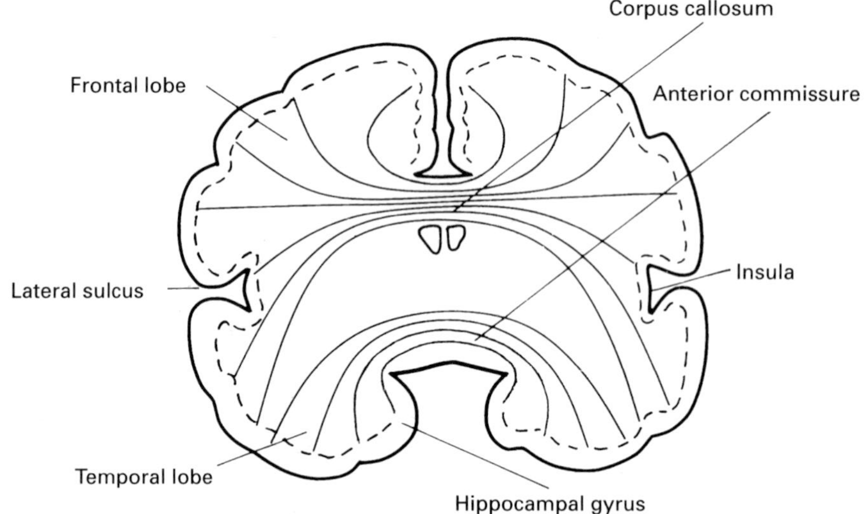

Fig. 2.24 Coronal section showing the two main commissures.

Partial transections of the corpus callosum in man have confirmed that the posterior portion is principally concerned with the transmission of visual information while the central portion transmits somatosensory information (Myers 196l, Sperry 1964, Ettlinger 1965). Earlier, Hoff put forward the interesting hypothesis that the different portions of the corpus callosum had different roles. The posterior parts were thought to integrate information, the anterior portions to separate functions, e.g. the independent functions of the two hands, while the middle parts of the corpus callosum were thought to allow 'for joint or independent activities of the hemispheres, as need for joint or independent operations may arise' (Gloning & Hoff 1969, p. 36). In recent times the projections of the corpus callosum in man have been traced by stimulating the corpus in different parts during operation and recording the resulting evoked potentials (Tan et al 1991).

The effects of commissure section or commissurotomy are detailed in Chapter 8.

Callosal fibres from the frontal and occipital poles and the medial aspects of these lobes take curved pathways known as the *anterior* and *posterior forceps* (Fig. 2.25). Where the fibres cross the floor of the interhemispheric fissure they form the roof of the lateral ventricles. Although most of the fibres in the corpus callosum unite corresponding or homologous areas, there are a small number of non-homologous fibres (Crosby et al 1962) (see Fig. 2.25).

The *anterior commissure* is a rounded compact bundle of fibres which crosses the midline just anterior to the anterior column of the fornix and just below the interventricular foramen. Its shape has been likened to bicycle handlebars (Carpenter 1972). Its main part connects regions of the inferior and middle temporal gyri while a smaller portion interconnects olfactory regions on the two sides (Fig. 2.24).

The *hippocampal commissure* is composed of transverse fibres which join the posterior columns of the fornix. Fibres arising in the hippocampus pass into the posterior columns of the fornix which sweep around the splenium of the

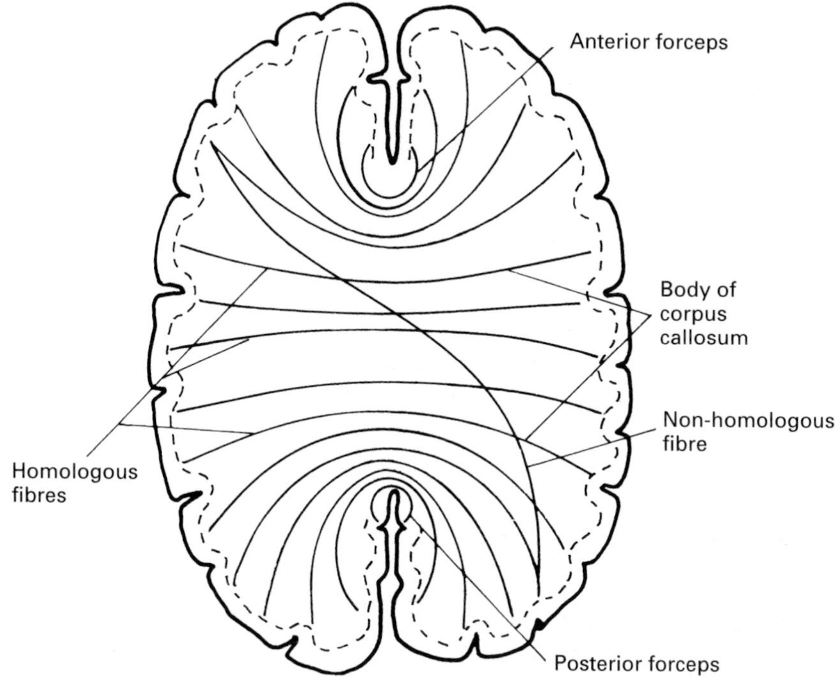

Fig. 2.25 Horizontal section showing commissural fibres.

corpus callosum approaching each other as they pass forward to join in the body of the fornix. The transverse fibres of the hippocampal commissure become shorter as the columns converge and the appearance of this portion gave rise to the name *psalterium* because of the resemblance to an ancient stringed instrument (Figs 2.16 and 2.26).

Projection fibres. The projection fibres are of two types, afferent and efferent. Afferent fibres convey impulses to the cortex while efferent fibres carry impulses away from it. The projection fibres are arranged as a radiating mass, the *corona radiata,* that converges towards the brain stem (Fig. 2.27). Near the upper part of the brain stem the fibres are arranged in a narrow area between medial and lateral nuclear collections and are known as the *internal capsule.* The *caudate nucleus* and *thalamus* flank the capsule on the medial side while the *putamen* and *globus pallidus* flank it laterally (Fig. 2.6). A horizontal section through the brain shows that the internal capsule has an anterior limb and a posterior limb.

The most posterior portion of the posterior limb of the internal capsule contains fibres of the *optic radiation* travelling from the lateral geniculate body to the calcarine sulcus in the occipital lobe.

The afferent fibres in the internal capsule arise mainly from the thalamus and project to nearly all areas of the cortex. Efferent fibres arise from various parts of the cortex. Among these are the important motor pathways which innervate the musculature of the opposite side of the body and whose disruption gives rise to contralateral paralysis since the fibres cross the midline lower down in the decussation of the pyramids.

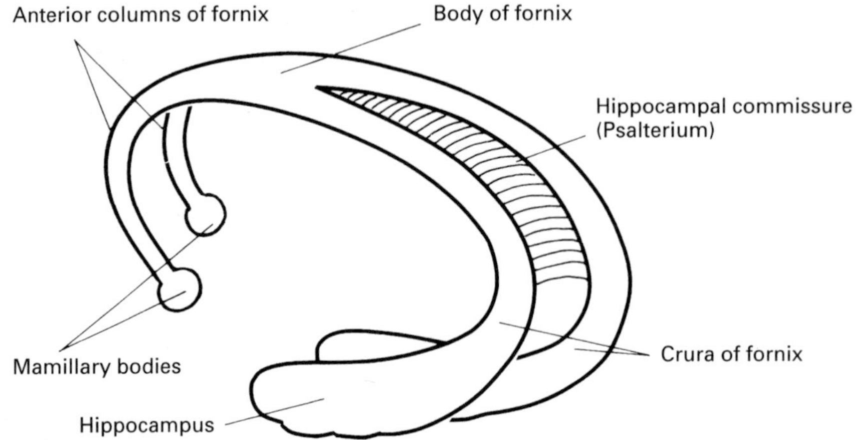

Fig. 2.26 Hippocampal commissure (psalterium).

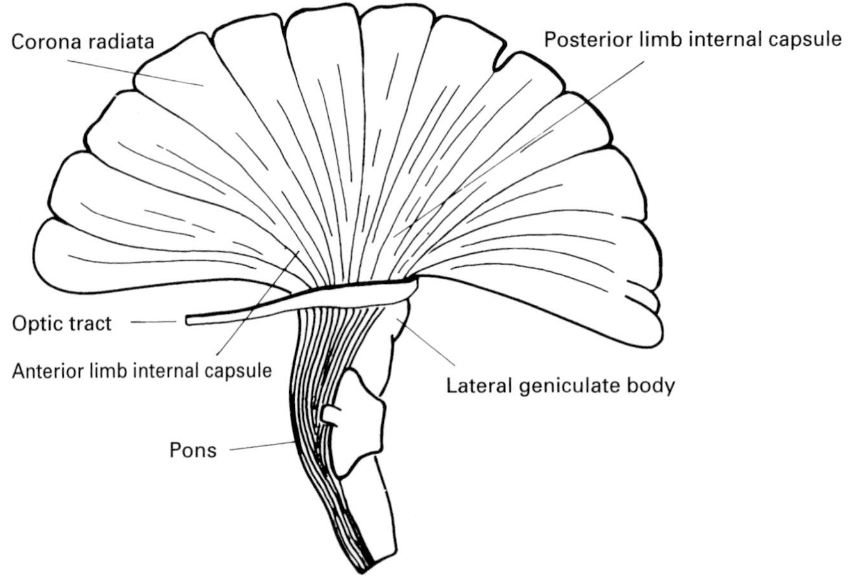

Fig. 2.27 Corona radiata.

BLOOD SUPPLY OF THE BRAIN

Since the central nervous system is one of the most metabolically active tissues in the body it requires a rich supply of oxygen. Some estimates put the nervous system's utilization of oxygen as high as one fifth of that of the whole body. If there is serious diminution in blood supply to nervous tissue for even a relatively short period, there is tissue death or necrosis. The importance of understanding the rudiments of the circulation can be seen when it is realized that impairment of blood supply is the most common cause of lesions in the central nervous system.

Apart from the physiology of the cerebral circulation, it is important to understand the distribution of the blood via the various branches, since regional interruption to the blood supply is often associated with characteristic neuropsychological signs and symptoms, and a careful examination of the higher functions in such cases may allow inferences to be made about the nature and location of vascular blockages, insufficiencies, haemorrhages or the like. As yet, insufficient investigation has been given by neuropsychologists to this field.

The blood supply to the brain comes from two pairs of arterial trunks: (i) the internal carotid arteries; and (ii) the vertebral arteries (Figs 2.28 and 2.29).

The internal carotid arterial system

The *internal carotid artery* enters the skull and, after making several sharp curves which form the *carotid siphon*, ascends lateral to the optic chiasma and breaks up into its major branches – the smaller anterior cerebral artery and the larger middle cerebral artery. The latter is often considered as the direct continuation of the internal carotid artery. On its way to this major bifurcation, the internal carotid artery sends off three important branches, one anterior and two posterior. The anterior branch is the *ophthalmic artery* which passes forward through the opening in the optic orbit to supply the eye. The two posterior branches are the anterior choroidal artery and the *posterior communicating artery* (Figs 2.28 and 2.29).

The *anterior choroidal artery* is usually of small calibre and passes backward across the optic tract and then laterally toward the anteromedial portion of the

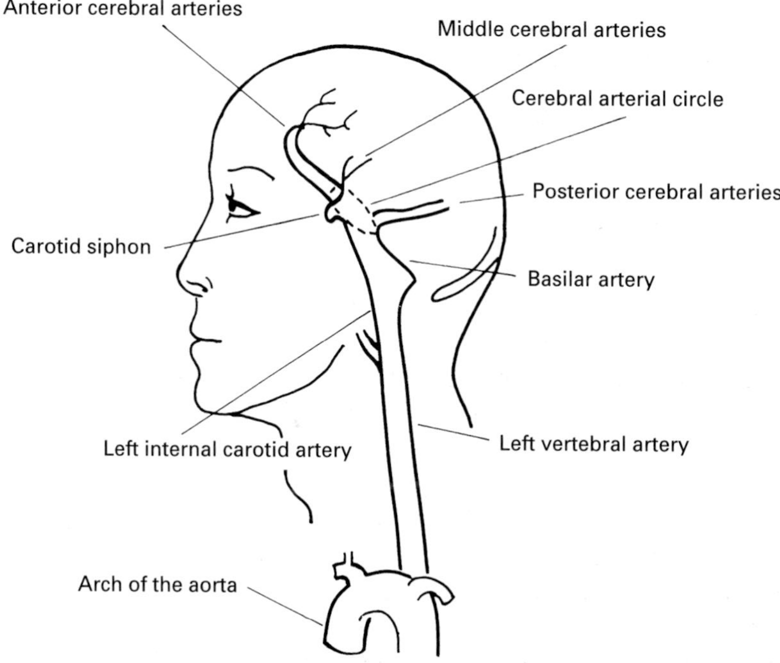

Fig. 2.28 The two arterial supply systems.

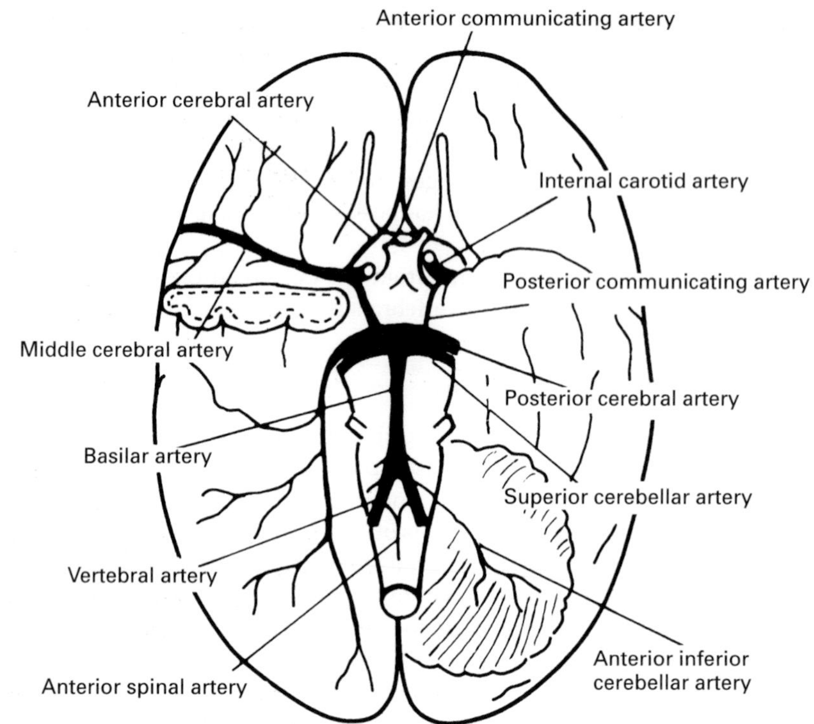

Fig. 2.29 Arteries at the base of the brain.

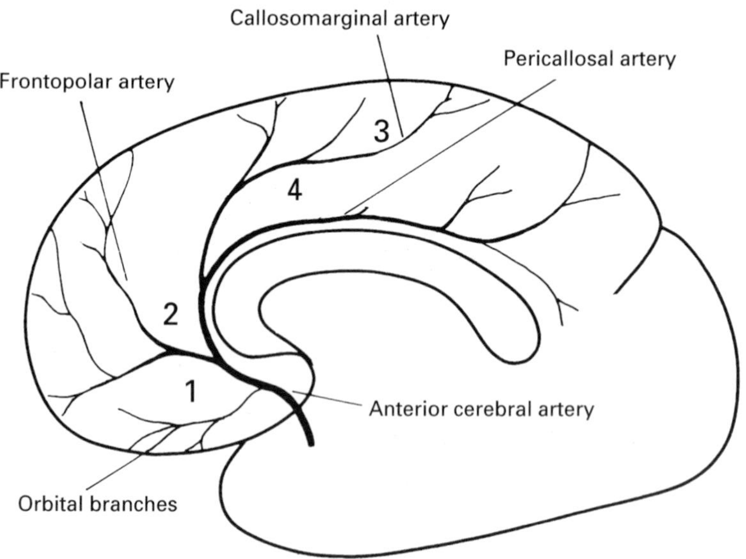

Fig. 2.30 The anterior cerebral artery.

temporal lobe. The artery enters the inferior or temporal horn of the lateral ventricle where it supplies the choroid plexus. As well as the choroid plexus the anterior choroidal artery supplies the hippocampal formation and other deeply placed structures such as parts of the amygdaloid complex, caudate nucleus, thalamus, globus pallidus, and internal capsule. As mentioned later, recent evidence has strongly implicated the hippocampus in the process of memory and for this reason a knowledge of the blood supply of this region becomes relevant to the neuropsychologist.

The *posterior communicating arteries* run backward to become joined to the proximal portions of the posterior cerebral arteries.

Anterior cerebral artery. The anterior cerebral artery (Fig. 2.30) passes dorsal to the optic nerve and approaches the anterior cerebral artery of the other side and is soon joined to it by the *anterior communicating artery*. The artery then enters the fissure between the two hemispheres, curves upward over the anterior portion (genu) of the corpus callosum and courses backwards on the medial surface of the cerebral hemisphere on the superior surface of the corpus callosum. It has a number of named branches: (1) orbital branches which supply the orbital regions; (2) the frontopolar artery which supplies medial parts of the frontal lobe and extends on to the convexity of the hemisphere; (3) the callosomarginal artery which supplies the paracentral lobule and parts of the cingulate gyrus; and (4) the pericallosal artery which lies along the dorsal surface of the corpus callosum (which it supplies in passing) to provide branches to the medial surface of the parietal lobe. The anterior cerebral artery also supplies the anterior columns of the fornix.

Middle cerebral artery. The middle cerebral artery passes laterally to enter the lateral cerebral fissure between the temporal lobe and the insula. It often breaks up into two stems which lie superficially in the lateral fissure (Fig. 2.31). The middle cerebral artery gives by far the largest supply to the cerebral hemispheres, accounting for some 75 per cent or more of the blood going to the hemispheres. It supplies branches not only to extensive areas of the cortex but

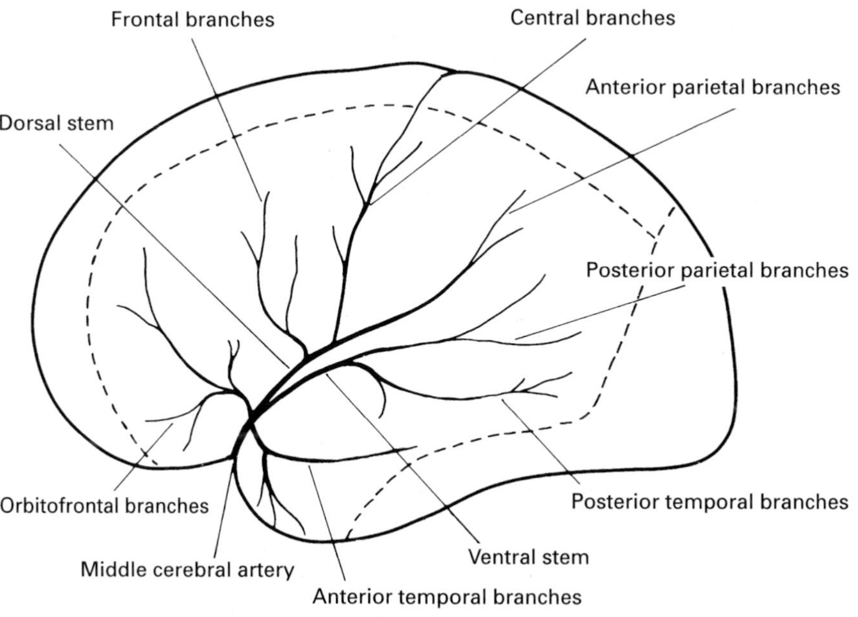

Fig. 2.31 Middle cerebral artery.

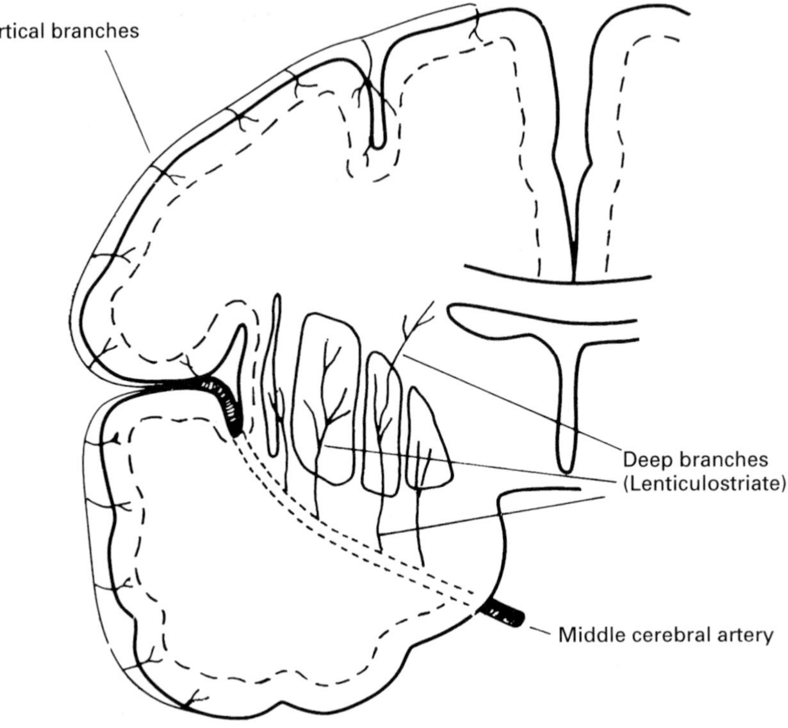

Fig. 2.32 Middle cerebral artery. Lenticulostriate branches.

also to the internal nuclear masses and internal capsule (Fig. 2.32). One of these branches, the lenticulostriate artery has been known as 'the artery of cerebral haemorrhage' because of the frequency with which it is involved in spontaneous haemorrhages or 'strokes'.

The cortical branches from the dorsal portion or stem of the middle cerebral artery supply the area above the lateral fissure, i.e. orbitofrontal, precentral and anterior parts, while the ventral stem provides anterior temporal, posterior temporal, and posterior parietal branches.

The vertebrobasilar arterial system

The *vertebral arteries* (Figs 2.28 and 2.29) enter the skull through the large opening, the *foramen magnum* through which the spinal cord becomes continuous with the brain stem. The two vertebral arteries rise along the anterolateral surfaces of the medulla and unite in the midline at the lower edge of the pons to form the basilar artery. Thus, this major supply is often termed the *vertebrobasilar system*. The vertebral arteries give branches to the spinal cord before their entry into the cranial cavity while the intracranial branches of the vertebrobasilar system supply the spinal cord, brain stem (medulla, pons, midbrain), cerebellum, posterior diencephalon, and towards the termination of the system, the basilar artery bifurcates to form the two posterior cerebral arteries which supply parts of the temporal and occipital lobes of the cerebral hemispheres.

The *posterior cerebral arteries* pass around the lateral aspect of the midbrain

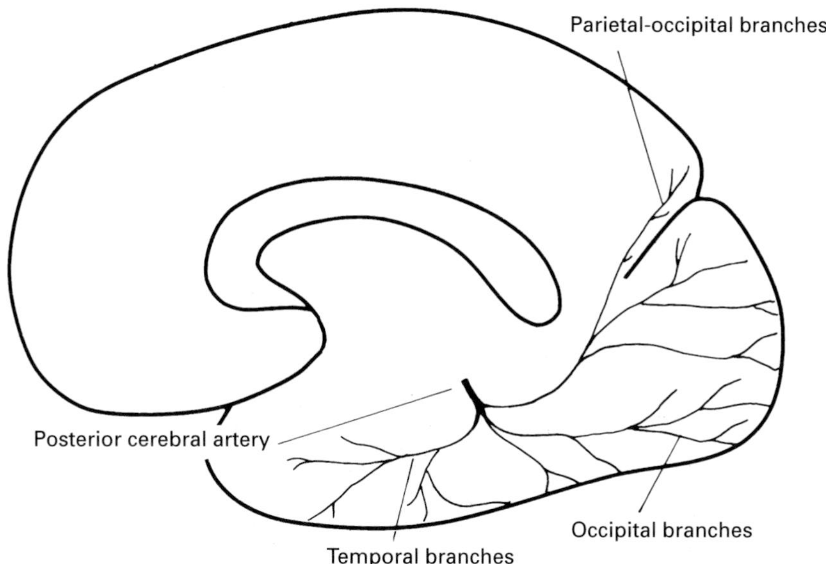

Fig. 2.33 Posterior cerebral artery.

and then pass dorsal to the tentorium cerebelli on to the inferior and medial surfaces of the temporal and occipital lobes (Figs 2.29 and 2.33). The posterior cerebral artery has three main branches: (i) the anterior temporal which supplies all the inferior surface of the temporal lobe with the exception of a small area of the tip which is supplied by the middle cerebral artery; (ii) the posterior temporal which supplies the posterior part of the inferior surface of the temporal lobe; and (iii) the largest or occipital which runs in the calcarine fissure and gives branches which supply the whole of the medial and a large part of the other surfaces of the occipital lobe including the visual cortex (see Ch. 7).

As the posterior cerebral artery passes around the cerebral peduncle it supplies the adjacent structures and provides the posterior choroidal branch which helps to supply the choroid plexus and the larger, posterior part of the hippocampus that is not supplied by the anterior choroidal. The arterial supply of the deeper structures of the brain is shown in Figure 2.34.

The cerebral arterial circle

The cerebral arterial circle (circle of Willis) is a ring of connecting blood vessels which encircles the optic chiasma and the region between the cerebral peduncles (Fig. 2.35). The circle is formed by vessels which link the two great arterial systems, the internal carotid and vertebrobasilar. In front of the optic chiasma the anterior cerebral arteries are joined by the usually short anterior communicating artery while the whole of the internal carotid system is joined to the basilar system by a pair of posterior communicating arteries which run back from the internal carotid arteries to join the proximal portions of each posterior cerebral artery.

There are variations both in the disposition and size of vessels which enter into the arterial circle in individual cases. A review of these variations is given

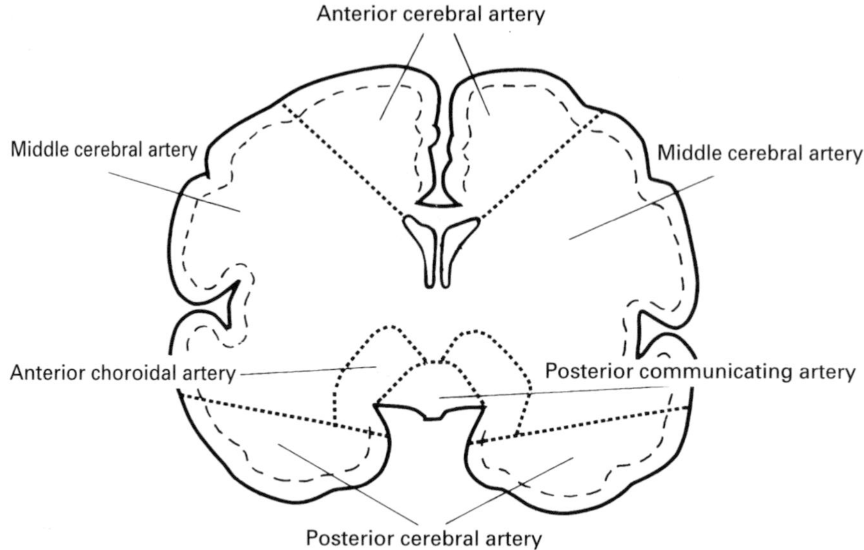

Fig. 2.34 Blood supply to deep structures.

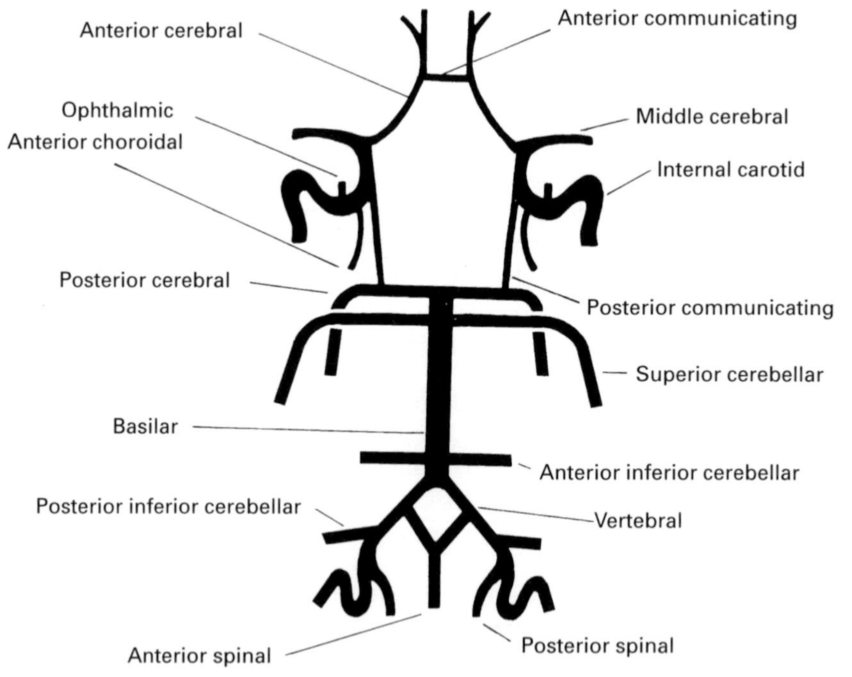

Fig. 2.35 The cerebral arterial circle (the circle of Willis).

in Lippert and Pabst (1985). The circle has been thought to equalize the distribution of blood flow throughout the brain but, with an equality of blood pressure, there is normally little or no exchange of blood either between the two sides of the circle or between the internal carotid and posterior cerebral vessels. However, when a blockage occurs at any portion of the circle, this may be bypassed through the other portions of the circle. The adequacy of this process will depend both on the calibre of the vessel occluded, the size and nature of the alternative circulation, and the rapidity or otherwise of the occlusion. Such 'alternative' pathways are known as *anastomoses*. They are defined by Zülch as 'intercommunications of a network character in one or between two or more functionally separate systems, allowing the possibility of draining blood from them. An auxiliary supply may result, usually after widening of the channel, and flow may result in any direction' (Zülch 1971, p. 107). Thus, the slow narrowing which occurs from the thickening of an artery (arteriosclerosis) may allow an anastomotic circulation to develop while a rapid occlusion by an embolus or clot may not.

Figure 2.36 provides a schematic representation of several possibilities of alternative supply with blockages in the vertebrobasilar system. Alternative routes for the flow of blood may be worked out for the points of occlusion indicated. For example, blockage of the right posterior cerebral artery at A will deprive the right occipital and basal temporal regions of their blood supply. Blockage at B will cause a loss of supply to the territory of both posterior cerebral arteries. Occlusion at such a 'bottleneck' will have serious consequences. On the other hand, even where both vertebral arteries are occluded (C and D) the effects may not be nearly so pronounced since an alternative supply may reach the brain via the patent branches which connect the anterior spinal artery with the vertebral arteries.

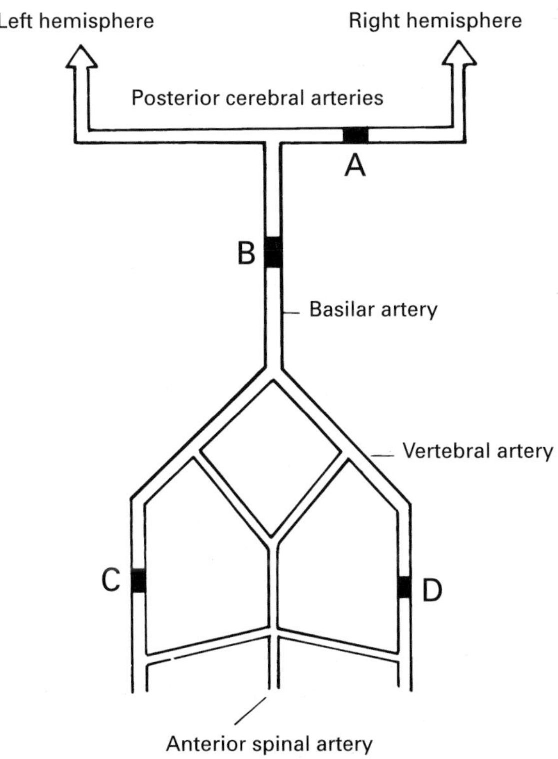

Fig. 2.36 Occlusions and alternative routes in the vertebrobasilar system.

Table 2.1 The arterial supply of the principal structures

Structure		Arterial supply
Frontal lobe		
Lateral surface	—	middle cerebral artery
Medial surface	—	anterior cerebral artery
Inferior surface	—	middle and anterior cerebral arteries
Temporal lobe		
Lateral surface	—	middle cerebral artery
Medial surface	—	middle cerebral, posterior cerebral, anterior choroidal, and posterior communicating arteries
Inferior surface	—	posterior cerebral artery
Parietal lobe		
Lateral surface	—	middle cerebral artery
Medial surface	—	anterior cerebral artery
Occipital lobe		
All surfaces	—	posterior cerebral artery
Corpus callosum	—	anterior cerebral artery
Hippocampus	—	anterior choroidal artery, posterior choroidal branches of posterior cerebral artery
Fornix		
Anterior columns	—	anterior cerebral artery
Body and crura	—	posterior choroid branches of posterior cerebral artery
Mamillary bodies	—	posterior cerebral and posterior communicating arteries

This oversimplified version of the supply pattern of the cerebral circulation can be expanded by the more extensive treatment by Zülch (1971), Kaplan and Ford (1966) and others. The arterial supply of the principal structures may be summarized as in Table 2.1.

References

Bowsher D 1970 Introduction to anatomy and physiology of the nervous system, 2nd edn. Blackwell, Oxford

Brodal A 1980 Neurological anatomy in relation to clinical medicine, 3rd edn. Oxford University Press, New York

Carpenter M B 1972 Core text of neuroanatomy. Williams and Wilkins, Baltimore

Crosby E C, Humphrey T, Lauer E W 1962 Correlative anatomy of the nervous system. Macmillan, New York

Ettlinger E G (ed) 1965 Functions of the corpus callosum. Churchill, London

Gloning K, Hoff H 1969 Cerebral localization of disorders of higher nervous activity. In: Vinken P J, Bruyn G W (eds) Handbook of clinical neurology. North-Holland, Amsterdam, vol 2, ch 3

Isaacson R L, Pribram K H (eds) 1976 The hippocampus. Vol 1. Structure and development. Vol 2 Neurophysiology and behavior. Plenum Press, New York

Kaplan H A, Ford D H 1966 The brain vascular system. Elsevier, Amsterdam

Krieg W J S 1963 Connections of the cerebral cortex. Brain Books, Evanston, Illinois

Lippert H, Pabst R 1985 Arterial variations in man. Classification and frequency. Springer Verlag, Heidelberg

Luria A R 1973 The working brain. Allen Lane, The Penguin Press, London

Myers R E 1961 Corpus callosum and visual gnosis. In: Fessard A et al (eds) Brain mechanisms and learning. Blackwell, Oxford

Papez J 1937 A proposed mechanism of emotion. Archives of Neurology and Psychiatry 38: 725–743

Seifert W (ed) 1983 Neurobiology of the hippocampus. Academic Press, New York
Sperry R W 1964 The great cerebral commissure. Scientific American 10: 4–5
Sunderland S 1940 The distribution of commissural fibres in the corpus callosum of the macaque monkey. Journal of Neurology and Psychiatry 3: 9–18
Tan Y L, Yang J D, Zhang J et al 1991 Localization of functional projections from corpus callosum to cerebral cortex. Chinese Medical Journal 104: 851–857
Wright M K 1959 Fibre systems of the brain and spinal cord, 2nd edn. Witwatersrand University Press, Johannesburg
Zülch K J 1971 Some basic patterns of the collateral circulation of the cerebral arteries. In: Zülch K J (ed) Cerebral circulation and stroke. Springer, New York

3

Elements of neurology

Neuropsychologists are most often psychologists by primary training. Whether engaged in research or acting as consultants concerning the patient's higher cerebral functions, they bring to the collaboration with other workers in the neurosciences a rather different background. Tallent (1963), points out that 'the psychologist and his associates are members of considerably different cultures'. These cultural differences may bring fresh information and orientations which will prove helpful but they also create barriers in understanding and communication. The present chapter is aimed at providing psychologists with the barest background to neurology, including some of its terms and methodology, so that they may begin to understand, albeit in a very rudimentary fashion, the majority of neurological conditions they are likely to encounter in the literature and in practice. Absorption of some of the medical culture, along with a sensible expression of their own, is likely to prove mutually rewarding. Perhaps the greatest contribution in any cultural interchange is an understanding of the other culture's language.

The selection of topics is biased in the direction of the issues which have been of concern to both neurology and neuropsychology in recent years.

Standard textbooks of neurology (e.g. Brain 1992, Adams & Victor 1993) will be needed to expand the psychologist's understanding of the field, while a briefer résumé such as that of Simon et al (1987) makes a useful addition to an office reference set. A comprehensive source is the *Handbook of Clinical Neurology* (Vinken & Bruyn 1969–1982, new series volume 45 onwards Vinken et al 1985). It is noteworthy that the first volume of the new series was devoted to neuropsychology. A concise coverage of the principal functional brain disorders with key references is provided by Hier et al (1987).

METHODS OF INVESTIGATION

The neurological examination

Neurological examination consists firstly of the taking of a detailed history from the patient and, often of paramount importance, from those around him.

Much valuable information about the types of neuropsychological tests to employ may be gained from a perusal of the patient's neurological case notes though, regrettably, many patients are still referred to the psychologist with a simple request 'for psychometric testing'. Where the anamnesis is insufficiently detailed, e.g. in questions relating to the patient's higher cerebral functions, the neuropsychologist should develop a routine of careful questioning.

A clinical neurological examination in itself is often an extensive, careful record of the patient's sensation, reflexes, movement and muscle tone, and clinical neuropsychologists will need to familiarize themselves with the details of the neurological examination and with the traditional interpretation of neurological symptoms and signs. Disturbances of integrative cerebral functions and the terminology in common use are described below.

Neurology has developed special methods in the investigation of disorders of the nervous system, and neuropsychologists will be better equipped to assist in the solution of neurological problems if they understand them. The remainder of the book is concerned with the most recently developed method, namely neuropsychological investigation, which is aimed at obtaining information on the changes in specifically human functions which occur with lesions in the nervous system so that this information may be added to the methods already in use for the diagnosis of the nature and location of the lesions. 'In this respect neuropsychology is merely the most complex and newest chapter of neurology, and without this chapter, modern clinical neurology will be unable to exist and develop' (Luria 1973). Clinical neuropsychology will be useful to the extent to which it provides added information to the data base on which decisions regarding diagnosis, management, and rehabilitation are made.

Radiological investigation

Progress in neuroradiology has been rapid over the past decade and the new methods have had a considerable impact on the practice of clinical neurology and neuropsychology. Some earlier methods, particularly pneumoencephalography, have practically disappeared in most centres. Neuropsychologists, particularly those whose practice includes patients with acute neurological disorders, need to be familiar with the basic nature of neuroradiological methods and the types of information which they are capable of providing.

Most radiographic methods rely on the detection of differences of electron density between the tissues for a differential effect on X-ray attenuation, which is then used to create a visual image. The procedures are referred to collectively as imaging techniques.

Computerized tomography (CT scan)

This technique was rapidly accepted as the standard for studying morphological changes in the brain. It is safe and easy to carry out, both on in-patient and out-patient cases. The technique was described by New et al (1974) and a number of comprehensive works are now available (e.g. Williams & Haughton 1985).

In essence, the procedure consists of scanning the head with a narrow beam of X-rays which allows the transmission of X-ray photons in the layer to be

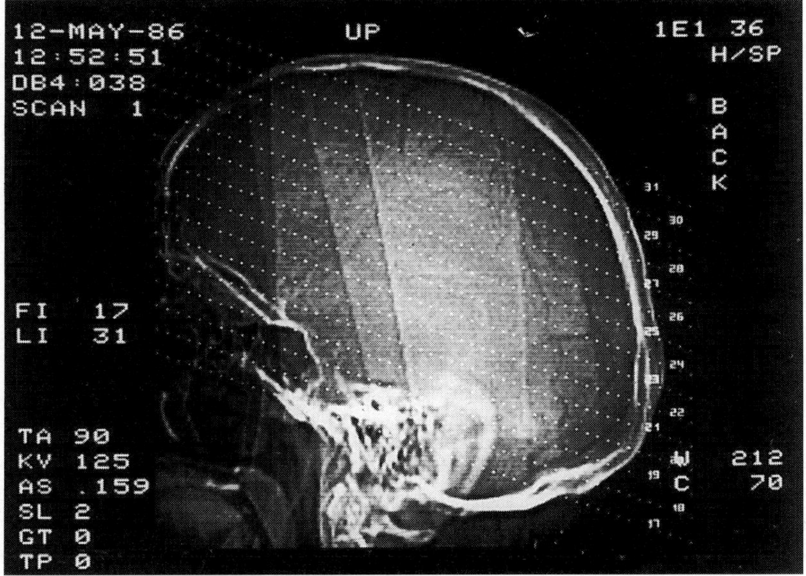

Fig. 3.1 Planes of sections with computerized tomography.

measured. A number of standard 'cuts' are made at successive levels (Fig. 3.1). The photon data is processed by a computer and the density information is converted to a visual image of the internal structure of the brain. Pathological processes are indicated by alterations of normal density and by deformation of brain structures. Several examples appear throughout the text.

The sensitivity of computerized tomography can be enhanced by the intravenous injection of iodine-containing material. Where there is a defect in the blood–brain barrier or increased vascularity, retention of the high density element results in increased contrast between normal and abnormal tissue (Fig. 3.2).

The great value of CT to neuropsychology lies in its clear delineation of the morphology of neurological lesions in vivo, against which behavioural indices may be correlated. In its first decade, CT scan information confirmed and greatly clarified the anatomical basis of neuropsychological disorders (e.g. see Kertesz 1983).

It must be remembered, however, that CT scan provides a static picture at the moment of evaluation. Serial scans provide further information, but are still restricted to demonstrating structural change (e.g. Pasquier et al 1997). It is apparent from assessment of function, e.g. by neuropsychological examination, that disruption of brain function may extend considerably beyond the changes seen on static scanning. Newer methods of imaging improve on the information provided, but these methods (see below) are not available in many centres.

Positron emission computed tomography (PET scan)

Like CT scanning, the positron emission scan provides a cross-sectional image of the brain, but, unlike the static nature of the former, PET scanning is capable of providing dynamic information on a wide range of cerebral functions such

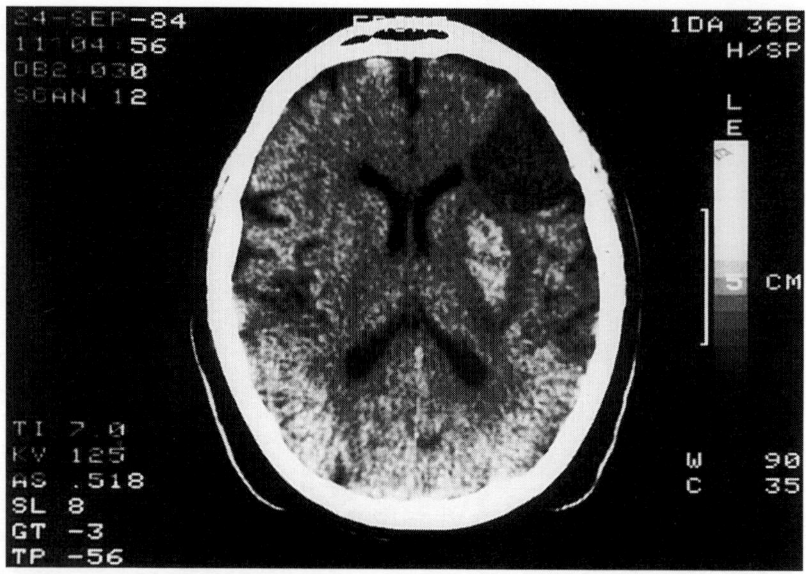

Fig. 3.2 Computerized tomography (CT scan) showing old frontal infarct (dark area) and new striatocapsular infarct (deep light area).

as local cerebral blood flow (LCBF) and local cerebral glucose and oxygen metabolism (LCMRGlc, LCMRO), as well as blood volume and other measures.

PET is a scanning method for producing an image of brain radioactivity following the intravenous injection of a labelled indicator; the biologically active compounds used include positron emitting isotopes of elements such as carbon, fluorine, nitrogen, and oxygen. It proved useful in demonstrating altered cerebral function of a lasting nature in tissues which appear normal with computed tomography (Kuhl et al 1980a, b, Phelps et al 1982, 1983). Some examples of the potential of PET investigation in neuropsychology are described by Benson et al (1983), with Watson (1997) providing a succinct summary. Although largely restricted by its cost to anatomico-pathological correlations in clinical cases, PET is beginning to provide studies of cognitive processes in normal as well as clinical cases. An example is the report of Heiss et al (1992), which clarifies the implication of networks related anatomically to the limbic system in the complex processes of memory, underlining the fact that the involvement of outlying 'association' areas depends on the nature of the material being processed. Similar fractionation of visual processing with discrete 'activations' for components of perception are emerging, exemplified by studies of visual motion detection (Watson et al 1993, Watson 1996). Such sophisticated medical techniques are contributing significantly to our understanding of the neuropsychological models underlying brain–behaviour relationships.

Single photon emission computed tomography (SPECT)

Because of the operational complexity and great cost of installation of PET, alternative imaging techniques have been developed for routine use in certain clinical areas. One of these is single photon emission tomography, SPECT

(Royal et al 1985). This consists of a gamma camera to record emissions after the injection of a radiotracer that is taken up differentially by normal and pathological tissue, and thus allows the recording of regional differences such as those of cerebral blood flow.

One of the most fruitful areas has been the study of epileptogenic foci, where there is the possibility of surgical excision of the affected area with cure or amelioration of the condition. In this instance comparison measurements are made between the interictal state of the brain and the activity during a period of electrical abnormality. Since the substances used, e.g. ^{99m}Tc-HMPAO, remain in the tissues for a considerable time after injection, the camera recording can be delayed, though the actual injection needs to be made in close temporal proximity to the change in brain activity (often signalled by a disturbance such as a complex partial seizure). In such cases the appearance is of hyperperfusion of the temporal lobe and hippocampus together with hypoperfusion of the lateral structures in the immediate postictal period. An example is shown in Figure 3.3. The patient suffered from complex partial seizures and the three phases of activity – interictal, ictal and postictal – are clearly shown.

The findings from SPECT are often correlated with other measures, particularly MRI (Duncan et al 1990, Adams et al 1992), EEG (Verhoeff et al 1992), and neuropsychological testing.

This technique, allowing as it does the study of larger numbers of patients and their comparison with normal subjects, lends itself nicely to studies of patients with other conditions such as Alzheimer's disease (Hunter et al 1989, Montaldi et al 1991, Bauer et al 1991, Dewan & Gupta 1992, Pearlson et al 1992), head injury (Oder et al 1992), and amnestic disorders (Hanyu et al 1992).

Arteriography

This is the technique for outlining the circulation by means of a rapid series of radiographs taken during the passage of radiopaque material which has been

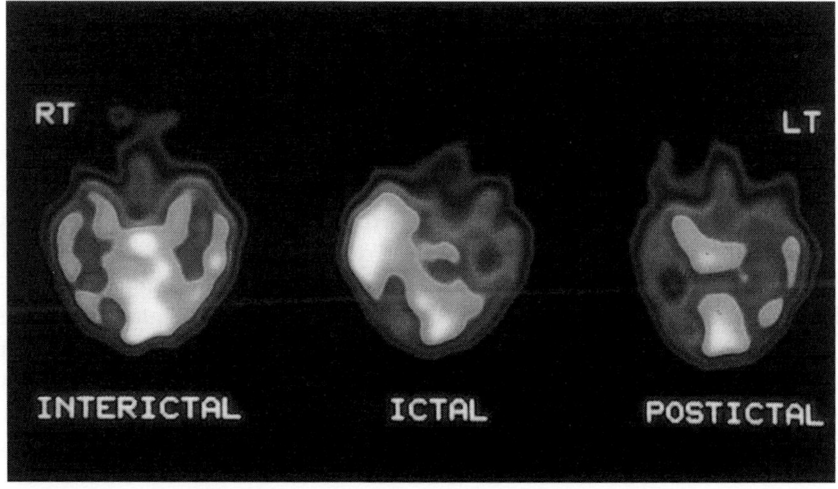

Fig. 3.3 SPECT measures taken between seizure periods, during a complex partial seizure and shortly after.

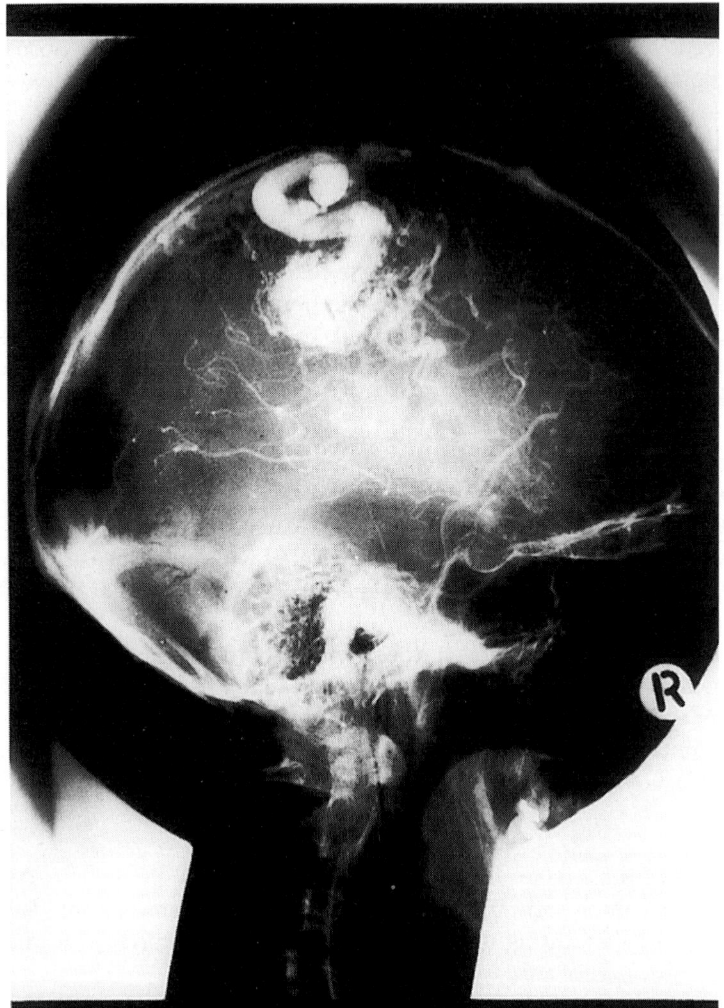

Fig. 3.4 Lateral arteriogram of the internal carotid circulation showing an arteriovenous malformation.

injected into the blood stream. The term 'cerebral angiography' is used to refer to the radiological investigation of both the arterial and venous channels of the brain and is often used interchangeably with the term arteriography. Formerly the injection was made directly into the artery, most commonly the internal carotid artery, but it is now customary to pass a catheter via the femoral artery. This allows injection of material into the arch of the aorta to display the origins of all vessels or selective catheterization of chosen vessels to study the extracranial and intracranial circulation. With the catheter in situ, separate injections can be made to visualize the circulation from lateral or anteroposterior orientations (Fig. 3.4). The presenting symptoms will determine whether the injection is made into the anterior (internal carotid, anterior and middle cerebral arteries and their branches) or the posterior circulation (vertebral, basilar, and posterior cerebral arteries).

Angiography is of particular value in the investigation of structural abnormalities of the blood vessels themselves, e.g. narrowing or ulceration of one or more vessels, intracranial aneurysms, or arteriovenous malformations. On the other hand, alteration in the shape and position of vessels may indicate the presence of a space occupying lesion such as a cerebral tumour.

In the Wada technique of sodium amytal ablation described in Chapter 5, an arteriogram is usually carried out to check the circulation prior to the injection of the drug.

Arteriography is not without risk, much of which has been associated with sensitivity to the injected radiopaque materials. These reactions have been greatly reduced in recent times with the introduction of more physiologically compatible contrast materials. The frequency of use of this technique has declined in some areas with the advent of newer imaging techniques.

Digital subtraction angiography

This later form of angiography consists of scanning the output from an X-ray image intensifying tube with a video camera. This video signal is then amplified and stored in digital form in the imager's memory. Further images are taken after the arrival of contrast material at the site. The first set of data, termed the 'mask image', is then subtracted by the computer to produce the final image.

The contrast material can be introduced intravenously so that it is possible to visualize either the extracranial or intracranial circulation on an out-patient basis with relative safety, avoiding the risks associated with intra-arterial injection. The technique can also be utilized with the intra-arterial injection of a much smaller quantity of material than traditionally used in cerebral angiography, with reduced risk (Little et al 1982). The method is of particular value in detecting extracranial vascular pathology such as stenosis, occlusion and ulceration, and thus performs a valuable role in the prevention of stroke.

Magnetic resonance imaging (MRI)

This technique, alternatively termed nuclear magnetic resonance (NMR) imaging, differs fundamentally from conventional radiographic techniques. It does not employ X-rays and does not require the injection of contrast media. Palmer (1985) gives the following succinct summary.

> When the nuclei of certain atoms – usually hydrogen protons – are placed in a high magnetic field, they align with the axis of spin in the direction of the field. A radiofrequency applied at right angles to the field changes the angle of spin, and the return to equilibrium when the radiofrequency pulse ceases is associated with the emission of a radiofrequency characteristic of the element and its physicochemical environment. In MRI, gradient magnetic fields in the three directions allow spatial detection of signal data and a two-dimensional image to be formed.

Further information can be found in Pykett (1982) and Tress et al (1985).

It is now possible to obtain images of the brain of outstanding quality and surprisingly realistic reconstructions (Fig. 3.5). Images are usually superior to those obtained with CT scanners, and the greater sensitivity of MRI in many neurological conditions coupled with its ability to produce images in all planes

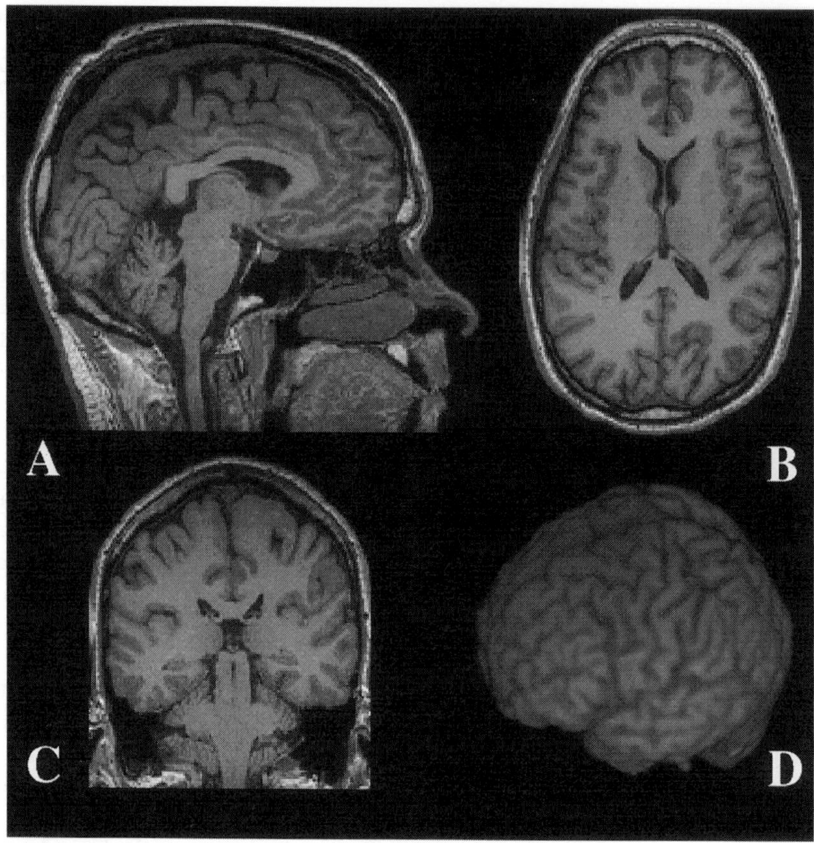

Fig. 3.5 Magnetic resonance imaging (MRI) scans: A, mid-sagittal; B, axial; and C, coronal slices from a volumetric acquisition oriented in the sagittal plane. D, high quality 3-dimensional reconstruction taken from the same series showing detailed lateral surface anatomy (after scalp is removed by segmentation).

(horizontal, coronal, sagittal), has made it the investigation of choice. The technique has wide applications and has been much used in studies of temporal lobe epilepsy (e.g. Lencz et al 1992, Kuzniecky 1997, Watson et al 1997); it has also proved valuable in head injury outcome studies (Wilson et al 1988).

MRI measures both structural and physiological abnormalities. Structural studies demonstrate anatomical relationships both within the brain between grey and white matter and cerebrospinal fluid spaces, and surface features when reconstructed and rendered as three-dimensional images (Fig. 3.5). Measurements of the volume of brain structures in both serial and cross-sectional studies have found correlations in many neurological conditions relevant to neuropsychology, e.g. Alzheimer's disease and amygdalo-hippocampal volume (Lehericy et al 1994, Frisoni et al 1996b), or frontotemporal dementia (Frisoni et al 1996a). Alignment of serial MRI studies in three dimensions (termed *co-registration*) may visualize early regional neurodegeneration (Freeborough et al 1996). Magnetic resonance angiography (MRA) provides rapid non-invasive depiction of vascular anatomy. MRI physiological studies use dynamic imaging techniques to measure markers of function in vivo.

Retarded diffusion of water molecules can detect probable irreversible ischaemic damage in acute strokes within minutes, whilst influx of injected contrast material can show blood perfusion, indicating further 'at risk' tissue (e.g. Barber et al 1998).

A recent MRI innovation with considerable potential for neuropsychology is *functional magnetic resonance imaging*, based on image signal intensity varying with regional blood volume, in which increases in neuronal activity can be visualized during specific cognitive tasks (Le Bihan 1996, Bandettini & Wong 1997). One technique, blood oxygenation level dependent (BOLD) contrast, uses paramagnetic properties intrinsic to deoxygenated haemoglobin to alter the MRI signal. Cognitive paradigms are constructed with at least two states, varying ideally by only one cognitive parameter, and steady state BOLD images from each state are compared to determine those areas which are uniquely 'active'. Such techniques have become extremely sophisticated as some recent research reports and reviews demonstrate (Latchaw et al 1995, Sakai et al 1995, Sereno et al 1995, Tootell et al 1995, Moseley et al 1996, Stern et al 1996, Courtney et al 1997). Function can also be measured at a chemical level using *magnetic resonance spectroscopy* (Kuzniecky 1997). Such studies offer many opportunities for, and would benefit from, neuropsychological collaboration.

Electrical investigation

Recording

One of the most widely used investigative techniques in neurology is *electroencephalography*. This is the technique of recording the electrical activity of the brain through the skull by means of electrodes placed on the scalp. The potential differences between two points on the skull produced by brain activity are very small and have to be amplified many times before they can be used to drive a recording device such as a pen or inkjet recorder. The mean amplitude of the brain's electrical activity is about one hundredth that of the heart. The brain potentials are recorded in wave form from 1 to 100 Hz, with an amplitude ranging from about 5 to several hundred microvolts.

The scalp electrodes are usually placed in a standard pattern (Fig. 3.6) and the activity between any pair of electrodes recorded as a single channel, of which there are usually about 16. The various areas being analysed at any one time, termed a 'montage', may be varied by switching the outputs between pairs of electrodes, for example in one period of examination eight channels might be devoted to the potential differences between Fp2–F8, F8–T4, T4–T6, T6–02 and the corresponding areas on the left side of the head. In a subsequent 'run' differences might be examined in the transverse direction, e.g. T3–C3, C3–Cz, Cz–C4, C4–T4 and other areas. In this way a thorough coverage of the brain can be achieved and the activity of the various areas compared. Newer digital systems allow recording from all sites at once, allowing transient changes to be viewed with different montages. Interpretation depends on an analysis of the principal characteristics of the wave activity, viz. the frequency, amplitude, form and distribution (see textbooks such as Niedermeyer & Lopes da Silva 1982).

For some time after the invention of the electroencephalograph it was hoped

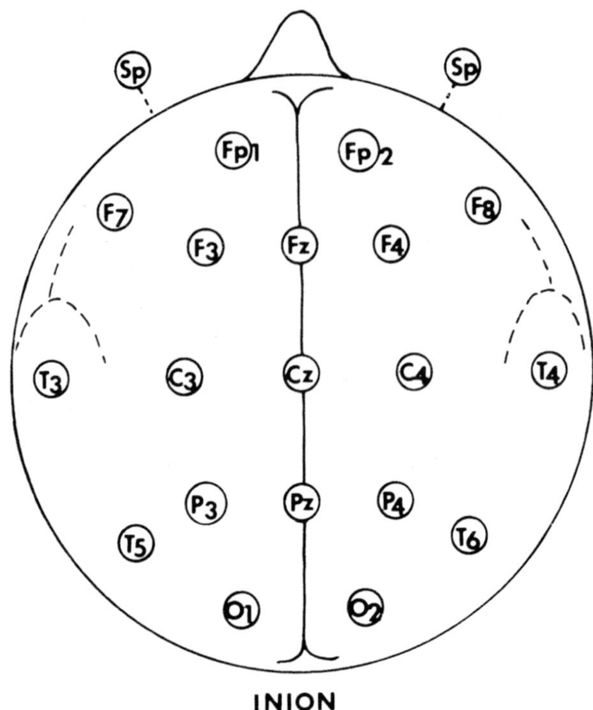

Fig. 3.6 Electrode placement in electroencephalogram.

by many that it would provide the tool to unlock many of the brain's secrets. The study of the relation between the EEG and higher mental functions has been singularly disappointing, though increasing sophistication in recording and analysing equipment, including computer analysis, may yet prove of value. The technique is, however, often valuable in neurological diagnosis. It is a safe and relatively simple procedure routinely used in most larger hospitals.

The EEG is of particular value in the investigation of epilepsy. Here abnormal electrical activity may be recorded in the period between the patient's clinical seizures – the interictal period. The observed abnormalities may be apparent in many of the channels or may be restricted to a clearly defined focus such as over one temporal lobe.

Unfortunately, any one EEG record taken from an epileptic patient may prove to be normal and serial recordings are often needed. Latent abnormalities may be brought out by using various activation procedures which may be effective in evoking the epileptic discharges so that they appear on the record, though the patient may not have any clinical manifestations. Commonly used activation techniques are: (i) recording during sleep; (ii) overbreathing for 2 or 3 minutes; (iii) photic stimulation in the form of repetitive light flashes; (iv) administration of drugs.

Recent advances in electronic technology have made it possible to record EEG activity in ambulatory patients in their normal environments for periods of 24 hours or more. The electrical signals are recorded from a small preamplifier attached to the scalp between a pair of silver chloride electrodes. With care in electrode application satisfactory recordings can be obtained even during vigorous activity or major seizures though movement artefact may prove troublesome. The method can be used for reliable quantification of seizure activity and frequency in the absence of an observer. Four channels have commonly been used but commercially available products now include eight or more. 'The technique has sufficient positive yield to be applied to any patient with epilepsy or a question of epilepsy in whom routine EEG has not provided sufficient information' (Bridgers & Ebersole 1985).

Recording from depth electrodes forms an essential part of the in-patient investigation in patients with intractable epilepsy in whom surgical treatment is proposed. The electrodes may remain in situ over many days, while recording is made from cable or radiotelemetry with concurrent video monitoring of the patient's behaviour.

Apart from its primary role in the study of epilepsy, the EEG is also of diagnostic value in the localization of organic lesions of the brain, such as cerebral tumours, abscess or infarction (see below), but is of much less value in determining the nature of the pathological process. It should also be borne in mind that negative findings do not rule out the presence of even major pathology since in some proven pathological lesions EEG recordings sometimes appear entirely normal. The more superficial the lesion the more reliable is the localization.

Like evidence from other specialized diagnostic procedures, the findings at electroencephalography must be examined in the light of the patient's history and clinical examination.

Stimulation

Electrical stimulation of nerve tissues is historically older than electrical recording techniques and, in many respects, is complementary to it. The value of both techniques has increased with the advance in sophistication of electronic equipment.

Modern electronic stimulators permit investigators to control such parameters of stimulation as the frequency, duration, shape and intensity of the pulses used.

Opportunities for study of human beings are restricted to patients undergoing neurosurgical procedures under local anaesthesia. Quite surprisingly, very few *positive* responses have been evoked with stimulation outside the primary motor and sensory areas. The major exception is the evocation of complex experiences from the temporal lobe described by Penfield and reported in Chapter 5. There is also great variability of response from patient to patient and in individual patients over time (e.g. Ojemann 1979).

On the other hand, negative responses, i.e. the disruption of functions, are much more common. A typical example would be the disruption of language functions, such as the ability to name objects when certain areas of the cortex are stimulated (Penfield & Rasmussen 1950, Penfield & Jasper 1954, Penfield 1958, Penfield & Roberts 1959, Fedio & Van Buren 1974, Ojemann & Mateer 1979a, b, Ojemann 1980, 1981) (Fig. 3.7). Less common are the reports of interference with non-language functions with cortical stimulation (Fedio 1980, Fried et al 1982).

The early work was largely associated with the neurosurgical treatment of epilepsy and thus was much concerned with the cerebral cortex. More recently,

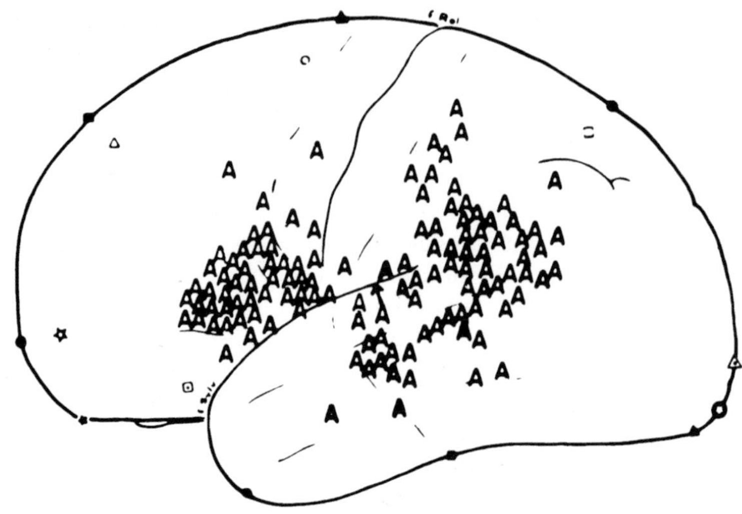

Fig. 3.7 Points at which stimulation produced aphasic responses (Fig. XIII–II: Penfield W & Roberts L 1959 Speech and brain mechanisms. Courtesy of Princeton University Press).

stereotactic operations in subcortical regions, particularly the thalamus, for the treatment of dyskinesias have revealed a specific dissociation of effects according to the side of stimulation. It is also clear that the timing of stimulation is crucial, for example stimulation at the time of input of information may actually enhance retrieval, whereas stimulation in the same sites at the time of retrieval may worsen performance compared with the normal state (for details see Ojemann & Fedio 1968, Ojemann 1971, Ojemann et al 1971, Fedio & Van Buren 1975, Ojemann 1977, 1979, Mateer & Ojemann 1983).

COMMON NEUROLOGICAL DISORDERS

Cerebral trauma

The functions of the brain can be seriously disturbed by physical injury. The effects of penetrating wounds of the brain resulting from high velocity projectiles such as bullets and shrapnel fragments have been studied intensively in large series of military cases, some of which have been followed up for one or more decades. These studies have contributed greatly to our understanding of neuropsychology. It is unfortunate that the drawings of such lesions, often pictured as a small dot on a map of the brain, tend to leave the reader with the impression that one is dealing with a small circumscribed lesion which affects the cortex at the point of entry only. The nature of the fibre connections severed and the effect of the shock wave produced in the very soft brain mass by the penetrating missile are seldom known with any degree of accuracy. These wounds are, of course, relatively uncommon in studies of civilian subjects.

On the other hand, craniocerebral injury from the rapid acceleration and deceleration of the head in motor vehicle accidents is an ever-increasing problem. Even where the skull is not fractured, the brain may sustain a wide variety of pathological lesions. These include generalized lesions scattered throughout the brain with or without localized damage such as contusion, laceration or haemorrhage. With this complexity of pathology, clinico-anatomical correlation might seem to be an unproductive exercise. However, the presence of residual neuropsychological deficits, particularly of memory and adaptive behaviour in many so-called recovered patients, and the proven relationship between lesions of the frontal and temporal regions of the brain and these disorders, tempts one to draw a causal relationship between the major locus of damage in closed head injury and such deficits. Before considering this possibility, readers should consult sources which convey the complexity of the pathology (Strich 1969, Adams 1975, Gurdjian 1975).

The advent of computerized tomography offered an opportunity to correlate the major focus of localized pathology and behavioural change in individual cases, but even this is unlikely to be sensitive to the diffuse microscopic lesions which occur in severe head injury and which are seen better on MRI. Nevertheless, the CT scan often provides dramatic confirmation for the local character of some lesions.

Briefly, cerebral damage may be defined as primary or secondary. Primary lesions are associated with the trauma itself. The principal forms are contusion, laceration or haemorrhage, though there is often a mixture of all three and contusion and laceration cannot be distinguished on clinical grounds. Secondary lesions arise from reduction of blood supply (*ischaemia*), reduction of oxygen to the tissues (*anoxia*), brain swelling (*oedema*), and intracranial haemorrhage.

Mechanism and sites of cerebral contusion

The exact mechanism of production of contusional lesions is still debated, though there is general agreement about the use of two descriptive terms. '*Coup*' injuries refer to damage beneath the site of impact, while '*contre-coup*' injuries refer to lesions at some distance from the site (Fig. 3.8). The mechanics of head injuries have been the focus of numerous studies using inert models, animals and man (Holbourn 1943, Lindenberg & Freytag 1960, Rowbotham 1964, Gurdjian et al 1966, Ommaya & Gennerelli 1974).

Though there is disagreement about what mechanical stresses produce the damage, there is no such disagreement about their location. Courville (1942) observed that the greatest zone of brain contusion following head injury was not invariably opposite to the impact. 'Essentially identical lesions of the subfrontal and anterior temporal regions result from contact of either the frontal region or the occipital region of the moving head and the fact that neither gross coup nor contrecoup lesions occur in the occipital region suggests that the anatomic relation of the brain and the portion of the skull proximate to it is essentially responsible for the nature and distribution of the lesion.' Speaking of the sudden deceleration of the head in motor vehicle injuries, Jamieson (1971, p. 31) likened the movement of the brain within the skull to the movement of objects within the motor vehicle: 'The soft brain then travels onward and crashes into the built-in dashboard that each of us owns, the knife-like sphenoidal ridges (complete with anterior clinoid projections), together with an unyielding fascia of front wall of middle fossa and a windscreen of rough orbital plates and frontal bone'. In modern motor accidents with high velocity deceleration, the damage to the anterior portion of the temporal lobe and sometimes the frontal lobe may be so great that it produces subdural haemor-

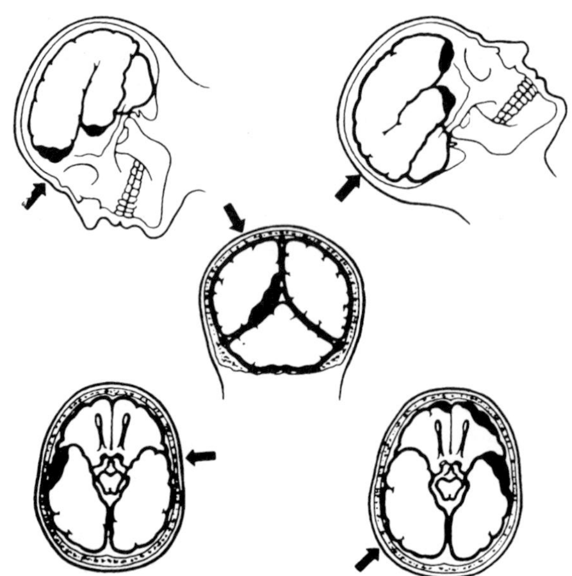

Fig. 3.8 Mechanism of cerebral contusion (Fig. 137: Courville C B 1945 Pathology of the nervous system. Courtesy of Pacific Press Publications).

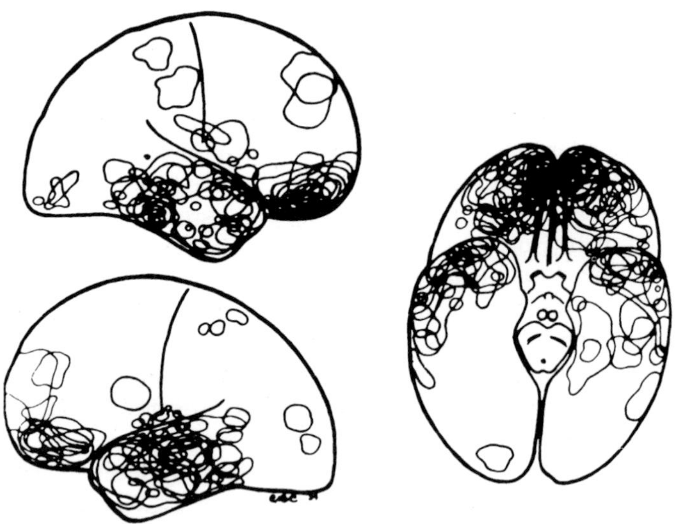

Fig. 3.9 Sites of cerebral contusion (Fig. 138: Courville C B 1945 Pathology of the nervous system. Courtesy of Pacific Press Publications).

rhage, brain contusion, laceration and intracerebral bleeding that has been termed the 'exploded pole' (Bottrell & Stewart, cited in Hooper 1966). The frontotemporal concentration of contusional injury has frequently been confirmed (Gurdjian et al 1943, Courville 1945, Gurdjian et al 1955, Lindenberg & Freytag 1957, Hooper 1966, 1969). Figure 3.9 provides a composite sketch from these sources.

An understanding of the mechanism of cerebral contusion is important for neuropsychology and it helps to explain why some patients after head injuries have psychological deficits which suggest damage to localized areas distant from the site of impact, e.g. the very frequent occurrence of 'frontal lobe' signs, such as uninhibited behaviour and lack of planned initiative, in patients who have sustained head injuries. The tendency to consider all cases of closed head injury as suffering only from the effects of diffuse brain insult is not supported by the evidence, and careful neuropsychological assessment may give valuable information about the location and extent of the damage which should prove useful in rehabilitation programmes.

Concussion

Prominent among the symptoms of head injury is impairment of consciousness. In a simple concussion there may be only a brief clouding of consciousness or a temporary loss. This temporary loss of consciousness is probably caused by injury to the brain stem reticular formation. The patient cannot remember the incident causing the concussion and has a loss of memory for events just preceding it. This is termed retrograde amnesia, which usually shrinks with time. There may also be a period of memory loss for the period subsequent to the injury which is termed *anterograde* or *post-traumatic amnesia.* Very early examination of football players after concussive injuries has found persisting neuropsychological deficits despite apparent neurological recovery (Maddocks & Saling 1996), and attempts at standardizing early assessment are emerging (McCrea et al 1997).

Measures of severity

Coma. The usefulness of employing length of coma as a measure of severity against which to correlate clinical and social sequelae was lessened by the variable and uncertain ways in which coma was defined in the early studies. This situation has been improved by the widespread adoption of the Glasgow Coma Scale, a simple standardized chart of eye opening, motor response and verbal response (Teasdale & Jennett 1974).

Post-traumatic amnesia (PTA). This measure was introduced by Russell and Nathan (1946), following an earlier study by Russell (1932). This used the length of time from injury to the time the patient became aware that he had regained consciousness. It corresponds to the time when the patient begins to retain a stable record of ongoing events. The definition of Russell and Nathan (1946) and the minor modification of Russell and Smith (1961) combine the length of unconsciousness with the period when the patient is awake and responding but not consolidating memories, i.e. coma plus the period of anterograde amnesia. Recently, Artiola i Fortuny et al (1980) have attempted to provide an objective assessment of PTA. This simple quantitative procedure correlated well with independent estimates made by experienced neurosurgeons. An extension of the Oxford scale with high inter-rater reliability that has proven easy to use in clinical practice has been under trial for several years in Australian hospitals with encouraging preliminary results (Shores et al 1986). This scale, the Westmead PTA Scale, demonstrated in a two-year follow-up study that such measures of PTA are superior to duration of coma in predicting outcome (Shores 1989). The Westmead scale differs from the Galveston Orientation and Amnesia Test (Levin et al 1979) in that both correct orientation and the ability to recall newly learned information are required to define the emergence from post-traumatic amnesia.

A detailed discussion of the relative merits of the two major measures, namely length of coma and PTA, is provided by Levin et al (1982), though there are few direct comparisons available. One of these (Brooks et al 1980) found that duration of coma as measured by the Glasgow Coma Scale bore little relation to cognitive outcome as measured by psychological tests, whereas duration of post-traumatic amnesia significantly predicted cognitive performance. Newcombe (1982) warns that the complexity of factors involved means that there will be no simple relationship between PTA and severity of defect. While a convincing general trend may be apparent in group data there are bound to be exceptions in both directions, some individuals with lengthy PTA having little impairment while others with shorter PTA are left with considerable deficit.

Traumatic haemorrhage

While small haemorrhages may occur in virtually any part of the brain after any form of head injury, more extensive haemorrhages occur from the laceration of blood vessels inside the skull; for example, a fracture of the skull may tear the middle meningeal artery which, by bleeding under considerable pressure into the space outside the covering of the brain, greatly compresses the cerebral hemisphere and later the basal portions of the brain. This *extradural* haematoma is a neurosurgical emergency and has little relevance for neuropsychology.

On the other hand, bleeding from blood vessels beneath the dura mater produces a *subdural* haematoma (Fig. 3.10), which may be less dramatic and, in elderly patients, may follow an injury so trivial that the patient does not even recall the incident.

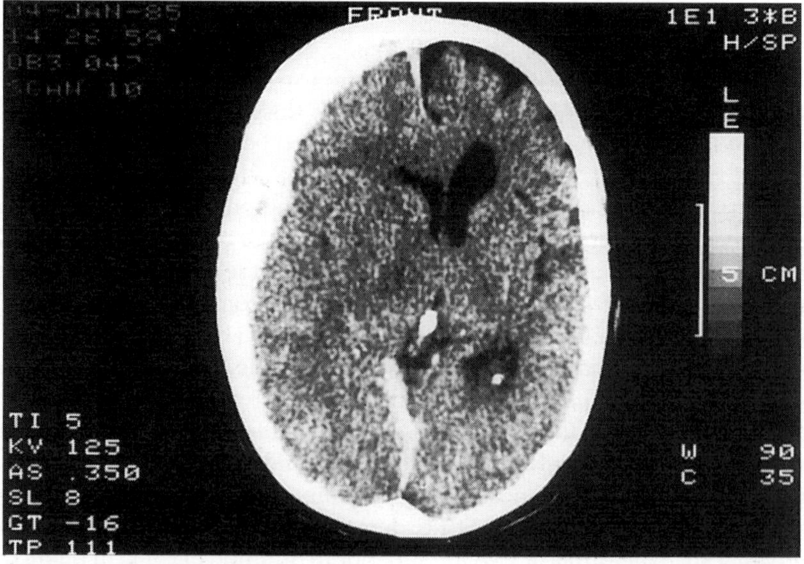

Fig. 3.10 CT scan showing right subdural haematoma extending over falx cerebri with midline shift and compression of right lateral ventricle.

This condition may produce changes which develop over days or even weeks after the injury, often simulating the picture of dementia with loss of concentration, episodes of confusion, and memory loss.

Intracranial tumours

The word tumour literally means a swelling. When referring to intracranial tumours, 'often erroneously labelled cerebral tumours' (Escourolle & Poirier 1973), the term usually means a neoplasm or new growth. Such a neoplasm has been defined as a 'mass of cells...resembling those normally present in the body, but arranged atypically, which grow at the expense and independently of the organism without subserving any useful purpose therein' (Handfield-Jones & Porritt 1949, p. 86).

These neoplasms in the brain may be benign or malignant. Benign neoplasms most frequently grow from the coverings of the brain. These coverings are termed *meninges* and tumours arising from them, *meningiomas*. Such benign tumours may grow slowly and attain a large size before they cause symptoms from their pressure effect on the brain or they may be symptomless and only be discovered at autopsy. They can be successfully removed in their entirety as they do not usually invade the brain substance.

Unfortunately, benign tumours are much less frequent than the malignant type which invades the tissue of the brain. The latter can rarely be completely removed by surgery because of the extent to which they infiltrate the surrounding tissue.

Most malignant brain tumours arise from the glial or supporting cells and not from the nerve cells or fibres themselves. They are termed *primary neoplasms*. The most common type, the *glioma*, which accounts for some 40% of adult brain tumours, is also the most malignant. A smaller proportion of brain tumours are called *secondary neoplasms*, since they multiply from cells of malignant tumours in other parts of the body. These cells of origin of cerebral secondary neoplasms have become detached from their parent tumours and been carried by the blood stream to lodge in the brain to begin independent growth there. Tumours of the lung and breast often give rise to such *metastatic* or secondary tumours.

Sometimes conditions that are not neoplastic may give rise to very similar signs and symptoms, e.g. an abscess in the brain. Though these may be diagnosed from signs which signal the presence of infection, their nature may not be discovered until an exploratory operation is carried out. For this reason tumours, abscesses, and other mechanically similar conditions are given the title of 'space occupying lesions'.

It can be seen from this short description that tumours within the skull may produce a multitude of symptoms which depend on their nature, location and growth. While most space occupying lesions will produce a set of general symptoms, each particular case will have specific features which depend on the interruption of connections between different parts of the brain. Thus, a small lesion in a strategic situation may have disastrous early effects because it interferes with vital centres or cuts a large number of interconnections between different areas of the brain, while a large lesion in another area may be almost silent for a relatively long period.

It is this failure to take into account the nature and location of cerebral lesions which defeated many earlier attempts to draw conclusions from psychological studies of heterogeneous populations of 'brain-damaged' people.

Cerebrovascular disorders

The term 'cerebrovascular disorder' can be taken to mean any disruption of brain function arising from some pathological condition related to the blood vessels. These produce an array of disorders of great complexity.

The vascular pathology may take many forms, e.g. lesions of the walls of the blood vessels themselves in the form of deposited material (atheroma) with or without ulceration, rupture of the vessel wall itself, narrowing (stenosis), or total occlusion of the lumen from thickening of the vessel wall or the presence of an obstructing clot (thrombus) or embolus, or changes in the characteristics of the blood itself.

While the types of cerebrovascular disease are numerous the majority of cases are due to cerebral *ischaemia* (deprivation of blood supply) or to haemorrhage. Ischaemia may be transient with symptoms that recover. Any prolonged ischaemia will lead to death of tissue or *infarction*. The most common cause of infarction is thromboembolism and this accounts for two-thirds of all cases of cerebrovascular disability. Some 15–25% of cases are caused by intracerebral or subarachnoid haemorrhage, while the remaining 5–10% result from less common causes.

Cerebral ischaemia

Transient ischaemic attacks (TIAs). This term refers to recurrent attacks of short-lived local neurological deficit produced by temporary ischaemia. By accepted definition, recovery should take place within 24 hours but is often complete within a much shorter time. Although the episodes take many forms they are often rather similar, even stereotyped, in the one individual. The patient experiences sudden loss of neurological function. This may be loss of power, which often begins distally, but may progress to affect the whole limb or an entire side. There may be sudden sensory loss, particularly loss of vision in one eye (amaurosis fugax, fleeting blindness), or loss of speech, memory or the functions referable to the cerebral hemisphere territories supplied by the internal carotid system. It is unusual for the brain and the eye to be affected simultaneously in one attack. When the vertebrobasilar system is compromised there may be symptoms such as ataxia and vertigo, signalling dysfunction in the cerebellum or brain stem. The attacks vary from infrequent (e.g. less than one a month) to very frequent (several times a day). During the attack the neurological signs will be indistinguishable from a developing infarct, but examination between the episodes will be normal.

Approximately a third of patients do go on to suffer obvious infarction. In keeping with the higher incidence of atherosclerosis in males than females and in hypertensive patients, some two thirds of those suffering from TIAs are male or hypertensive or both. Another third will continue to have attacks without any apparent permanent disability, while the remainder will have attacks which cease spontaneously. It is currently impossible to predict the outcome, though newer MRI techniques may assist (Barber et al 1998).

In transient ischaemic attacks it is generally assumed that ischaemia has occurred without actual death of neurons, though this may not necessarily be the case, and the apparent absence of findings may represent the insensitivity of functional measures as well as the relatively 'silent' location of the affected territory. Careful neuropsychological examination sometimes reveals that lasting deficits of higher function are present in some of these cases even when they appear to be neurologically intact between episodes.

Surgical treatment. Two major types of surgical procedure have been devised to prevent strokes and ischaemic attacks by reconstituting the arterial blood flow. The most common is the operation of *endarterectomy,* which aims at correction of stenosis, removal of atheromatous plaques, or removal of an organized thrombus and other conditions compromising the circulation. It is sometimes necessary to remove totally a diseased segment of artery and replace it with a vein graft. The operations are carried out at the sites of predilection for atheroma formation, e.g. at the origin of the internal carotid artery. The indication for operation is usually the presence of transient ischaemic attacks in the territory distal to a radiologically demonstrated high grade stenotic or ulcerated lesion (Paddock-Eliasziw et al 1996). Surgery for asymptomatic lesions remains controversial.

Cerebral infarction

The basic pathological process. The most common basic pathological process in infarction is *atherosclerosis*. This is not a uniform process but one which affects certain parts of the arterial system more than others. The deposition of material, mostly cholesterol, causes plaques which narrow the artery and thus restrict the flow. This may progress to complete occlusion of the affected vessel. Whether infarction occurs depends upon whether there is a collateral source of supply for the affected region (see below). In general, however, the size of an infarct depends to a large extent on the size of the vessel occluded – this may range from the minute to massive death of a large part of the hemisphere from sudden occlusion of an internal carotid artery.

There are certain sites of predilection in the formation of atheromatous plaques, mostly where arteries branch or bifurcate. The most common sites are the origin of the internal carotid artery, the upper end of the vertebrals and the lower portion of the basilar, the stem of the middle cerebral, and the posterior cerebral, though other vessels are also commonly affected. The plaques may ulcerate and the debris which collects, e.g. platelets, fibrin and cholesterol, may detach in the form of emboli and travel further afield to block smaller vessels.

The other common cause of cerebral embolism is thrombi forming in the heart because of arrhythmias or myocardial infarction.

A dramatic embolic phenomenon is *amaurosis fugax*. The term literally means 'fleeting blindness' and the condition is most commonly caused by emboli blocking retinal arterioles. The sudden transient loss is unilateral and often takes the characteristic form of a blind or curtain coming down (or ascending) over the visual field. The ensuing blindness may last up to 5 minutes, but is often much shorter. Full vision is usually restored within 5 to 15 minutes, often in a manner reverse from its onset. The emboli come most frequently from ulcerated plaques in the internal carotid artery (Glaser 1978).

Cerebral haemorrhage

Bleeding within the cranial cavity may result from a large number of causes (see Adams & Victor 1977, p. 536), however three conditions account for the majority of cases. In each condition the severity may vary from a small, almost symptomless bleed to a massive haemorrhage leading to sudden death.

1. *Hypertensive intracerebral haemorrhage.* This is the most common form of haemorrhage, with extravasation, or bursting out, of blood into the substance or parenchyma of the cerebral hemisphere. The bleeding destroys brain tissue and, if it continues, causes pressure effects on neighbouring tissue by compression or displacement. Large haemorrhages may so displace vital centres that they lead to death. Less serious pressure may disrupt the function of adjacent or nearby tissue without destroying it and this accounts for the partial, though often considerable, recovery of function after the acute stages. While the onset of symptoms is rapid, hence the term 'stroke', the full development of the clinical picture may take an appreciable time, sometimes hours, depending on the rate of bleeding and its final cessation. When bleeding stops there is no recurrence from the same site, a situation unlike that of bleeding from aneurysms. While the bleeding may commence in the brain's substance, it breaks into the ventricular system and thus into the cerebrospinal fluid in a high proportion of cases.

The brunt of symptomatology with intracerebral haemorrhage tends to be on neurological rather than behavioural features, since the cortex is often relatively spared. Sites of primary haemorrhage in decreasing order of frequency are the basal ganglia, thalamus, cerebellar hemispheres, pons and subcortical areas. Haemorrhages arise mainly from the penetrating branches of the middle cerebral, posterior cerebral and basilar arteries.

2. *Ruptured aneurysm.* These thin-walled protrusions are most common on the vessels which form the arterial circle (circle of Willis) or their major branches. They are assumed to be developmental defects in the arterial walls and are prone to rupture. Over 90% are found on vessels of the internal carotid system, only a few on the vertebrobasilar system. The most frequent sites of rupture are the anterior communicating region and the middle cerebral bifurcation, accounting for nearly half the cases. Sometimes the aneurysms are multiple.

In rupturing, blood may be spurted into the subarachnoid space or into the adjacent brain substance, producing an intracerebral haematoma. Bleeding into the cerebral substance is particularly prone to occur at the two most common locations mentioned. The territories of vessels in the areas often show infarction – this is possibly related to arterial vasospasm since at autopsy the vessels may be patent.

The clinical symptoms and signs are those related to blood under pressure in the subarachnoid space: usually excruciating headache and collapse, followed in survivors by those of local disruption of function by local pressure from extracerebral blood clot, intracerebral haemorrhage and infarction.

3. *Ruptured arteriovenous malformation (AVM).* These developmental malformations vary from a small localized abnormality of a few millimetres to a large mass of vessels occupying considerable space, often in the form of a wedge extending from the cortex to the ventricle. An example is shown in Figure 3.4. The blood vessels forming the mass interposed between the feeding arteries and the draining veins are pathologically thin-walled and liable to rupture.

Rupture of the larger malformations may produce intracerebral as well as subarachnoid bleeding. Like saccular aneurysms, AVMs have a tendency to recurrent bleeding. Hydrocephalus is a complication in some cases. Symptoms and signs are thus extremely varied.

Degenerative disorders

The anatomical organization of the present text does not lend itself readily to a consideration of disorders which are based on widespread pathology. The very common occurrence of dementing disorders, however, requires some treatment. The topic is taken up in more detail in the companion text (Walsh 1991), which also gives a number of case illustrations. Even in the so-called dementias, symptoms with the characteristics of *localized* disorders are to be found (see frontotemporal dementia, below).

Dementia

Dementia is a generic term which refers to a complex set of changes of known or unknown aetiology, which are reflected in widespread dissolution of human mental capabilities and social functions. 'The presence of dementia should be suspected whenever mental changes of insidious onset emerge without sufficient situational stress and gradually interfere with the daily living activities that are appropriate for age and background. Dementia can be reversible or irreversible, precipitously progressive or indolent, bristling with multiple cognitive deficits, or characterized almost exclusively by disturbances of affect, motivation, and personality' (Mesulam 1985, p. 2559).

The dementias have been divided into primary types, caused by parenchymatous cerebral degeneration, and secondary types, associated with known conditions. The secondary dementias may be further divided into those associated with systemic or neurological disease. In the primary type, of which *Alzheimer's disease* is by far the most common, the dementia is the only evidence of disease, while in the secondary type features of neurological or other systemic disorder may manifest themselves before the onset of intellectual decline. Many of the causes of dementia can now be identified (Table 3.1). A brief description of several of the most common is given below. More extensive treatment can be found in texts such as Cummings and Benson (1983) and Pitt (1987), as well as standard texts of psychiatry and neurology.

Alzheimer's disease

This primary degenerative disease of unknown aetiology accounts for about half of all cases of dementia. The condition was first described in a 51-year-old woman, but such cases show the same changes as are seen in what was formerly called 'senile dementia' (Newton 1948). Females are affected nearly twice as frequently as males. The condition is steadily progressive, though the rate of progression varies from individual to individual; commonly only a few years elapse between the first signs, usually memory loss and disorientation, and gross intellectual dissolution. This intellectual loss is accompanied by personality changes, disappearance of insight, and worsening difficulties with the tasks of everyday living. The deterioration in self-care is often the most notable

Table 3.1 Diagnosis in 417 patients fully evaluated for dementia (from Wells 1979)

Diagnosis	%
Dementia of unknown cause	47.7
Alcoholic dementia	10.0
Multi-infarct dementia	9.4
Normal pressure hydrocephalus	6.0
Intracranial masses	4.8
Huntington's chorea	2.9
Drug toxicity	2.4
Post-traumatic	1.7
Other identified diseases	6.7
Pseudodementia	6.7
Uncertain	1.7

feature. As with most ill understood conditions it is possible that subtypes of Alzheimer's disease exist (Price et al 1993).

The most important factor in diagnosis of the condition is the personal history (see Roth 1981, Strub & Black 1981, Walsh 1991). It will also become apparent very often that changes have been taking place for a considerable time before professional attention is sought. As means of arresting if not reversing the disorder emerge (Knapp et al 1994, Knopman & Morris 1997), early detection and differentiation will become paramount.

Frontotemporal dementia (FTD)

From 1892, Pick noted instances of circumscribed cerebral atrophy, and in 1906 he described a form of presenile dementia which was characterized by localized frontotemporal atrophy and clinical features which, in retrospect, we recognize as being predominantly associated with anterior lesions, e.g. loss of social grace, disinhibition or apathy and, frequently, aphasia. The specific pathology was described later by Alzheimer, who also derived the term 'Pick's disease' and made other contributions to the separation of different forms of dementia. The assumption that Pick made such a contribution is unfounded.

In recent years it has become apparent that a significant number of cases of presenile dementia show atrophy principally in the frontal and temporal regions, however only some of these display characteristic Pick bodies (see Brun 1987). The other cases have come to be classified as frontotemporal dementia (FTD), though histopathological findings are increasingly being regarded as transitional (Brun et al 1994, Schmitt et al 1995, Brun & Passant 1996). The clinical picture of this larger subgroup is consistent from centre to centre (Hagberg & Gustafson 1985, Neary et al 1986, 1987, 1988, Gustafson 1987, Johanson & Hagberg 1989, Brun & Passant 1996). The disorder usually presents in the presenium and has remarkably few neurological signs and an insidious onset: the first signs are usually a set of changes which can be subsumed under the rubric of alteration in mood and personality and which has a characteristic 'frontal' flavour. There is loss of interest in usual activities, including work, with a bland indifference that is soon followed by loss of self-care together with emotional unconcern identical to the 'apragmatic' form of Pick's disease (Tissot et al 1985). A disregard for others with unaccustomed rudeness is sometimes what first alerts those around to the changes. When these are mentioned the patient shows both lack of concern and lack of insight. There may be periods of crude jocularity or unwarranted euphoria despite a lowering of spontaneity and initiative. Occasionally the patient appears depressed, and he or she is usually refractory to therapy. Self-neglect is often a prominent feature (Orrell et al 1989).

Another feature which clearly distinguishes the group from Alzheimer's disease is the relative preservation of orientation and memory for a considerable period after the onset of the personality changes. Neary (1990) states 'memory disturbance is variable and idiosyncratic. Patients remain oriented as to time and place and can often give detailed accounts of current and historical events of personal significance. However, *they are forgetful and require reminding in a fashion suggestive to relatives of a perverse amnesia to the patients' apparent benefit*' (italics added). Forgetfulness often fluctuates as a function of lack of attention, and for quite some time formal testing reveals preserved ability to learn some new material. In keeping with this Knopman et al (1989) found a relative preservation of memory in six cases of Pick's disease despite marked impairment of executive functions usually considered to be dependent on the integrity of the frontal lobes (see Ch. 4). Visuospatial abilities also remain largely normal for a considerable time (Mendez et al 1996). The most typical neurobehavioural change is progressively reduced speech and language with stereotypy, but frank aphasia does not appear in the early stages. There is a progression later in some cases to mutism. In their psychometric analysis, Johanson and Hagberg (1989) found expressive speech changes to be the most characteristic finding. As with other frontal lesions, associative verbal fluency tasks are particularly sensitive, showing a paucity of generation with response repetition and rule-breaking. There may be a strikingly poorer performance for initial letter than semantic category verbal fluency (see Ch. 4). In some cases this is at marked variance with the apparent sparing of intellectual functions based on well practised skills.

Though scores on tests such as the Wechsler Adult Intelligence Scale may remain in the so-called normal range for some time, patients with this disorder may prove difficult to examine because of their personality changes. They may evince a cavalier attitude and be casual, inattentive and perseverative and they frequently desist as testing progresses, rendering doubtful the validity of any quantitative evaluation. Nevertheless, this test behaviour only serves to reinforce that obtained at clinical interview of a 'frontal' syndrome. Those tests with a high loading on so-called executive functions or adaptive behaviour, which are so useful in all disorders with suspected frontal involvement, also prove very sensitive in this disorder (Walsh 1991, Mendez et al 1996). No case of suspected dementia should be cleared on the basis of preservation of appropriate levels on standard psychometric tests. Early detection through sensitive examination will allow planning for the patient's future and may avoid social disasters through anticipation.

Occasionally the features may suggest the diagnosis of a catatonic syndrome, which may be compelling if the case arises at an early age. Buisson (1989) presents such a case and reminds us that, in their studies of Pick's disease, Henri Ey and associates had pointed out this possibility in 1950.

Although the mean age of FTD onset is around 55, cases at earlier and later ages certainly occur. A family history of a similar disorder is present in as many as half the relatives (e.g. Passant et al 1993). In the elderly population self-neglect is a not uncommon problem and with the apparent preservation of intellect and memory it is probable that many elderly patients with frontal lobe wasting fail to come under neurological or neuropsychological scrutiny (Orrel et al 1989). This latter group has recently pointed to the fact that self-neglect is one of the common deciding factors in admission of the elderly to psychiatric facilities (Orrell & Sahakian 1991). No doubt health professionals will now look more closely at such referrals with the growing knowledge of the frontal degenerative syndrome.

Investigations

The differentiation between Alzheimer's and Pick's diseases is greatly improved by CT and MRI scanning, and made even clearer by positron emission tomography (PET) (Szelies & Karenberg 1986, Kamo et al 1987, Heiss et al 1989, Salmon & Franck 1989). With the growing interest in frontotemporal dementia, studies of blood flow and of glucose and oxygen metabolism using PET and SPECT have typically shown a differential fall-off in the anterior brain regions compared with the parietal and occipital lobes in such cases, while the reverse has been true in patients with Alzheimer's disease (Chase et al 1987, Risberg 1987, Neary et al 1988, Weinstein et al 1989, Kitamura et al 1990, Miller et al 1991, Talbot et al 1995). The correlation of imaging findings with clinical neurological and neuropsychological evaluations will further delineate the disorder (or disorders).

Histological changes appear to be very similar in FTD and Pick's disease, with the same regional differentiation noted in the imaging studies (Englund & Brun 1987). Moreover, epidemiological and neuropathological similarities have been noted between FTD and several other degenerative conditions, specifically primary progressive aphasia (Neary et al 1993), motor neurone disease with dementia (Bergmann et al 1996), and an akinetic-rigid syndrome called *cortico-basal ganglionic degeneration* (Black 1996). These conditions demonstrate similar pathological changes, though initially in different regions of the brain, and not infrequently can occur in the same person, or in first degree relatives (Neary et al 1993). An underlying common genetic defect is reported in some cases (Basun et al 1997, Wilhemsen 1997), though the conditions may still be heterogeneous (see Kertesz 1997, Neary 1997). Another 'focal cortical dementia' termed *posterior cortical atrophy* (Benson et al 1988, see Black 1996 for review), is clinically and pathologically distinct, commonly showing isolated parieto-occipital Alzheimer pathology (Ross et al 1996).

It has been known for some time that, in contrast to patients with Alzheimer's disease, the EEG tends to be normal in the FTD group.

Dementia with Lewy bodies (DLB)

New neuropathological antibody-based staining techniques have led to the differentiation of this entity from other dementias. Pathologically, DLB is distinguished by the presence of ubiquitin positive cortical neuronal inclusions, termed *Lewy bodies* (McKeith et al 1996). These inclusions are similar to those seen in typical Parkinson's disease within cells of the substantia nigra in the midbrain, though staining less noticeably with older histological stains.

Clinically, DLB patients may have prominent attentional disturbances, with fluctuating confusion over minutes, hours, days, or longer. These dominate test performances, and may lead to highly variable results both within and between test sessions. Memory deficits may also be highly variable. Vivid visual hallucinations are common, and at times the patient may act in such a strange manner towards these visions as to suggest delusional ideation. Motor features resembling those seen in Parkinson's disease occur, but these may commence after the onset of cognitive changes. Some patients appear to have co-existing Alzheimer pathology, contributing to mixed clinical presentations and confusion over nomenclature (McKeith et al 1996); neuropsychologists should be aware of this possibility since these patients may resemble patients with Alzheimer's disease.

Ischaemic vascular dementia (IVD)

This is the term for intellectual loss brought about by multiple cerebral infarctions, formerly called *multi-infarct dementia*. Its incidence is variable, mainly because of differences in definition (Tatemichi et al 1992a, Wetterling et al 1996), though it has been stated to be the second most common cause of dementia in the elderly. Recent conceptions emphasize 'strategic infarctions', each of which causes specific recognizable deficits but whose summed disability fulfills criteria for dementia (Tatemichi 1990, Tatemichi et al 1992b). Unlike the steadily progressive course of Alzheimer's disease, IVD is characterized by sudden onset followed by a stepwise decline which is often marked by remissions and exacerbations. The frequent presence of focal neurological symptoms and signs and the absence of personality deterioration is unlike Alzheimer's disease. Unfortunately, in clinical practice, differentiation between these two common types of dementia in the elderly is obscured by the presence of 'mixed' cases which show clear evidence of both vascular and degenerative pathology (Tomlinson et al 1968, Todorov et al 1975, Jellinger 1976, Tomlinson 1977). There have been recent attempts to establish an agreed set of criteria for the diagnosis of IVD to facilitate differentiation from other forms of dementia, particularly Alzheimer's disease, and to provide a base for research into the causes and treatment of vascular dementia (Chui et al 1992, Wetterling et al 1996).

The infarctions of IVD may be either predominantly cortical or subcortical, or a combination of the two: the clinical picture may thus vary widely (see Loeb & Meyer 1996). The relation between the lesions and the deterioration still remains unclear. This is highlighted by the relative preservation of patients who show numerous lacunae on imaging. The term 'leuko-araiosis' refers to variable periventricular changes on imaging (Chimowitz et al 1992), associated with age, Alzheimer's disease and hypotension (Jorgensen el al 1995, Tarvonen-Schroder et al 1996), and whose contribution alone to cognitive deficits is controversial, though probably including attentional deficits (Ylikoski et al 1993). A cross section of reading should include: Fisher 1968, 1982; Hachinski et al 1974; Wells 1978; Cummings and Benson 1983; and Tatemichi 1990.

DISRUPTION OF HIGHER CEREBRAL FUNCTIONS

The following section presents an outline of the disorders of higher mental functions which have formed the focus of the bulk of neuropsychological studies in man. They are reviewed here in general terms only, each topic being dealt with in greater detail in the remainder of the text. The localization of lesions which produce aphasia is covered in detail in several chapters of Kertesz (1983), while a concise and very clear account of the various forms of language disorder can be found in Benson (1979).

Aphasia

The term aphasia refers to an acquired impairment in the reception, manipulation or expression of the symbolic content of language due to brain damage. Such definitions normally exclude perceptual, learning and memory difficulties and purely sensory or motor deficits, unless they specifically involve language symbols.

Speech difficulties caused by interference with the peripheral speech mechanisms, larynx, pharynx and tongue, are termed *dysarthria*.

In general, the various forms of aphasia develop as a result of lesions in the so-called dominant hemisphere.

The importance of aphasia lies in its great localizing value in diagnosis, and no neuropsychological examination is complete without a careful examination of the patient's language functions. More recently, and perhaps more correctly, the term *dysphasia* has been used to denote any disorder, however mild, of the patient's normal symbolic function, though current usage favours aphasia.

The dramatic quality of certain symptoms in individual patients has led some authors to give a variety of different descriptive labels to a large number of aphasias. More systematic study in recent decades has emphasized the fact that aphasia may show itself in various guises but that pure forms of any of the many aphasias described in the earlier literature are extremely rare, and some may be a function of the author's abstracting an entity and giving it a name. This is not to imply that a careful detailed analysis of the language disturbance should not be carried out, rather that we should not continue to multiply labels which have few or no implications for the nature or location of the lesions which produce the disabilities or the types of treatment that might be employed to assist patients with these difficulties.

Aphasic disturbances have usually been classified under two principal headings: (i) motor aphasia; and (ii) sensory aphasia.

Motor aphasia or Broca's aphasia. This generally results from a lesion in the posterior part of the inferior frontal convolution (Fig. 3.11), though cases have been reported where complete removal of Broca's area has led to only transient aphasia. The disability may vary from a complete loss of speech to a mild deficit in which the patient's sole difficulty may be finding the appropriate word. Where the difficulty is great, the patient may become extremely distressed and the examination of the aphasic patient is never an easy task. With the less severe disability, the patient's language may be characterized by a restriction in the range of vocabulary, and the patient may use words repetitively with long pauses between words or phrases.

Patients with motor aphasia often have difficulty with grammatical construction and tend to use sentences of very simple structure, with a predominance of nouns and verbs and a paucity of adjectives, adverbs and joining words (functors), which gives their speech a telegraphic style. This disorder has been referred to as non-fluent speech or *agrammatism*. Comprehension of grammatically complex or unusual constructions is also commonly impaired, hence use of the term 'expressive aphasia' is misleading and not recommended.

It has been commonly believed that in persons who have learned more than one language, the more recently acquired patterns of speech are more readily disturbed than speech in the native tongue. While this may occur on some occasions it is usually true that in aphasia all the patient's languages are equally impaired. This misconception rests in many cases on the examiner's own lack of fluency in the other language so that he fails to recognize the extent of the deficit. The use of an intelligent interpreter in doubtful cases is essential, since the alterations of language may be of a subtle nature and thus may not be evident in simple conversation. Functional MRI studies have recently examined regions that are active in bilingual subjects, finding that later age of acquisition of the second language correlated with differing sub-regions within Broca's area, but no difference in Wernicke's area (Kim et al 1997).

Difficulty commonly also extends to written language where the aphasic patient shows the same difficulty as in verbal expression. On rare occasions this *agraphia* has been described in cases with no obvious difficulties of verbal expression. The second frontal gyrus has been implicated in some of these cases (Aimard et al 1975).

Sensory aphasia. This generally results from a lesion in the region of Wernicke's area of the dominant hemisphere (Fig. 3.11). The prime difficulty is a loss of the association between words and their meaning, particularly for spoken nouns and verbs, but often for the written word as well. Thus, two major forms of sensory aphasia may be distinguished, an auditory receptive aphasia, usually related to lesions in the superior temporal convolution, and a visual receptive aphasia related to more posteriorly placed parieto-temporal lesions.

Patients with *auditory receptive aphasia* have trouble in understanding what is

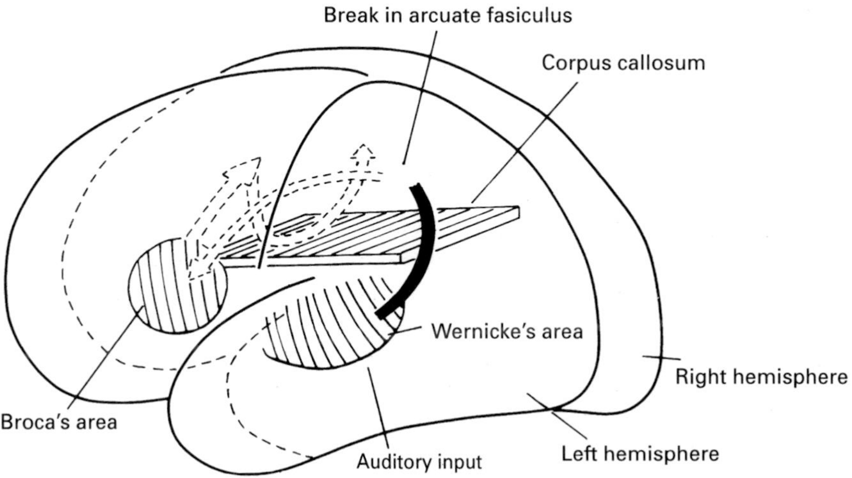

Fig. 3.11 Conduction aphasia caused by a lesion disrupting the arcuate fasciculus.

said to them. The problem is caused by a failure in comprehension, since auditory acuity as tested by audiometry remains adequate. The common presence also of expressive difficulties manifested by errors in word or phrase selection (*paraphasias*) in these patients again points to the undesirability of retaining rigid categories of classification.

Unlike the patient with motor aphasia, the sensory aphasic's verbalizations may be grammatically fluent, without apparent hesitancy, and, in fact, the individual may be unusually voluble. However, the patient's language is often unintelligible. Since they are not capable of monitoring their own verbal expression because of difficulty in auditory comprehension, they may be unaware of the inappropriateness of their utterances. Verbal confusion and the paraphasias may result in a very disjointed form of speech disorder termed *jargon aphasia.*

In *visual receptive* aphasia the understanding of written language is impaired. This difficulty is referred to as *alexia* or sometimes 'word blindness' (*dyslexia* is usually used to denote developmental reading difficulties). While patients may be able to identify individual letters, they are unable to perceive words as meaningful wholes. Alexia may occur together with difficulty in recognizing objects in the syndrome of *visual object agnosia.* On the other hand, a syndrome of alexia without agraphia has long been recognized. Sometimes the alexia is also accompanied by an inability to name colours (*colour anomia*), and the ability to read numbers may be preserved while the ability to read letters and words is lost. Geschwind's (1965) masterly analysis of the syndrome of alexia without agraphia forms a fine example of the use of the concept of the disconnection syndrome in analysing disorders of higher cerebral processes (Ch. 7), though other explanations are reported (Benito-León et al 1997). It utilizes Wernicke's notion of the importance of the connections between different parts of the brain in the building up of complex activities. An example of the disconnection syndrome as the anatomical basis of the aphasias concludes this section.

Global or mixed aphasia. This refers to cases where both motor and sensory elements are present. These cases are usually severe in their symptoms and present extensive lesions on pathological examination.

Amnestic, amnesic, anomic or nominal aphasia. This is characterized by the patient's inability to identify people or objects by their proper names. If shown a hairbrush, the patients will be unable to evoke the name 'brush' though they will demonstrate both with words and actions that they are well aware of the nature of the object and will recognize the correct word when it is given (*one-way anomia*). This ability to recognize the correct word when it is provided is not seen in patients with sensory aphasia (*two-way anomia*). This form of aphasia is quite different from motor aphasia. It does not have a precise localization within the peri-sylvian language areas, though the lesion is usually behind the central sulcus. It is the association between the object and its particular noun that is lost. If the deficit is marked, speech may be greatly reduced. When unable to find the correct word, the patients may substitute colloquialisms and employ circumlocutions and periphrastic expressions to convey their meaning.

Some authors consider amnestic aphasia to be essentially a form of sensory aphasia, and the responsible lesion is usually found in the posterior region of the superior temporal convolution on the dominant side.

The anatomical disconnection model. Geschwind (1969) has extended the anatomical model, first put forward by Wernicke, to provide understanding of the various forms of aphasia.

1. With a lesion in Wernicke's area, incoming auditory information will not be understood and, since a lesion in this region may interrupt the passage of visual information travelling forward from the visual association cortex, isolating this information from the anterior speech area, patients will be unable to describe in words what they see. Furthermore, since visual forms no longer arouse auditory ones because of the disconnection, the patients no longer understand written language.

2. A lesion in the principal connecting link between the comprehension area and the expressive area, the *arcuate fasciculus*, leads to abnormality in speech with the preservation of comprehension of both written and spoken speech. Such a disorder is termed *conduction aphasia* (Fig. 3.11). Since Wernicke's area is intact, patients can understand what is said to them. On the other hand, with Broca's area also intact they will be able to speak spontaneously. The speech is often copious but is abnormal because of the isolation between the two major areas. Since the connection has been broken between the receptive area and the motor speech area, patients will be unable to repeat what the examiner says. This disproportionate difficulty in repetition is said to be the principal characteristic of this disorder.

Furthermore, in order for the patient to carry out movements on command, the information needs to go forward from Wernicke's area to the motor area and so the patient is unable to carry out such commands. As the pathway in the diagram shows, a lesion in the arcuate fasciculus will lead to bilateral difficulty in carrying out verbal commands since these are prevented from reaching the appropriate motor areas of either hemisphere.

3. When a lesion damages the left visual cortex and the posterior portion of the corpus callosum known as the splenium, the patient is still able to see stimuli in the left visual field corresponding to the intact right visual cortex though not in the right visual field. However, the information perceived by the right hemisphere can no longer reach the left hemisphere language areas so that patients cannot understand written language though, with the preservation of both Broca's and Wernicke's areas, they can both comprehend and speak spontaneously. This disorder is termed pure alexia or agnosic alexia.

4. Sometimes even extensive lesions in the hemispheres may spare both Broca's and Wernicke's areas, isolating them from the rest of the brain. Speech production and comprehension are both impaired, but the ability to repeat spoken words is preserved. Such a disability is termed *mixed transcortical aphasia*. Anterior lesions beyond the inner peri-sylvian language area can cause motor speech difficulties with preservation of comprehension and repetition (*transcortical motor aphasia*), whilst posterior lesions can cause comprehension deficits and circumlocution without motor or repetition difficulties (*transcortical sensory aphasia*).

Further examples of the use of the anatomical model are given elsewhere and, despite limitations, this model 'most closely meets the criteria of efficiency in explaining the known data, efficiency in predicting new phenomena, or in design of important experiments and susceptibility to refinements that can be checked by observation or experiment' (Geschwind 1969). Modern imaging techniques have lent support to the 'classical' anatomical theory (Kertesz 1979, 1983), though other explanations based on specialized centres within a distributed language network also exist (Benito-León et al 1997).

Agnosia

It is a useful generalization to consider all the cortical territory behind the central sulcus as being concerned with getting to know the world around us. In line with the early name for the central sulcus – the fissure of Rolando – lesions in this region are still frequently referred to as retrorolandic lesions. In Luria's terms (Luria 1973) this is the second major unit of the higher nervous system, the one concerned with the reception, analysis and storage of information. It is divided into three major types of cortex:

Primary projection areas are modality-specific, i.e. they serve only one sense modality such as vision, audition or bodily sensation. Each of these areas is laid out in a somatotopic manner as described in Chapter 2.

Projection-association cortex is adjacent to a primary projection area and, while still concerned with only one sensory mode, organizes the incoming information into meaningful wholes.

An area of cortex which is concerned with the integration of information from all sensory channels and, in this integrative sense, is supramodal. This cortex, which is specific to man, is found at the confluence of the parietal, temporal and occipital areas in the region of the supramarginal gyrus.

The major divisions of the postcentral or retrorolandic cortex are shown in Figure 3.12.

Lesions of the postcentral area give rise to simple or complex sensory or

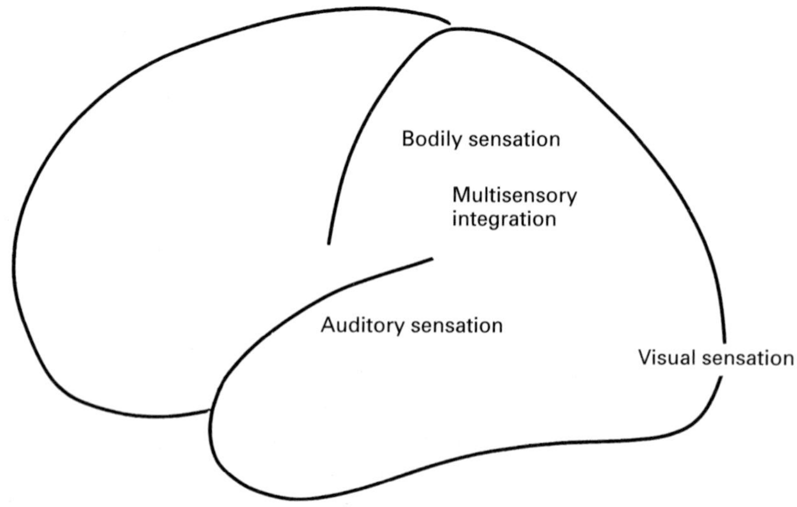

Fig. 3.12 The posterior or retrorolandic cortex and sensory systems.

perceptual disturbances, and affect one or more modalities, according to their location. Since, with the possible exception of some penetrating missile wounds, cerebral lesions are seldom discrete, individual cases usually show a mixture of symptoms.

Agnosia refers to a failure to recognize familiar objects perceived via the senses where the inability does not rest on sensory impairment, intellectual deterioration or other cause. Where it is associated with only one modality, e.g. visual agnosia, an object may be recognized through other senses such as touch, or a person may not be recognized until he or she speaks.

The many types or forms of agnosia reported in the medical literature are probably not separate entities and the difficulties raised by the multiplication of labels mentioned above with regard to aphasia apply equally here. The very concept of agnosia has been attacked by a number of workers. The term is so common, however, that the following notes on the various described forms may familiarize the beginning student with the terminology likely to be encountered.

Auditory agnosia is the term used to refer to the inability to recognize speech. The failure to recognize melodies is referred to as *sensory amusia*. A careful analysis by Vignolo and others of patients' difficulties with different types of auditory material has led to a valuable distinction between semantic-associative difficulties on one hand, and auditory-discriminative difficulties on the other (Ch. 5). As these difficulties show double dissociation with respect to the left and right temporal lobes they should prove of value as a diagnostic aid. Both forms of auditory agnosia occur without audiometric loss.

Visual agnosia has been classified according to the class of visual perceptual material with which the patient has difficulty. There may be *visual object agnosia*, where the patient without disturbances of visual acuity or visual field defects fails to recognize the object for what it is, or may be unable to recognize pictorial representations of objects. The patient can see individual features but 'cannot combine these individual features into complete forms' (Luria 1973, p. 116). Visual object agnosia is a rare clinical entity. However, the careful examination of a case by Taylor and Warrington (1973) showed clear cut dissociation between primary apprehension of the object via the visual modality (apperception) and the association of the object with meaning. This is close to the distinction made by Hebb some years ago between figural unity and figural identity (Hebb 1949).

A particular difficulty in recognizing familiar faces is referred to as *prosopagnosia*. Patients may not only fail to recognize familiar faces such as those of family members, but may be unable to recognize their own reflection in the mirror. There may be *agnosia for colours* which, when associated with alexia, has special localizing significance. These and other visual agnosias are treated in Chapter 7.

Spatial agnosia. Sometimes referred to as visual or spatial disorientation. Patients are unable to find their way around in a familiar environment such as their own district or even their own home, though they may recognize separate objects in the home quite well. There may also be defects in visual and topographical memory, so that patients with this disorder are unable to find their way on a map or, if asked to draw a map, will produce one with topographical distortions and omissions.

Tactile agnosia or *astereognosis* refers to inability to recognize objects by feeling them. The relation of tactile agnosia to sensory defects is discussed in relation to lesions of the parietal lobes in Chapter 6.

The neglect syndrome

Subsumed under this term are a number of clinical presentations which have received increased attention in recent years (for review see Heilman et al 1985). 'A patient with the neglect syndrome fails to report, respond, or orient to novel or meaningful stimuli presented to the side opposite a brain lesion' (Heilman 1979).

Four major forms have been distinguished:

1. *Unilateral spatial neglect*, also termed *hemispatial neglect, hemispatial agnosia* and *visuospatial agnosia*. When asked to perform tasks in space, patients neglect the half of space contralateral to the lesion; for example, when asked to bisect a line they may neglect the presence of one side and thus move their bisection point some distance to the side of the lesion, or they may fail to cross out lines on one side of a page which has lines scattered randomly over it (Albert 1973). In everyday life, patients with neglect may fail to eat food on one side of the plate and bump into objects to one side which they appear not to notice. This topic is dealt with in Chapter 6.
2. *Hemi-inattention* overlaps with the former description and refers to a failure to report stimuli of various kinds presented unilaterally. Obviously it may be difficult to distinguish unilateral inattention from hemianopia or hemianaesthesia (i.e. loss of the visual half field, or loss of sensation on one side of the body). However, the subject with hemi-inattention may be able to detect the stimulus with relative ease if attention is directed specifically to its presence.
3. *Sensory inattention, sensory extinction, sensory suppression* or *perceptual rivalry* denotes a failure to appreciate a stimulus when a similar stimulus is applied to a corresponding part of the body or to both halves of the visual field simultaneously. The patient is quite able to see and recognize things in any part of the visual field when they are presented alone or to report a tactile stimulus from either side of the body. It is only when the stimuli are presented simultaneously that the disorder comes to light. The method is termed *double simultaneous stimulation*. The inattention is for the stimulus opposite the side of the lesion. This phenomenon has been reviewed by Critchley (1949), Bender (1952) and Denny-Brown et al (1952), and has been the object of numerous studies in the past decades. These attest to the existence of the phenomena in a wide variety of sense modalities, e.g. vision, audition, pain, touch, temperature, pressure, taste, kinaesthesia and vibration. The range of explanations is almost as wide ranging as the phenomena themselves, though that of Weintraub and Mesulam (1987) has gained experimental support (Corbetta et al 1993, Gitelman et al 1996).
4. Some patients with unilateral lesions may show a slowing of movement or an inability or delay in initiating movement of the limb contralateral to the lesion, a condition called *akinesia*. Attempts at bilateral movement may worsen the contralateral limb akinesia, a condition akin to sensory extinction and actually termed 'motor extinction' by Valenstein and Heilman (1981).

Body agnosia

Body agnosia, corporeal agnosia or *autotopagnosia* is a lack of awareness of the body's topography, an inability to recognize or localize parts of the patient's own body. A special form of autotopagnosia is *finger agnosia*, where the patient cannot point to, or show the examiner the various fingers of each hand. It forms one of the four classical features of Gerstmann's syndrome which, because of its important bearing on the notion of cerebral dominance or lateralization, is discussed at length in Chapter 8. Body agnosia is also often associated with lack of awareness of disease or disability known as *anosognosia*, e.g. the patient fails to perceive or denies that the arm and leg are paralysed. Anosognosia also accompanies other serious disorders such as cerebral blindness (see Ch. 7).

Discussion of other disorders of the body schema may be found in Frederiks (1985).

Apraxia

Apraxia is the inability to carry out purposive or skilled acts because of brain damage and not as a result of the numerous other reasons which may result in imperfectly executed movements, e.g. failure to comprehend what to do, weakness or paralysis, or sensory loss.

In the first of a number of works on apraxia or 'motor asymboly', Liepmann (1900) commented on the case of an individual who had suffered a stroke and who acted 'with his right extremities as if he were a total imbecile, as if he understands neither questions nor commands, as if he could neither understand the value of objects nor the sense of printed or written words, yet prove by an intelligent use of his left extremities that all of those seemingly absent abilities were in reality present'. Liepmann termed this 'unilateral apraxia'. The patient was globally aphasic and as a result of his lack of correct responses also had been considered to be demented. Liepmann's description of his examination is a paradigm for insightful evaluation and the derivation of conclusions from clinical observation.

Prior to the work of Liepmann, this disorder was thought to be secondary to agnosia. Through the work of Liepmann and his contemporaries, a number of types were soon described: (i) motor or limb-kinetic apraxia; (ii) ideomotor or ideokinetic apraxia; and (iii) ideational apraxia. Later, the word 'apraxia' was added to other terms, e.g. constructional apraxia, dressing apraxia, although in the strict sense of the term these conditions are not true apraxias. However, the usage has remained. Perhaps nowhere else in the realm of neuropsychological disorders has classification been so confusing (see Heilman et al 1983, Geschwind & Damasio 1985). Apraxia is strongly associated with lesions of the left hemisphere (and two forms may be described in the same patient). Apraxia is therefore often associated with aphasia. Ajuriaguerra et al (1960) reported the occurrence of the various forms of motor apraxia in *left* posterior (retrorolandic) lesions but none in their 151 right-sided cases.

Motor apraxia is believed to be caused by loss of the kinaesthetic memory patterns or engrams necessary for the performance of the skilled act, as first suggested by Liepmann (1908). This form of apraxia usually affects the finer movements of one upper extremity – movements such as doing up buttons, opening a safety pin, placing a letter in an envelope. Where there is associated weakness, the clumsiness of the movement is out of all proportion to the loss of power. This form of apraxia usually results from a lesion of the precentral gyrus contralateral to the side of the body affected.

Ideomotor apraxia is the most common type of motor apraxia. It is a condition in which the patient finds it difficult to carry out an action on verbal command with either hand but may do so automatically or almost fortuitously. Patients are usually unable to imitate actions that are demonstrated to them. The kinetic engram is preserved but is not available to the patient's voluntary recall. This form of apraxia is usually associated with a lesion in the posterior part of the left or dominant hemisphere, particularly in the region of the supramarginal gyrus.

The concept of the disconnection syndrome is also useful in understanding the anatomical basis of the apraxias. In the case of carrying out a skilled movement on verbal command there is a complex chain of events. Firstly, the auditory information is organized in Wernicke's area, i.e. the left superior temporal region if we are considering a right-handed patient. From here the information travels to the motor association cortex in the frontal lobe and thence to the motor cortex which sends impulses to the appropriate muscle groups on the right side of the body to execute the command. If the patient is asked to carry out the action with his left hand, the sequence will have to be the same with the important addition that the information will have to travel from the left motor association area to that on the right, since the right motor region commands the left hand. Consequently a lesion of the anterior part of the corpus callosum, which carries these fibres between the left and right hemispheres, will render the patient incapable of carrying out verbal commands with the left hand while still able to carry them out with the right (Fig. 3.13). This disorder has

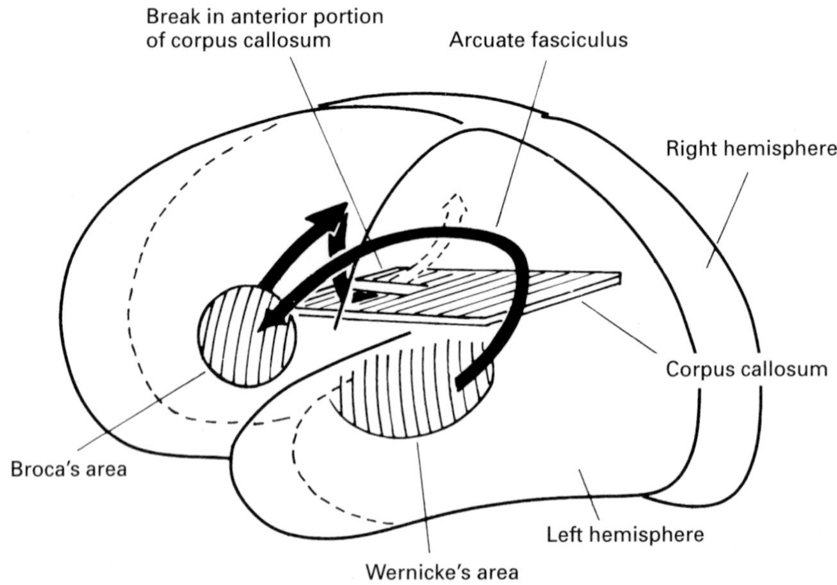

Fig. 3.13 Left-sided or callosal apraxia produced by an anterior lesion of the corpus callosum.

been termed *left-sided apraxia, unilateral limb apraxia* or *callosal apraxia*. In essence it is a unilateral ideomotor apraxia.

Ideational apraxia is the difficulty in executing the correct sequence of steps which makes up a complex act though the individual component acts may be successfully carried out. It is a disruption of the total programme of the required acts. Patients may show no difficulty in imitating sequences, i.e. where the programme is provided for them. The disorder may look like an extreme absent-mindedness. It is often associated with difficulty in using objects correctly. The patient seems to be unaware of what the object was designed to do, akin to an agnosia of utilization. Ideational apraxia is associated with dominant hemisphere parietal lobe lesions and is thus often accompanied by fluent aphasia and elements of Gerstmann's syndrome (Ch. 6). Ideational apraxia is also seen with bilateral lesions.

Constructional apraxia is a 'higher' disorder which has received much more attention from neuropsychologists than the three major forms already outlined. Perhaps the major difference between constructional apraxia and other forms of praxic disorder is that special tests, albeit simple, are usually necessary to elicit it, while other forms are clinically apparent. With constructional apraxia the patient is unable to put together parts to make a whole. A detailed account of methods of testing for constructional apraxia is given by Critchley (1953), and later reviews by Warrington (1969) and Benton (1969) examined most aspects of the disorder and its implications for localization. The deficit is discussed later in relation to parietal lobe dysfunction (Ch. 6). A few examples of the patient's difficulties will suffice here.

On block design tests such as that of the Wechsler Adult Intelligence Scale (Wechsler 1958), patients often have difficulty with the earliest and simplest designs and generally perform at a much lower level than other patients on this test. A poor level of performance on block design tests is not pathognomonic of the disorder since many patients with lesions in various parts of the brain perform poorly on this test for a variety of reasons, however an examination of the quality of performance shows that patients with constructional apraxia have a greater number of constructional deviations in their attempts (Ben-Yishay et al 1971). Simple drawing tests, such as copying geometric designs of varying complexity (Benton 1962) or drawing common objects such as a house, will elicit the difficulty, though more complex tasks such as constructing a copy of a three dimensional model with blocks may have to be employed (Benton & Fogel 1962).

Finally, so-called *dressing apraxia* is the condition in which the patient is unable to clothe himself properly, more commonly leaving the left side partly or wholly unclad. It appears to be a reflection of the patient's neglect of part of his body mentioned above and is seen more frequently with parietal lesions of the non-dominant hemisphere. It should be considered as part of the neglect syndrome rather than as a disorder of skilled movement.

Though apraxia may be seen in isolation, it often accompanies other defects such as agnosia, aphasia and impairment of memory, and, despite the separation used here, it may be difficult to decide in individual patients how much the defect of action is due to a lack of awareness, a lack of skilled movements, or some degree of weakness or ataxia of the affected limb.

Amnesia

Memory disorders are a frequent accompaniment of cerebral disorders and have given rise to countless studies reported in the literature. An overall review such as that of Whitty and Zangwill (1977) can be updated from the major specialist journals in neuropsychology. Major subdivisions of this vast subject are covered in several of the later chapters.

Terminology

Clinical reports often refer to two principal terms, which have derived from the study of memory disorders following cerebral insult. *Anterograde amnesia* is characterized by an inability to retain (or at least report spontaneously) ongoing events. It is synonymous with a new learning difficulty. Material which is clearly apprehended, as measured by the ability of the patient to repeat it immediately, cannot be reported a short time later. It is common after cerebral trauma for this condition to improve with the passage of time but lesions in certain anatomical sites may lead to a lasting memory impairment. *Retrograde amnesia* refers to the difficulty in recalling events which occurred prior to the injury. With the passing of time retrograde amnesia shrinks so that, while a few days after the injury patients may not recall events that happened weeks or even months before, they may later be able to recall events much closer to the injury; the gap left in their memory may thus be very short.

Post-traumatic amnesia (PTA) is the period from the time of injury to the time when the patient begins to report ongoing events, i.e. when anterograde amnesia stops. Its duration has been used as a guide to the severity of the damage: the longer the period of PTA, the more severe the damage is likely to be, although there are some striking exceptions (for further discussion see Walsh 1991).

Types of memory disorder

Amnesic syndromes may accompany neurological or psychological disorders, they may be transient or lasting, and they may be specific or general.

Two major forms of memory disturbance of a non-organic nature are *hysterical fugue* and *psychogenic amnesia*. A hysterical fugue consists of a series of events whereby the patient often may remove himself from his current situation, which is almost invariably disagreeable, and move to another. This may involve travel to distant parts and even a change from a customary occupation. The behaviour is often described as a dissociation and patients may appear to be unaware of their past while in the fugue state, i.e. they have a total amnesia and on return to their 'former self' will be amnesic for the period occupied by the fugue. Behaviour appears to be fairly well integrated and consistent in each of the states.

Less striking memory disorders may appear as the sole complaint in other neurotic disorders, particularly those termed sick role enactments (Walsh 1991). Such *psychogenic amnesias* or pseudoneurological amnesias may mimic those of a neurological aetiology but can be differentiated by their lack of concordance with the characteristics of the organic varieties.

Of the neurological amnesic disorders some are transient while others are lasting. *Transient global amnesia* (TGA) was the term used by Fisher and Adams

(1964) for a sudden loss or difficulty with memory unaccompanied by any major neurological signs and followed shortly after by a return of normal memory function. Characteristically, the period extends over several hours and the patient is permanently amnesic for the duration of the attack. The aetiology is commonly agreed to be vascular. TGA was reviewed by Caplan (1985) and an up-to-date review is given in Chapter 5.

Lasting amnesia is much more common than TGA and may be divided into general and specific amnesic disorders.

The principal lasting amnesic syndrome is called by a number of names. Where the unqualified term *the amnesic syndrome* is used in the literature this can be taken to be synonymous with the general amnesic syndrome described by Korsakoff as the major feature of the syndrome which bears his name. A translation of his classic paper of 1887 was published by Victor and Yakovlev (1955).

Korsakoff's amnesic syndrome shows (i) an almost complete inability to learn new material despite (ii) an adequate immediate memory as tested by repetition, with (iii) retrograde amnesia, and (iv) preservation of early established skills and habits. A more detailed description of the general amnesic syndrome and its congeners appears under the generic term 'diencephalic amnesia' in Chapter 9.

While the characteristic pathology of the general amnesic syndrome is bilateral damage to certain structures around the central core or axis of the brain, *material specific amnesias* are caused by *unilateral* lesions. The crucial areas are the same structures which are affected in general amnesic syndromes, namely parts of the hippocampus–fornix–mamillary body complex (Fig. 3.14), however the amnesia is restricted to one class of material, either verbal or non-verbal, and this follows the rule of hemispheric specialization of function. Dominant hemisphere lesions affect verbal memory but spare the non-verbal, while non-

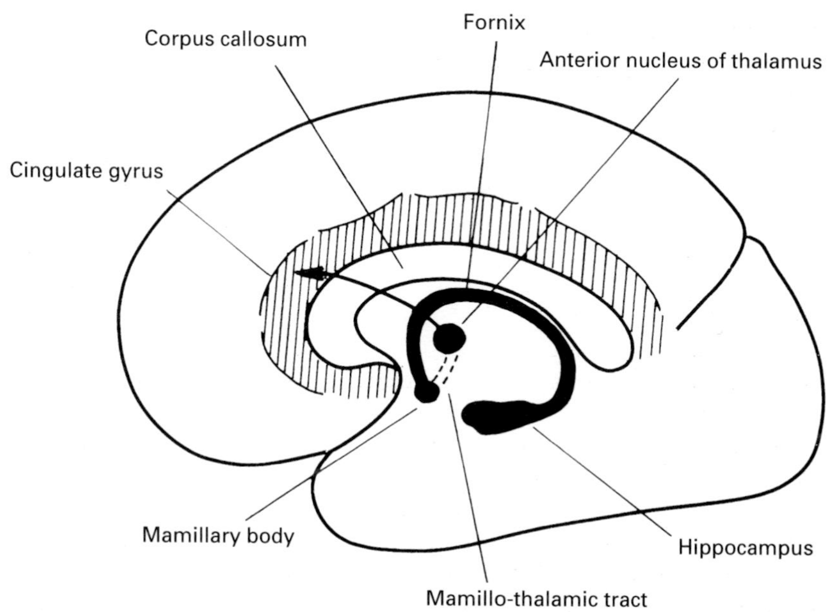

Fig. 3.14 Hippocampus–fornix–mamillary body complex.

dominant lesions produce the reverse pattern. Again, these material specific amnesias are discussed further in Chapter 5.

EPILEPSY

This condition has been left until this stage since it cuts across numerous divisions of our subject matter.

The term epilepsy means a seizure, i.e. a sudden disruption of the patient's senses, and, because it manifests itself in a great variety of ways, it is difficult to define more clearly in a short space. The problem is aggravated by the vast array of terms which has been, and continues to be, used to define the same or very similar conditions.

Clinical classification

In 1969, The Commission on Classification and Terminology of the International League Against Epilepsy introduced a classification which has received widespread, though by no means universal, support (Gastaut 1970). Later (1981) the Commission attempted further to refine this generally useful classification though there were those (e.g. Parsonage 1983) who felt that the newer classification was premature and that the 1969 system should stand until we have considerably more knowledge.

The Commission recognized a distinction between *epileptic seizures* (Table 3.2) and the *epilepsies* (Table 3.3). For further detail readers are referred to general reviews (Gastaut & Broughton 1972, Aird et al 1984). More recently the Commission has set out yet another proposal for further revision of the classification of epilepsies and epileptic syndromes (Commission on Classification of the ILAE 1989).

Generalized seizures

The principal feature of many generalized seizures is disordered muscular

Table 3.2 Types of epileptic seizures (condensed from the international classification)

Generalized seizures (bilaterally symmetrical and without local onset)
- Tonic-clonic seizures (*grand mal*)
- Absences (*petit mal*)
- Other forms (includes akinetic, atonic, tonic, clonic, bilateral myoclonic, etc.)

Partial seizures (seizures beginning locally)
- Partial seizures with elementary symptomatology (generally without impairment of consciousness)
- With motor symptoms
- With sensory or somatosensory symptoms
- With autonomic symptoms

Partial seizures with complex symptomatology (generally with impairment of consciousness, temporal lobe or psychomotor seizures)
- With impairment of consciousness only
- With cognitive or affective or psychosensory or psychomotor symptomatology

Unilateral seizures

Unclassified

Table 3.3 International classification of the epilepsies

Generalized epilepsies
Primary (includes petit and grand mal seizures)
Secondary
Undetermined
Partial (focal, local) epilepsies (includes jacksonian, temporal lobe and psychomotor seizures)
Unclassified epilepsies

contraction. The term *tonic-clonic* seizure describes the two main phases of the paroxysm which were previously termed *grand mal* seizures. In the tonic phase the muscles contract and the subject often falls to the ground. Contraction of respiratory muscles may produce a grunt or cry. Swallowing is lost and the patient becomes cyanosed from lack of oxygen. Contraction of muscles often produces incontinence of urine and, less commonly, of faeces. The clonic phase follows after a brief time (a few seconds to a minute) and is marked by rhythmic contractions of limb and trunk muscles. After a variable time the clonic phase ceases and the patient passes from stupor, through confusion, to a normal conscious state. On some occasions one generalized seizure may follow another in rapid succession, the so-called *status epilepticus*.

Generalized seizures may be primary or may be precipitated from a localized focus. The primary form of epilepsy was often referred to as *centrencephalic* epilepsy. The term *centrencephalon* was introduced by Penfield to refer to those neural systems which are centrally placed in the upper brain stem and symmetrically connected with both cerebral hemispheres and which serve to co-ordinate their functions (Fig. 3.15). Although generalized seizures are now thought to arise from the cortex, this concept has persisted.

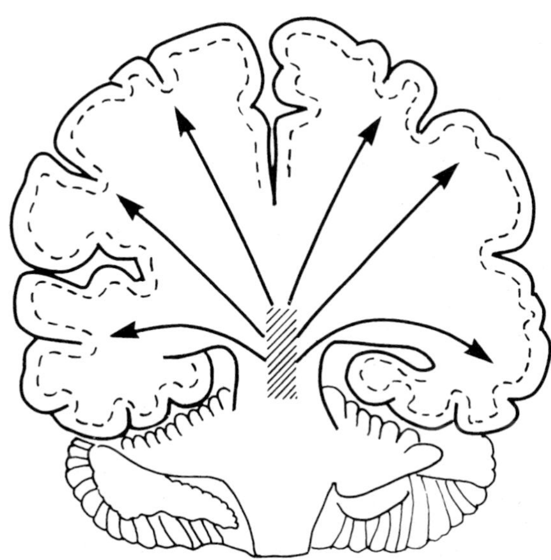

Fig. 3.15 Schematic representation of the spread of excitation from the centre of the brain.

The second form is the *absence*, formerly termed *petit mal* seizures. This is largely a disorder of childhood, its prolongation into adult life being rare. The attacks are characteristically brief, usually only a few seconds, with an abrupt onset and termination. The patient's ongoing activity is disturbed with interruption of mental functions and sudden resumption of activity after the absence. The EEG shows a characteristic 'spike and wave' pattern during the attacks and often bursts of such activity can be seen in the record even when no disturbance of ongoing activity is to be seen clinically. About one third of children with absences also have tonic-clonic seizures.

Partial seizures

These seizures have also been termed focal seizures, since they reflect a neuronal discharge which is more or less localized to one area of the brain. They are divided into two main types (a) those with elementary, and (b) those with complex symptomatology. The former type characteristically occur without any loss of consciousness, while some impairment of the conscious state is found with complex partial seizures.

Simple partial seizures. Motor symptoms may take many forms and point to the localization, mainly in portions of the region in front of the central or *rolandic fissure*, though the focal abnormality may lie in the temporal or parietal region, e.g. when *aphasia* is brought about by the epileptic or ictal discharge.

Sensory symptoms may take the form of any of the sense modalities, i.e. somatosensory phenomena or sensations referable to the special senses of vision, audition and olfaction in particular. There may be a fine line between the designation of a symptom as a simple sensory seizure, a sensory illusion or even a sensory hallucination, but a careful examination may be of value in localization. Patients differ a good deal in their ability to describe their symptoms, and carefully phrased questions will help.

Symptoms of autonomic disturbance rarely occur without other symptoms.

Complex partial seizures. Since these seizures present so frequently with symptoms of disruption of higher mental functions, they have become of increasing interest to neuropsychologists.

Certain characteristics of the seizure may suggest that the focus of abnormal excitation lies in one of the neocortical association areas and so may be used as localizing signs. Frequently, the onset of the seizures or aura as it is usually called, is signalled by a subjective feeling or behaviour referable to a particular area, and tables of the relation between the clinical type of seizure and localization have been in use for some time.

Though many attacks may recur frequently in the same manner in some patients, there are other cases where the initial warning symptoms or auras vary from one seizure to the next, so that care must be taken in using the signs and symptoms associated with any single attack as localizing indications.

Where the lesion is fairly well circumscribed, it may lend itself to surgical removal. This has been particularly successful in certain refractory cases of lesions restricted to the temporal lobes, where the removal of a portion of the temporal lobe (temporal lobectomy) may completely cure or greatly ameliorate the condition. The very frequent reference in the past two decades to studies of various higher functions in populations of patients with temporal lobe seizures before and after lobectomy makes it mandatory for the psychologist to have a clear understanding of the complex symptomatology of this group of seizures.

The portions of the cortex which may be involved in complex partial seizures are the frontal, temporal and parietal neocortex, and the subcortical structures associated with them. The clinical features which distinguish the subgroups mentioned below are often present in the same patient, either in the one attack or at different times, and may be accompanied by impaired consciousness which may obscure the picture. The main types can be grouped as follows.

1. Cases where impairment of consciousness is the principal or even the sole symptom.
2. Psychomotor attacks where the principal symptoms are confusion and automatic behaviour. Confusional automatisms may be merely a 'mechanical' prolongation of the behaviour in which the patient was engaged at the onset of the attack, or the automatisms may represent new behaviour beginning during the attack. Many forms of automatisms have been given descriptive labels, e.g. ambulatory automatisms, in which the patient may carry out co-ordinated movements of some complexity during the attack and for a varying time after the seizure, verbal automatisms, gestural automatisms, and the like.
3. Seizures with sensory illusions or hallucinations. The nature of these seizures varies with the region of cortex which is the site of discharge. Where the primary projection areas of the cortex are mainly affected, the phenomena are simpler sensory experiences or alteration of the perception of present stimuli, while excitation of the association areas appears to give rise to integrated perceptual experiences which, since they occur in the absence of appropriate stimuli in the environment, have earned the title 'hallucinations'.

Once again, a careful examination of the patient's experience may point to the affected area. The illusions may be related to a specific sense modality, i.e. visual, auditory, olfactory, somaesthetic illusions, or, when the discharge affects the borderland between the parietal, temporal and occipital areas, compound illusions may result.

A special form of alteration in sense experience occurs with some temporal lobe seizures, so that present experience is interpreted in a manner quite different from usual. New situations or objects may be perceived as having been seen or heard before (*déjà vu, déjà entendu*) or familiar ones as not having been experienced before (*jamais vu, jamais entendu*).

An early description of an olfactory hallucination associated with a temporal lobe lesion was given by Hughlings Jackson (1890). The following account was provided by the patient and her sister.

> The patient was a cook. In the paroxysm the first thing was tremor of the hands and arms; she saw a little black woman who was always very actively engaged in cooking; the spectre did not speak. The patient had a very horrible smell (so-called 'subjective sensation' of smell) which she could not describe. She had a feeling as if she was shut up in a box with a limited quantity of air. She would stand with her eyes fixed and then say, 'What a horrible smell!'. The patient did not, so her sister reported, lose consciousness, but remembered everything that happened during the attack; she turned of a leaden colour. The patient told us that she passed her

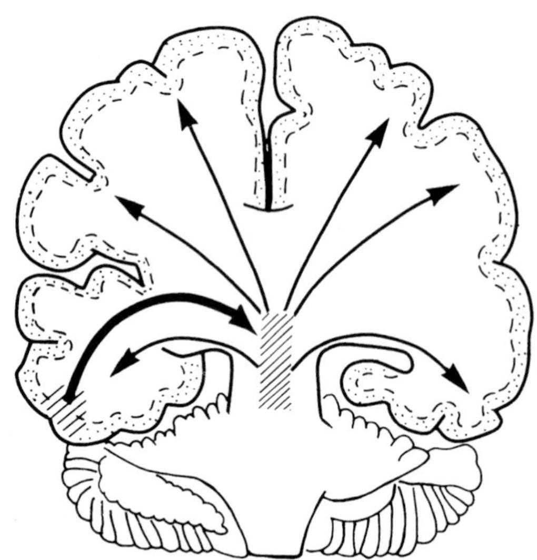

Fig. 3.16 Temporal lobe focus giving rise to a generalized seizure.

urine in the seizures. There was no struggling, and the tongue was not bitten. She never believed the spectre to be a real person.

After leaving her kitchen work she had paroxysms with the smell sensation but no spectre. At autopsy a tumour 'the size of a tangerine orange' was found occupying the anterior portion of the temporal lobe.

4. Some partial seizures may produce sudden alteration in the emotional state, usually in the form of fear.
5. Disturbances of memory and thought processes may occur during temporal lobe seizures.

Finally, it is common for simple symptomatology to be followed by the more complex or there may be an admixture of both. Epilepsy associated with temporal lobe pathology is discussed in more detail in Chapter 5.

Partial seizures may at times progress to generalized seizures (Fig. 3.16).

Unilateral seizures

In this type of disorder the discharge, while spread over a wide area, is restricted to one hemisphere and demonstrates itself by clinical phenomena on the opposite (*contralateral*) side of the body. The excessive neuronal discharge causing the seizure may arise in the *centrencephalon* whence it spreads exclusively or mainly to the hemisphere on one side, or the discharge may originate in a local region of the cerebral cortex of one hemisphere and spread to the centrencephalon from which it projects in turn to the whole of that hemisphere.

The reason for considering these unilateral seizures as separate from partial seizures is that there are no signs in the periods between the seizures of clinical or EEG features of localized brain impairment, and such seizures may alternate from side to side from one attack to another, or even during the course of a single attack. As with generalized seizures, unilateral seizures have been classified into a number of subtypes according to the symptomatology.

References

Adams C, Hwang P A, Gilday D L et al 1992 Comparison of SPECT, EEG, MRI, and pathology in partial epilepsy. Pediatric Neurology 8: 97–103

Adams J H 1975 The neuropathology of head injuries. In: Vinken P J, Bruyn G (eds) Handbook of clinical neurology, vol 23. North-Holland, Amsterdam, ch 3, p 35

Adams R D, Victor M 1977 Principles of neurology. McGraw-Hill, New York

Adams R D, Victor M 1993 Principles of neurology, 5th edn. McGraw-Hill, New York

Aimard G, Devic M, Lebel M, Trouillas P, Boisson D 1975 Pure (dynamic?) agraphia of frontal origin. Revue Neurologique 131: 505–512

Aird R B, Masland R L, Woodbury D M (eds) 1984 The epilepsies: A critical review. Raven Press, New York

Ajuriaguerra J de, Hécaen H, Angelergues R 1960 Les apraxies, variétés cliniques et latéralisation lésionelle. Revue Neurologique 102: 494–566

Albert M L 1973 A simple test of visual neglect. Neurology 23: 658–664

Artiola i Fortuny L, Briggs M, Newcombe F, Ratcliff G, Thomas C 1980 Measuring the duration of post-traumatic amnesia. Journal of Neurology, Neurosurgery and Psychiatry 43: 377–379

Bandettini P A, Wong E C 1997 Magnetic resonance imaging of human brain function. Principles, practicalities, and possibilities. Neurosurgery Clinics of North America 8: 345–371

Barber P A, Darby D G, Desmond P M et al 1998 Prediction of stroke outcome with echoplanar perfusion- and diffusion-weighted magnetic resonance imaging. Neurology 51: 416–426

Basun H, Almkvist O, Axelman K et al 1997 Clinical characteristics of a chromosome 17-linked rapidly progressive familial frontotemporal dementia. Archives of Neurology 54: 539–544

Bauer J, Stefan H, Feistel H et al 1991 Ictal and interictal 99mTc-HMPAO SPECT studies in temporal lobe epilepsy with unilateral EEG focus. Nervenarzt 62: 745–749

Ben-Yishay Y, Diller L, Mandelberg I, Gordon W, Gerstman L J 1971 Similarities and differences in Block Design performance between older normal and brain-injured persons. A task analysis. Journal of Abnormal Psychology 78: 17–25

Bender M B 1952 Disorders in perception. Thomas, Springfield, Illinois

Benito-León J, Sánchez-Suárez C, Díaz-Guzmán J, Martínez-Salio A 1997 Pure alexia could not be a disconnection syndrome. Neurology 49: 305–306

Benson D F 1979 Aphasia, apraxia and agraphia. Churchill Livingstone, New York

Benson D F, Metter E J, Kuhl D E, Phelps M E 1983 Positron-computed tomography in neurobehavioral problems. In: Kertesz A (ed) Localization in neuropsychology. Academic Press, New York, pp 121–139

Benson D F, Davis R J, Snyder B D 1988 Posterior cortical atrophy. Archives of Neurology 45: 789–793

Benton A L 1962 The visual retention test as a constructional praxis task. Confinia Neurologica 22: 141–155

Benton A L 1969 Constructional apraxia; some unanswered questions. In: Benton A L (ed) Contributions to clinical neuropsychology. Aldine, Chicago, ch 5

Benton A L, Fogel M L 1962 Three dimensional constructional praxis. Archives of Neurology 7: 347–354

Bergmann M, Kuchelmeister K, Schmid K W, Kretzschmar H A, Schroder R 1996 Different variants of frontotemporal dementia: a neuropathological and immunohistochemical study. Acta Neuropathologica 92: 170–179

Black S E 1996 Focal cortical atrophy syndromes. Brain & Cognition 31: 188–229

Brain W R 1992 Brain and Bannister's Clinical neurology, 7th edn. Oxford University Press, Oxford

Bridgers S L, Ebersole J S 1985 The clinical utility of ambulatory cassette EEG. Neurology 35: 166–173

Brooks D N, Aughton M E, Bond M R, Jones P, Rizvi S 1980 Cognitive sequelae in relationship to early indices of severity of brain damage after severe blunt head injury. Journal of Neurology, Neurosurgery and Psychiatry 43: 529–534

Brun A 1987 Frontal lobe degeneration of non-Alzheimer type. I. Neuropathology. Archives of Gerontology and Geriatrics 6: 193–208

Brun A, Passant U 1996 Frontal lobe degeneration of non-Alzheimer type. Structural characteristics, diagnostic criteria and relation to other frontotemporal dementias. Acta Neurologica Scandinavica (suppl) 168: 28–30
Brun A, Englund B, Gustafson L, Passant U, Mann D M A, Neary D, Snowden J S 1994 Clinical and neuropathological criteria for frontotemporal dementia. Journal of Neurology, Neurosurgery and Psychiatry 57: 416–418
Buisson G 1989 A propos d'un cas d'état démentiel précoce: maladie de Pick ou schizophrenie? Annales Medico-Psychologiques 147: 121–124
Caplan L B 1985 Transient global amnesia. In: Vinken P J, Bruyn G W, Klawans H L (eds) Handbook of clinical neurology. New series l, vol 45. Elsevier, Amsterdam, pp 205–218
Chase T N, Burrows G H, Mohr E 1987 Cortical glucose utilisation in primary degenerative dementias of the anterior and posterior type. Archives of Gerontology and Geriatrics 6: 289–298
Chimowitz M I, Estes M L, Furlan A J, Awad I A 1992 Further observations on the pathology of subcortical lesions identified on magnetic resonance imaging. Archives of Neurology 49: 747–752
Chui H C, Victoroff J I, Margolin D, Jagust W, Shankle R, Katzman R 1992 Criteria for the diagnosis of ischemic vascular dementia. World Neurology 7: 12–13
Commission on Classification and Terminology of the International League Against Epilepsy 1989 Proposal for revised classification of epilepsies and epileptic syndromes. Epilepsia 30: 389–399
Corbetta M, Miezin F M, Shulman G L, Petersen S E 1993 A PET study of visuospatial attention. Journal of Neuroscience 13: 1202–1226
Courtney S M, Ungerleider L G, Keil K, Haxby J V 1997 Transient and sustained activity in a distributed neural system for human working memory. Nature 386: 608–611
Courville C B 1942 Coup-contrecoup mechanism of cranio-cerebral injuries: some observations. Archives of Surgery 55: 19–43
Courville C B 1945 Pathology of the nervous system, 2nd edn. Pacific Press, Mountain View, California
Critchley M 1949 The phenomenon of tactile inattention with special reference to parietal lesions. Brain 72: 538–561
Critchley M 1953 The parietal lobes. Edward Arnold, London
Cummings J L, Benson D F 1983 Dementia: A clinical approach. Butterworth, Boston
Denny-Brown D, Meyer J S, Horenstein S 1952 The significance of perceptual rivalry resulting from parietal lesions. Brain 75: 433–471
Dewan M J, Gupta S 1992 Toward a definite diagnosis of Alzheimer's disease. Comprehensive Psychiatry 33: 282–290
Duncan R, Patterson J, Hadley D M et al 1990 CT MR and SPECT imaging in temporal lobe epilepsy. Journal of Neurology, Neurosurgery and Psychiatry 53: 11–15
Englund E, Brun A 1987 Frontal lobe degeneration of non-Alzheimer type. IV. White matter changes. Archives of Gerontology and Geriatrics 6: 235–243
Escourolle R, Poirier J 1973 Manual of basic neuropathology. Saunders, Philadelphia
Fedio P 1980 Thalamo-cortical mediation of perception and memory in man. Proceedings of the International Union of Physiological Sciences 14: 111
Fedio P, Van Buren J M 1974 Memory deficits during electrical stimulation of the speech cortex in conscious man. Brain and Language 1: 29–42
Fedio P, Van Buren J M 1975 Memory and perceptual deficits during electrical stimulation in the left and right thalamus and parietal subcortex. Brain and Language 2: 78–100
Fisher C M 1968 Dementia in cerebral vascular disease. In: Toole J F, Sickert R G, Whisnant J P (eds) Cerebral vascular disease. Sixth Princeton Conference. Grune and Stratton, New York
Fisher C M 1982 Lacunar strokes and infarcts: a review. Neurology 32: 871–876
Fisher C M, Adams R D 1964 Transient global amnesia. Acta Neurologica Scandinavica 40 (suppl 19): 1–83
Frederiks J A M 1985 Disorders of the body schema. In: Vinken P J, Brúyn G W, Klawans H L (eds) Handbook of clinical neurology, revised series 1, vol 45. Elsevier, Amsterdam, pp 373–393
Freeborough P A, Woods R P, Fox N C 1996 Accurate registration of serial 3D MR brain images and its application to visualizing change in neurodegenerative disorders. Journal of Computer Assisted Tomography 20: 1012–1022

Fried I, Mateer C, Ojemann G, Wohns R, Fedio P 1982 Organization of visuospatial functions in the human cortex. Brain 105: 349–371
Frisoni G B, Beltramello A, Geroldi C, Weiss C, Bianchetti A, Trabucchi M 1996a Brain atrophy in frontotemporal dementia. Journal of Neurology, Neurosurgery and Psychiatry 61: 157–165
Frisoni G B, Beltramello A, Weiss C, Geroldi C, Bianchetti A, Trabucchi M 1996b Linear measures of atrophy in mild Alzheimer disease. American Journal of Neuroradiology 17: 913–923
Gastaut H 1970 Clinical and electroencephalographical classification of epileptic seizures. Epilepsia 11: 102–113
Gastaut H, Broughton R 1972 Epileptic seizures. Clinical and electrographic features, diagnosis and treatment. Thomas, Springfield, Illinois
Geschwind N 1965 Alexia and colour-naming disturbance. In: Ettlinger G (ed) Functions of the corpus callosum. Churchill, London, pp 95–101
Geschwind N 1969 Problems in the anatomical understanding of the aphasias. In: Benton A L (ed) Contributions to clinical neuropsychology. Aldine, Chicago
Geschwind N, Damasio A 1985 Apraxia. In: Vinken P J, Bruyn G W, Klawans H L (eds) Handbook of clinical neurology. New series 1, vol 45. Elsevier, Amsterdam, pp 423–432
Gitelman D R, Alpert N M, Kosslyn S, Daffner K, Scinto L, Thompson W, Mesulam M M 1996 Functional imaging of human right hemispheric activation for exploratory movements. Annals of Neurology 39: 174–179
Glaser J S 1978 Neuro-ophthalmology. Harper and Row, New York
Gurdjian E S 1975 Impact head injury. Thomas, Springfield, Illinois
Gurdjian E S, Webster J E, Arnkoff H 1943 Acute craniocerebral trauma. Surgery 13: 333–353
Gurdjian E S, Webster J E, Lissner H R 1955 Observations on the mechanism of brain concussion, contusion and laceration. Surgery, Gynaecology and Obstetrics 101: 680–690
Gurdjian E S, Lissner H R, Hodgson V R, Patrick L M 1966 Mechanisms of head injury. Clinical Neurosurgery 2: 112–128
Gustafson L 1987 Frontal lobe degeneration of non-Alzheimer type. II. Clinical picture and differential diagnosis. Archives of Gerontology and Geriatrics 6: 209–223
Hachinski V C, Lassen N A, Marshall J 1974 Multi-infarct dementia: a cause of mental deterioration in the elderly. Lancet 2: 207–210
Hagberg B, Gustafson L 1985 On diagnosis of dementia: psychometric investigation and clinical psychiatric evaluation in relation to psychiatric diagnosis. Archives of Gerontology and Geriatrics 14: 321–332
Handfield-Jones R M, Porritt A E 1949 The essentials of modern surgery. Livingstone, Edinburgh
Hanyu H, Abe S, Arai H et al 1992 1231-IMP SPECT study on patients with amnestic syndrome. Kaku Igaku 29: 691–694
Hebb D O 1949 The organization of behavior. Wiley, New York
Heilman K M 1979 Neglect and related disorders. In: Heilman K M, Valenstein E (eds) Clinical neuropsychology. Oxford University Press, New York, pp 268–307
Heilman K M, Rothi L, Kertesz A 1983 Localization of apraxia-producing lesions. In: Kertesz A (ed) Localization in neuropsychology. Academic Press, New York, pp 371–390
Heilman K M, Valenstein E, Watson R T 1985 The neglect syndrome. In: Vinken P J, Bruyn G W, Klawans H L (eds) Handbook of clinical neurology. Revised series 1, vol 45. Elsevier, Amsterdam, pp 153–183
Heiss W-D, Herholz K, Pawlik G, Klinkhammer P, Szelies B 1989 Positron emission findings in dementia disorders: contributions to differential diagnosis and objectivizing of therapeutic effects. Keio Journal of Medicine 38: 111–135
Heiss W-D, Pawlik G, Holthoff V, Kessler J, Szelies B 1992 PET correlates of normal and impaired memory functions. Cerebrovascular and Brain Metabolism Reviews 4: 1–27
Hier D B, Gorelick P B, Shindler A G 1987 Topics in behavioral neurology and neuropsychology. Butterworths, London
Holbourn A H S 1943 Mechanisms of head injuries. Lancet 2: 438–441
Hooper R 1969 Patterns of acute head injury. Edward Arnold, London
Hooper R S 1966 Head injuries – past, present and future. Medical Journal of Australia 2: 45–54
Hunter R, McLuskie R, Wyper D et al 1989 The pattern of function-related regional cerebral

blood flow investigated by single photon emission tomography with 99mTc-HMPAO in patients with Alzheimer's disease and Korsakoff's psychosis. Psychological Medicine 19: 847–855

Jackson J H 1890 Case of tumour of the right temporosphenoidal lobe bearing on the localization of the sense of smell and on the interpretation of a particular variety of epilepsy. Brain 12: 346–357

Jamieson K G 1971 A first notebook of head injury, 2nd edn. Butterworth, Sydney

Jellinger K 1976 Neuropathological aspects of dementias resulting from abnormal blood and cerebrospinal fluid dynamics. Acta Neurologica Belgica 76: 83–102

Johanson A, Hagberg B 1989 Psychometric characteristics in patients with frontal lobe degeneration of non-Alzheimer type. Archives of Gerontology and Geriatrics 8: 129–137

Jorgensen H S, Nakayama H, Raaschou H O, Olsen T S 1995 Leukoaraiosis in stroke patients. The Copenhagen stroke study. Stroke 26: 588–592

Kamo H, McGeer P L, Harrop R et al 1987 Positron emission tomography and histopathology in Pick's disease. Neurology 37: 439–445

Kertesz A 1979 Aphasia and associated disorders: taxonomy, localization and recovery. Grune and Stratton, New York

Kertesz A 1983 Localization in neuropsychology. Academic Press, New York

Kertesz A 1997 Frontotemporal dementia, Pick disease, and corticobasal degeneration: one entity or 3? 1. Archives of Neurology 54: 1427–1429

Kim K H, Relkin N R, Lee K M, Hirsch J 1997 Distinct cortical areas associated with native and second languages. Nature 388: 171–174

Kitamura S, Araki T, Sakamoto S, Iio M, Terashi A 1990 Cerebral blood flow and cerebral oxygen metabolism in patients with dementia of frontal type. Rinsho Shinkeigaku 30: 1171–1175

Knapp M J, Knopman D S, Solomon P R, Pendlebury W W, Davis C S, Gracon S I, for the Tacrine Study Group 1994 A 30-week randomized controlled trial of high-dose tacrine in patients with Alzheimer's disease. Journal of the American Medical Association 271: 985–991

Knopman D S, Morris J C 1997 An update on primary drug therapies for Alzheimer disease. Archives of Neurology 54: 1406–1409

Knopman D S, Christensen K J, Schut L J et al 1989 The spectrum of imaging and neuropsychological findings in Pick's disease. Neurology 39: 362–368

Kuhl D E, Engel J, Phelps M E, Selin C 1980a Epileptic patterns of local cerebral metabolism and perfusion in man determined by emission computed tomography of 18 FDG and 13 NH3. Annals of Neurology 8: 348–360

Kuhl D E, Phelps M E, Kowell A P et al 1980b Effects of stroke on local cerebral metabolism and perfusion: Mapping by emission computed tomography of 18 FDG and 13 NH3. Annals of Neurology 8: 47–60

Kuzniecky R 1997 Magnetic resonance and functional magnetic resonance imaging: tools for the study of human epilepsy. Current Opinion in Neurology 10: 88–91

Latchaw R E, Ugurbil K, Hu X 1995 Functional MR imaging of perceptual and cognitive functions. Neuroimaging Clinics of North America 5: 193–205

Le Bihan D 1996 Functional MRI of the brain: principles, applications and limitations. Journal of Neuroradiology 23: 1–5

Lehericy S, Baulac M, Chiras J et al 1994 Amygdalohippocampal MR volume measurements in the early stages of Alzheimer disease. American Journal of Neuroradiology 15: 929–937

Lencz T, McCarthy G, Bronen R A et al 1992 Quantitative magnetic resonance in temporal lobe epilepsy: relationship to neuropathology and neuropsychological function. Annals of Neurology 31: 629–637

Levin H S, O'Donnell V M, Grossman R G 1979 The Galveston orientation and amnesia test: A practical scale to assess cognition after head injury. Journal of Nervous and Mental Disease 167: 675–684

Levin H S, Benton A L, Grossman R G 1982 Neurobehavioral consequences of closed head injury. Oxford University Press, New York

Liepmann H 1900 The syndrome of apraxia (motor asymboly) based on a case of unilateral apraxia. Monattschrift für Psychiatrie und Neurologie 8: 15–44. Translated in: Rottenberg D A, Hochberg F H (eds) 1977 Neurological classics in modern translation. Hafner Press, New York

Liepmann H 1908 Drei Aufsatze aus dem Apraxiegebiet. Karger, Berlin
Lindenberg R, Freytag E 1957 Morphology of cortical contusions. Archives of Pathology 63: 23–42
Lindenberg R, Freytag E 1960 The mechanisms of cerebral contusions. A pathologic-anatomic study. Archives of Pathology 69: 440–469
Little J R, Furlan A J, Medic M T, Weinstein M A 1982 Digital subtraction angiography in cerebrovascular disease. Stroke 13: 557–566
Loeb C, Meyer J S 1996 Vascular dementia: still a debatable entity? Journal of the Neurological Sciences 143: 31–40
Luria A R 1973 The working brain. Allen Lane, The Penguin Press, London
Maddocks D, Saling M 1996 Neuropsychological deficits following concussion. Brain Injury 10: 99–103
Mateer C A, Ojemann G A 1983 Thalamic mechanisms in language and memory. In: Segalowitz S J (ed) Language functions and brain organization. Academic Press, New York, pp 171–191
McCrea M, Kelly J P, Kluge J, Ackley B, Randolph C 1997 Standardized assessment of concussion in football players. Neurology 48: 586–588
McKeith I G, Galasko D, Kosaka K et al for the Consortium on Dementia with Lewy Bodies 1996 Consensus guidelines for the clinical and pathologic diagnosis of dementia with Lewy bodies (DLB): report of the consortium on DLB international workshop. Neurology 47: 1113–1124
Mendez M F, Cherrier M, Perryman K M, Pachana N, Miller B L, Cummings J L 1996 Frontotemporal dementia versus Alzheimer's disease: differential cognitive features. Neurology 47: 1189–1194
Mesulam M M 1985 Dementia: its definition, diagnosis, and subtypes. JAMA 253: 2559–2561
Miller B L, Cummings J L, Villanueva-Meyer J et al 1991 Frontal lobe degeneration: clinical, neuropsychological, and SPECT characteristics. Neurology 41: 1374–1382
Montaldi D, Brooks D N, Wyper D, Patterson J, Barron E, McCulloch J 1991 Measurements of regional cerebral blood flow and cognitive performance in Alzheimer's disease. Journal of Neurology, Neurosurgery, and Psychiatry 53: 33–38
Moseley M E, de Crespigny A, Spielman D M 1996 Magnetic resonance imaging of human brain function. Surgical Neurology 45: 385–391
Neary D 1990 Dementia of frontal lobe type. Journal of the American Geriatrics Society 38: 71–72
Neary D 1997 Frontotemporal degeneration, Pick disease, and corticobasal degeneration: one entity or 3? 3. Archives of Neurology 54: 1425–1427
Neary D, Snowden J S, Bowen D M et al 1986 Neuropsychological syndromes in presenile dementia due to cerebral atrophy. Journal of Neurology, Neurosurgery and Psychiatry 49: 163–174
Neary D, Snowden J S, Shields R A et al 1987 Single photon emission tomography using 99mTc-HMPAO in the investigation of dementia. Journal of Neurology, Neurosurgery and Psychiatry 50: 1101–1109
Neary D, Snowden J S, Northen B, Goulding P 1988 Dementia of frontal lobe type. Journal of Neurology, Neurosurgery and Psychiatry 51: 353–361
Neary D, Snowden J S, Mann D M 1993 Familial progressive aphasia: its relationship to other forms of lobar atrophy. Journal of Neurology, Neurosurgery and Psychiatry 56: 1122–1125
New P F J, Scott W R, Schnur J A, Davis K R, Taveras J M 1974 Computerized axial tomography with the EMI scanner. Radiology 110: 109–123
Newcombe F 1982 The psychological consequences of closed head injury. Assessment and rehabilitation. Injury 14: 111–136
Newton R D 1948 The identity of Alzheimer's disease and senile dementia and their relationship to senility. Journal of Mental Science 94: 225–249
Niedermeyer E, Lopes da Silva F H 1982 Electro-encephalography: Basic principles, clinical applications and related fields. Urban and Schwarzenberg, Baltimore
Oder W, Goldenberg G, Spatt J, Podreka I, Binder H, Deecke L 1992 Behavioural and psychosocial sequelae of severe closed head injury and regional cerebral blood flow: a SPECT study. Journal of Neurology, Neurosurgery 55: 475–480
Ojemann G 1971 Alteration in nonverbal short-term memory with stimulation in the region of the mamillothalamic tract in man. Neuropsychologia 9: 195–201

Ojemann G 1977 Asymmetric function of the thalamus in man. Annals of the New York Academy of Science 299: 380–396
Ojemann G 1979 Altering human memory with human ventrolateral thalamic stimulation. In: Hitchcock E, Ballantine H, Myerson B (eds) Modern concepts in psychiatric surgery. Elsevier, Amsterdam, pp 103–109
Ojemann G 1980 Brain mechanisms for language: observations during neurosurgery. In: Lockhard J, Ward A A (eds) Epilepsy: a window to brain mechanisms. Raven, New York, pp 243–260
Ojemann G 1981 Interrelationship in the localization of language, memory and motor mechanisms in human cortex and thalamus. In: Thompson R (ed) New perspectives in cerebral localization. Raven, New York, pp 157–175
Ojemann G, Fedio P 1968 Effect of stimulation of the human thalamus and temporal white matter on short term memory. Journal of Neurosurgery 29: 51–59
Ojemann G, Mateer C 1979a Human language cortex: localization of memory, syntax, and sequential motor-phoneme identification systems. Science 205: 1401–1403
Ojemann G, Mateer C 1979b Cortical and subcortical organization of human communication: evidence from stimulation studies. In: Steklin H, Raleigh M (eds) The neurobiology of social communication in primates. Academic Press, New York, pp 111–131
Ojemann G, Blick K, Ward A 1971 Improvement and disturbance of short-term verbal memory with ventrolateral thalamic stimulation. Brain 94: 225–240
Ommaya A K, Gennerelli TA 1974 Cerebral concussion and traumatic unconsciousness. Correlation of experimental and clinical observations of blunt head injuries. Brain 97: 633–654
Orrell M W, Sahakian B J 1991 Dementia of frontal lobe type. Psychological Medicine 21: 553–556
Orrell M W, Sahakian B J, Bergmann K 1989 Self-neglect and frontal lobe dysfunction. British Journal of Psychiatry 155: 101–105
Paddock-Eliasziw L M, Elizszie M, Barr H W K, Barnett H J M 1996 Long-term prognosis and the effect of carotid endarterectomy in patients with recurrent ipsilateral ischemic events. Neurology 47: 1158–1162
Palmer J 1985 Advances in imaging technology and their applications. Medical Journal of Australia 142: 3–4
Parsonage M 1983 The classification of epileptic seizures (ILAE). In: Rose F C (ed) Research progress in epilepsy. Pitman, London, pp 22–38
Pasquier F, Hamon M, Lebert F, Jacob B, Pruvo J P, Petit H 1997 Medial temporal lobe atrophy in memory disorders. Journal of Neurology 244: 175–181
Passant U, Gustafson L, Brun A 1993 Spectrum of frontal lobe dementia in a Swedish family. Dementia 4: 160–162
Pearlson G D, Harris G J, Powers R E et al 1992 Quantitative changes in mesial temporal volume, regional cerebral blood flow, and cognition in Alzheimer's disease. Archives of General Psychiatry 49: 402–408
Penfield W 1958 The cerebral cortex in man. Archives of Neurology and Psychiatry 40: 417–442
Penfield W, Jasper H 1954 Epilepsy and the functional anatomy of the human brain. Little, Brown, Boston
Penfield W, Rasmussen A T 1950 The cerebral cortex of man. Macmillan, New York
Penfield W, Roberts L 1959 Speech and brain mechanisms. Princeton University Press, Princeton, New Jersey
Phelps M E, Mazziotta J C, Huang S C 1982 Study of cerebral function with positron computed tomography. Journal of Cerebral Blood Flow and Metabolism 2: 113–162
Phelps M E, Schelbert H R, Mazziotta J C 1983 Studies of cerebral function and dysfunction. Annals of Internal Medicine 98: 339–359
Pick A 1892 Ueber die Beziehungen der senilen Hirnatrophie zur Aphasie Prager. Medizinische Wochenschrift 17: 165–167 Translated in: Rottenberg D A, Hochberg F H (eds) 1977 Neurological classics in modern translation. Hafner Pres, New York
Pick A 1906 Ueber einen weiteren Symptomenkomplex im Rahmen der Dementia senilis, bedingt durch umschriebene stärkere Hirnatrophie (gemischte Apraxie). Monattschrift für Psychiatrie und Neurologie 19: 97–108
Pitt B 1987 Dementia. Churchill Livingstone, Edinburgh

Price B H, Gurvit H, Weintraub S, Geula C, Leimkuhler E, Mesulam M 1993 Neuropsychological patterns and language deficits in 20 consecutive cases of autopsy-confirmed Alzheimer's disease. Archives of Neurology 50: 931–937
Pykett I J 1982 NMR imaging in medicine. Scientific American 246: 78–88
Risberg J 1987 Frontal lobe degeneration of non-Alzheimer type. III. Regional cerebral blood flow. Archives of Gerontology and Geriatrics 6: 225–233
Ross S J M, Graham N, Stuart-Green L, Prins M, Xuereb J, Patterson K, Hodges J R 1996 Progressive biparietal atrophy: an atypical presentation of Alzheimer's disease. Journal of Neurology, Neurosurgery and Psychiatry 61: 388–395
Roth M 1981 The diagnosis of dementia in late and middle life. In: Mortimer J A, Schuman L M (eds) The epidemiology of dementia. Oxford University Press, New York
Royal H D, Hill T C, Holman L 1985 Clinical brain imaging with isopropyl iodoamphetamine and SPECT. Seminars in Nuclear Medicine 15: 357–376
Rowbotham G F 1964 Acute injuries of the head, 4th edn. Livingstone, Edinburgh
Russell R W 1932 Cerebral involvement in head injury. Brain 55: 549–503
Russell R W, Smith A 1961 Post-traumatic amnesia in closed head injury. Archives of Neurology 5: 4–17
Russell W, Nathan P 1946 Traumatic amnesia. Brain 69: 280–300
Sakai K, Watanabe E, Onodera Y et al 1995 Functional mapping of the human colour centre with echo-planar magnetic resonance imaging. Proceedings of the Royal Society of London – Series B 261: 89–98
Salmon E, Franck G 1989 Positron emission tomographic study in Alzheimer's disease and Pick's disease. Archives of Gerontology and Geriatrics, suppl 1: 241–247
Schmitt H P, Yang Y, Förstl H 1995 Frontal lobe degeneration of non-Alzheimer type and Pick's atrophy: lumping or splitting? European Archives of Psychiatry & Clinical Neuroscience 245: 299–305
Sereno M I, Dale A M, Reppas J B et al 1995 Borders of multiple visual areas in humans revealed by functional magnetic resonance imaging. Science 286: 889–893
Shores E A 1989 Comparison of the Westmead PTA Scale and Glasgow Coma Scale following extremely severe head injury. Journal of Neurology, Neurosurgery and Psychiatry 52: 126–127
Shores E A, Marosszeky J E, Sandanam J, Batchelor J 1986 Preliminary validation of a clinical scale for measuring the duration of post-traumatic amnesia. Medical Journal of Australia 144: 569–572
Simon R P, Aminoff M J, Greenberg D A 1987 Clinical neurology. Appleton and Lange, East Norwalk, Connecticut
Stern C E, Corkin S, Gonzalez R G et al 1996 The hippocampal formation participates in novel picture encoding: evidence from functional magnetic resonance imaging. Proceedings of the National Academy of Sciences of the USA 93: 8660–8665
Strich S J 1969 The pathology of brain damage due to blunt head injuries. In: Walker A E, Caveness W F, Critchley M (eds) The late effects of head injury. Thomas, Springfield, Illinois
Strub R I, Black F W 1981 Organic brain syndrome: an introduction to neurobehavioral disorders. Davis, Philadelphia
Szelies B, Karenberg A 1986 Disorders of glucose metabolism in Pick's disease. Fortschritte der Neurologie und Psychiatrie 5: 393–397
Talbot P R, Snowden J S, Lloyd J J, Neary D, Testa H J 1995 The contribution of single photon emission tomography to the clinical differentiation of degenerative cortical brain disorders. Journal of Neurology 242: 579–586
Tallent N 1963 Clinical psychological consultation. Prentice Hall, Englewood Cliffs, New York
Tarvonen-Schroder S, Roytta M, Raiha I, Kurki T, Rajala T, Sourander L 1996 Clinical features of leuko-araiosis. Journal of Neurology, Neurosurgery and Psychiatry 60: 431–436
Tatemichi T K 1990 How acute brain failure becomes chronic: a view of the mechanisms of dementia related to stroke. Neurology 40: 1652–1659
Tatemichi T K, Desmond D W, Mayeux R et al 1992a Dementia after stroke: baseline frequency, risks, and clinical features in a hospitalized cohort. Neurology 42: 1185–1193
Tatemichi T K, Desmond D W, Prohovnik I, Cross D T, Gropen T I, Mohr J P, Stern Y 1992b Confusion and memory loss from capsular genu infarction: a thalamocortical disconnection syndrome? Neurology 42: 1966–1979

Taylor A M, Warrington E K 1973 Visual discrimination in patients with localized cerebral lesions. Cortex 9: 82–93

Teasdale G, Jennett B 1974 Assessment of coma and impaired consciousness: A practical scale. Lancet 2: 81–84

Tissot R, Constantinidis J, Richard J 1985 Pick's disease. In: Frederiks J A M (ed) Handbook of Clinical Neurology 2 (46): 233–246

Todorov A B, Go R C, Constantinidis J et al 1975 Specificity of the clinical diagnosis of dementia. Journal of the Neurological Sciences 26: 81–98

Tomlinson B E 1977 The pathology of dementia. Contemporary Neurology Series 15: 113–153

Tomlinson B E, Blessed G, Roth M 1968 Observation on the brains of non-demented old people. Journal of Neurological Sciences 7: 331–356

Tootell R B, Reppas J B, Kwong K K et al 1995 Functional analysis of human MT and related visual cortical areas using magnetic resonance imaging. Journal of Neuroscience 15: 3215–3230

Tress B M, Stimac G K, Brant-Zawadski M 1985 Nuclear magnetic resonance imaging. Applications in the diagnosis of cerebrospinal diseases. Medical Journal of Australia 142: 25–28

Valenstein E, Heilman K M 1981 Unilateral hypokinesia and motor extinction. Neurology 31: 445–448

Verhoeff N P, Weinstein H C, Aldenkamp A P et al 1992 Focus localization in patients with partial epilepsy with 99mTc-HMPAO SPECT under continuous surface EEG monitoring. Nuclear Medicine Communications 13: 123–126

Victor M, Yakovlev P I 1955 S.S. Korsakoff's psychic disorder in conjunction with peripheral neuritis. A translation of Korsakoff's original article with brief comments on the author and his contribution to clinical medicine. Neurology 5: 394–406

Vinken P J, Bruyn G W (eds) 1969–1982 Handbook of clinical neurology. North-Holland, Amsterdam

Vinken P J, Bruyn G W, Klawans H L (eds) 1985 Handbook of clinical neurology. Revised series 1, vol 45 forward. Elsevier, Amsterdam

Walsh K W 1991 Understanding brain damage. A primer of neuropsychological evaluation, 2nd edn. Churchill Livingstone, Edinburgh

Warrington E 1969 Constructional apraxia. In: Vinken P J, Bruyn G W (eds) Handbook of clinical neurology. North-Holland, Amsterdam, vol 4, ch 4

Watson C, Jack C R, Cendes F 1997 Volumetric magnetic resonance imaging: clinical applications and contributions to the understanding of temporal lobe epilepsy. Archives of Neurology 54: 1521–1531

Watson J D 1996 Functional imaging studies of human visual cortex. Clinical & Experimental Pharmacology & Physiology 23: 926–930

Watson J D 1997 Images of the working brain: understanding human brain function with positron emission tomography. Journal of Neuroscience Methods 74: 245–256

Watson J D, Myers R, Frackowiak R S et al 1993 Area V5 of the human brain: evidence from a combined study using positron emission tomography and magnetic resonance imaging. Cerebral Cortex 3: 79–94

Wechsler D 1958 The measurement and appraisal of human intelligence. Williams & Wilkins, Baltimore

Weinstein H C, Hijdra A, van Royen E A, Derix M M 1989 Determination of cerebral blood flow by SPECT: a valuable tool in the investigation of dementia? Clinical Neurology and Neurosurgery 91: 13–19

Weintraub S, Mesulam M-M 1987 Right cerebral dominance in spatial attention: further evidence based on ipsilateral neglect. Archives of Neurology 44: 621–625

Wells C E 1978 Role of stroke in dementia. Stroke 9: 1–3

Wells C E 1979 Diagnosis of dementia. Psychosomatics 20: 517–522

Wetterling T, Kanitz R-D, Borgis K-J 1996 Comparison of different diagnostic criteria for vascular dementia (ADDTC, DSM-IV, ICD-10, NINDS-AIREN). Stroke 27: 30–36

Whitty C W M, Zangwill O L 1977 Amnesia, 2nd edn. Butterworth, London

Wilhemsen K C 1997 Frontotemporal dementia is on the MAP tau. Annals of Neurology 41: 139–140

Williams A L, Haughton V M 1985 Cranial computed tomography. Mosby, St Louis

Wilson J T L, Wiedmann K D, Hadley D M, Condon B, Teasdale B, Brooks D N 1988 Early

and late magnetic resonance imaging and neuropsychological outcome after head injury. Journal of Neurology, Neurosurgery and Psychiatry 51: 391–396
Ylikoski R, Ylikoski A, Erkinjuntti T, Sulkava R, Raininko R, Tilvis R 1993 White matter changes in healthy elderly persons correlate with attention and speed of mental processing. Archives of Neurology 50: 818–824

4

The frontal lobes

ANATOMY AND FUNCTIONAL ORGANIZATION

The frontal lobes are the most recently developed parts of the brain. In man they make up about one third of the mass of the cerebral hemispheres. It is only in the past few decades or so that we have begun to come to an understanding of the basic role which the frontal lobes play in many forms of human behaviour, especially with regard to the regulation of complex activities. Much of this work has been greatly advanced by Aleksandr Luria and his Russian colleagues, and the brief summary in this section owes much to this source (Luria 1969, Luria 1973a, b). Other contributions are dealt with in later sections of this chapter.

The frontal lobes lie anterior to the central sulcus and may be subdivided into four major subdivisions: (i) the motor area, which occupies the precentral gyrus; (ii) the premotor area, which lies anterior to the motor area and includes Brodmann's area 6 and part of area 8; (iii) the prefrontal area (9, 10, 45, 46); and (iv) the basomedial portion of the lobes (9 to 13, 24, 32). These latter two divisions are often considered together as one 'prefrontal' region.

A specialized area termed the *frontal eye field* is situated in the middle zone of the dorsolateral surface, taking in prefrontal as well as premotor cortex (parts of areas 9, 8, and 6, Fig. 4.1). Stimulation, particularly in area 8, causes eye movements, most often to the contralateral side. The area is thought to be the mediator of voluntary and involuntary eye movements and it is strategically situated to receive information from the prefrontal (planning) cortex for relay to the motor system. It has been visualized in man using MRI (Darby et al 1996).

In Chapter 2 mention was made of the study of cytoarchitecture. This leads to a distinction in terminology which is often used in relation to the frontal regions. Some anatomists have grouped the finer subdivisions of cytoarchitecture, as depicted by workers such as Brodmann, into a small number of fundamental types which share common characteristics. Departure from the 'typical' six-layered cortex allows a broad division first of all into cortex in which the granular layers (layers II and IV) are either well represented or markedly absent. Cortex termed *agranular cortex* shows a lack of granular layers II and IV,

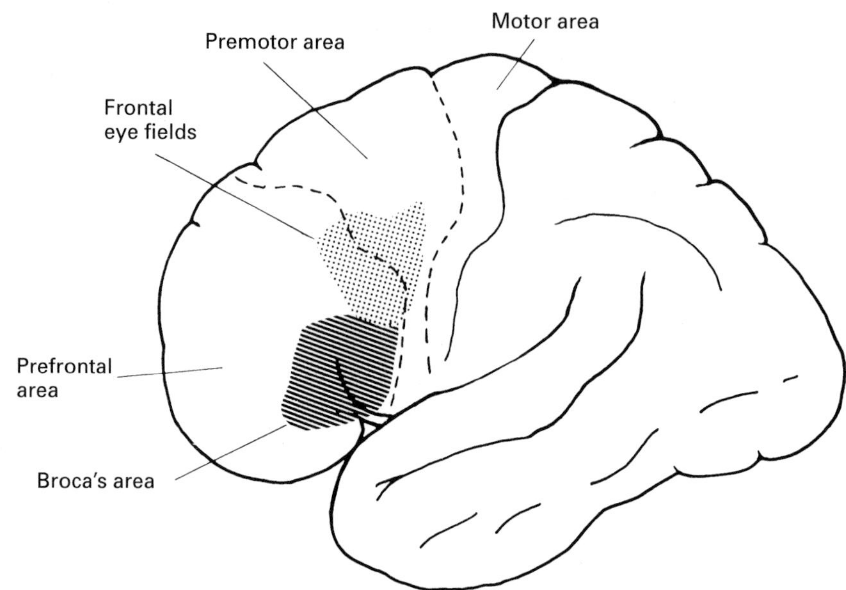

Fig. 4.1 Dorsolateral frontal cortex with functional areas.

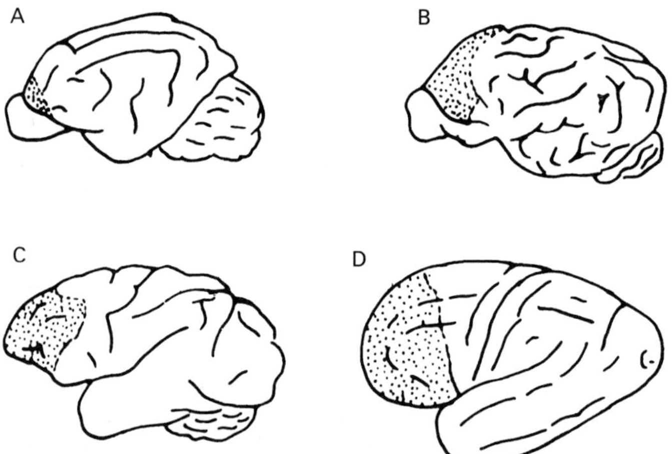

Fig. 4.2 Frontal granular cortex. A, cat; B, dog; C, Rhesus monkey; D, man (not drawn to scale).

whereas layers III and V are very well developed. This agranular cortex is seen in the posterior parts of the frontal lobes anterior to the central sulcus and is characteristic of the motor cortex. Areas 4 and 6, together with portions of Brodmann's areas 8 and 44, belong to this type. Anterior to this the cortex may be divided into a number of fundamental types, but as the granular layers are present in varying degree it might loosely be characterized as *frontal granular cortex*. This term gave its name to a symposium in 1964, and studies of frontal granular cortex might be said to be concerned with those frontal lobe functions which are not purely motor. The relative development of this type of cortex in different species is shown in Figure 4.2.

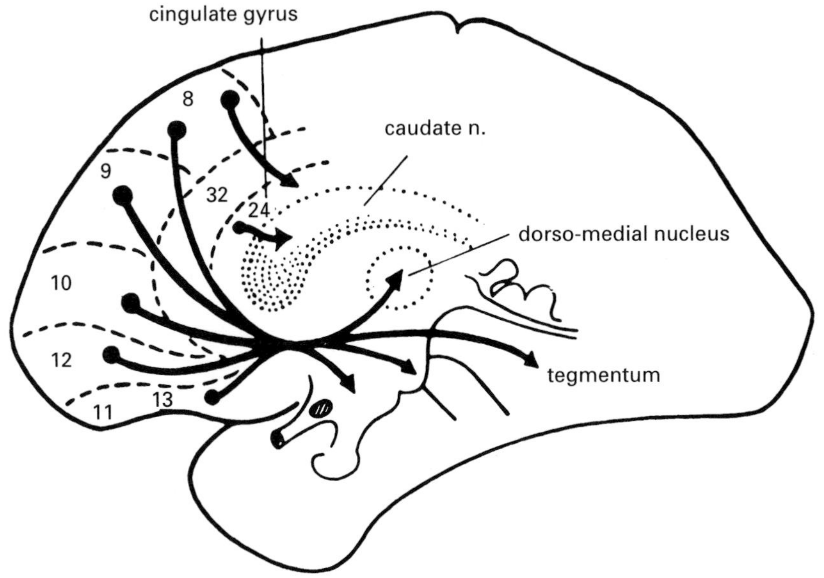

Fig. 4.3 Efferent connections in the frontal region (from Walsh E G Physiology of the nervous system, courtesy of Churchill Livingstone. Figure has been modified by LeGros Clark The Lancet 1948; by courtesy of the editors).

The frontal regions have well-developed systems of efferent nerve cells leading from the cortex to lower brain centres and peripheral parts of the nervous system. The efferent projections from the frontal areas pass to the ventral and dorsomedial nuclei of the thalamus as well as to numerous other structures (Fig. 4.3). Afferent fibres reach the frontal cortex over the thalamo-frontal radiation (Fig. 4.4).

Parallel to his division of the posterior zones into primary (sensory), secondary (association), and tertiary (supramodal or integrative) cortex, Luria perceived the organization of the frontal regions in a similar hierarchical arrangement, viz. motor cortex, premotor cortex (motor organization), and prefrontal cortex (higher integration). This leads to the concept of two types of syndrome: (i) premotor; and (ii) prefrontal. This chapter is principally concerned with the latter.

Luria also pointed out that the prefrontal regions serve as tertiary zones for the limbic system as well as for the motor system. They have rich connections with (i) the upper parts of the brain stem and thalamus, and (ii) all other cortical zones. The richness of these connections is shown in Figure 4.5. Through the first set of connections the prefrontal areas, particularly the basal and medial aspects of the lobes, are intimately concerned with the state of alertness of the organism, while the rich connections with the posterior receptor areas and motor cortex allow the lateral prefrontal regions to organize and execute the most complex of man's goal-directed or purposive activities.

From a clinical point of view the division of prefrontal cortex into lateral and basomedial (orbitomedial) regions may serve as a useful first approximation in the search for brain-behaviour relationships. This would accord well with the known projections from the thalamus. The medial part of the dorsomedial

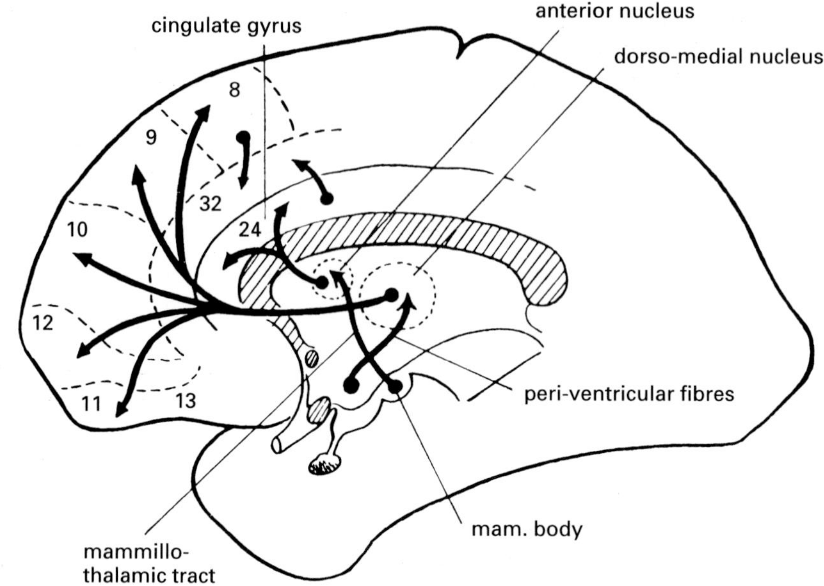

Fig. 4.4 Afferent connections in the frontal region (from Walsh E G Physiology of the nervous system, courtesy of Churchill Livingstone. Figure has been modified by LeGros Clark The Lancet 1948; by courtesy of the editors).

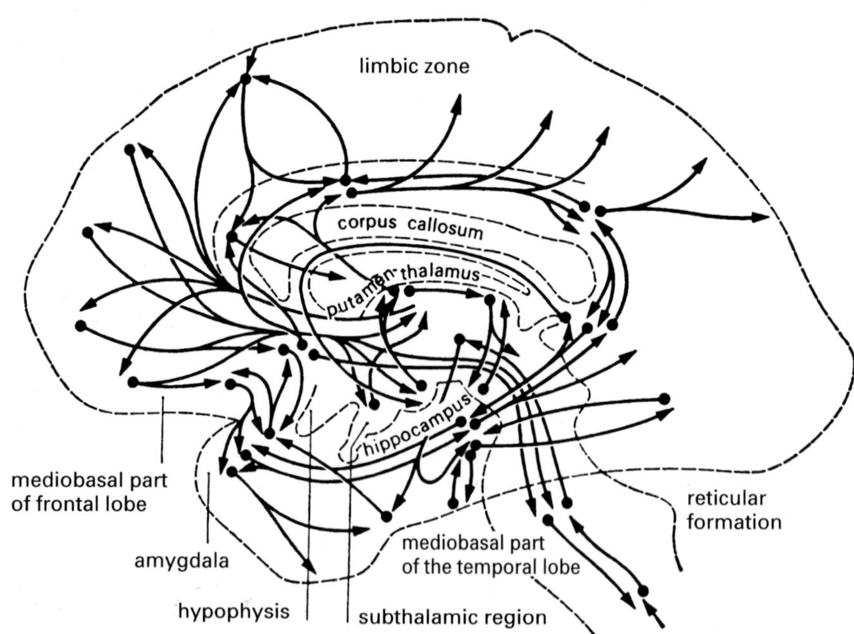

Fig. 4.5 Complete ramification of frontal lobe connections, after Polyakov (from Luria A R 1973b The working brain. Allen Lane Penguin. Courtesy of VAAP, Moscow).

nucleus projects to the ventromedial aspects of the prefrontal cortex while the lateral part projects to the dorsolateral aspect.

In the lateral (convexity) portions of the frontal lobes the character of the disturbances alters according to the placement of the lesions in the anteroposterior direction. With posterior frontal lesions adjacent to the motor cortex the disturbances are those of the organization of movements. As the lesions move forward they lead firstly to the disintegration of motor programmes and then to a disturbance of comparison of motor behaviour with its original plan. This latter disruption reminds us that not only must a programme of movement be organized and initiated, it must also be continuously monitored and necessary adjustments made in the light of feedback from the activity for the sequence to be smooth and effective. 'All these disturbances are particularly marked in patients with lesions of the lateral zones of the left (dominant) frontal lobe which are closely connected with the cerebral organization of speech, and the disorganization of *speech activity* and of those *behavioural acts* which are especially dependent upon the participation of speech for their regulation' (Luria 1973b, p. 222).

Speech disorders are particularly associated with lesions of the lower parts of the lateral cortex of the dominant hemisphere. Disturbance of speech from lesions of the posterior inferior area (Broca's area) is termed motor aphasia. Though the term *Broca's area* has been widely used, it is impossible to define its limits precisely from the early descriptions and material of Broca. It approximates to Brodmann's area 44 and part of 45.

There are other speech disturbances of a more subtle nature found with lesions anterior to Broca's area which are seen in patients who are not considered clinically to be suffering from aphasia. Reference is made to these in later parts of this chapter. Luria included the following in such disorders of the left inferolateral frontal cortex: (i) inability to make a spontaneous discursive statement; (ii) difficulty in expressing a thought in discursive speech; and (iii) 'verbal adynamia' or 'frontal dynamic aphasia' (see below).

In the other major functional subdivision, the basomedial frontal cortex, the disorders are related to the state of activation of the subject and his or her affective responses. Luria (1973a, b) pointed to the research of the British and Russian workers on 'expectancy waves' in the electroencephalogram which, together with other evidence, shows 'that the frontal parts of the brain-cortex play an essential role in the regulation of the state of activation that arises as a result of some task given to the subject' (1973b, p. 6). Extensive experience with psychosurgical lesions isolating the basomedial areas has confirmed earlier thought that these areas are concerned with the emotional life of the individual and with the control of inhibition. A complete account of the functional anatomy of the prefrontal cortex is given in the texts by Stuss and Benson (1986) and Fuster (1989).

THE FRONTAL LOBE CONTROVERSY

Perhaps the most vexatious question regarding the frontal lobes has been whether they are more important for man's intellectual life than other portions of the brain. Much evidence has accumulated on both sides since the introduction of psychological tests in the area of brain impairment around the 1930s. This evidence is worth reviewing since it provides a number of lessons about making inferences based on incomplete information.

In view of the great development of the prefrontal regions in man, it seemed natural to some that these regions should be concerned with the highest integrative functions. Many neurologists in the era before the introduction of psychological testing had supported the notion of the paramount importance of the frontal lobe (Jackson 1874, Phelps 1897, Dana 1915, Goldstein & Gelb 1918, Dew 1922, Papez 1929, Worster-Drought 1931) though there were those who were opposed to this notion (Feuchtwanger 1923, Jefferson 1937). Jefferson's six cases of frontal lobectomy not only appeared to demonstrate no apparent loss after operation but an improvement in some cases '...those who showed no mental alteration before the operation were unaffected by partial removal of the anatomical frontal lobe...those who had mental symptoms were much better after the lobe had been excised'. Jefferson was opposed to the notion that the higher functions were 'localized' within the confines of the frontal lobes.

The care which must be exercised in making inferences from clinical material with 'presumptive' evidence of localization is exemplified by a case reported several times by Brickner (1934) and one on which he based an interpretation of frontal lobe function. This patient, who had undergone a partial bilateral frontal lobectomy for a meningioma, was found at autopsy very much later to have had multiple meningiomas including a very large parieto-occipital tumour. Brickner's case was also important as the author claimed that the patient did not appear to show any marked impairment of abstract thought, one of the higher intellectual functions which some writers, particularly Kurt Goldstein, felt was most likely to be affected by lesions in the frontal lobes. Commenting on Brickner's case, Goldstein (1944) pointed to an important distinction which should be borne in mind. 'The underlying reason for this difference is seen in the fact that Brickner considered the use of abstract words as an expression of the ability to think in abstract terms or as a sign of the abstract attitude. This is an assumption made very often, and I, myself, had the greatest difficulty in differentiating abstract thinking on the one hand and the concrete use of words with abstract meaning on the other'. Goldstein (1936a) had also been at pains to point out that the changes seen with frontal damage may be elusive to traditional examinations.

> ...the personality changes characteristic of the frontal lobes are of a definite type and may easily be overlooked, because the methods of examination usually employed are unsuited to disclosing them...For these reasons the greater part of the literature is useless for answering the questions whether psychic disturbances occur in cases of lesions of the frontal lobe and if so, what these disturbances are.

The first large study of intellectual changes with frontal lesions was that of Rylander (1939), who examined 32 cases of partial excision for either tumour or abscess. The tests of higher intellectual function, which included some which would be classified as tests of abstract thinking, were also given to 32 control subjects. There were highly significant differences between the operated subjects and the controls on most measures. The intellectual changes occurred in 21 of the 32 cases. This underlines the importance of not basing conclusions on a single case or small samples, though it does provoke the question of why some patients showed changes while others did not. In a second study of 16 cases with brain resections in the temporal, parietal and occipital lobes, Rylander (1943) found very few of the symptoms described in an earlier report, e.g. there were no difficulties with 'abstract thinking, the power of combination, and acts involving judgment'. At a time when psychosurgical procedures were becoming popular, Rylander warned of the risk of mental invalidism after extensive frontal surgery, particularly in those doing intellectual or other complicated work.

An early study of Halstead (1940) on the sorting behaviour of patients with frontal versus non-frontal locations disclosed a poorer performance on the part of frontal subjects.

Against this emerging support for the importance of the frontal lobes, Hebb accumulated impressive evidence that frontal patients were not in fact inferior on tasks when compared with those with posterior lesions (Hebb 1939, 1941, 1945, Hebb & Penfield 1940). The cases were made up of two right frontal cases, four left frontal cases, and one with extensive bilateral frontal lobectomy. Examination of the latter case (Hebb & Penfield 1940) before and after operation failed to show postoperative deficits, in fact there was a striking improvement both clinically and psychometrically in this patient as well as lack of the traditional frontal lobe signs. They commented: 'It becomes evident that human behaviour and mental activity may be more greatly impaired by the positive action of an abnormal area of brain than by the negative effect of its complete absence' (p. 431). Hebb (1945) considered that there was evidence in some of the reported cases showing deficits after frontal lobe surgery that 'the deterioration they describe(d) may have been due to pathological complication and not to surgical lesion at all'. While not denying that loss of frontal tissue might have important effects on behaviour, Hebb felt that such changes had not been adequately demonstrated (Hebb 1949). Another worker, Goldstein, felt that the frontal lobes were the structures which were most concerned with that complex set of behaviours which he termed taking up the abstract attitude. There is extensive controversy over abstract thinking and brain damage, and it is dealt with separately below. Speaking of Hebb's cases Goldstein remained sceptical. 'However, I think these cases are not convincing because in none of them are such tests used by which the characteristic frontal lobe symptom can be disclosed' (Goldstein 1944). Although we have learned a good deal about the frontal lobe syndrome in the ensuing five decades, it remains a truism of clinical practice that patients with frontal lobe lesions often appear essentially normal until they are examined with appropriate tests. Hebb's counterclaim (1945) was that Goldstein was placing emphasis on supporting cases while disregarding those which were opposed.

In 1947 Halstead published his theory of 'biological intelligence'. This was based on factor analysis of a number of tests which appeared sensitive to the effects of cerebral impairment. One of the factors was that of abstraction. Among the tests in Halstead's battery, the Category Test had a particularly high loading on this factor. In keeping with earlier claims of lowered abstract ability after frontal lesions, Halstead and colleagues reported that abstraction loss in the form of high error scores on the Category Test was indeed greater with frontal involvement (Halstead 1947, Shure & Halstead 1958). Neither of these sources presents strong evidence upon which to make the general claims that were put forward. The first study presented only a small amount of data, and both studies accepted levels of significance well short of those which have become conventional. An examination of Shure and Halstead's data shows that it is largely derived from Shure (1954) and that a direct test of the effect of size of lesion, laterality and locus of lesion (frontal versus non-frontal) in this original study revealed that all three main effects failed to reach significance in a 2×2×2 analysis of variance. Using Shure and Halstead's data, Chapman and Wolff (1959) employed their own method for re-estimating the mass of tissues removed in the 1958 study. To this they added other cases of their own where the extent and site of tissue removed could be clearly specified and where each case was restricted to one of the lobar divisions of the brain and where there was neither evidence of progressive disease nor other disorders. The findings showed that 'impairment was independent of site or side of the defect in the cerebral hemispheres but was directly related to the mass of hemisphere tissue loss. No one category of higher functions was significantly or predictably impaired in relation to the site of defect, whereas all functions were progressively impaired with increasing mass of defect'.

During the 1950s Teuber and associates accumulated a good deal of data, mainly but not exclusively, on penetrating missile wounds, concerning the relative performance with frontal versus posterior lesions. Deficits were greater in frontal cases for a small number of visual tasks discussed below but the remainder of the tasks showed equal or greater impairment with posterior lesions. These visual tasks comprised: (i) complex visual tasks including sorting tasks (Teuber et al 1951, Weinstein et al 1955); (ii) complex tactual tasks (Semmes et al 1954, Teuber & Weinstein 1954); (iii) visual and tactile discrimination learning (Battersby et al 1955); (iv) practical problem solving (Battersby et al 1953); and (v) the Army General Classification Test, a general intelligence test (Weinstein & Teuber 1957, Teuber & Weinstein 1958, Teuber 1959). The poorer performance of the posterior lesion group could not be explained on the basis of primary visual defects. Much of this and other evidence is comprehensively summarized in Teuber (1964). Supporting evidence against the preeminence of the frontal lobes in intellectual functions came from Birkmayer (1951) and Pollack (1960). Later, Black (1976) confirmed Teuber's findings using subjects with penetrating missile wounds with the damage presumably restricted to one frontal lobe. The principal measures employed were the Wechsler intelligence and memory scales.

A good deal of insight into the reasons for the contradiction in the literature was provided by the two well designed studies reported by Reitan (1964). The studies used a wide variety of psychological measures and included the Halstead–Reitan group of tests, an Aphasia Screening Test, Reitan's Trail Making Test, an examination for sensory imperception, and the Wechsler–Bellevue Intelligence Scale. These tests were administered to 64 patients with focal lesions and 48 with diffuse cerebral involvement. The first study required the psychologist to draw inferences from the psychological data in the absence of the neurological diagnosis. These inferences concerned the questions: (i) is the disorder focal or diffuse? and (ii) what is the location of the lesion? (left anterior, right anterior, left posterior, right posterior, diffuse). There was a fairly satisfactory degree of concurrence between the psychological and neurological ratings. For the purposes of the present section this means that the psychological test results must have been differentially influenced by the locus of the lesion, e.g. frontal versus non-frontal, as well as the laterality and other factors.

The second study looked at the local damage cases only and employed the formal comparison of test results between the known groups, i.e. intergroup mean comparisons using analysis of variance. Virtually no important differential features were revealed by this analysis. Reitan commented: 'Since the results of Study 1 could not have occurred unless the necessary information for the inferences was present in the data, the conclusion seems inescapable that the analysis was inadequate in Study 2'. It follows that the failure of other studies to show differential features between frontal and non-frontal patients cannot be taken to mean that such differential features do not exist. More sophisticated statistical techniques such as multiple discriminant function analysis or cluster analysis may prove of greater value since they permit the most advantageous use of the pattern of results. On the other hand, such methods are probably less flexible than the use of qualitative features of the patient's behaviour on specially selected tests, some of these features being almost pathognomonic of lesions in particular locations. The features which appear to be most characteristic of frontal behaviour are discussed in the remaining sections of this chapter.

THE FRONTAL LOBE SYNDROME

Changes in personality after brain injury are most often noted after damage to the frontal lobes. These changes have been reported for well over a century and no description of what has come to be called the frontal lobe syndrome would be complete without reference to the case of Phineas Gage. The following summary, which has appeared in many places, is quoted by Kimble (1963).

> Phineas P. Gage, an 'efficient and capable' foreman, was injured on September 13, 1848, when a tamping iron was blown through the frontal region of his brain. He suffered the following change in his personality according to the physician, J.M. Harlow, who attended him. 'He is fitful, irreverent, indulging at times in the grossest profanity (which was not previously his custom), manifesting but little deference to his fellows, impatient of restraint or advice when it conflicts with his desires, at times pertinaciously obstinate yet capricious and vacillating, devising many plans for future operation which no sooner are arranged than they are abandoned in turn for others appearing more feasible. His mind was radically changed so that his friends and acquaintances said that he was no longer Gage.'

Such gross changes are usually seen only with severe bilateral frontal damage, but the lack of inhibition, impulsivity and lack of concern of such patients can be seen to a lesser degree in others whose injury is less severe. In its milder forms it could be taken to be within the extreme range of 'extraversion' if the examiner were not familiar with the patient's prior personality. Another of the characteristic features of the frontal syndrome is the mania for making puerile jokes referred to as 'Witzelsucht'.

Many of these signs seen in the early months after head injuries fade with the passage of time, though the more severe the injury the more likely it is that some personality change will remain. Besides the all-too-common effects of road trauma, both war injuries (Hillbom 1960) and psychosurgery have provided potent evidence of the personality changes which accompany bilateral frontal damage.

The complex set of changes with bilateral frontal damage which comprise the frontal lobe syndrome was concisely expressed by Benton (1968). The first set of changes is related to what may be loosely termed personality: 'diminished anxiety and concern for the future; impulsiveness, facetiousness and mild euphoria; lack of initiative and spontaneity. (However, it may be noted that, while they are not mentioned prominently in group studies, anxiety states have been described occasionally in clinical case reports as a presenting symptom in patients with frontal lobe disease.)'

Related to complex impairments of motivation and social behaviour is the appearance of stereotyped and ritualistic behaviour without signs of anxiety. This may sometimes be termed obsessive-compulsive behaviour. A recent case following head injury (Donovan & Barry 1994) highlights two features: firstly, the likelihood that the symptoms may be more common than anticipated because they are not reported by the patient due to apathy; secondly, as in similar cases (Eslinger & Damasio 1985), neurological and neurocognitive examinations were normal. In 1933 Minski reported the symptoms with cerebral tumours, and one of the present authors has seen two cases of frontal neoplasm where these 'obsessional' features had led to a first diagnosis of obsessive-compulsive disorder. Baxter's 1992 review of brain-imaging studies shows evidence in many cases of lesions in the orbitofrontal cortex.

The second set of changes may be termed intellectual: 'impaired integration of behaviour over a period of time, a deficit which for want of a better term has been called impairment in 'recent memory'; loss of the capacity to think in abstract terms; finally, inability to plan and follow through a course of action and to take into account the probable future consequence of one's actions, a deficit which is perhaps closely related to some of the observed personality changes as well as to the impairment in recent memory' (Benton 1968, p. 53). These two sets of changes will be considered separately in the sections which follow, though there is obviously a good deal of interaction between them. There is some evidence from lesion studies both in animals and man that there is at least a partial dissociation between the two major groups of symptoms (Warren & Akert 1964). This is supported by the extensive literature on psychosurgery suggesting that the intellectual changes are more associated with damage to the dorsolateral connections, while the personality changes are more associated with damage to the orbitomedial (or basomedial) regions (Walsh 1960, Girgis 1971).

A third set of changes may be seen in association with lesions of the mesial aspects of the frontal lobes. Since these latter are relatively well protected compared with the basal and lateral regions, the changes are seen most clearly not with trauma but with obstruction or haemorrhage of the anterior cerebral arteries which supply the region. The principal clinical feature is an *adynamia* and this may evidence itself in a complete or relative lack of verbal or overt behaviour (see below).

Thus the term frontal lobe syndrome has broad connotations implying the presence of all three sets of changes or some combination of subsets. Rather than refer to *the* frontal lobe syndrome it might be preferable to refer clinically to the presence of a frontal lobe syndrome and to specify which set of changes is prominent in the individual case. This specification might assist in pointing up the features, for example, which will require the design of appropriate rehabilitation procedures. Other terms such as the dysexecutive syndrome (Baddeley 1986) which attempt to encapsulate a major part of the so-called *frontal* features without begging the question of their origin in frontal pathology have not yet found wide acceptance. This may come with further analysis in the discipline of cognitive neuropsychology.

Confabulation

Confabulation refers to the tendency of the patient to produce erroneous material on being questioned about the past, either recent or remote. Fisher (1989) points out that the frequent use of the term to connote 'fabrication of ready answers and experiences without regard to the truth, is misleading'. It may accompany amnesia associated with a wide variety of pathological disorders, e.g. Korsakoff's psychosis, hypoxic brain damage, post-traumatic states, normal pressure hydrocephalus and anterior communicating artery aneurysms. Though closely associated with amnesia it is obviously not caused by the memory loss alone since the majority of amnesic patients do not confabulate. Certainly, confabulation appears to be more common in the early stages, disappearing as the particular condition becomes chronic (Moll 1915, Weinstein 1987). Our own experience agrees with that of Zangwill (1978, personal communication) that the presence of confabulation in Korsakoff's disorder appears to be inversely related to the presence of insight. It was earlier thought to be a necessary part of the diagnosis but this is no longer considered to be the case (Victor et al 1971).

Many writers have remarked on the close association of confabulation with denial or lack of awareness of dysfunction (anosognosia), particularly blindness in Anton's syndrome (see Ch. 7). Fisher (1989) put the matter succinctly '...It is my experience that patients who are aware of their memory loss...do not confabulate, but rather that unawareness is a necessary precondition (for confabulation)'.

In his literature review and study of cases of confabulation in Korsakoff patients and an unselected group with dementia, Berlyne (1972) pointed to the distinction between two forms of confabulation, a division made many years before by Bonhoeffer (1904). The first and more common type, termed *momentary confabulation* consists of the production of autobiographical material, often of an habitual nature (e.g. war service or occupation), in response to questioning. The responses are brief but not stereotyped. This type has also been termed 'transient' or 'provoked' confabulation. The second type is much less common and consists of material around a grandiose theme, often arising spontaneously and frequently repeated. It bears no relation to prior experience. Again after Bonhoeffer, Berlyne termed this *fantastic confabulation*. A similar distinction between spontaneous and provoked confabulation is made by Kopelman (1987).

Spontaneous, impulsive confabulation appears to be related to the loss of the subject's self-critical faculty, with inability to inhibit responses. Earlier studies (Mercer et al 1977, Stuss et al 1978, Kapur & Coughlan 1980) strongly suggested that the common factor was frontal lobe disorder. The most common association appeared to be with perseveration of response set which was frequently accompanied by such 'frontal' signs as inability to inhibit incorrect responses, and faulty self-monitoring (Shapiro et al 1981). Recent studies (De Luca 1992, 1993, Fischer et al 1995) appear to demonstrate that 'spontaneous' confabulation occurs with simultaneous damage to the mesial forebrain as well as frontal cognitive systems. Such cases show both frontal and amnesic disorders. More limited lesions may result in 'transient' or 'provoked' confabulatory responses. The presence of executive function disorders appears to be greater in the spontaneous than in the provoked form (Fischer et al 1995).

The role of the thalamus seems most important. Of 21 patients with amnesia following posterior cerebral artery infarction, five exhibited confabulation and each had a lesion in the thalamic region while none of the remaining 16 without confabulation had a thalamic lesion (Servan et al 1994). On the other hand a patient with an acute Korsakoff disorder with severe amnesia and confabulation showed SPECT signs in both the frontal (orbital and medial) and medial diencephalic regions in the acute stage, but later, when the frontal perfusion had returned to normal, the confabulation had disappeared but the amnesia remained with no improvement in the SPECT for the diencephalic region (Benson et al 1996).

That spontaneous and provoked confabulation are separate disorders rather than merely a difference of degree is supported by the double dissociation shown in the examination of 16 patients by Schnider et al (1996). A qualitatively different form of confabulation may be seen in schizophrenia and may also result from the difficulty in inhibiting inappropriate responses as in organic cases (Nathaniel-James & Frith 1996).

Utilization behaviour

In 1983 Lhermitte employed this term to describe a form of behaviour in which patients with a frontal lesion gave an instrumentally appropriate but exaggerated response to objects that were introduced to them. At first this behaviour was described in terms of clinical examinations but was later described in detail with two patients in a wide variety of environmental situations (Lhermitte 1986). In the presence of objects, and without direct instruction, the patients appeared constrained to carry out sequences of behaviour commonly associated with them. Lhermitte et al (1986) examined 75 patients who showed utilization behaviour or its early stage, termed imitation behaviour. A high proportion of these had involvement of the inferior part of the anterior half of one or both frontal lobes, an area thought by some to be responsible for the lifting of control in frontally damaged patients. The condition has been described in association with a number of pathological conditions affecting this region (Aimard et al 1983, Cambier et al 1985), and also with thalamic lesions (Eslinger et al 1991, Fukui et al 1993, Hashimoto et al 1995), suggesting that a disconnection or diaschisis or deafferentation effect may be at work. Shallice and colleagues (1989) have made a distinction between 'induced utilization', where objects are presented directly, and 'incidental utilization' where the objects are nearby though the patient's attention is not directed to them. These authors remind us that psychologists have long been aware that a person's behaviour may be affected by implicit as well as by explicit cues. Orne (1962) termed these features the 'demand characteristics' of a situation. They clearly influence the behaviour even of those without brain lesions (Orne & Scheibe 1964). Patients with utilization behaviour appear to have an extreme form which Lhermitte (1986) called the 'environment dependency syndrome'. This author has recently described imitation and utilization behaviour in major depression with patients showing underactivity in the frontal regions on PET scan (Lhermitte 1993).

Lesion studies and cognitive change

Abstract thinking

The question of the importance of the frontal lobes for abstract thinking is intimately connected with the controversy over whether these regions are more crucial than others for the highest integrative functions of man. The summary on theoretical formulations of abstraction in the monograph by Pikas (1966) would form an excellent background to research and reading in this area. This work also provided a summary of empirical studies to that time.

The central questions appear to be whether damage to the cerebrum leads to qualitative versus quantitative changes in what we might loosely term abstract thought processes and, if so, whether these are exclusive to frontal lobe involvement.

The foremost advocate of the qualitative position was Kurt Goldstein who, in numerous publications, put forward the notion that there exist two qualitatively different modes of thought and behaviour, the abstract and the concrete. The normal person is said to be capable of exercising both modes according to the demands of the situation, while many brain impaired patients are restricted to use of the concrete (Goldstein 1936a, b, 1939a, b, 1940, 1942a, b, 1943, 1944, 1959, Goldstein & Scheerer 1941, Hanfmann et al 1944). Several of these publications put forward the claim that impairment of abstraction was maximal with lesions of the frontal lobe.

Goldstein's central concept was that of taking up the 'abstract attitude'. The notion of concrete and abstract attitudes was seen as a dichotomy, although there are instances where Goldstein admits to degrees of abstraction and concreteness. For example, we read: 'In the concrete attitude we experience and recognize a given thing or situation immediately. Our thinking and acting are directly determined by the present claims upon us. In the abstract attitude we go beyond the current claims of objects or of sense impressions. Specific properties or situations are overlooked. We are oriented in our actions by a conceptual point of view which takes into consideration the demands of the entire situation' (Goldstein 1943). Or, again '...abstraction is separate in principle from concrete behaviour. There is no gradual transition from one to the other. The assumption of an attitude toward the abstract is not more complex merely through the addition of a new factor of determination; it is a totally different activity of the organism' (Goldstein 1940). 'There is a pronounced line of demarcation between these two attitudes which does not represent a gradual ascent from more simple to more complex mental sets. The greater difficulty connected with the abstract approach is not simply one of greater complexity, measured by the number of separate, subservient functions involved. It demands the behaviour of the new emergent quality, generically different from the concrete' (Goldstein & Scheerer 1941, p. 22).

Operationally the 'abstract attitude' was defined by performance on a series of tests. These included the Weigl Colour-Form Sorting Test, and an object sorting test, together with a block design test of the Kohs type and the Goldstein-Scheerer Stick Test. In the monograph which gives the method of administration of the tests (Goldstein & Scheerer 1941), Goldstein presented a detailed definition of the term abstract attitude.

> The abstract attitude is the basis for the following *conscious* and *volitional* modes of behaviour:
>
> 1. To detach our ego from the outer world or from inner experiences.
> 2. To assume a mental set.
> 3. To account for acts to oneself; to verbalize the account.
> 4. To shift reflectively from one aspect of the situation to another.
> 5. To hold in mind simultaneously various aspects.
> 6. To grasp the essential of a given whole; to break up a given whole into parts, to isolate and to synthesize them.
> 7. To abstract common properties reflectively; to form hierarchic concepts.
> 8. To plan ahead ideationally; to assume an attitude towards the 'mere possible' and to think or perform symbolically. Concrete behaviour has not the above mentioned characteristics (Goldstein & Scheerer 1941, p. 4).

A reading of the examples provided in the monograph to explain these eight modes of behaviour reveals that Goldstein incorporated under one term many of the features of frontal behaviour which are considered under other headings in the remainder of the chapter. As some of these are considered characteristic of frontal behaviour by other workers it is regrettable, as Battersby (1956) pointed out, that 'Even in a comprehensive monograph describing details of the sorting test (and other allied procedures), no quantitative data were presented which would enable the reader to compare the relative effects of cerebral lesions in different locations'.

There is also a fundamental theoretical difficulty involved.

> The question of whether a more abstract level of functioning is only a quantitative extension of a more concrete level, and the two levels are hence continuous... or is so qualitatively different from the more concrete functioning that it is discontinuous from it... is indeed an old and yet unresolved one. It is, among other questions, the problem of reductionism versus holism, or relatedly of quantity versus quality, issues with which psychology – indeed all of science – has spent much effort.... (Harvey et al 1961).

Quantitative versus qualitative change. A number of studies by Reitan and colleagues addressed themselves to the question of qualitative versus quantitative changes following brain damage. Reitan (1955) established the presence of striking group differences between brain damaged and control subjects on the ten tests of Halstead's Impairment Index and the Wechsler-Bellevue Scale. He felt that 'if different kinds of abilities were used by the brain damaged subjects, the interrelationships or correlations between various tests would differ from the interrelationships between tests shown by the group without brain damage' (Reitan 1958). Correlation coefficients were computed between each pair of variables for each group. A correlation of 0.85 was obtained between the matrices for brain damaged and control groups. Thus, while the brain damaged subjects showed definite impairment, their abilities remained essentially of the same kind as non-damaged subjects. In a second study, Reitan (1959), using the Halstead Category Test, found no significant differences in kind of response to subtests between the two groups though there was a clear difference in the mean error scores. This finding was extended by Doehring and Reitan (1962), again using the Category Test. Taking the ratio of errors on each subtest to total errors on the test they found no difference in the pattern of responding between left hemisphere, right hemisphere and control groups. Earlier Simmel and Counts (1957), in examining the errors of temporal lobe cases and control subjects on the Category Test, had reported that both groups reacted essentially alike to the stimulus material, choosing the erroneous alternatives in much the same way.

Goldstein G et al (1968) pointed out that a difficulty with Kurt Goldstein's (qualitative) and Reitan's (quantitative) positions has been their failure to evaluate the possibility that both observations may be correct, depending upon the kind of brain damaged patients and the abilities being evaluated. They employed concept identification problems, both simple and complex, of the type reported in Bourne (1966). They comment:

> The issue of quantitative vs. qualitative impairment of abstract reasoning in the brain damaged is not independent of the subject's status, perhaps particularly his age, type of deficit, locus of lesion and problem to be solved. Some brain damaged individuals behave as do the patients in Goldstein and Scheerer's case presentations. They seem to be completely incapable of adopting the abstract attitude. Others behave as did the typical subject in the 1959 Reitan study. They can apparently adopt the abstract attitude, but not as effectively as the non-brain damaged individual.

It is obviously important in the resolution of this problem to take the suggested factors into consideration. While the study just cited supported the importance of age and task complexity, the role of location of the lesion has been insufficiently explored.

Frontal locus and abstraction. There is a good deal of evidence that patients with frontal lesions perform poorly on so-called tests of abstraction. Many studies after psychosurgery in the 1940s and 1950s showed such loss on a variety of tests (Fleming 1942, Kisker 1944, Rylander 1947, Malmo 1948, Yacorzynski et al 1948, Petrie 1949, Grassi 1950). That these changes might be more subtle with less radical operations has already been mentioned. One large study (Mettler 1949, Landis et al 1950) reported only transient loss after psychosurgery.

Studies based on the examination of cases with other frontal lesions, including excision of small and large portions of the frontal lobes, have often described poor abstract ability defined by poor performance on one or more tests (Goldstein 1936a, 1939a, 1944, Rylander 1939, Halstead 1947, Shure 1954, Shure & Halstead 1958, Milner 1963). These studies have often concentrated on the behaviour of individuals with frontal lesions without any comparable examination of patients with lesions in other locations or, where this has been done, e.g. in the Halstead studies, the evidence of a major difference is unconvincing. Teuber (1964) cited several studies where patients with posterior lesions performed at least as poorly as frontal patients, even where sorting or categorizing tests were used.

The unsatisfactory nature of this area of research lies in the nature of many of the tests used and the unwarranted assumptions which have been made about the abilities which are felt to be central to their solution. A *patient may fail on a test of abstract thinking for a number of reasons other than alteration in the ability to think abstractly*. Milner's argument that the frontal patient may fail because of an inability to inhibit preferred modes of responding would appear to account for many of the failures described in the literature. When one looks at a complex test such as the Category Test one is not surprised at the failure of brain damaged patients in general since so many factors appear to be crucial for good performance on this test. This point of view is supported by studies such as that of Messerli et al (1979). One of their tasks required the subject to abstract the rule underlying the presentation of series using coloured counters, e.g. Red Green Red Green (RGRG); RRGG; RGGRGG. Frontal patients were significantly poorer than all other lesion groups on complex 'asymmetrical' series such as RGGRGG but individual subjects failed for different reasons. Some perseverated by adhering to an earlier successful programme while others persevered with a newly devised hypothesis even though it proved obviously wrong. Some gave two or more successful sequences and then disregarded the rule. Yet others could verbalize the rule but not execute it.

While the present authors feel that there is little doubt about the frontal patient's poor performance on abstraction tasks, it is inaccurate to ascribe the reason for failure solely to loss of abstract ability.

Planning and problem-solving

One of the most helpful of Luria's contributions to neuropsychology lies in his conception of the frontal lobes at the summit of the brain's hierarchy. This point of view is nowhere more clearly expressed than in The Working Brain (1973b):

> Man not only reacts passively to incoming information, but creates *intentions*, forms *plans* and *programmes* of his actions, inspects their performance, and regulates his behaviour so that it conforms to these plans and programmes; finally, he verifies his conscious activity, comparing the effects of his actions with the original intentions and correcting any mistakes he has made (pp. 78–80).

This higher form of man's activity has been referred to in other areas of psychology, largely under the heading of thought processes, e.g. 'Thinking is a form of problem-solving behaviour which involves the correlation and integration of critical events in time and space. It is characterized by (a) a period of preliminary exploration, (b) a pre-solution period of search, (c) a period of vicarious testing of tentative solution, (d) an act of closure and registry of a memory trace, and (e) appropriate action' (Halstead 1960). It has been the task of neuropsychology to demonstrate the dependence of each of these major steps upon the integrity of the frontal lobes. This is not to say that there were no early contributions of worth, merely that converging lines of evidence in recent years have given us a better total picture of the complex functioning of the prefrontal regions. Some of the complexity can be gained from an examination of three areas: (i) maze behaviour; (ii) visuo-constructive activities; and (iii) problem solving. This is merely a convenient illustrative sample, since planning and programming activities permeate virtually everything which man does. Frontal patients seem to have particular difficulty in laboratory or everyday life tasks which have multiple subgoals necessary for successful completion (Shallice & Burgess 1991, Dimitrov et al 1996), even in cases where performance on standard neuropsychological tests is adequate (Goldstein et al 1993).

Maze behaviour. As far back as 1914, in the days when mental testing was in its infancy, Porteus introduced a set of pencil and paper maze problems which have been in widespread use since that time (Fig. 4.6). One of the reasons for the continued use of the test must be that it measures some characteristic which is basic to man's intelligent behaviour. Porteus himself referred to this in a number of ways, e.g. as 'planfulness', 'planning capacity', or at another time as 'prehearsal', i.e. a mental rehearsal of the act that the individual is about to perform. If we retain the simple term 'planning', it was this which Porteus considered was measured by the Maze Test and which he felt was a *prerequisite to every intelligent act* (Porteus 1950, 1958, 1959, 1965). Moreover, he was to come to the conclusion, based on his own studies and those of others, that this factor was maximally represented in the frontal lobes. In one of the earliest reports of extensive frontal lobectomy it is remarked 'In so far as final conclusions from the first two cases…are justifiable it may be stated that maximal amputation of right or left frontal lobe has for its most detectable sequel impairment of those mental processes which are requisite to planned initiative' (Penfield & Evans 1935).

The advent of psychosurgery allowed Porteus to validate his longstanding claim that the Mazes were a measure of planfulness. Patients undergoing classical lobotomy procedures showed a clear loss in this area when investigated clinically. Such patients also showed loss on the Mazes (Porteus & Kepner 1944, Porteus & Peters 1947). This finding was soon confirmed by others (Malmo 1948, Mettler 1949, 1952, Petrie 1949, 1952a, 1952b, Robinson & Freeman 1954). The failure of some workers to demonstrate such losses may have depended not only on the smaller size of the lesion but also on the well known practice effect in such tests. This would account for findings such as those of Fabbri (1956), who demonstrated a slight *increase* in the quantitative score after transorbital lobotomy as well as a marked decrease in qualitative errors.

That losses on the Maze Test are dependent on the location of the lesion within the frontal lobe has been shown by Crown (1952) and Lewis and colleagues (1956). These authors demonstrated that posterior and superior lesions affected performance on the tests more consistently than did lesions in other sites. The work of Robinson on the other hand suggested that the extent of the loss might be related to the amount of the frontal lobe disconnected.

A different type of maze test which appeared sensitive to cerebral impairment was introduced by Elithorn (1955). Examples of different degrees of difficulty are shown in Figure 4.7. The subject is instructed to find the way from the bottom to the top, passing through the maximum number of dots, this

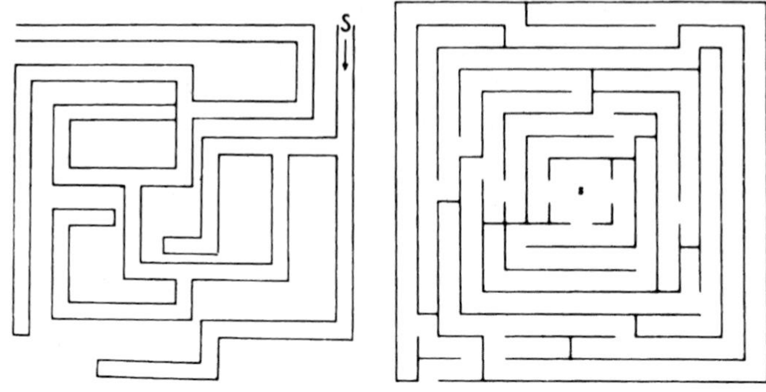

Fig. 4.6 Two examples from the Porteus Maze Test (by kind permission of D. Hebden Porteus).

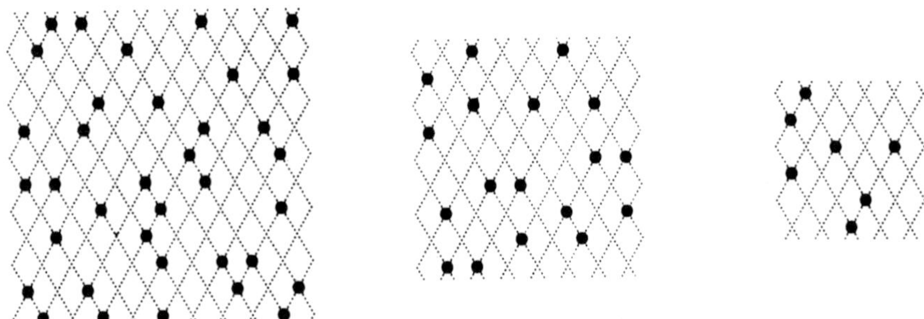

Fig. 4.7 Examples of the Elithorn Maze Test.

number being printed on the form. The subject is instructed to keep to the dotted lines and is told not to cross the white diamonds and that reversing direction is not permitted. Though a later study showed the sensitivity of the Elithorn Maze Test to brain damage there was no indication that frontal patients were differentially impaired (Benton et al 1963). However we have noted that same disregard for the rules in the face of their correct repetition by the subject and admonition by the examiner when employing an electrical stylus maze. A binary form of the maze for experimental work was developed by Elithorn et al (1963), while Gregson and Taylor (1975) used a computer programme to generate a series of similar mazes where the dot density in the lattice has been controlled.

Visuoconstructive activities. These tasks are often performed poorly by patients with brain impairment. Perhaps the most frequently used has been the Block Design task of the Kohs type, which has found its way into popular aggregate measures of intelligence such as the Wechsler Scales. The Block Design Test failed to live up to expectation as a universal indicator of brain damage, but recent reappraisal would suggest that careful analysis of qualitative features of the patient's performance could reveal valuable indicators of brain impairment if the lesion is situated in the frontal or parietal regions.

Constructional difficulties are often all loosely referred to as 'constructional apraxia' (Ch. 6). In posterior lesions the difficulties arise because of a loss of spatial organization of the elements. Luria and Tsvetkova (1964) have demonstrated that frontal constructional difficulties arise through disruption of one or more of the steps mentioned at the beginning of this section, namely, *intention, programming, regulation, or verification*. Lhermitte, Derouesné and Signoret (1972) provided confirmation of this viewpoint by demonstrating how the performance of the frontal lobe patient may be facilitated by means of a programme provided by the examiner. As in the case cited in the later section on psychosurgery, a patient who was unable to execute a block design problem could do so immediately and without error when presented with a model or design where each constituent block was clearly delimited. In the words of Barbizet (1970), the examiner is here acting as the patient's frontal lobes by generating part of the programme for solution.

Other tasks are also improved when partial programmes are provided for frontal patients. This does not appear to be the case with lesions in other parts of the brain.

Lhermitte et al also employed the Complex Figure of Rey (Fig. 4.8, Rey 1941, 1959, Osterrieth 1944). The frontal patients' copying was much more adequate than reproduction from memory. This was not, however, caused by a primary disorder of memory. Following their poor reproduction from memory, the patients were given a structured sequence of the figure to copy. This began with copying the basic rectangle. They then had to copy a version consisting of the rectangle plus other features, and more and more complete figures were given until the full figure was reached. The patients copied each of the more and more complete versions from the beginning so that, by the time they had reached the full design, they had experienced a sequential programme for its execution on a number of occasions. Their later reproduction from memory was much improved. The improvement appears to result more from the provision of a programme than from the sheer weight of practice. This is borne out by our own experience where the provision of extra experience alone leads to little or no improvement. Moreover, the patient is just as poor with any new

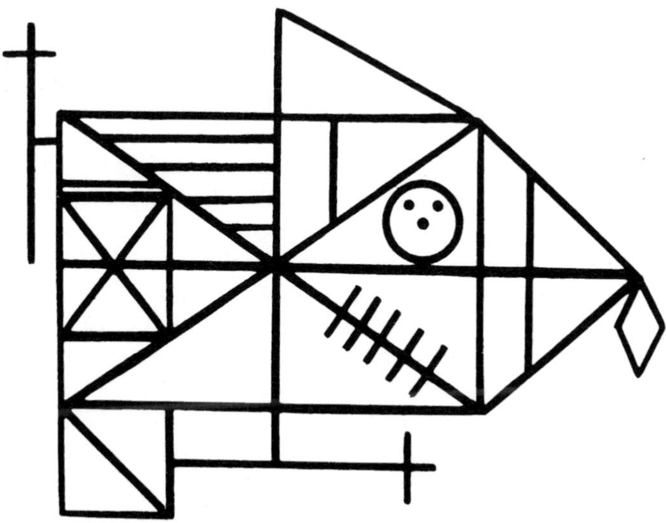

Fig. 4.8 The Complex Figure of Rey (Rey 1959, courtesy of Les Editions du Centre de Psychologie Appliquée).

figure for which a programme had not been established. It is painfully evident that one can teach frontal patients specific programmes, but not how to generalize from them, even to activities which seem to the observer to be very similar.

Superficially, the Rey Figure copies of frontal patients look like constructional apraxia. However, the spatial relationships of many key elements are preserved, e.g. the crossed hatched lines on the diagonal are at right angles, the lines in the upper left quadrant are horizontal, and other features are correctly reproduced (Messerli et al 1979). It is the failure to organize or integrate the components into the whole which is at fault.

Arithmetical problem solving. With frontal lobe lesions there do not appear to be significant disturbances of well established operations such as addition and subtraction and none of the 'spatial' mathematical difficulties seen in parietal patients (Ch. 6). The essential difficulties are better described as those of problem solving or of 'discursive intellectual activity' (Christensen 1975). Once again, patients may be able to repeat the problem but their actions suggest a form of amnesia. They seem to have forgotten how to generate and execute even a simple two or three step programme which would have presented no difficulty prior to their lesion. As in other areas of behaviour much of their difficulty arises through incomplete analysis and an inability to inhibit the first tendency aroused by the problem (Luria 1966). A detailed analysis of the arithmetical problem solving ability of patients with frontal (and other) lesions is given in the French monograph of Luria and Tsvetkova (1967). Three sample problems likely to elicit difficulties are as follows (from Luria 1966):

A. There were 18 books on two shelves, and there were twice as many books on one as on the other. How many books were on each shelf?
B. A son is 5 years old; in 15 years his father will be twice as old as he. How old is the father now?
C. A pedestrian takes 30 minutes to reach the station, while a cyclist goes 3 times as fast. How long does the cyclist take?

Christensen gives a succinct summary of the behaviour of the frontal patient confronted with these problems. 'The patient only grasps one particular fragment of the problem; he does not make any plans but starts to carry out disconnected arithmetical operations with this fragment. The whole process of solution may be transformed into a series of impulsive, fragmentary arithmetical operations, frequently unconnected with the ultimate goal' (p. 188).

The patient often construes 'twice as many' and similar expressions as meaning 'multiply' without any regard for the context and so arrives at what appear ludicrous answers, e.g. in problem C (termed 'conflict' problems by Christensen) he arrives at the answer 90 minutes for the cyclist.

Another problem solving task which is performed more poorly by frontal patients than any other group is cognitive estimation (Shallice & Evans 1978). Here subjects must generate a plan and execute it while checking it against their store of common knowledge. Examples are: 'What is the length of the average man's spine?'; 'What is the length of a five pound note?' Frontal patients produced numerous bizarre estimates, i.e. those which exceeded the estimates of all or most normal subjects. Frontal subjects have also shown difficulty in estimating the frequency of recurrence of items in a presented series, right frontal subjects having more difficulty than left (Smith & Milner 1988). These authors considered that the difficulty might be due to poor memory searching, poor cognitive estimation, or both.

Error utilization. One of the major changes in behaviour with frontal lobe cases is the apparent lack of full awareness of deficits. Luria has referred to this as a 'lack of self-criticism' or 'lack of critical attitude towards one's own action' (Luria & Homskaya 1963, 1964) and felt that this could be regarded 'as the result of a general loss of some feedback mechanism, a disturbance in signals of error, or an inadequate evaluation of the patient's own action. It can be reduced to a deficit in matching of action carried out with the original intention...' (Luria & Homskaya 1964, p. 355). In discussing their patient's inability to carry out compounded or symbolic instructions, Luria, Pribram and Homskaya (1964) stress what has been pointed out several times already, namely that the failure is not one of understanding what is required, 'These incapacities seem not to depend on any difficulty in apprehending the instructions per se: they may however, be related to an inability, shown by our patient, to evaluate errors, especially self-produced errors' (p. 278).

A most important contribution to conceptualizing the nature of the frontal defect has been made by Konow and Pribram (1970). They describe a patient who made errors and, at the same time, gave clear indication that she was aware of making them. She was not, however, able to correct them. 'We therefore confronted her with a test in which one of us carried out the commands of the other, sometimes correctly and sometimes erroneously. The patient usually had no difficulty in spotting our errors. This was true even when they were embedded in rather complex serial performances' (p. 490). The important feature was the patient's inability to use such information to modify her ongoing programme of action. This analysis leads to an important distinction which should have marked implications for attempts to rehabilitate patients with frontal injury, i.e. the distinction between error recognition and *error evaluation* on one hand and *error utilization* on the other. The latter term is a clear expression of the dissociation between thought and action mentioned by many neuropsychologists in a variety of ways, e.g. the 'dissociation between knowing and doing'. One study has pointed to the similarity of such behaviour with that of non-human primates with frontal damage (Rolls et al 1994).

The problem of error utilization can be subtle but very disruptive and can be easily overlooked unless appropriate tests are used. We have found it a common disability after closed head injury and in chronic alcoholism. Serial maze learning of the length and complexity of the Milner pathway (Milner 1965) using the Austin Maze (Walsh 1991) or similar apparatus brings out the difficulty very well. The subject may rapidly learn the general plan of the maze, reducing errors to a small number in a few trials, only to have difficulty in eradicating errors completely. Even when the subject has reached an errorless trial, subsequent trials may show recurrence of errors. This highlights the point that measures such as trials to criterion (e.g. one errorless trial) may be quite misleading as a measure of the patient's capacity to work effectively. Wherever there is suspicion of frontal lobe involvement the criterion of learning should be the execution of a stable *error-free performance*. One has only to think of the consequences of even one error in the programme of operating machinery, preparing a recipe, or flying a plane to see the importance of excluding the difficulty of error utilization when examining patients for rehabilitation.

Luria argued that the basic factor contributing to the frontal patient's difficulties was lack of the 'verbal regulation of behaviour'. In other words the patients' verbalizations (both internal and external) do not command their actions. Drewe (1975a, b) specifically tested this proposition and found that while it might fit some of the findings it was unable to explain a good deal of the experimental findings in frontal subjects.

The 'Tower of London' problems. This set of problems is the first of a series of tasks intended by the originator (Shallice 1982) to examine frontal lobe processes. The test has the great advantage that it is derived from the author's general model for thought and action, which will allow predictions about frontal deficits to be examined systematically. There are a series of novel problems of graded difficulty in which the most efficient solution depends on breaking down the goal into subgoals which must then be tackled in an appropriate order. Figure 4.9 illustrates a problem of moderate difficulty. On each problem the subject is presented with a standard array of coloured beads on sticks and must achieve a given arrangement *in a stated number of moves* by shifting the beads one at a time from stick to stick.

In the seminal study, patients with left anterior lesions showed a specific

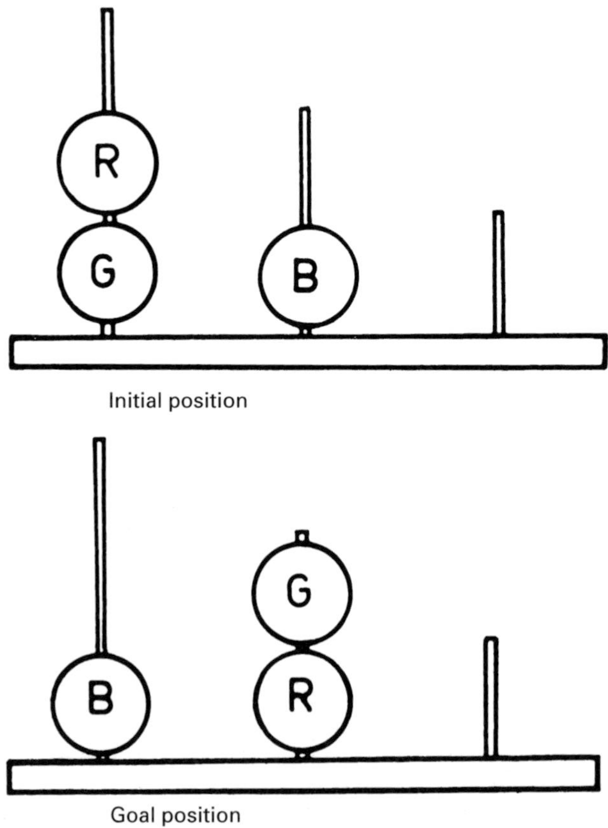

Fig. 4.9 One of the Tower of London problems (Shallice 1982).

deficit compared with right anterior and both posterior groups. A recent study of normal subjects on the test employing single photon emission computerized tomography (SPECT) showed not only an increased perfusion in the left prefrontal region, but also a higher measure in those who took more planning time for their moves (Morris et al 1993), while another SPECT study with volunteers showed bilateral frontal activation with the Tower problems, and also a number of other planning tasks, but not the Porteus Maze (Rezai et al 1993). The pattern of activation varied from test to test.

The 'Tower' problems seem more highly loaded on a planning factor than most others in common use and are a welcome addition to research and clinical method. Their sensitivity is confirmed by studies such as that of Owen et al (1990) who showed that while initial thinking time was not impaired compared with controls, frontal subjects had significantly prolonged thinking time in subsequent moves. This accords well with our clinical experience.

While frontal patients undoubtedly perform badly on *planning* tests, Goel and Grafman (1995) suggest that the difficulty may not be one of 'looking ahead', as is often assumed, but may result from a difficulty in resolving goal-subgoal conflicts which arise in the performance of these tasks.

The findings cited in this section agree well with the opinion of Delis et al (1992) who examined a variety of deficits in frontal and other groups on a new sorting task. The frontal patients showed 'a wide spectrum of deficits in abstract thinking, cognitive flexibility, and use of knowledge to regulate behavior' which impaired their abstract thinking. As in other areas throughout the text, the use of imaging is beginning to clarify the relation between specific parts of the frontal systems and specific subcomponents of cognitive processes (e.g. Owen et al 1996).

Rigidity and cerebral impairment

One of the most frequently mentioned features of the behaviour of brain impaired patients is a lack of flexibility in their approach to many situations. This has been noted in both clinical and psychological test situations. Particular studies express this in different ways, e.g. (i) lessening of the ability to shift from one concept to another when compared with normal subjects (Goldstein & Scheerer 1941, Weigl 1941, Aita et al 1947, Ackerly & Benton 1948, Gleason 1953, Halstead 1959, Milner 1963, 1964); (ii) inflexibility, rigidity, perseveration or stereotyped behaviour (Nichols & Hunt 1940, Rosvold & Mishkin 1950, Appelbaum 1960, Allison 1966, Mackie & Beck 1966, Allison & Hurwitz 1967); (iii) sensitivity to the effect of set or *Einstellung* (Kauffman 1963). This list is by no means exhaustive but points to the common occurrence of a mode of behaviour we will term inflexible. There is no convincing evidence that all these descriptions refer to a unitary disability.

This condition has been described most frequently in association with tests of abstract thinking, but has been found also in a variety of other test situations involving learning and problem solving as well as being reflected in the patient's everyday behaviour. Among the various tests which have brought out the brain impaired subject's inflexibility have been the Goldstein-Scheerer tests, parts of the Halstead battery, the Wisconsin Card Sorting Test, stylus maze problems, pegboard discrimination, paired associate learning, problem solving, and word association tests. The notion of inflexibility of behaviour finds one of its clearest and most extensive expressions in the monograph of Goldstein and Scheerer (1941).

One fruitful experimental approach which has received little attention is to examine flexibility under the paradigm of negative transfer. The only direct examination appears to be that of Gleason (1953), who defined negative transfer as 'retardation in the acquiring of an activity as a result of being engaged in a prior activity'. Gleason found support for an increase in negative transfer in brain damaged subjects on several tasks, e.g. a pegboard discrimination task, a card sorting task and a rotated stylus maze, demonstrating that there was 'an application of old responses in new situations where such responses are inappropriate'.

There is considerable evidence that inflexibility is particularly marked after lesions of the prefrontal regions (Nichols & Hunt 1940, Halstead 1947, Ackerly & Benton 1948, Rosvold & Mishkin 1950, Luria 1963, 1965, 1966, 1973b, Luria & Homskaya 1963, Luria et al 1964, Milner 1963, 1964). Milner's findings suggest that such deficits may be more associated with lesions affecting the dorsolateral aspect of the frontal lobes rather than the orbitomedial regions. Such a finding may be in keeping with the reports of a number of psychosurgical studies which show little or no intellectual alteration when division of fibre pathways is restricted to the ventromedial quadrant of the frontal lobes (Malmo 1948, Petrie 1952b, McIntyre et al 1954, Bradley et al 1958, Smith & Kinder 1959, Walsh 1960, Hohne & Walsh 1970). However, a more recent study of patients with ventral damage to the frontal lobes showed a tendency to continue to make inappropriate responses on discriminative tasks to a previously rewarded stimulus (Rolls et al 1994).

Despite this accentuation of the frontal lobe, there is clear evidence that inflexibility is also found with lesions in other parts of the brain (Critchley 1953, Allison 1966, Allison & Hurwitz 1967). The latter authors point out that perseveration 'is not an occasional accompaniment of aphasia but... occurs in the majority of cases'. In fact 16 out of their 24 patients showed the symptom. The perseveration was linked to each patient's specific deficit, being elicited by tests related to the deficit but not by tests related to preserved language functions. Like many authors they comment that perseveration was facilitated by anxiety but was also seen in its absence. They also noted that, in their series, absence of spontaneous talk was a frequent accompaniment of perseveration. In line with what is said below on the verbal adynamia with frontal lesions, one might suspect that the frontal lobes were affected in at least some of these cases. However, in a few cases where autopsy proof was available, perseveration also existed in temporal lesions. With Critchley's observation of perseveration with parietal lesions, one can be sure that inflexible behaviour is not seen solely with frontal lesions. In a recent study (Owen et al 1991), frontal patients showed a dissociation between shifting set to a previously irrelevant dimension, which they found difficult, but not to new instances of a previously relevant dimension. Thus care should be taken in interpreting data in the light of the role that 'novelty' plays in the situation. Patients with temporal lobe resections had no difficulty with either paradigm.

Perseveration or inflexibility appears to be most prominent when the task is difficult or the patient is fatigued. This is not surprising since these are the conditions under which such lapses are likely to appear in normal adults. It is when it becomes constant and pervasive that it provides one of the most valuable signs of cerebral impairment.

In a number of communications Luria provided evidence of motor perseveration with frontal lobe damage (Luria 1963, 1965, 1966, 1973b, Luria & Homskaya 1963, Luria et al 1964) and hypothesized two kinds of 'frontal' perseveration associated with two different neuronal systems. The first type involves compulsive repetition of a movement that has been initiated but the patient is able to shift from one action to another. The second type represents what Luria terms an inertia of the programme of action itself '... the patient, having once performed the required task, is incapable of switching to the fulfilment of any other task but continues even when instructed otherwise, to perform the first task on which he has 'stuck' (p. 1). Type 1 is thought to be associated with deep seated lesions of the premotor zones involving the subcortical ganglia, while the second type is associated with massive involvement of the anterior or basomedial portions of the frontal lobes. 'The only significant difference is that, whereas in lesions of the premotor zones the pathological inertia extends only to the effector components of the action, and performance of the programme as a whole is undisturbed, in massive lesions of the frontal lobes it extends to the scheme of the action itself, with the result that performance of the programme becomes impossible' (1973b, p. 206). The validity of Luria's 'premotor syndrome' as a separate distinct entity has been strongly supported by the study of Derouesné (1973) of five cases of frontal tumour restricted largely to the rolandic/prerolandic area. Luria makes it clear that patients who perseverate when given a verbal instruction do not fail through lack of understanding but because the verbal instruction does not regulate their behaviour as it does with normal subjects '... it is not a matter of forgetting the instructions (the patient can reproduce its correct wording) but rather the loss of its regulatory role and replacement of the required programme by an inert motor stereotype' (1973b, p. 206). This apparent disregard of instructions has already been mentioned. An extensive and detailed description of the tasks designed by Luria to elicit this behaviour, together with examples of a typical patient's responses, is provided in Luria et al (1964). Luria's complete neuropsychological examination with explanatory texts was prepared by Christensen (1975).

As mentioned above, the question of inflexibility has been inextricably interwoven with the question of abstract thinking. A striking confirmation of the difficulty which frontal patients have with conceptual shifts was provided by Milner (1963). Using the Wisconsin Card Sorting Test (WCST), she examined patients with static lesions in the frontal and temporal regions before and after cortical excision for the relief of epilepsy. Patients with dorsolateral frontal excisions were more impaired in their ability to shift than those with temporal excisions or those with orbitofrontal excisions even when combined with temporal lobectomy. There were no laterality effects shown in this study, but a long term follow-up (Milner 1975) showed more lasting and consistent deficits on the WCST after left frontal lesions than with right, such deficits being dissociable from language functions. Teuber et al (1951), using the same task, had found that anterior missile wound patients were less impaired than posterior patients, though in this study Teuber did not allow the prior mode of responding to be built up strongly before alternating the principle, so that Milner's study is more conclusive for the effect of perseveration or inability to dissolve a prior mental set. As early as 1948 Grant and Berg showed that the 'amount of perseveration' shown on the WCST is a function of the amount of reinforcement of original modes of response. Since then numerous studies have shown the effects of reinforcement on reversal learning, i.e. alteration of response set. It must also be remembered that behaviour on complex tasks of abstract thinking is determined by a number of factors, some of which are affected more by frontal and others by posterior lesions. Milner (1964) has commented:

> It would be a mistake to attribute the failure of the frontal lobe patients on the sorting task to a defect of abstract thought. Such patients frequently surprise the examiner by telling him that there are three possibilities: 'color, form and number', yet seem unable to recognize the possibility of change, once a particular mode of responding has become established. Thus they show a curious dissociation between their ability to verbalize the requirements of the test and the ability to use the verbalization as a guide to action. (p. 86)

She considers that the difficulty of the frontal patients on the WCST should perhaps be regarded as a special instance of a more general inability to change response set readily in accordance with varying environmental signals' (1964, p. 323). The recent study of Ricci and Blundo (1990) tends to support this contention by showing that patients with difficulty in shifting on the WCST also showed perceptual perseveration, requiring significantly more prompts before recognizing the second of two aspects of a set of ambiguous figures.

The performance of frontal patients on related tests is consistent with the hypothesis that they find it difficult to suppress inappropriate hypotheses (Cicerone et al 1983).

Malmo (1974) extended Milner's (1963) findings, and others have confirmed the presence of poorer performance with more perseverative errors on the WCST (Nelson 1976, Robinson et al 1980). Nelson's modified version of the test has removed ambiguities from the administration and made it more widely acceptable to patients. Vilkki (1988) also confirmed the difficulty of frontal patients compared with others on a very similar task, though not finding more perseverative errors for the frontal group.

Despite fairly wide acceptance of the notion that set shifting difficulty is characteristic of brain impaired subjects, particularly with frontal lesions, the nature of the difficulty has remained unclear. Johnson et al (1973) suggest that this is largely due to the use of tasks varying in complexity both of stimulus and response, as well as different types of abstraction task such as the Weigl Sorting Test (see above) or the reversal shift paradigm, as exemplified by the study of Phelan and Gustafson (1968). Their study suggests the need to study attentional and other general factors which may influence the performance of patients on tests used to elicit inflexible behaviour.

Intellectual loss and inflexibility. It has often been inferred that intelligence and behavioural inflexibility may be more closely related among brain impaired subjects than among normals. Mackie and Beck (1966) examined this proposition in a study employing 20 brain damaged subjects and an equal number of controls. Their results showed that a brain damaged subject may suffer intellectual loss without increased inflexibility and that inflexibility may exist in brain impaired subjects without general intellectual loss.

No examination of test inflexibility in patients would be complete without taking into consideration factors which have been shown to influence the nature, extent and frequency of such behaviour in normal subjects. Goldstein (1943), in offering a comprehensive treatment of the problem of rigidity, emphasized that it is a normal phenomenon and distinguished two types: (i) primary rigidity, where the stimulus aroused a response system so strongly that the individual became incapable of altering response set; and (ii) secondary rigidity, when the subjects were faced with a situation with which they could not cope, and which enabled them to avoid difficult tasks which gave an overwhelming feeling of helplessness – the so-called 'catastrophic reaction' (Goldstein 1936b). Goldstein's stress on the fact that rigidity simply becomes exaggerated with brain damage seems to refer to both these reactions. If these two areas are to be evaluated, then not only must we study traditional learning theory which examines factors influencing primary rigidity, but also study the effects of the individuals' perceptions of their successes and failures as exemplified in studies such as those of Feather (1966) and Nuttin and Greenwald (1968).

Inflexibility, general considerations. The psychological literature on rigidity or inflexibility should form a background for its study in impaired subjects. Reviews of aspects of rigidity are given by Cattell et al (1954), Chown (1959), Fisher (1949), and Schaie (1955, 1958). Baer's (1964) factor analysis of a number of rigidity scales and other personality, perceptual and aptitude tests suggested that rigidity cannot be represented by a unitary factor. This multidimensionality of the concept of rigidity is discussed in detail by Chown who cites the following definitions.

> The difficulty with which old established habits may be changed in the presence of new demands. (Cattell & Tiner 1949)
>
> The inability to change one's set when the objective conditions demand it. (Rokeach 1948)
>
> Resistance to shifting from old to new discriminations. (Buss 1952)
>
> Adherence to a present performance in an inadequate way. (Goldstein 1943)
>
> Lack of variability of response. (Werner 1946)

Chown points out that while tests of rigidity can be classed under general headings, e.g. (i) tests of *Einstellung* or set, (ii) concept formation tests, (iii) tests of personality rigidity or dispositional rigidity, and (iv) tests of perceptual rigidity, there is a need for a study of the relationship between tests in these areas, especially as a good deal of overlap between some measures is apparent.

Since the presence of these several factors has been neglected or overlooked in many neuropsychological studies, it is not surprising that the relation between brain impairment and inflexible behaviour is yet to be clarified. Its presence has been noted frequently in cases of dementia, particularly those with anterior pathology (Ames et al 1994). A broad review of perseverative and stereotyped behaviour is provided by Ridley (1994).

Frontal amnesia

Clinical writers have stressed the frequency of memory impairment in patients with tumours of the frontal lobes. This is generally considered to be more marked for recent memory. Hécaen (1964) recorded an incidence of 20% of isolated memory disorder in a series of 131 frontal tumours, while a survey of the literature revealed figures ranging from 29–73% in other series. Unfortunately, there is little if any psychometric detail provided in this material, nor is there adequate information about the presence of memory disorder with regard to the relative location of the lesion within the frontal lobe. With the increase in knowledge of the neuropathology of memory disorders reported in the next chapter, it seems possible that some of the memory defects seen with frontal lesions may be caused by encroachment on connections between the frontal regions and the limbic or 'axial' structures. Certainly some patients with frontal lesions appear to have difficulty with learning new verbal paired associates, though a true Korsakoff type of amnesia is rare (Hécaen 1964).

Some writers consider that there is no true amnesia in frontal patients, i.e. no inability to register or to retrieve material given the proper conditions. In their views the memory disorder is only apparent, and the poor performance of frontal patients on some memory tasks is better seen as a disruption of complex forms of behaviour which reflects itself in numerous ways. Luria was one of the foremost advocates of such a theory: 'a lesion of the frontal lobes leads to gross disturbances of the formation of intentions and plans, disturbance of the formation of behaviour programmes and disturbances of the regulation of mental activity and the verification of its course and results. In other words, while leaving the operative part intact, it leads to a profound disturbance of the whole structure of human conscious activity' (Luria 1973b, p. 300). Thus the features of 'frontal amnesia' can be readily distinguished from amnesic disorders associated with temporal lobe lesions (Luria et al 1967b). In these latter cases the whole programme or general meaning is preserved so that 'patients who are unable to retain separate elements often can grasp the general meaning of a sentence or paragraph'. Frontal patients, on the other hand, suffer from a change in the total structure of behaviour, which Luria (1971) believed was due to 'high distractibility on one hand and pathological inertia (of traces) on the other', resulting in a loss of programmed forms of activity. In such cases, there is no true amnesia, general or partial, and good retention of a series of items in any modality after 'free' intervals of two minutes or more is seen. 'The defect of retrieval in these patients results from *an inability to create a stable intention to remember with failure to "shift" their recall from one group of traces to another*' (Luria 1971, pp. 372–373).

Other writers have commented on the atypical nature of the memory difficulty of the frontal patient; Benton (1968) calling it 'impaired integration of behaviour over a period of time, a deficit which for want of a better term has been called impairment in "recent memory" . . .'. Barbizet (1970) agreed that simple registration and recall of both visual and verbal material was largely unaffected by 'frontal lesions'. 'In fact, only by means of memory tests in which the frontal patient must retain several facts simultaneously before he can accomplish a specific task are difficulties in recall and learning revealed, and these are often severe . . .' (Barbizet 1970, p. 83). The frontal patient, while possessing the information necessary to solve a problem, often acts as if the (correct) way to proceed has been forgotten. Barbizet recounts the following difficulty in a patient with resection of portion of the right frontal lobe for trauma.

Q. What is the length of one quarter of the Eiffel Tower?
A. After long hesitation, he said he did not know.
Q. What is the height of the Eiffel Tower?
A. 300 meters.
Q. What is half of 300?
A. 150
Q. What is half of 150?
A. 75.
Q. What is the length of one quarter of the Eiffel Tower, which measures 300 meters?
A. (after long cogitation) …200 meters (and despite many attempts he failed each time. (Barbizet 1970, pp. 84–85)

Barbizet considered the frontal memory defect to be of a specific type, affecting particularly the use of previously acquired information. There is also a great similarity to the description of the disorder given by Luria. 'The evidence seems to suggest that frontal lesions suppress the programs that govern the execution of the mental strategies that bring recall and memorization into play during the operation of any new task, whether it be the resolution of a problem or the learning of a piece of poetry' (Barbizet 1970, p. 87).

Frontal patients seem to have difficulty with voluntary learning or memorizing, but when they are made to repeat material frequently by the examiner they show that they are quite able to acquire new information which they can also retain.

One specific study has enquired whether frontal patients, like retrorolandic patients, have specific short term memory deficits. Ghent et al (1962) found consistent negative results for frontal patients when they compared them with control and non-frontal cases on a number of tasks with both immediate recall and delayed recall after 15 seconds. There were no significant differences between frontal and control subjects on conventional tasks in the form of recall of digits or recall of simple visual geometric forms or on specially devised memory for position tasks. These latter were created in an attempt to find, for use with human subjects, suitable tasks which might create an analogous situation to the delayed response paradigm which has presented such striking difficulty for frontal monkeys. With this in mind, stimulus material was chosen which 'could not be categorized readily with reference to a verbal or other framework'. Once again the frontal patients were not significantly different from controls.

Milner (1965) studied the effects of visually guided maze learning in patients with variously located lesions, both unilateral and bilateral. This stylus maze approximates the 'visible path, invisible stops' type of maze devised many years ago by Carr (Woodworth & Schlosberg 1954). The problem is to find the way from start to finish by touching the boltheads with a stylus, moving one step at a time, errors being signalled by a click from the error counter. After working across the board once, the patient was required to repeat the procedure in blocks of 25 trials twice daily until the criterion of three successive errorless trials had been met. Parietal and left temporal groups were close to the performance of normal subjects, but the right temporal, right parieto-temporo-occipital and frontal groups were markedly impaired. It is highly likely that these various groups performed poorly on this task for quite different reasons.

Although the frontal patients were not more impaired on this task than some other groups, certain aspects of test behaviour were specific to the frontal lobe group. They acted on occasion as if they were unaware of the test instructions by frequently breaking the rules, such as failing to return to the previous correct choice after making an error, moving diagonally against repeated instructions and back tracking towards the starting point. This latter type of behaviour led to frontal patients making the same error on the one trial. These qualitative differences may reflect the frontal patient's difficulty in inhibiting aroused response tendencies, but it is interesting to note that Milner described a dissociation in some of her frontal patients on the WCST (above) and the stylus maze. One patient had many 'qualitative' errors on the maze but showed normal flexibility on the card sorting task. Two other frontal patients gave the reverse pattern.

In an earlier study, Walsh (1960) had used a very similar maze in an examination of patients who had undergone modified frontal leucotomy in the orbito-medial quadrant. One of the most frequently reported changes reported after classical prefrontal lobotomy had been the inability of the patients to benefit from past experience. This was noticed not only in the clinical and social settings but had been remarked many times in studies using the Porteus Maze Test. 'Patients tended to make the same mistake repeatedly after the operation which did not happen before the operation, suggesting a loss in the ability to learn from errors' (Petrie 1952b). 14 clinically improved patients tested over a year after modified leucotomy were significantly inferior to an equal number of control subjects on both the stylus maze and the Porteus Mazes. The operated patients also had a greater number of the qualitative errors described by Milner though this comparison failed to reach significance.

Since the study mentioned above there have been many opportunities to observe this disregard of instruction on various forms of the stylus maze which have been used in our clinic. They are seen to a marked degree only in frontal cases and are particularly evident after frontal trauma, particularly if this is bilateral.

Finally, the whole question of the relation of frontal damage to amnesia is made more complex by cases such as that described in detail by Baddeley and Wilson (1988) where an amnesia partaking of most of the features of a diencephalic type of general amnesia (see Chapter 9) was accompanied by features of difficulty with the execution of behaviour classically described with frontal lesions. Since a general amnesic syndrome is seen also alone after trauma it may be that some cases of amnesia accompanying frontal disturbances may be due to lesions in two separate functional systems, and the absence of *obvious* central lesions does not rule out this possibility. The improvement in imaging techniques may help to clarify the question. In brief, patients with frontal lesions, particularly after trauma, may have one or both types of disturbance of their learning and memory functions.

The association of frontal features with specific memory disturbance in thalamic lesions is taken up in Chapter 9.

Verbal behaviour

Two major forms of aphasia occur with frontal lobe lesions. These are Broca's aphasia and transcortical motor aphasia. Treatment of aphasic disorders is beyond the scope of the present text and readers are referred to standard texts on the subject (e.g. Benson 1979, Kertesz 1979). However, there are certain verbal disorders which may be observed in the frontal patient who is not demonstrably aphasic and which should be familiar to the neuropsychologist.

Repetition and verbally directed behaviour. Patients with lesions of the left frontal lobe often appear to have intact speech on superficial examination. However, careful examination will often bring out evidence of perseveration or, in severe cases, echolalia. Since some of the features may come out only on detailed examination, it is advisable to follow a regular programme of examination in non-aphasic patients suspected of having localized cerebral pathology. Detailed descriptions of such examination have been given in Luria et al (1964), Lhermitte et al (1972), and Christensen (1975). The following précis is taken from these sources.

Patients typically have no difficulty in repeating isolated words or simple sentences and may also manage quite well with an unconnected series of words but often have much more difficulty if the word order is changed, e.g. they may repeat the set CAT – FOREST – HOUSE but have difficulty with the rearranged sets CAT – HOUSE – FOREST and FOREST – HOUSE – CAT, showing perseveration of the earlier order. When asked to name objects the patient will name single objects readily but may have difficulty if the objects to be named are presented in various pairings, e.g. the series WATCH–PEN, SCISSORS–THERMOMETER, WATCH–THERMOMETER, SCISSORS–PEN may produce perseveration of earlier elements as the test proceeds. Such difficulties are exaggerated if the pairs are presented with only a small temporal separation.

Such difficulties are also frequently coupled with reduction of 'verbal fluency', described in the next section, and with difficulties in what Luria has termed the verbal regulation of behaviour. These latter are brought out most clearly when a sequence of behaviour is called for. Two examples will suffice.

1. The patient is instructed to place in a line one black counter followed by two white counters and to continue doing this. Two attempts from a patient with a left frontal meningioma are shown (from Luria et al 1964).

B.W.W.B.B.W.W.W.W.W.W…
B.W.W.B.W.B.W.W.B.W.

These incorrect attempts were made despite the fact that the patient was able to repeat the instructions perfectly. Though appearing to understand, neither the patient's own internal language nor the verbal behaviour of others was capable of regulating behaviour.

2. Particular difficulty may arise where there is apparent conflict in the instructions, e.g. 'Tap your hand once on the table when I tap twice and tap twice when I tap once'. The patient may be unable to do so or may begin correctly only to deteriorate rapidly into producing a random series or, more commonly, a rigid stereotype of tapping irrespective of the number of taps given by the examiner. However, there is no difficulty with echopraxis, i.e.

simple repetition of movements in imitation of the examiner and, again, the ability to repeat the instructions is retained signifying comprehension of the task.

Verbal fluency. Frontal patients' behaviour is often characterized by a general lack of spontaneity and voluntary action to which the term 'adynamia' has been applied. There is frequently an associated impoverishment of spontaneous speech and a reduction in the patient's conversational replies which often shrink to passive responses to questions. These responses often have an echolalic quality, e.g. 'Have you had your lunch?' 'Yes, I've had my lunch.' This verbal adynamia is often more marked after left prefrontal damage than elsewhere in the brain, including the right frontal region. Luria (1973b) felt that this form of reduction of speech should not be regarded as an aphasic disorder.

Milner (1964) employed Thurstone's Word Fluency Test in a comparison of left frontal, right frontal, and left temporal lobectomies. This test requires the patient to write as many words as possible in five minutes which begin with the letter S and then as many four-letter words which begin with C. Milner found that left frontal cases were much poorer than the other two groups. Since there was a marked difference between the left frontal and left temporal groups the effect would appear to be specific to the left frontal region and not due solely to involvement of the left (language dominant) hemisphere. Moreover, she found a double dissociation between the left frontal and left temporal groups on the task of verbal fluency versus two tasks of verbal recall. Left frontal patients performed poorly on verbal fluency but adequately on verbal recall of prose passages and paired associates while the reverse was true of the left temporal patients.

Benton (1968) confirmed and expanded these findings. His test of verbal associative fluency has been used in other studies and has become part of the Standardized Neurosensory Center Comprehensive Examination for Aphasia (Spreen & Benton 1969). The patient is asked to say as many words as possible in one minute for each of the letters F, A, and S with the proviso that names and other capitalized words are to be avoided and words with different endings but the same stem are not acceptable, e.g. eat, eaten, eating. Benton restricted his examination to the frontal regions, the lesions being mainly tumours classified in three groups, left frontal, right frontal and bilateral. On the verbal fluency test, left frontal and bilateral cases were both inferior to right frontal cases, though there was no significant difference between the first two groups. Benton pointed out that the left hemisphere patients were 'ostensibly non-aphasic' and felt that, since the impairment was seen in speaking as well as in writing (Milner 1964), it was a rather general higher level language loss. Ramier and Hécaen (1970) confirmed the verbal fluency loss with left frontal lesions. They felt that the defect depended on 'the interaction of 2 factors: frontal lobe damage (defective initiation of an action) and left-sided lateralization of the lesion (verbal domain)'. There is now strong support for the usefulness of scores on verbal fluency tests as an indicator of frontal lobe dysfunction (Pendleton et al 1982, Miller 1984).

Benton Word Fluency Test

'F'	'A'	'S'
force	add	skin

fool	a	scoot
fiddle	alphabet	school
fink	adjective	skin (I said skin)
find	account	skittle
fool	advance	sun
Friday		
fink	animal	sound
fool		skin
find		skittle
fink		sun
fool		
Friday		

The preceding case from our files shows the responses of a young woman of good education who had suffered severe left hemisphere damage with major accent on the frontal region. There were no obvious clinical signs of aphasia at the time of this examination.

The case typifies the frequent occurrence of difficulty in this form of word finding together with perseverations and failure to comply with the instructions. Lhermitte et al (1972) point out that the semantic and morphological perseverations which characterize the performance of frontal patients on this task are also seen in their attempt to define words.

Luria and co-workers (1967a) described a case with a deep left mesial frontal tumour which was also affecting the right side. In this case a disturbance of language became more evident as the tumour increased in size and the authors suggest that careful examination in the early stages of such tumours might reveal certain 'pre-aphasic' signs. One of these is that psychological processes lose what the above authors termed their selective character. When asked to reproduce a sentence or word series, patients will intrude additional associations which they are unable to inhibit. They also have difficulty in naming objects. Luria et al comment '...the naming of an object is a complex process, which includes singling out some leading features of the article, and also assignment to a certain category. This process necessarily includes the suppression of inappropriate alternatives, and a selective choice of proper designations...Often this symptom showed itself in a certain excess of detail in the replies indicating an impairment of inhibition of extraneous associations' (p. 111).

The present authors have frequently observed this symptom in post-traumatic cases along with other obvious signs of frontal involvement. It is nicely demonstrated during psychological testing where a vocabulary test, such as that in the WAIS, is used. Here the patient has to give an appropriate definition of a series of words. If one can consider that in order to produce the correct definition the patient must at the same time inhibit competing response tendencies, the impairment of inhibition leads to many inappropriate responses. To the untrained observer these may appear to have the idiosyncratic quality of some psychotic verbalizations. However patients may demonstrate during the examination that they are well aware of the correct definition, the difficulty being the inability to inhibit the competitors, some (but not all) of which may appear on association by sound with the word to be defined, i.e. what are referred to in the psychiatric literature as 'clang' associations. The inability to inhibit aroused response tendencies is often evident in other aspects of the patient's behaviour. The following vocabulary responses are taken from one of the authors' post-traumatic cases. The patient also showed impulsiveness, facetiousness and fluctuating euphoria.

DESIGNATE	blow up something (detonate)
REMORSE	woman singing a real sad song and she starts crying
CALAMITY	man is overcome with stone, rocks, everything
FORTITUDE	where all the soldiers are all going back to the fortitude because all the Indians attack.
(Patient laughs)	
TIRADE	here the patient gave a long rambling description of disaster at sea, shipwreck etc. and finished by announcing…'and this was all about a tirade wave'.
(Patient again laughs)	

Many of this patient's other responses were perfectly acceptable.

Perret (1974) extended and clarified Ramier and Hécaen's hypothesis, utilizing the concept of loss of control of inhibition. This study reported left frontal patients as being significantly poorer than other patients both on a word fluency test and on a modified version of the Stroop Test (Stroop 1935), where the subject must make a response in which one category of response is pitted against another, e.g. name the colour in which a word is printed, the word itself being the name of a colour. The words BLUE, GREEN, RED and YELLOW were presented randomly in this way with the print in blue, green, red or yellow ink.

Right frontal patients performed more poorly than right posterior patients on the modified Stroop Test, though the difference was small. The sensitivity of the Stroop Test to frontal lesions has been confirmed in other studies (Golden 1976).

Perret considered that the basic difficulty which accounted for the exceedingly poor response by left frontal patients lay in the fact that for successful performance the patient must resist the habit of using words according to their meaning. In the word fluency test the subject is asked to search for words according to the beginning letter and not to the usual method of word finding related to meaning. 'Thus the tests may not have measured the ability to find words, but rather to *suppress the habit of using words according to their meaning*.' 'These results corroborate the hypothesis of the role of the frontal lobe in the adaptation of behaviour to unusual situations, the left frontal lobe being of fundamental importance when verbal factors are involved' (pp. 323–324).

Despite this strong evidence, Vilkki & Holst (1994) found no significant difference on word fluency and category alternation tasks between a group of 29 patients with anterior lesions and 31 with posterior lesions. As with other tests, verbal fluency tasks may require more than one ability and thus different reasons for passing or failing. The 'switching' component seems very vulnerable to frontal lesions (Troyer et al 1997).

Anterior alexia. This term has been used to describe what some consider to be a separate syndrome (Benson 1977, 1979, Kirshner & Webb 1982, Rothi et al 1982). Benson (1977) used the term *the third alexia* to distinguish it from the other two major forms which occur with centrally placed and occipital lesions respectively. More detailed treatment of the alexias is given by Greenblatt (1983) and Benson (1985).

Patients with anterior alexia most often have a non-fluent aphasia and right-sided hemiplegia or hemiparesis. Other signs of posterior involvement, such as hemianopia and auditory comprehension difficulty, are characteristically absent. Anterior alexics may be able to read some words, particularly nouns and action verbs, but are unable to read some words, such as prepositions and terms of relationship, which are syntactically important. They are also unable to read single letters even where they can read the whole word. Thus this form of reading difficulty has been termed syntactic or literal alexia. The syntactic difficulty has been studied as part of the investigation of non-fluent aphasia (Zurif et al 1972, Caramazza & Berndt 1979, Samuels & Benson 1979). The establishment of a separate alexia syndrome is still incomplete because of the variability of the lesions and the frequent accompanying non-fluent aphasia.

Perceptual difficulties

In 1861 Aubert described the following phenomenon which bears his name. When subjects are asked to align a luminescent rod to the vertical in a dark room they are usually able to do so with a fair degree of accuracy. However, if the subject's head (or both head and body) is tilted the perceived vertical is displaced to the side opposite to the direction of body tilt and in proportion to the degree of head or body tilt.

Teuber and Mishkin (1954) examined the Aubert effect in subjects with penetrating missile wounds in various locations. They found a 'double dissociation' on this task with regard to anterior (frontal) and posterior (parieto-occipital) lesions. Frontal patients had difficulty in setting the rod to the vertical with their head and body tilted (the visual–postural condition, Fig. 4.10). Posterior lesion subjects had little difficulty on this task. On the other hand, posterior subjects performed much more poorly on a visual–visual condition where they were required to set a black thread to the apparent vertical against an interfering background of visual stripes while their body was upright. On the simple visual condition for setting the rod and also on a simple postural task where patients had to set their own chair to the vertical there were no major group differences.

Visual search and analysis of complex material. Teuber's laboratory was also the first to demonstrate experimentally a 'subtle but lasting deficit in visual searching' (Teuber et al 1949). Patients were required to point as quickly as possible to the matching stimulus when one of the 48 stimuli was displayed on a circular centre area (Fig. 4.11). Frontal patients were much poorer on this task than either control subjects or non-frontal lesion cases. Unilateral frontal cases, unlike the other subjects, also were disproportionately slower in finding objects on the side opposite the lesion.

An analysis of eye movements in frontal subjects appeared in a number of publications. Luria et al (1966) examined eye movements in a patient with a large right frontal tumour and demonstrated a disturbance in the complex process of exploration of complex pictures. Chedru et al (1973) reported increased identification time for pictures in the contralateral visual half-field but found that the searching activity was similar in the two visual half-fields.

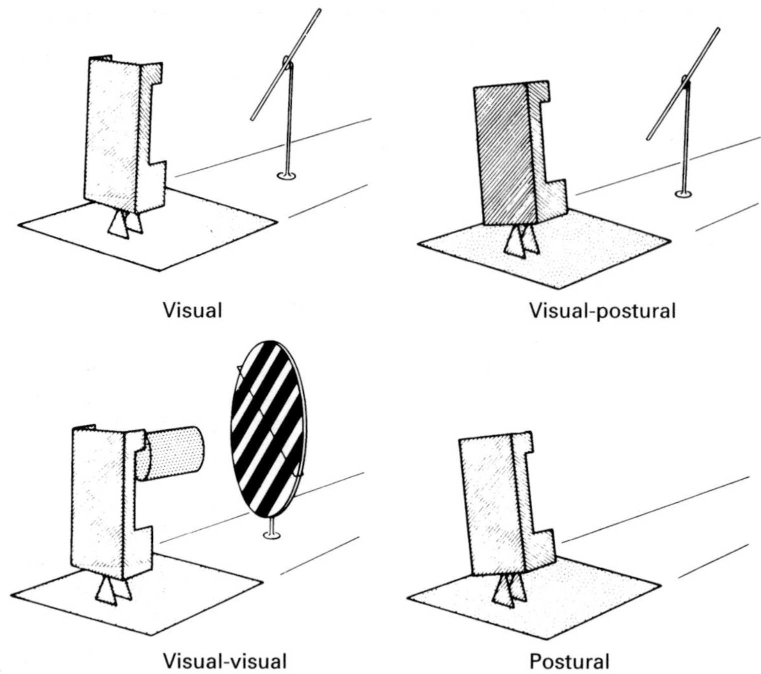

Fig. 4.10 Aubert experiments (Fig. 20.6: Teuber 1964. In: Warren J M, Akert J (eds) The frontal granular cortex and behavior. Used with permission of McGraw-Hill Book Company).

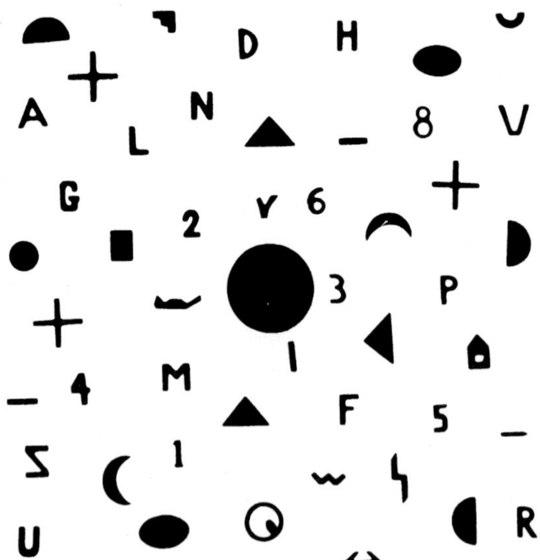

Fig. 4.11 Field of search test (Fig. 20.4: Teuber 1964. In: Warren J M, Akert J (eds) The frontal granular cortex and behavior. Used with permission of McGraw-Hill Book Company).

They considered that the longer identification time might be accounted for by assuming that some alerting value was lost on the affected side by an alteration or disruption of occipitofrontal connections, an explanation similar to the disconnection hypothesis invoked elsewhere. Eye movements of the four patients studied were normal on verbal command and in following a moving target but differed from normals when complex pictorial material was used. Here preliminary visual exploration was reduced and almost compulsive fixation given to one or two details required for answering specific questions about the picture.

Luria (1973b) saw the failure of preliminary analysis as a basic reason why frontal patients fail to grasp the meaning of 'thematic' pictures. The type of behaviour deficit shown by frontal patients in this situation is very similar to that provoked by other problem solving situations. 'To understand the meaning of such a picture the subject must distinguish its details, compare them with each other, formulate a definite hypothesis of its meaning, and then test this hypothesis with the actual contents of the picture, either to confirm it or to reject it, and then resume the analysis' (pp. 213–214). Frontal patients will form an 'hypothesis' based on very little preliminary analysis, what Luria calls the 'impulsive hypothesis' and, since they fail to complete the other steps in the programme of action, will also be satisfied with their explanations, e.g. they do not carry out further exploration which would bring forth added information which would then confirm or disconfirm an hypothesis. Luria points out that the recording of eye movements in normal subjects reveals an alteration in the searching process when the subject is asked to answer different questions about a thematic picture such as the period of the picture, the age of the people depicted, their relationship to each other and so on. The frontal patient fixes on any point and impulsively gives the first hypothesis which comes to mind. The non-analytical nature of the patient's behaviour is reflected graphically in the eye movement record.

This type of behaviour with thematic pictures is often seen on the Picture Arrangement sub-test of the Wechsler intelligence scales. In this test the subject is given in random order a number of cards which, when placed in the correct sequence, will tell a logical story.

We have observed frontal patients to be uncritical in their arrangement, making few alterations in the positions of the cards and then telling a loosely connected story in which only one or two salient features are mentioned and the logical links between elements of the picture series are missing. On occasion the patient may be quite satisfied with the presented random order and then proceeds to tell a story which lacks the richness one would expect from the background or from an estimate of the patient's intelligence based on tests of stored information which are relatively resistant to cerebral insult. At other times the person describes some salient features of each card as though it were a separate unit and not part of a series. McFie and Thompson (1972) analyzed the Picture Arrangement test in 143 adults with circumscribed cerebral lesions and found that, while patients with variously located lesions performed poorly on this test, the tendency to leave pictures in the presented order (in whole or in part) occurred more frequently with frontal than with non-frontal lesions, particularly on the right side. They felt that this tendency reflected 'a specific inability to correct a response in spite of evidence that it is wrong' (p. 551).

There is little doubt that Luria's explanation of the frontal patient's difficulty with thematic pictures would apply equally well to performance on the Picture Arrangement test.

Recently, similar exploration tasks termed 'content-based' exploration or curiosity, have been reported to show little decrement in people with uncomplicated ageing, despite declines in other eye movement parameters (Daffner et al 1991). Patients with probable Alzheimer's disease showed abnormalities reminiscent of Luria's frontal patients (Daffner et al 1994).

Reversible perspective. Cohen (1959), working in Teuber's laboratory with penetrating missile cases, found that unilateral frontal cases experienced far fewer reversals of a double Necker cube (Fig. 4.12) than patients with lesions in other areas, though all unilateral brain damaged individuals were inferior to controls. The average number of reversals was smallest for the right frontal group. Rather unexpectedly, bilateral frontal cases showed the reverse phenomenon, reporting many more reversals than normal control subjects. The significance of these findings is uncertain.

Laterality and the frontal lobes

As far back as Jackson (1874), some writers remarked on the greater disturbance of behaviour by left frontal lesions than by right, though some studies, e.g. Rylander (1939), have found no difference associated with the laterality of lesion. Zangwill (1966) pointed out that Feuchtwanger and Kleist had described certain higher level verbal difficulties in left frontal lesions which were not seen in right-sided cases. In summary these were: '(1) a certain loss of spontaneity of speech in the absence of articulatory disorder; (2) difficulty in evoking appropriate words or phrases, amounting on occasions to frank agrammatism; (3) in some cases, definite impairment of verbal thought processes'. More recently, attention has been addressed to the question of whether the asymmetry of function of the two hemispheres is reflected in the frontal lobes as it is in the posterior parts of the brain (Ch. 8.). A large study of unilateral frontal tumour cases by Smith (1966), using the Bellevue-Wechsler Scale, appeared at first to agree with Teuber's evidence that frontal lesions have less effect on test intelligence than lesions in other areas. 31 frontal cases had a mean IQ of 95.55, whereas 68 posterior cases had a mean IQ of 91.46. However, a division into left frontal (14 cases) and right frontal (17 cases) revealed a significant mean IQ difference between the left (90.1) and right (99.5) cases. Smith re-examined Pollack's data on the Wechsler-Bellevue Scale for the latter's reported tumour cases and found a mean IQ of 86.25 for 4 left frontal cases and a mean IQ of 103.5 for 6 right frontal cases. Thus, by grouping together all frontal cases, one important difference had been concealed.

Smith also examined the ages of left and right frontal cases reported in

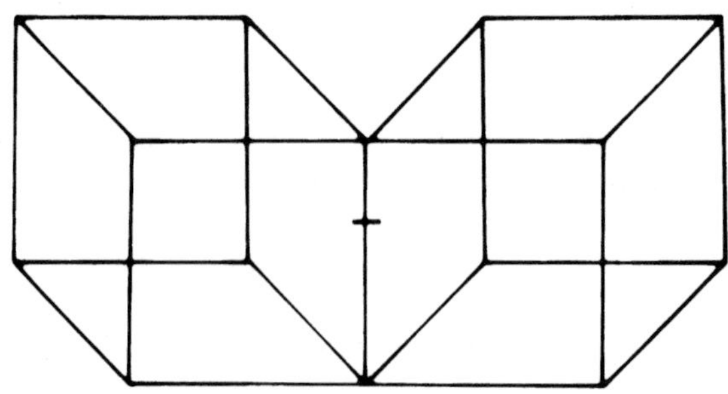

Fig. 4.12 Reversible double Necker cube.

several studies (Rylander 1939, Halstead 1947, McFie & Piercy 1952a, b), and found consistently younger ages for those with left frontal tumours. Together with clinical evidence that left frontal tumours appear to declare themselves earlier than right frontal tumours, Smith finds this a strong argument against the proposition that the disruptive effect of frontal tumours can be attributed to their larger size since the most disruption clearly comes from those of earlier onset, i.e. left frontal.

Benton (1968) looked at the question of laterality effects in frontal lesions by utilizing tests meaningfully related to evidence of hemispheric asymmetry. The following tests were used:

1. two 'left hemisphere' tests: (i) verbal associate fluency (see below); and (ii) paired associate verbal learning
2. two 'right hemisphere' tests: (i) three-dimensional constructional praxis test (Benton & Fogel 1962, Ch. 6); and (ii) copying designs (Benton Visual Retention Test)
3. two 'bilateral' tests: (i) Gorham Proverbs; and (ii) temporal orientation.

Although only a small sample was available (8 right, 10 left and 7 bilateral cases) the findings strongly suggest that interhemispheric differences are reflected in the frontal lobes. Left frontal patients were inferior to right on the word fluency test, while right frontal patients were inferior to left frontal on both the constructional praxis and copying tasks. Somewhat unexpectedly, the right frontal group was inferior to the left on the proverbs task.

While the data on verbal fluency has been interpreted as showing poorer performance by left frontal cases, Jones-Gotman and Milner (1977) found a right frontal bias on their test of design fluency in which subjects had to generate nonsense designs. The nature of the task and particularly its evaluation has made this finding difficult to replicate.

The care that must be taken in interpretation of unequal test performance of two lesion groups is shown by the experiments on recency judgements carried out by Milner's group. Two early studies (Milner 1971, 1974) asked subjects to judge which of two stimuli inserted in a series had been presented more recently. Patients with left frontal lesions were impaired on verbal material but not on non-verbal material (representational drawings and abstract designs), while those with right frontal lesions were impaired on all three tasks, their performance on the verbal task being nearly as poor as the left frontal group. Similarly Làdavas et al (1979) found a material specific recency effect for patients with epileptic foci in the left frontal region.

In a second set of experiments (Milner 1982, Petrides & Milner 1982), despite the use of similar material, there was a strong bias towards poorer performance by the left frontal group when subjects were required to choose their own order of responding. The finding comports well with data which argues for a greater role for the left hemisphere in planning and programming behaviour. The recent study of Wiegersma et al (1990) supports Milner's proposition that frontal subjects are deficient on subject-ordered tasks.

Finally, it is not inconsistent with clinical findings that patients with left frontal lobectomy demonstrate impulsive behaviour on a cognitive risk-taking task, and are impaired in solving such tasks (Miller 1992).

Frontal adynamia

This condition is seen predominantly with bilateral lesions affecting the medial aspects of the frontal lobes and hence may be seen most clearly with lesions of the anterior cerebral arteries. It ranges from a mild state, where the patient is less active than usual with little spontaneous speech, to the fully blown *akinetic mutism* which accompanies bilateral anterior cerebral artery infarction. In reporting three such cases, Freemon (1971) described that condition as 'a disorder of consciousness characterized by unresponsiveness but with the superficial appearance of alertness. The patient's eyes are open but he neither speaks nor moves, nor is the examiner able to communicate with the patient' (p. 693). The sister of one of our patients, noting the apparent alertness, felt that her brother simply did not want to speak to her.

Akinetic mutism of frontal origin is seen with bilateral cingulate gyrus lesions (Nielsen & Jacobs 1951, Buge et al 1975, Jurgens & Von Cramon 1982) but the disorder is also seen with peri-aqueductal lesions.

The milder cases may be described as placidity (Poeck & Kerschensteiner 1975) and those in our experience have certain common features. Patients are generally akinetic and they will remain in one situation for long periods of time. No spontaneous conversation or comment is proffered, but they will reply cogently to others' conversation and carry out actions without any difficulty, even where these are of a high level of complexity. On several occasions we have found that, despite their adynamia, patients may show a normal reaction time even to a long series of signals occurring randomly over several minutes.

Frontal adynamia presents a serious impediment to rehabilitation since, while patients may respond normally to direct external stimuli, they lapse back into inactivity on their withdrawal. The problem appears to lie in an inability to generate and sustain one's own motivation, a defect of the *voluntary* regulation of arousal brought about by a break between the neocortical and brain stem components of arousal mechanisms.

PSYCHOSURGERY

Prefrontal lobotomy and its congeners

The first report of brain surgery in psychiatric disorders was that of Burckhardt in 1891. This surgery took the form of small topectomies, and the author abandoned the treatment some five years later (for review see Joanette et al 1993). The birth of modern psychosurgery, however, is considered to be in November 1935, this being the date when Egas Moniz and Pedro Almeida Lima made the first attempt to alleviate mental suffering by operating on the human frontal lobes (Moniz 1937, 1954). For various reasons, there was at first little interest shown in this new therapy by the medical profession as a whole, and the advent of World War II no doubt contributed to the slow progress made in this field during the ensuing years in Europe.

Following the publication by Freeman and Watts of their book *Psychosurgery* (1942), general interest in these techniques increased rapidly. The classical lobotomy of Freeman and Watts became the standard procedure in most centres, and their finding that the dorsomedial nucleus of the thalamus degenerated when the frontal lobe was isolated provided an interesting and important connection between this work and the suspicions of earlier workers that connections between the frontal lobe and the thalamus provided 'for the addition within the prefrontal fields of affective impulses of thalamic origin' (Herrick 1963).

The standard early lobotomy consisted of very radical division of the white matter of the frontal lobes in a more or less vertical plane just anterior to the tip of the frontal horn of the lateral ventricle (Fig. 4.13).

The extent of destruction of tissue can be seen in Figure 4.14, taken from Freeman and Watts (1948). The term lobotomy used by American and other writers means literally an incision into the lobe. English writers on the other hand preferred the term leucotomy, meaning a cutting of the white matter. The two terms can be taken to be synonymous though care should be taken in reading the literature to ascertain the placement and extent of the lesion in any given series.

Neurosurgeons and psychiatrists very soon became aware, following the early radical operations, that a percentage of patients showed a post-lobotomy syndrome which had many undesirable features. Indeed, in many cases where such a syndrome existed after operation, the second state of the patient appeared to be worse or less desirable than the pre-morbid one. Moreover, the mortality rate was considerable in some series, as was the incidence of postoperative epilepsy and intellectual deterioration. All this led to an abandonment of the procedure by some, and a search by others for a modified form of operation which would preserve any therapeutic value while minimizing the risk of unwanted changes.

In England, Dax and Radley Smith (1945) developed a modified operation

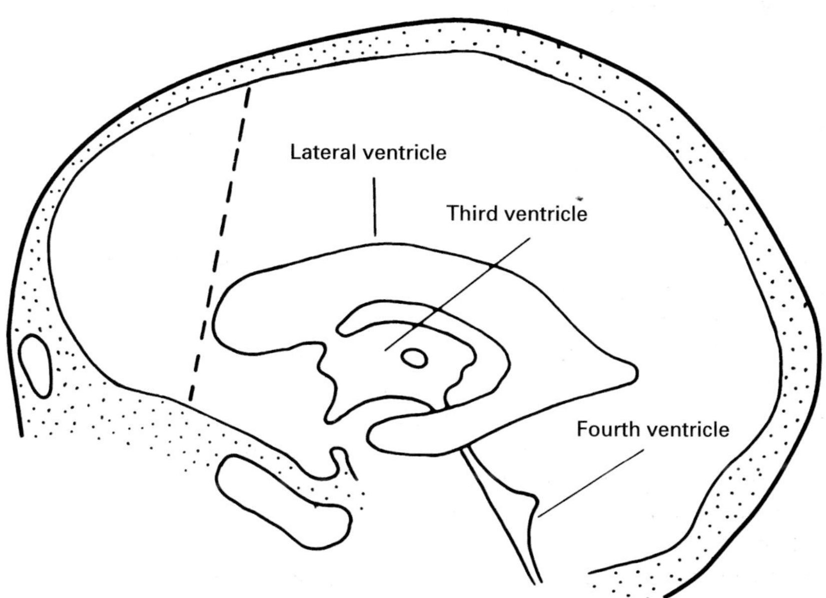

Fig. 4.13 Plane of section in classical prefrontal lobotomy.

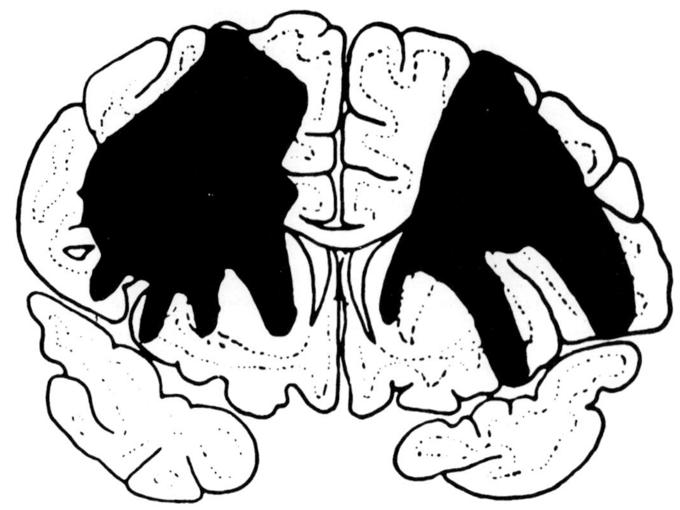

Fig. 4.14 Extensive lobotomy incisions (from Freeman & Watts 1948).

termed ventromedial leucotomy which used a special instrument (the MacGregor-Crombie leucotome). In these operations the upper, middle and lower portions of the frontal lobe were severally divided by sections in a plane parallel to the coronal suture. Other workers also reported that sectioning only the inferior quadrants produced equally good results as those obtained in the more extensive Freeman & Watts operation. From the early forties, the number and types of surgical intervention rapidly multiplied; the accumulation of evidence however seemed to suggest that the more important thalamo-frontal fibres to be severed were those in close proximity to the tip of the frontal horn of the lateral ventricle, and it was a minor variation of the lower section operation first performed by Dax and Radley Smith which formed the operative technique for a series reported by the present author (Hohne & Walsh 1970, Walsh 1976).

This operative method would appear to be concerned with the destruction of much the same fibre pathways as the subsequent method of coagulation by Grantham (1951), which also placed its circumscribed lesion just anterior to the frontal horn of the ventricle, in the lower medial quadrant of the frontal lobe. The procedure was described in detail by Bradley et al (1958). The placement of the lesions is shown in Figures 4.15 and 4.16.

These procedures had much to recommend them. The absence of a large cortical scar minimized the danger of postoperative epilepsy. Secondly, if it was felt that further isolation of frontal cortex was necessary, a second operation could be performed to extend the lesion at another time. Thirdly, such operations seemed to be almost free of the type of postoperative change often referred to as the chronic frontal lobe syndrome, while producing equally effective symptomatic relief.

It would seem that if division of this bundle of thalamo-frontal fibres was the most important mechanism in producing symptomatic relief, then one would expect most forms of leucotomy to have certain features in common, since the majority of operations interrupted part or all of this radiation.

Since this book is concerned with neuropsychological aspects of lesion stud-

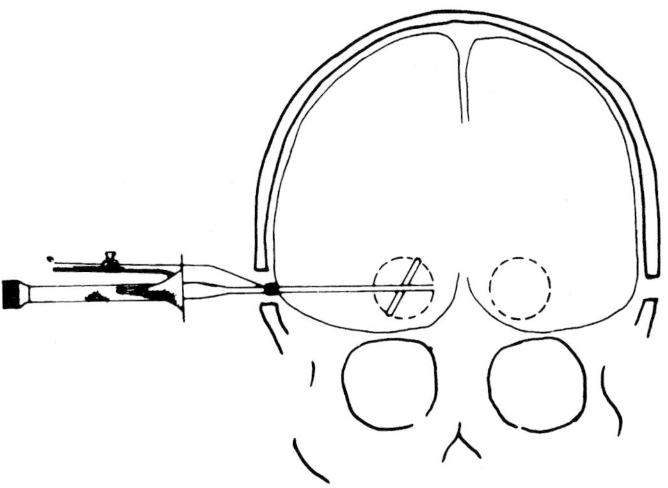

Fig. 4.15 Position of section in orbitomedial leucotomy (from Hohne & Walsh 1970).

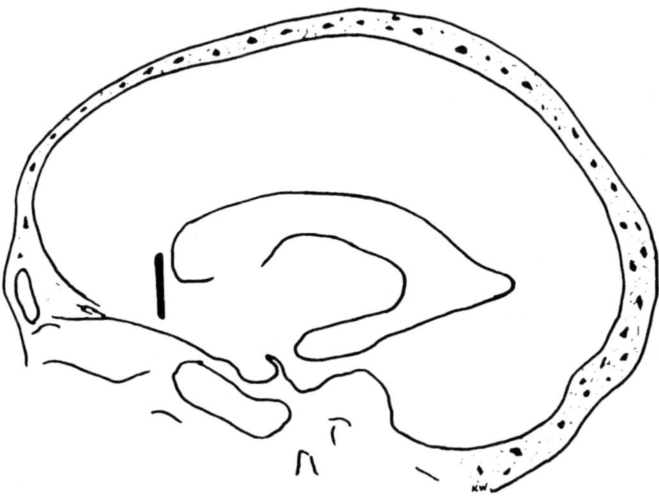

Fig. 4.16 Position of section in orbitomedial leucotomy (from Hohne & Walsh 1970).

ies, the reader interested in the clinical effects of the countless psychosurgical operations may refer to the numerous books and reviews which have appeared on the subject over the past four decades, of which the following is a sample (Mettler 1949, Freeman & Watts 1950, Greenblatt et al 1950, Mettler 1952, Petrie 1952a, Freeman 1953a, b, Robinson & Freeman 1954, Tow 1955, Freeman 1958, Robin 1958, Tooth & Newton 1961, McKenzie & Kaczanowski 1964, Hohne & Walsh 1970, Laitinen & Livingston 1973).

Some operations aimed at largely sparing the thalamo-frontal radiation. Operations which isolated only parts of the frontal cortex have reported good results. The restricted orbital undercutting of Area 13 and part of Area 14 appears to have been as successful as many more radical procedures (Knight & Tredgold 1955, Sykes & Tredgold 1964). During the 1960s, numerous attempts were made to reduce the size of the lesion and to localize it more accurately by means of stereotactic surgery. This included the use of electrodes, probes used for freezing, and the implantation of radioactive seeds. The latter method was introduced by Knight in 1965 and replaced his previous surgical method, while placing the lesion in the same anatomical site. Results were reported by Knight (1965), Strom-Olsen and Carlisle (1971) and Knight (1972).

In a brief but excellent review of psychosurgery, Sweet (1973) commented on the operations. 'On the assumption that some cerebral component of the limbic system was the appropriate target, lesions have been made in the gyrus cinguli, in the white matter of the posteromedial orbital cortex just below the head of the caudate nucleus'. Beginning at about this time, stereotactic limbic leucotomy, a focal and accurate procedure, became popular and continues to be used sparingly at the present time; a particular indication being obsessive-compulsive disorders intractable to other treatments. Recent reviews include those of Poynton (1993), Cosgrove and Rauch (1995), Cumming et al (1995) and Kitchen (1995).

THE FRONTAL LOBES AND PERSONALITY

One of the charges most frequently brought against psychosurgery was the lack of proper scientific rationale. Part of this stems from the relative absence of detailed psychological studies of the effects of such operations on the person's internal organization or self. A review of the literature shows that the relatively few studies which have concerned themselves with psychological assessment limit this to an investigation of the effectiveness of operation in reducing anxiety or depression, or to a demonstration that psychosurgery, in its 'modified' forms, does not have an adverse effect upon aggregate measures of intelligence such as the Wechsler scales. Remarkably few studies have been addressed to the question of the relation between personality change and a rationale for operation. In 1950 Freeman said: 'In order to establish a satisfactory result by psychosurgery, it is necessary to change the personality of the patient from his preoperative one or even his premorbid one' (Freeman & Watts 1950). A study of such changes might then not only increase our understanding of brain-behaviour relationships in the sphere of personality, but also provide a better understanding of indication and contraindication for psychosurgery.

Early in our own series, the rationale for selection was based on the belief that leucotomy becomes the treatment of choice in a patient with the symptom complex of what Arnot (1949) termed 'a fixed state of tortured self-concern', where this has been unrelieved over a long period by other measures. The concept of 'self-concern' as a favourable indication had also been referred to by others (Poppen 1948, Freeman & Watts 1950). With this background and knowledge derived from our early cases, a certain picture of the most suitable candidates for leucotomy gradually crystallized, and a constellation of personality features emerged, almost all of which were related to the patients' preoccupation with their self-concept. This was reflected in referrals in numerous ways. Thus, one patient might be referred as suffering 'somatic delusions', of 'hypochondriasis' or even 'paraphrenia', while others were referred for 'persistent painful rumination' or 'anxious depression'. We agree with Robinson and

Freeman (1954) that these are all aspects of concern over the self, the continuity of which can be modified by psychosurgery so that guilt-laden rumination about the past and fearful anticipation of the future are reduced in the direction of living more fully and contentedly in the immediate present. In an attempt to assess the personality changes that followed operation, the Minnesota Multiphasic Personality Inventory was administered to 100 consecutive cases before and after operation. The clinical scales of the inventory showed a marked decrease in group means after operation. This effect was differential, the most marked alterations being in the Depression, Hysteria, Psychasthenia and Schizophrenia scales (beyond 0.001 significance level).

Against the generally favourable improvement on the MMPI, one scale moved in an adverse direction. This was the Ego Strength (Es) scale, which had been derived from the MMPI by Barron (1953) who felt that this scale reflected the ego strength or latent capacity for integration in the personality, the potential of the personality for coping with situations. The decrease in this scale after operation might support the frequently made claim that leucotomy may lead to a lessening of constructive forces within the personality. It is a reminder that even modified operations may not be carried out with complete immunity. An item analysis showed that many items moved in the 'improved' direction following treatment. The most frequent improvement was in those items related to self-concern expressed either as general painful rumination, brooding or worrying, or related to specific areas of dysfunction, most notably concern about mental health or concern over somatic complaints. Accompanying these changes was an improvement in items reflecting introversion. Items expressing depressive mood also showed marked improvement.

If these changes were the principal cause of improvement there should have been an overlap between the most frequently changed items and those taken from the most improved cases. This was the case, the items being those which expressed the central themes of self-concern, introversion and depressed psychological mood in the most unambiguous manner.

Item analysis related to particular symptoms showed that anxieties, phobias and painful rumination were most affected, obsessions improved to a lesser degree, and hallucinations and delusions remained unchanged.

Since the main principle of selection was centred around the notion of tortured rumination about the self, it follows that we would anticipate alteration in self-concern in successful cases. A comparison of 14 'most improved' with 14 'least improved' cases, using Robinson's three tests of self-continuity (Robinson & Freeman 1954), showed a highly significant difference on all measures when the patients were examined 1–2 years after operation. Those cases classed as improved showed significantly lower scores on the measures of self-concern than those classed as unimproved. One can conclude that a reduction in the capacity for the feeling of self-continuity may be regarded as a central mechanism of psychosurgery.

These findings have several implications:

i. It is only where the particular personality changes described are likely to lead to a better overall state for the patient that a rationale exists for operation.

ii. Not only are major frontal sections which produce more drastic changes unjustified, even modified operations may be inimical where decreased self-concern might aggravate rather than help the patient's condition.

iii. Selection should be based on symptomatology rather than nosology.

The latter point seems particularly important. Reliance on traditional diagnostic categories in selection often led to disappointing results, since the symptom complex most likely to be favourably affected was not highly represented in the cases. The failure of frequently cited 'controlled' studies to show significant improvement after operation is misleading when an examination of the type of case operated shows a remarkable absence of rational principles of selection (Robin 1958, Vosburg 1962, McKenzie & Kaczanowski 1964).

Follow-up studies in series like our own suggested that operation was successful to the degree that the symptom complex of tense rumination was present. Where such symptoms formed only part of the clinical picture, e.g. in what has been termed pseudoneurotic schizophrenia, only part of the condition was helped. It would not be logical to expect otherwise.

Finally, the present author had the opportunity of following a small number of patients for almost two decades. Clinical examination supplemented by psychological examination (including the MMPI in a few cases) demonstrated that the changes brought about by operation were still apparent.

The principal feature of modified leucotomy appears to be a modification of the personality in the direction of lessened self-concern. It is probable that this is the central factor by which various forms of prefrontal operation bring about relief of symptoms.

COGNITIVE CHANGES WITH MODIFIED LEUCOTOMY

While cognitive changes appeared to be minor with modified operations and did not trouble the patient in everyday life even in demanding occupations, they are of some theoretical significance in the light of more recent studies.

It was the general opinion that it was encroachment on the dorsolateral frontal regions which led to intellectual deficit following radical lobotomy (Malmo 1948, Petrie 1952a, Smith & Kinder 1959). Hamlin (1970) showed that the long term losses of 'superior topectomy' patients (upper frontal lesions) on intelligence measures were appreciable, whereas orbital topectomy cases examined after the same postoperative period of 14 years showed scores 'remarkably comparable to those of nonoperated controls' (p. 307). Operations of all types confined to the orbitomedial area seem to have been relatively free of intellectual loss, at least as measured by standardized tests. This is now understandable since such tests are greatly dependent upon long-stored information and skills. Most of them are not of the sort to elicit the subtle changes in the regulation of behaviour by the initiation and monitoring of appropriate plans of action which have been described above.

Frontal planning difficulties in some of our cases were well brought out by the Kohs block designs. Though this is a complex task that is also failed by patients with lesions in retrorolandic regions, an examination of the type of performance shows some pathognomonic features in frontal patients. Lhermitte et al (1972) pointed out that a number of steps are necessary in the solution of the block design problems, namely, preliminary analysis, generation of a programme, implementation and control of the programme and final comparison. Patients with frontal damage may fail at any stage, often being blocked in their attempts at solution at the stage of preliminary analysis: '*il faut en effet, decomposer le modèle en ses cubes constitutifs de façon a pouvoir choisir le nombre et les faces correctes des ces cubes. Sans cette analyse préalable, la reproduction des modèles est tout a fait impossible*' (Lhermitte et al 1972, p. 429). That is, to be successful one has to break down the design mentally into its component parts and without this preliminary work the task is impossible.

The Goldstein and Scheerer (1941) version of the block design test was given to 14 of our operated subjects and a matched control group. If subjects could not complete the design with the small pictured example they were given a design equal in size to the four blocks utilized in construction. If this was failed, they were given a design with the lines of the edges of the blocks superimposed on the design, either in a reduced size or a larger version equal to the size of four blocks. No control subject needed any of this assistance, whereas the operated subjects often needed a partial programme for the solution, the divided diagram being of particular assistance to most subjects (Fig. 4.17). Design 10 shown in the diagram presented marked difficulty for 9 of the 14 subjects. Qualitative differences were seen in the experimental group. Several subjects expressed puzzlement that a particular design could be reproduced and even after completing the design exhibited uncertainty about it. Several other subjects successfully copied a design, expressed dissatisfaction, broke up the design and commenced again. Subject 14 had no difficulty up to design 7. After great trouble with this design she was given assistance in the form of a large undivided design, then a smaller divided design but still failed. After a long time she succeeded with the aid of the large divided design, but volunteered the remark 'You're sure it is possible to get the other one right?'. She could see no apparent connection between the original design and the 'assisted' versions which followed. In view of the position and relatively small size of lesions in our series and the apparent preservation of the patients' intelligence, these signs take on added significance. They appear identical in nature to, though less pronounced than, those described with massive frontal lesions. Design 10 also proved difficult for the patient described by Luria and Tsvetkova (1964).

The second area of difficulty was seen on two maze problems. There was a

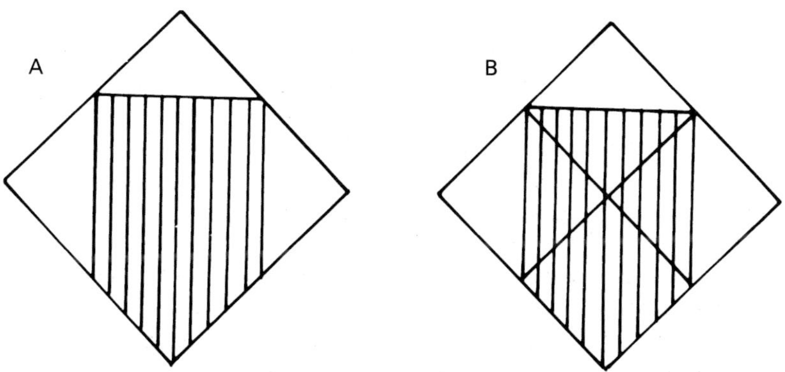

Fig. 4.17 Block design: A, undivided; B, divided design.

slightly poorer performance by operated subjects than controls on the Porteus Maze Test. Such a loss has been reported frequently with frontal lesions and needs no further documentation. On a second type of maze, an electrical stylus maze (Walsh 1960), the patients showed more of the qualitative types of error described by Milner (1965) in the section above, though the difference between leucotomy and control subjects failed to reach significance. These errors reflected frequent failure to comply with the test instructions, though patients showed very clearly on questioning that they understood the rules. Moreover, the knowledge of their errors did not modify the patients' subsequent behaviour or, at least, did not do so as quickly as it did in control subjects. Similarly, the patients often failed on problems of the Porteus Maze Tests by repeatedly entering the incorrect alley while often remarking that their choice *was going to be incorrect*. In a minor way this seems to reflect the difficulty which frontal damaged patients have in inhibiting response tendencies once they have been aroused.

The final example of cognitive impairment comes from the Colour-Form Sorting Test. In this test no control subject experienced difficulty. Again, qualitative differences were noted in the experimental group. Only one of the experimental subjects gave a spontaneous verbal account of the correct groupings. Four others were able to complete the two groupings and showed evidence when questioned that they had successfully classified the pieces and were able to shift from one group to the other. All the remaining subjects required further assistance.

Three of the experimental subjects were only able to shift to the second of the groupings after a considerable amount of verbal assistance and a demonstration of the second group by the tester. Two others were able to perform both groupings after explanation as well as documentation of both colour and form groupings. Three subjects were unable to complete either sorting, irrespective of the amount of instruction and assistance given.

The difficulties of scoring such material can be seen in Subject 1, who placed similar forms together and described them in terms of common objects. The request to sort them differently resulted in another grouping described as everyday objects. The subject was then presented with the proper colour groupings. Her response was: 'They don't fit just like that. They don't fit into a pattern according to size. You could have numbers, size, colours'. Despite this verbalization of an apparently high order of abstraction, she was unable to perform the colour groupings, and resorted to several form groupings, the last of which comprised three groups of forms placed in a row. She explained that the pieces were ordered according to length. Several other examples will demonstrate how difficult it may be to quantify these changes in behaviour.

Subject 9 first grouped forms together and gave a correct account. Asked to do it a second way, she persisted in separating the forms, but used them to represent concrete objects. Shown the colour groupings and asked to account for them, she replied: 'One of each shape in each group'.

E: 'What do they have in common?'
S: 'Shape in common. The number in the group.'
E: 'What would you call that group?' (pointing to green pieces)
S: 'The right-hand corner. There are two (groups) in the right-hand corner and two in the left.'

Subject 4 began by turning over the four squares to their white sides to represent a 'tile'. The four circles were placed together as 'rings' while the triangles were 'going to make an octagon; but I need another one'. The request to sort the pieces another way resulted in a more complex pattern. The demonstration of colour sorting seemingly made no sense to her, while the form sorting with the white sides up evoked the following response:

E: 'Does that make sense?'
S: 'Only that you are sorting them out…into one colour…white.'

Such subjects cannot be said to have lost all ability to categorize or abstract, yet they appear to have great difficulty with a task which normal individuals perform readily. The relatively poor performance of patients on these tasks is in sharp contrast to the fact that these were clinically improved subjects coping with their occupations at their preoperative level. However, Goldstein (1944) pointed out that in everyday life much thinking runs in such familiar ways, i.e. learned patterns of responses, that frontal impairment may not be evident to the patient's physician or friends.

In the early part of the eighties, the Boston group studied extensively 16 schizophrenics subjected to prefrontal leucotomy over 25 years previously and compared their results with non-operated schizophrenics and control subjects (Benson et al 1981, Benson & Stuss 1982, Stuss & Benson 1983, 1984, Stuss et al 1981a, b, 1982a, b, 1983). The lesions were variable in size and extent, as well as sometimes being asymmetrical. Although the lesions were described as orbitofrontal, it is apparent from the data provided that many of them must have severed portions of the thalamo-frontal radiation, thus isolating considerable sections of the dorsolateral cortex. The nature of the preoperative psychiatric disorder is also vastly different from that in those patients subjected to modified leucotomy.

Nevertheless, the general tenor of the Boston results compares well with the summaries in this chapter. The operated subjects differed in being more concrete in their responses, with a difficulty in shifting set and maintaining sequences of correct responses, and a dissociation between verbalization and action. These changes were independent of IQ measures from the WAIS. While there was no deficit on one of the abstraction tasks used, the Metaphor Test of Winner and Gardner (1977), the content of the test was familiar and the use of the content not sufficiently demanding to test the 'abstract attitude' in the sense described earlier.

A 10 year follow-up of obsessive-compulsive patients subjected to modified operations showed a poor performance only on the Wisconsin Card Sorting test, with general intellectual preservation (Hay et al 1993).

Finally, even 40 years after surgery, there appeared to be no interaction between the cognitive effects of surgery and ageing effects in schizophrenic patients (Harvey et al 1993).

FRONTAL LOBE SYNDROME: ONE OR MANY?

It will now be apparent that the term *frontal lobe syndrome* is a very general term indeed, covering as it does the disruption of a vast geographic area, with areas which are probably both histologically and functionally distinct, and the matter is not likely to be clarified without a good deal of correlative work on discrete cases which, for obvious reasons, will be slow in coming. As Mesulam (1986) commented: 'The specific pattern of the behavioural deficits in an individual patient is probably determined by the site, size, laterality, nature, and temporal course of the lesion and perhaps even by the past personality of the patient and age of onset' (p. 323).

Major texts which have attempted to cover this vast topic have differed significantly in the ways in which they have partitioned the task (compare Stuss & Benson 1986 with Fuster 1989).

In an earlier symposium, nicely entitled 'The riddle of frontal lobe function in man', in speaking of his wide experience with the study of frontal lesion cases, Teuber (1964) remarked: 'I started out by trying to find a unitary concept, but as I moved along, it became clear that no single-factor hypothesis could carry one far enough to cover all the manifestations of frontal lesions. And yet the thing that is so tempting to me after this symposium is to think that there may be a family resemblance among symptoms, even among those which seem in part dissociable'.

As in other areas, the nature of the clinical material available has hindered the development of a theory of the contribution of different frontal areas, despite the known anatomic specificity (Hécaen & Albert 1978). Few unique cases with localized pathology have been studied carefully with appropriate neuropsychological methods. Even the deliberately inflicted lesions of psychosurgery are noted for their variability. Coupled with this, and in order to test the complex functions of the frontal lobes, many of the tests which have been used are themselves complex. This means that there can be sundry reasons for individual failures.

One theoretical system which appears to be capable of incorporating the manifold aspects of frontal lobe dysfunction, both in man and animals, is that of Fuster who sees the prefrontal cortex as a kind of superordinate functional system much along the lines of the earlier formulations of Luria. This system is responsible for 'the formation of temporal structure of behavior with a unifying purpose or goal' (Fuster 1980, p. 126). The *temporal structures* endow the organism to deal with the four major characteristics of behaviour if this is to be adaptive: (i) changing demands; (ii) novelty; (iii) complexity; and (iv) integration over time. Fuster sees these component processes as served by the synthetic role of the prefrontal cortex. To be successful the system must be able to anticipate (plan) future outcomes and retain the scheme or plan with the elements executed to date until the goal is attained, and must be able to avert interfering influences that threaten to disrupt it.

References

Ackerly S S, Benton A L 1948 Report of a case of bilateral frontal lobe defect. Research Publications, Association for Research in Nervous and Mental Disease 27: 479–504

Aimard G, Robert H, Boisson D, Confavreux C, Devic M 1983 Utilization behavior during the course of a progressive multifocal leukoencephalopathy. Revue Neurologique 139: 307–308

Aita J A, Armitage S G, Reitan R M, Rabinowitz A 1947 The use of certain psychological tests in the evaluation of brain injury. Journal of General Psychology 37: 25–44

Allison R S 1966 Perseveration as a sign of diffuse and focal brain damage. British Medical Journal 2: 1095–1101
Allison R S, Hurwitz L J 1967 On perseveration in aphasics. Brain 90: 429–448
Ames D, Cummings J L, Wirshing W C, Quinn B, Mahler M 1994 Repetitive and compulsive behavior in frontal lobe degenerations. Journal of Neuropsychiatry and Clinical Neurosciences 6: 100–113
Appelbaum S A 1960 Automatic and selective processes in the word associations of brain damaged and normal subjects. Journal of Personality 28: 64–72
Arnot R E 1949 Clinical indications for prefrontal lobotomy. Journal of Nervous and Mental Disease 109: 267–269
Baddeley A 1986 Working memory. Oxford University Press, London
Baddeley A, Wilson B 1988 Frontal amnesia and the dysexecutive syndrome. Brain and Cognition 7: 212–230
Baer D J 1964 Factors in perception and rigidity. Perceptual and Motor Skills 19: 563–570
Barbizet J 1970 Human memory and its pathology. Freeman, San Francisco
Barron F 1953 An ego strength scale which predicts response to therapy. Journal of Consulting Psychology 17: 327–333
Battersby W S 1956 Neuropsychology of higher processes: cerebral damage and visual perception. In: Progress in clinical psychology. Grune and Stratton, New York
Battersby W S, Teuber H L, Bender M B 1953 Problem solving behavior in men with frontal or occipital brain injuries. Journal of Psychology 35: 329–351
Battersby W S, Krieger H P, Bender M B 1955 Visual and tactile discriminative learning in patients with cerebral tumors. American Journal of Psychiatry 70: 703–712
Baxter L R 1992 Neuroimaging studies of obsessive compulsive disorder. Psychiatric Clinics of North America 15: 871–884
Benson D F 1977 The third alexia. Archives of Neurology 34: 327–331
Benson D F 1979 Aphasia, alexia and agraphia. Churchill Livingstone, Edinburgh
Benson D F 1985 Alexia. In: Vinken P J, Bruyn G W, Klawans H L (eds) Handbook of clinical neurology. New Series 1, vol 45. Elsevier, Amsterdam
Benson D F, Stuss D T 1982 Motor abilities after frontal leukotomy. Neurology 32: 1353–1357
Benson D F, Stuss D T, Naeser M A, Weir W S, Kaplan E F, Levine H L 1981 The long-term effects of pre-frontal leucotomy. Archives of Neurology 38: 165–169
Benson D F, Djenderedjian A, Miller B L, Pachana N A, Chang L, Itti L, Mena I 1996 Neural basis of confabulation. Neurology 46: 1239–1243
Benton A L 1968 Differential behavioral effects of frontal lobe disease. Neuropsychologia 6: 53–60
Benton A L, Fogel M L 1962 Three dimensional constructional praxis. Archives of Neurology 7: 347–354
Benton A, Elithorn A, Fogel M, Kerr M 1963 A perceptual maze test sensitive to brain damage. Journal of Neurology, Neurosurgery and Psychiatry 26: 540–544
Berlyne N 1972 Confabulation. British Journal of Psychiatry 120: 31–39
Birkmayer W 1951 Hirnverletzungen Mechanismus, Spaetkomplitationen Funktions Wandel. Springer, Vienna
Black F W 1976 Cognitive deficits in patients with unilateral war-related frontal lobe lesions. Journal of Clinical Psychology 32: 366–372
Bonhoeffer K 1904 Der Korsakowsche Symptomenkomplex in seinen Beziehungen zu den verschieden Krankheitsformen. Allgemeine Zeitschrift für Psychiatrie 61: 744–752
Bourne L E 1966 Human conceptual behavior. Allyn and Bacon, Boston
Bradley K C, Dax E C, Walsh K W 1958 Modified leucotomy: report of 100 cases. Medical Journal of Australia 1: 133–138
Brickner R 1934 An interpretation of frontal lobe function based upon the study of a case of partial bilateral frontal lobectomy. Research Publications, Association for Research in Nervous and Mental Disease 13: 259–351
Buge A, Escourolle R, Rancurel G, Poisson M 1975 Mutisme akinétique et ramollissement bi-cingulaire. Revue Neurologique 131: 121–137
Buss A H 1952 Some determinants of rigidity in discrimination reversal learning. Journal of Experimental Psychology 44: 222–227
Cambier J, Masson M, Viader F, Limodin J, Strube A 1985 Frontal syndrome of progressive supranuclear palsy. Revue Neurologique 141: 528–536

Caramazza A, Berndt R S 1979 Semantic and syntactic processes in aphasia. A review of the literature. Psychological Bulletin 85: 898–918

Cattell R B, Tiner L B 1949 The varieties of structural rigidity. Journal of Personality 17: 321–341

Cattell R B, Dubin S S, Saunders D K 1954 Verification of hypothesized factors in one hundred and fifteen objective personality tests. Psychometrika 19: 209–230

Chapman L F, Wolff H F 1959 The cerebral hemispheres and the highest integrative functions of man. Archives of Neurology 1: 357–424

Chedru F, Leblanc M, Lhermitte F 1973 Visual searching in normal and brain-damaged subjects (contribution to the study of unilateral inattention). Cortex 9: 94–111

Chown S H 1959 Rigidity – a flexible concept. Psychological Bulletin 56: 195–223

Christensen A L 1975 Luria's neuropsychological investigation. Munksgaard, Copenhagen

Cicerone K D, Lazar R M, Shapiro W R 1983 Effects of frontal lobe lesions on hypothesis sampling during concept formation. Neuropsychologia 21: 513–524

Cohen L 1959 Perception of reversible figures after brain injury. Archives of Neurology and Psychiatry 81: 765–775

Cosgrove G R, Rauch S L 1995 Psychosurgery. Neurosurgery Clinics of North America 6: 167–176

Critchley M 1953 The parietal lobes. Arnold, London

Crown S 1952 An experimental study of psychological changes following prefrontal lobotomy. Journal of General Psychology 47: 3–41

Cumming S, Hay P, Lee T, Sachdev P 1995 Neuropsychological outcome from psychosurgery for obsessive-compulsive disorder. Australian and New Zealand Journal of Psychiatry 29: 293–298

Daffner K R, Scinto L M, Weintraub S, Mesulam M-M 1991 Diminished curiosity in patients with probable Alzheimer's disease as measured by exploratory eye movements. Neurology 41 (suppl 1): 235

Daffner K R, Scinto L M, Weintraub S, Guinnessey J, Mesulam M-M 1994 The impact of aging on curiosity as measured by exploratory eye movements. Archives of Neurology 51: 368–376

Dana C L 1915 Textbook of nervous diseases, 8th edn. Wood, New York

Darby D G, Nobre A C, Thangaraj V, Edelman R, Mesulam M-M, Warach S 1996 Cortical activation in the human brain during lateral saccades using EPISTAR functional magnetic resonance imaging. Neuroimage 3: 53–62

Dax E C, Radley Smith E J 1945 Prefrontal leucotomy with reference to indications and results. Proceedings of the Royal Society of Medicine 39: 448

Delis D C, Squire L R, Bihrle A, Massman P 1992 Componential analysis of problem-solving ability: performance of patients with frontal lobe damage and amnesic patients on a new sorting test. Neuropsychologia 30: 683–697

De Luca J 1992 Cognitive dysfunction following aneurysm of the anterior communicating artery. Journal of Clinical and Experimental Neuropsychology 14: 924–934

De Luca J 1993 Predicting neurobehavioral patterns following anterior communicating artery aneurysm. Cortex 29: 639–647

Derouesné C 1973 Le syndrome 'pré-moteur'. Revue Neurologique 128: 353–363

Dew H R 1922 Tumours of the brain: Their pathology and treatment; an analysis of 85 cases. Medical Journal of Australia 1: 515–521

Dimitrov M, Grafman J, Hollnagel C 1996 The effects of frontal lobe damage on everyday problem solving. Cortex 32: 357–366

Doehring D G, Reitan R M 1962 Behavioral consequences of brain damage associated with homonymous visual field defects. Journal of Comparative and Physiological Psychology 54: 489–492

Donovan N J, Barry J J 1994 Compulsive symptoms associated with frontal lobe injury. 151: 618

Drewe E A 1975a Go-No-Go learning after frontal lobe lesions in humans. Cortex 11: 8–16

Drewe E A 1975b An experimental investigation of Luria's theory on the effects of frontal lobe lesions in man. Neuropsychologia 13: 421–429

Elithorn A 1955 A preliminary report on a perceptual maze test sensitive to brain damage. Journal of Neurology, Neurosurgery and Psychiatry 18: 287–292

Elithorn A, Kerr M, Jones D 1963 A binary perceptual maze. American Journal of Psychology 76: 506–508

Eslinger P J, Damasio A R 1985 Severe disturbance of higher cognition after bilateral frontal lobe ablation: patient EVR. Neurology 35: 1731–1741
Eslinger P J, Warner G C, Grattan L M, Easton J D 1991 "Frontal lobe" utilization behavior associated with paramedian thalamic infarction. Neurology 41: 450–452
Fabbri W 1956 Leucotomia transorbitaria di Fiamberti e rispetto della personalità individuale nei rilievi psicometrici con il test di Porteus. Note e Riviste di Psichiatria 45: 311–332
Feather N T 1966 Effects of prior success and failure on expectations of success and subsequent performance. Journal of Personality and Social Psychology 3: 287–298
Feuchtwanger E 1923 Die Funktionen des stirnhirnes, ihre Pathologie und Psychologie. Springer, Berlin
Fischer R S, Alexander M P, D'Esposito M, Otto R 1995 Neuropsychological and neuroanatomical correlates of confabulation. Journal of Clinical and Experimental Neuropsychology 17: 20–28
Fisher C M 1989 Neurologic fragments. II. Remarks on anosognosia, confabulation, memory, and other topics; and an appendix on self-observation. Neurology 39: 127–132
Fisher S 1949 An overview of trends in research dealing with rigidity. Journal of Personality 17: 342–351
Fleming G W T H 1942 Some preliminary remarks on prefrontal leucotomy. Journal of Mental Science 88: 282–284
Freeman W 1953a Level of achievement after lobotomy: a study of 1000 cases. American Journal of Psychiatry 110: 269–276
Freeman W 1953b Hazards of lobotomy: report on 200 operations. Archives of Neurology and Psychiatry 69: 640–643
Freeman W 1958 Frontal leucotomy and its congeners. Diseases of the Nervous System 19: 11–15
Freeman W, Watts J W 1942 Psychosurgery. Thomas, Springfield, Illinois
Freeman W, Watts J W 1948 The thalamic projection to the frontal lobe. Research Publications, Association for Research in Nervous and Mental Disease 27: 200–209
Freeman W, Watts J W 1950 Psychosurgery, 2nd edn. Thomas, Springfield, Illinois
Freemon F R 1971 Akinetic mutism and bilateral anterior cerebral artery occlusion. Journal of Neurology, Neurosurgery and Psychiatry 34: 693–698
Fukui T, Hasegawa Y, Sugita K, Tsukagoshi H 1993 Utilization behavior and concomitant motor neglect by bilateral frontal lobe damage. European Neurology 33: 325–330
Fuster J M 1980 The prefrontal cortex. Raven, New York
Fuster J M 1989 The prefrontal cortex, 2nd edn. Raven, New York
Ghent L, Mishkin M, Teuber H L 1962 Short-term memory after frontal lobe injury in man. Journal of Comparative and Physiological Psychology 55: 705–709
Girgis M 1971 The orbital surface of the frontal lobe of the brain. Acta Psychiatrica Scandinavica, Supplementum 222: 1–58
Gleason W J 1953 Rigidity and negative transfer effects in patients with cerebral damage. Unpublished doctoral dissertation, Northwestern University
Goel V, Grafman J 1995 Are the frontal lobes implicated in "planning" functions? Interpreting data from the Tower of Hanoi. Neuropsychologia 33: 623–642
Golden C J 1976 Identification of brain disorders by the Stroop color and word test. Journal of Clinical Psychology 32: 654–658
Goldstein G, Neuringer C, Olson J 1968 Impairment of abstract reasoning in the brain-damaged: Qualitative or quantitative? Cortex 4: 372–388
Goldstein K 1936a The significance of the frontal lobes for mental performance. Journal of Neurology and Psychopathology 17: 27–40
Goldstein K 1936b The modification of behavior consequent to cerebral lesions. Psychiatric Quarterly 10: 586–610
Goldstein K 1939a Clinical and theoretical aspects of lesions of the frontal lobes. Archives of Neurology and Psychiatry 41: 865–867
Goldstein K 1939b The organism. American Book, New York
Goldstein K 1940 Human nature. Harvard University Press, Cambridge, Massachusetts
Goldstein K 1942a After effects of brain injuries in war. Grune and Stratton, New York
Goldstein K 1942b The two ways of adjustment of the organism to central defects. Journal of the Mount Sinai Hospital 9: 504–513
Goldstein K 1943 Brain concussion: Evaluation of the after effects by special tests. Diseases of the Nervous System 4: 3–12

Goldstein K 1944 Mental changes due to frontal lobe damage. Journal of Psychology 17: 187–208
Goldstein K 1959 Functional disturbances in brain damage. In: Arieti S (ed) American handbook of psychiatry. Basic Books, New York, vol 1, ch 39
Goldstein K, Gelb A 1918 Psychologischen Analysen Hirnpathologischer Falle auf Grund von Untersuchungen Hirnverletzer. Zeitschrift für die gesamte Neurologie und Psychiatrie 41: 1
Goldstein K, Scheerer M 1941 Abstract and concrete behavior: An experimental study with special tests. Psychological Monographs 43: 1–151
Goldstein L H, Bernard S, Fenwick P B, Burgess P W, McNeil J 1993 Unilateral frontal lobectomy can produce strategy application disorder. Journal of Neurology, Neurosurgery and Psychiatry 56: 274–276
Grant A D, Berg E A 1948 A behavioral analysis of degree of reinforcement and ease of shifting to new responses in a Weigl-type card sorting. Journal of Experimental Psychology 38: 404–411
Grantham E C 1951 Prefrontal lobotomy for the relief of pain with a report of a new operative technique. Journal of Neurosurgery 8: 405
Grassi J R 1950 Impairment of abstract behavior following bilateral prefrontal lobotomy. Psychiatric Quarterly 24: 74–88
Greenblatt M, Arnold R, Solomon H C 1950 Studies in lobotomy. Grune and Stratton, New York
Greenblatt S H 1983 Localization of lesions in alexia. In: Kertesz A (ed) Localization in neuropsychology. Academic Press, New York, pp 323–356
Gregson R A M, Taylor G M 1975 An administrative manual for the Patterned Cognitive Impairment Test Battery. University of Canterbury, New Zealand
Halstead W C 1940 Preliminary analysis of grouping behavior in patients with cerebral injury by the method of equivalent and non-equivalent stimuli. American Journal of Psychology 96: 1263–1294
Halstead W C 1947 Brain and intelligence. University of Chicago Press, Chicago
Halstead W C 1959 The statics and the dynamics. In: Beck S J, Molish H B (eds) Reflexes to intelligence. The Free Press, Glencoe, Illinois
Hamlin R M 1970 Intellectual function 14 years after frontal lobe surgery. Cortex 6: 299–307
Hanfmann E, Rickers-Ovsiankina M, Goldstein K 1944 Case Lanuti extreme concretization of behavior of the brain cortex. Psychological Monographs 57, no 4, whole no 264
Harvey O J, Hunt D E, Schroeder D M 1961 Conceptual systems and personality organization. Wiley, New York
Harvey P D, Mohs R C, Davidson M 1993 Leukotomy and aging in chronic schizophrenia: a follow up study 40 years after psychosurgery. Schizophrenia Bulletin 19: 723–732
Hashimoto R, Yoshida M, Tanaka Y 1995 Utilization behavior after right thalamic infarction. European Neurology 35: 58–62
Hay P, Sachdev P, Cumming S et al 1993 Treatment of obsessive-compulsive disorder with psychosurgery. Acta Psychiatrica Scandinavica 87: 197–207
Hebb D O 1939 Intelligence in man after large removals of cerebral tissue: report of four left frontal lobe cases. Journal of General Psychology 21: 73–87
Hebb D O 1941 Human intelligence after removal of cerebral tissue from the right frontal lobe. Journal of General Psychology 25: 257–265
Hebb D O 1945 Man's frontal lobes: a critical review. Archives of Neurology and Psychiatry 54: 10–24
Hebb D O 1949 The organization of behavior. Wiley, New York
Hebb D O, Penfield W 1940 Human behavior after extensive bilateral removal from the frontal lobes. Archives of Neurology and Psychiatry 44: 421–438
Hécaen H 1964 Mental symptoms associated with tumors of the frontal lobe. In: Warren J M, Akert K (eds) The frontal granular cortex and behavior. McGraw Hill, New York, ch 16
Hécaen H, Albert M L 1978 Human neuropsychology. Wiley, New York
Herrick C J 1963 Brains in rats and men. (Reprinted from 1926) University of Chicago Press, Chicago
Hillbom E 1960 After effects of brain injuries. Acta Psychiatrica Neurologica Scandinavica 35, Supplementum 142: 5–195
Hohne H H, Walsh K W 1970 Surgical modification of the personality. Mental Health

Authority, Victoria, Special Publications no 2. Victorian Government Printer, Melbourne
Jackson J H 1864, 1874, 1876 See: Taylor J (ed) Selected writings of John Hughlings Jackson. Basic Books, New York, 1958
Jefferson G 1937 Removal of right or left frontal lobes in man. British Medical Journal 2: 199–206
Joanette Y, Stemmer B, Assal G, Whitaker H 1993 From theory to practice: The unconventional contribution of Gottlieb Burckhardt to psychosurgery. Brain and Language 45: 572–587
Johnson G, Parsons O A, Holloway F A, Bruhn P 1973 Intradimensional reversal shift performance in brain-damaged and chronic alcoholic patients. Journal of Consulting and Clinical Psychology 40: 253–258
Jones-Gotman M, Milner B 1977 Design fluency: the invention of nonsense drawings after focal cortical lesions. Neuropsychologia 15: 653–674
Jurgens U, Von Cramon D 1982 On the role of the anterior cingulate cortex in phonation: a case report. Brain and Language 15: 234–248
Kapur N, Coughlan A K 1980 Confabulation and frontal lobe dysfunction. Journal of Neurology, Neurosurgery and Psychiatry 43: 461–463
Kauffman I 1963 Some aspects of brain damage as related to Einstellung. Journal of Neuropsychiatry 4: 143–148
Kertesz A 1979 Aphasia and associated disorders: taxonomy, localization and recovery. Grune and Stratton, New York
Kimble D P 1963 Physiological psychology. Addison-Wesley, Reading, Massachusetts
Kirshner H S, Webb W G 1982 Word and letter reading and the mechanism of the third alexia. Archives of Neurology 39: 84–87
Kisker G W 1944 Abstract and categorical behaviour following therapeutic brain surgery. Psychosomatic Medicine 6: 146–150
Kitchen N 1995 Neurosurgery for affective disorders at Atkinson Morley's Hospital 1948–1994. Acta Neurochirurgica Supplementum (Wien) 64: 64–68
Knight G 1965 Stereotactic tractotomy in the surgical treatment of mental illness. Journal of Neurology, Neurosurgery and Psychiatry 28: 304–310
Knight G 1972 Psychosurgery today. Proceedings of the Royal Society of Medicine 65: 1099–1108
Knight G, Tredgold R F 1955 Orbital leucotomy. A review of 52 cases. Lancet 1: 981–985
Konow A, Pribram K H 1970 Error recognition and utilization produced by injury to the frontal cortex in man. Neuropsychologia 8: 489–491
Kopelman M D 1987 Two types of confabulation. Journal of Neurology, Neurosurgery and Psychiatry 50: 1482–1487
Laitinen L V, Livingston K E (eds) 1973 Surgical approaches to psychiatry. Medical and Technical, Lancaster
Landis C, Zubin J, Mettler F A 1950 The functions of the human frontal lobe. Journal of Psychology 30: 123–138
Làdavas E, Umiltà C, Provinciali L 1979 Hemisphere-dependent cognitive performances in epileptic patients. Epilepsia 20: 493–502
Lewis N D C, Landis C, King H E 1956 Studies in topectomy. Grune and Stratton, New York
Lhermitte F 1983 'Utilization behaviour' and its relation to lesions of the frontal lobes. Brain 106: 237–255
Lhermitte F 1986 Human autonomy and the frontal lobes. Part II. Patient behavior in complex and social situations: the "environmental dependency syndrome". Annals of Neurology 19: 335–343
Lhermitte F 1993 Imitation and utilization behavior in major depressive states. Bulletin de l'Académie Nationale de Médicine 177: 890–892
Lhermitte F, Derouesné J, Signoret J L 1972 Analyse neuropsychologique du syndrome frontal. Revue Neurologique 127: 415–440
Lhermitte F, Pillon B, Serdaru M 1986 Human autonomy and the frontal lobes. Part I. Imitation and utilization behavior: a neuropsychological study of 75 patients. Annals of Neurology 19: 326–334
Luria A R 1963 Restoration of function after brain injury. Macmillan, New York
Luria A R 1965 Two kinds of motor perseveration in massive injury of the frontal lobes. Brain 88: 1–10

Luria A R 1966 Higher cortical functions in man. Basic Books, New York
Luria A R, Homskaya E D, Blinkov S M, Critchley M 1967a Impaired selectivity of mental processes in association with a lesion of the frontal lobe. Neuropsychologia 5: 105–117
Luria A R, Solokov E N, Klimkovsky M 1967b Towards a neuro-dynamic analysis of memory disturbances with lesions of the left temporal lobe. Neuropsychologia 5: 1–12
Luria A R 1969 Frontal lobe syndromes in man. In: Vinken P J, Bruyn G W (eds) Handbook of clinical neurology. North-Holland, Amsterdam, vol 2, ch 23
Luria A R 1971 Memory disturbances in local brain lesions. Neuropsychologia 9: 367–376
Luria A R 1973a Towards the mechanisms of brain disturbance. Neuropsychologia 11: 417–421
Luria A R 1973b The working brain. Allen Lane, The Penguin Press, London
Luria A R, Homskaya E D 1963 Le trouble du role regulateur de langage au cours des lésions du lobe frontal. Neuropsychologia 1: 9–26
Luria A R, Homskaya E D 1964 Disturbance in the regulative role of speech with frontal lobe lesions. In: Warren J M, Akert K (eds) The frontal granular cortex and behavior. McGraw Hill, New York, ch 17
Luria A R, Tsvetkova L D 1964 The programming of constructive activity in local brain injuries. Neuropsychologia 2: 95–108
Luria A R, Tsvetkova L S 1967 Les troubles de la résolution des problèmes. Analyse neuropsychologique. Gauthier-Villars, Paris
Luria A R, Pribram K H, Homskaya E D 1964 An experimental analysis of the behavioral disturbance produced by a left frontal arachnoidal endothelioma (meningioma). Neuropsychologia 2: 257–280
Luria A R, Karpov B A, Yarbuss A L 1966 Disturbances of active visual perception with lesions of the frontal lobes. Cortex 2: 202–212
Luria A R, Sokolov E N, Klimkovsky M 1967 Towards a neuro-dynamic analysis of memory disturbances with lesions of the left temporal lobe. Neuropsychologia 5: 1–12
Mackie J B, Beck E C 1966 Relations among rigidity, intelligence, and perception in brain-damaged and normal individuals. Journal of Nervous and Mental Disease 142: 310–317
Malmo H P 1974 On frontal lobe functions: psychiatric patient controls. Cortex 10: 231–237
Malmo R B 1948 Psychological aspects of frontal gyrectomy and frontal lobotomy in mental patients. Research Publications, Association for Research in Nervous and Mental Disease 27: 537–564
McFie J, Piercy M F 1952a Intellectual impairment with localized cerebral lesions. Brain 75: 292–311
McFie J, Piercy M F 1952b The relation of laterality of lesions to performance on Weigl's Sorting Test. Journal of Mental Science 98: 299–305
McFie J, Thompson J A 1972 Picture arrangement: A measure of frontal lobe function? British Journal of Psychiatry 121: 547–552
McIntyre H D, Mayfield F H, McIntyre A P 1954 Ventromedial quadrant coagulation in the treatment of the psychoses and neuroses. American Journal of Psychiatry 111: 112–120
McKenzie K G, Kaczanowski G 1964 Prefrontal leucotomy. A five year controlled study. Canadian Medical Journal 91: 1193–1196
Mercer B, Wapner W, Gardner H, Benson D F 1977 A study of confabulation. Archives of Neurology 34: 429–433
Messerli P, Seron X, Tissot P 1979 Quelques aspects de la programmation dans le syndrome frontal. Archives Suisses de Neurologie, Neurochirurgie et de Psychiatrie 125: 23–35
Mesulam M-M 1986 Frontal cortex and behavior. Annals of Neurology 19: 320–325
Mettler F A (ed) 1949 Selective partial ablation of the frontal cortex. Hoeber, New York
Mettler F A (ed) 1952 Psychosurgical problems. Blakiston, New York
Miller E 1984 Verbal fluency as a function of a measure of verbal intelligence and in relation to different types of cerebral pathology. British Journal of Clinical Psychology 23: 53–57
Miller L A 1992 Impulsivity, risk-taking, and the ability to synthesize fragmented information after frontal lobectomy. Neuropsychologia 30: 69–79
Milner B 1963 Effects of different brain lesions on card sorting. Archives of Neurology 9: 90–100
Milner B 1964 Some effects of frontal lobectomy in man. In: Warren J M, Akert K (eds) The frontal granular cortex and behavior. McGraw Hill, New York, ch 15

Milner B 1965 Visually-guided maze learning in man: effects of bilateral hippocampal, bilateral frontal and unilateral cerebral lesions. Neuropsychologia 3: 317–338

Milner B 1971 Interhemispheric difference in the localization of psychological processes in man. British Medical Bulletin 27: 272–277

Milner B 1974 Hemispheric specialization scope and limits. In: Schmitt F O, Worden F G (eds) The neurosciences third study. MIT Press, Cambridge, Massachusetts, ch 8

Milner B 1975 Report on section on the "Frontal Lobes" at the 17th International Symposium of Neuropsychology. Neuropsychologia 13: 129–133

Milner B 1982 Some cognitive effects of frontal lobe lesions in man. Philosophical Transactions of the Royal Society of London. Series B: Biological Sciences 298: 211–226

Minski 1933 The mental symptoms associated with 58 cases of cerebral tumour. Journal of Neurology and Psychopathology 13: 330–343

Moll J M 1915 The amnestic or 'Korsakov's syndrome' with alcoholic aetiology: an analysis of thirty cases. Journal of Mental Science 61: 424–443

Moniz E 1937 Prefrontal leucotomy in the treatment of mental disorders. Reprinted 1994 in: American Journal of Psychiatry 151 (6 suppl): 236–239

Moniz E 1954 How I succeeded in performing the prefrontal leucotomy. Journal of Clinical and Experimental Psychopathology 15: 373–379

Morris R G, Ahmed S, Syed G M, Toone B K 1993 Neural correlates of planning ability: frontal lobe activation during the Tower of London test. Neuropsychologia 31: 1367–1378

Nathaniel-James D A, Frith C D 1996 Confabulation in schizophrenia: evidence of a new form? Psychological Medicine: 26: 391–399

Nelson H E 1976 A modified card sorting test sensitive to frontal lobe deficits. Cortex 12: 313–324

Nichols I C, Hunt J McV 1940 A case of partial bilateral frontal lobectomy: A psychopathological study. American Journal of Psychiatry 96: 1063–1087

Nielsen J, Jacobs L 1951 Bilateral lesions of the anterior cingulate gyri. Bulletin of the Los Angeles Neurological Society 16: 231–234

Nuttin J, Greenwald A G 1968 Reward and punishment in human learning. Academic Press, London

Orne M T 1962 On the social psychology of the psychological experiment: with particular reference to demand characteristics and their implication. American Psychologist 17: 776–783

Orne M T, Scheibe K E 1964 The contribution of nondeprivation factors in the production of sensory deprivation effects: the psychology of the panic button. Journal of Abnormal and Social Psychology 68: 3–12

Osterrieth P A 1944 Le test de copie d'une figure complexe. Archives de Psychologie 30: 206–353

Owen A M, Downes J J, Sahakian B J, Polkey C E, Robbins T W 1990 Planning and spatial working memory following frontal lobe lesions in man. Neuropsychologia 28: 1021–1034

Owen, A M, Roberts A C, Polkey C E, Sahakian B J, Robbins T W 1991 Extra-dimensional versus intra-dimensional set shifting performance following frontal lobe excisions, temporal lobe excisions or amygdalo-hippocampectomy in man. Neuropsychologia 29: 993–1006

Owen A M, Doyon J, Petrides M, Evans A C 1996 Planning and spatial working memory: a positron emission tomography study in human beings. European Journal of Neuroscience 8: 353–364

Papez J W 1929 Comparative neurology. Crowell, New York

Pendleton M G, Heaton R K, Lehman R A W, Hulihan D 1982 Diagnostic utility of the Thurstone word fluency test in neuropsychological evaluation. Journal of Clinical Neuropsychology 4: 307–317

Penfield W, Evans J 1935 The frontal lobe in man: a clinical study of maximum removals. Brain 58: 115–133

Perret E 1974 The left frontal lobe of man and the suppression of habitual responses in verbal categorical behavior. Neuropsychologia 12: 323–330

Petrides M, Milner B 1982 Deficits on subject-ordered tasks after frontal- and temporal-lobe lesions in man. Neuropsychologia 20: 249–262

Petrie A 1949 Preliminary report of changes after prefrontal leucotomy. Journal of Mental Science 95: 449–455

Petrie A 1952a Personality and frontal lobes. Routledge and Kegan Paul, London
Petrie A 1952b A comparison of the psychological effects of different types of operation on the frontal lobes. Journal of Mental Science 98: 326–329
Phelan J A, Gustafson C W 1968 Reversal and nonreversal shifts in acute brain-injured with injury diffusely organized. Journal of Psychology 70: 249–259
Phelps C 1897 Traumatic injuries of the brain and its membranes. Appleton, New York
Pikas A 1966 Abstraction and concept formation. Harvard University Press, Cambridge, Massachusetts
Poeck K, Kerschensteiner M 1975 In: Zülch K (ed) Cerebral localization. Springer-Verlag, Heidelberg
Pollack M 1960 Effect of brain tumor on perception of hidden figures, sorting behavior and problem solving performances. Dissertation Abstracts 20: 3405–3406
Poppen J L 1948 Prefrontal lobotomy: technique and general impression based on results in 470 patients subjected to this procedure. Digest of Neurology and Psychiatry 17: 403–408
Porteus S D 1950 The Porteus Maze Test and intelligence. Pacific, Palo Alto, California
Porteus S D 1958 What do the Maze Tests measure? Australian Journal of Psychology 10: 245–256
Porteus S D 1959 Recent maze test studies. British Journal of Medical Psychology 32: 38–43
Porteus S D 1965 Porteus Maze Test: fifty years' application. Pacific, Palo Alto, California
Porteus S D, Kepner R De M 1944 Mental changes after bilateral prefrontal lobotomy. Genetic Psychology Monographs 29: 3–115
Porteus S D, Peters H N 1947 Psychosurgery and test validity. Journal of Abnormal and Social Psychology 42: 473–475
Poynton A M 1993 Current state of psychosurgery. British Journal of Hospital Medicine 50: 408–411
Ramier A M, Hécaen H 1970 Role respectif des atteintes frontales et de la latéralization lésionelle dans le déficits de la fluence verbale. Revue Neurologique 123: 17–22
Reitan R M 1955 Investigation of the validity of Halstead's measures of biological intelligence. Archives of Neurology and Psychiatry 73: 28–35
Reitan R M 1958 Qualitative versus quantitative changes following brain damage. Journal of Psychology 46: 339–346
Reitan R M 1959 Impairment of abstraction ability in brain damage: Quantitative versus qualitative changes. Journal of Psychology 48: 97–102
Reitan R M 1964 Psychological deficits resulting from cerebral lesions in man. In: Warren J M, Akert K (eds) The frontal granular cortex and behavior. McGraw Hill, New York, ch 14
Rey A 1941 L'examen psychologique. Archives de Psychologie 28: 112–164
Rey A 1959 Le test de copie de figure complexe. Editions Centre de Psychologie Appliquée, Paris
Rezai K, Andreasen N C, Alliger R et al 1993 The neuropsychology of the prefrontal cortex. Archives of Neurology 50: 636–642
Ricci C, Blundo C 1990 Perception of ambiguous figures after frontal lesions. Neuropsychologia 28: 1163–1173
Ridley R M 1994 The psychology of perseverative and stereotyped behaviour. Progress in Neurobiology 44: 221–231
Robin A A 1958 A controlled study of the effects of leucotomy. Journal of Neurology, Neurosurgery and Psychiatry 21: 262–269
Robinson A L, Heaton R K, Lehman R A, Stilson D W 1980 The utility of the Wisconsin Card Sorting Test in detecting and localizing frontal lobe lesions. Journal of Consulting and Clinical Psychology 48: 605–614
Robinson M F, Freeman W 1954 Psychosurgery and the self. Grune and Stratton, New York
Rokeach M 1948 Generalized mental rigidity as a factor in ethnocentrism. Journal of Abnormal and Social Psychology 43: 259–278
Rolls E T, Hornak J, Wade D, McGrath J 1994 Emotion-related learning in patients with social and emotional changes associated with frontal lobe damage. Journal of Neurology, Neurosurgery and Psychiatry 57: 1518–1524
Rosvold H E, Mishkin M 1950 Evaluation of the effects of prefrontal lobotomy on intelligence. Canadian Journal of Psychology 4: 122–126
Rothi L J, McFarling D, Heilman K M 1982 Conduction aphasia, syntactic alexia and the anatomy of syntactic comprehension. Archives of Neurology 39: 272–275

Rylander G 1939 Personality changes after operations on the frontal lobes: clinical study of 32 cases. Acta Psychiatrica et Neurologica Scandinavica, Supplement 20: 5–81
Rylander G 1943 Mental changes after excision of cerebral tissue. Acta Psychiatrica et Neurologica Scandinavica, Supplement 25
Rylander G 1947 Psychological tests and personality analysis before and after frontal lobotomy. Acta Psychiatrica et Neurologica Scandinavica Supplement 147: 383–398
Samuels J A, Benson D F 1979 Some aspects of language comprehension in anterior aphasia. Brain and Language 8: 275–286
Schaie K W 1955 A test of behavioral rigidity. Journal of Abnormal and Social Psychology 51: 604–610
Schaie K W 1958 Rigidity-flexibility and intelligence. Psychological Monographs 72, no. 9, whole no. 462
Schnider A, von Daniken C, Gutbrod K 1996 The mechanisms of spontaneous and provoked confabulations. Brain 119: 1365–1375
Semmes J, Weinstein S, Ghent L, Teuber H L 1954 Performance on complex tactual tasks after brain injury to man: analyses by locus of lesion. American Journal of Psychology 67: 220–240
Servan J, Verstichel P, Catala M, Gutbrod K 1994 Amnestic syndromes and confabulation in infarction of the posterior cerebral artery area. Revue Neurologique 150: 201–208
Shallice T 1982 Specific impairments of planning. Philosophical Transactions of the Royal Society of London 298: 199–209
Shallice T, Burgess P W 1991 Deficits in strategy application following frontal lobe damage in man. Brain 114: 727–741
Shallice T, Evans M E 1978 The involvement of the frontal lobes in cognitive estimation. Cortex 14: 294–303
Shallice T, Burgess P W, Schon F, Baxter D M 1989 The origins of utilization behaviour. Brain 112: 1587–1598
Shapiro B E, Alexander M P, Gardner H, Mercer B 1981 Mechanisms of confabulation. Neurology 31: 1070–1076
Shure G H 1954 Intellectual loss following excision of cortical tissue. Unpublished doctoral dissertation, University of Chicago
Shure G H, Halstead W C 1958 Cerebral localization of intellectual processes. Psychological Monographs 72, whole no. 465
Simmel M B, Counts S 1957 Some stable response determinants of perception, thinking and learning. A study based on the analysis of a single test. Genetic Monographs 56: 3–157
Smith A 1966 Intellectual functions in patients with lateralized frontal tumors. Journal of Neurology, Neurosurgery and Psychiatry 29: 52–59
Smith A, Kinder E F 1959 Changes in psychological test performances of brain-operated schizophrenics after eight years. Science 129: 149–150
Smith M L, Milner B 1988 Estimation of frequency of occurrence of abstract designs after frontal or temporal lobectomy. Neuropsychologia 26: 297–306
Spreen O, Benton A L 1969 Neurosensory Centre examination for aphasia. Neuropsychology Laboratory, University of Victoria, Canada
Strom-Olsen R, Carlisle S 1971 Bi-frontal stereotactic tractotomy. British Journal of Psychiatry 118: 141–154
Stroop J R 1935 Studies of interference in serial verbal reactions. Journal of Experimental Psychology 18: 643–662
Stuss D, Benson D F 1983 Frontal lobe lesions and behavior. In: Kertesz A (ed) Localization in neuropsychology. Academic Press, New York
Stuss D T, Benson D F 1984 Neuropsychological studies of the frontal lobes. Psychological Bulletin 95: 3–28
Stuss D T, Benson D F 1986 The frontal lobes. Raven, New York
Stuss D T, Alexander M P, Lieberman A, Levine H 1978 An extraordinary form of confabulation. Neurology 28: 1166–1172
Stuss D T, Benson D F, Kaplan E F, Weir W S, Della Malva C 1981a Leucotomized and nonleucotomized schizophrenics: Comparison on tests of attention. Biological Psychiatry 16: 1085–1100
Stuss D T, Kaplan E F, Benson D F, Weir W S, Naeser M A, Levine H L 1981b Long-term

effects of prefrontal leucotomy – an overview of neuropsychologic residuals. Journal of Clinical Neuropsychology 3: 13–32
Stuss D T, Kaplan E F, Benson D F 1982a Long-term effects of prefrontal leucotomy: Cognitive functions. In: Malatesha R N, Hartlage L C (eds) Neuropsychology and cognition. Martinus Nijhoff, The Hague, vol 2, pp 252–271
Stuss D T, Kaplan E F, Benson D F, Weir W S, Chiuli S, Sarazin F F 1982b Evidence for the involvement of orbitofrontal cortex in memory functions: An interference effect. Journal of Comparative and Physiological Psychology 6: 913–925
Stuss D T, Benson D F, Kaplan E F, Weir W S, Naeser M A, Lieberman I, Ferrill D 1983 The involvement of orbitofrontal cerebrum in cognitive tasks. Neuropsychologia 21: 235–248
Sweet W H 1973 Treatment of medically intractable mental disease by limited frontal leucotomy justifiable? New England Journal of Medicine 289: 1117–1125
Sykes M K, Tredgold R F 1964 Restricted orbital undercutting. British Journal of Psychiatry 110: 609–640
Teuber H L 1959 Some alterations in behavior after cerebral lesions in man. In: Bass A D (ed) Evolution of nervous control from primitive organisms to man. American Association for the Advancement of Science, Washington
Teuber H L 1964 The riddle of frontal lobe function in man. In: Warren J M, Akert K (eds) The frontal granular cortex and behavior. McGraw Hill, New York, ch 20
Teuber H L, Mishkin M 1954 Judgement of visual and postural vertical after brain injury. Journal of Psychology 38: 161–175
Teuber H L, Weinstein S 1954 Performance on a formboard task after penetrating brain injury. Journal of Psychology 38: 177–190
Teuber H L, Weinstein S 1958 Equipotentiality versus cortical localization. Science 127: 241–242
Teuber H L, Battersby W S, Bender M B 1949 Changes in visual searching performance following cerebral lesions. American Journal of Physiology 159: 592 abstract
Teuber H L, Battersby W S, Bender M B 1951 Performance of complex visual tasks after cerebral lesions. Journal of Nervous and Mental Disease 114: 413–429
Tooth G C, Newton M P 1961 Leucotomy in England and Wales, 1942–1954. HMSO, London
Tow P M 1955 Personality changes following frontal leucotomy. Oxford University Press, London
Troyer A K, Moscovitch M, Winocur G 1997 Clustering and switching as two components of verbal fluency: evidence from younger and older healthy adults. Neuropsychology 11: 138–146
Victor M, Adams R D, Collins G F 1971 The Wernicke-Korsakoff syndrome. Davis, Philadelphia
Vilkki J 1988 Problem solving deficits after focal cerebral lesions. Cortex 24: 119–127
Vilkki J, Holst P 1994 Speed and flexibility on word fluency tasks after focal brain lesions. Neuropsychologia 32: 1257–1262
Vosburg R 1962 Lobotomy in Western Pennsylvania: looking back over ten years. American Journal of Psychiatry 119: 503–510
Walsh K W 1960 Surgical modification of the personality. Unpublished Master's thesis, University of Melbourne
Walsh K W 1976 Neuropsychological aspects of modified leucotomy. In: Sweet W H (ed) Neurosurgical treatment in psychiatry, pain, and epilepsy. University Park Press, Baltimore, ch 11
Walsh K W 1991 Understanding brain damage. A primer of neuropsychological evaluation, 2nd edn. Churchill Livingstone, Edinburgh
Warren J M, Akert K 1964 The frontal granular cortex and behavior. McGraw Hill, New York
Weigl E 1941 On the psychology of the so-called process of abstraction. Journal of Abnormal and Social Psychology 36: 3–33
Weinstein E A 1987 The functions of confabulation. Psychiatry 50: 88–89
Weinstein S, Teuber H L 1957 Effects of penetrating brain injury on intelligence test scores. Science 125: 1036–1037
Weinstein S, Teuber H L, Ghent L, Semmes J 1955 Complex visual test performance after penetrating brain injury in man. American Psychologist 10: 408
Werner H 1946 The concept of rigidity: a critical evaluation. Psychological Review 53: 43–52

Wiegersma S, van der Scheer E, Human R 1990 Subjective ordering, short-term memory, and the frontal lobes. Neuropsychologia 28: 95–98
Winner E, Gardner H 1977 The comprehension of metaphor in brain-damaged patients. Brain 100: 717–729
Woodworth R S, Schlosberg H 1954 Experimental psychology, 3rd edn. Methuen, London
Worster-Drought C 1931 Mental symptoms associated with tumours of the frontal lobes. Proceedings of the Royal Society of Medicine 24: 1007
Yacorzynski G K, Boshes B, Davis L 1948 Psychological changes produced by frontal lobotomy. Research Publications, Association for Research in Nervous and Mental Disease 27: 642–657
Zangwill O 1966 Psychological deficits associated with frontal lobe lesions. International Journal of Neurology 5: 395
Zurif E B, Caramazza A, Myerson R 1972 Grammatical judgments of agrammatic aphasics. Neuropsychologia 10: 405–417

5

The temporal lobes

INTEGRATIVE FUNCTIONS OF THE TEMPORAL LOBE

The organization of the temporal lobes is very complex. It is related to the sense systems of olfaction and audition, whose primary projection areas and areas of perceptual elaboration lie within its boundaries. It is also related to the visual system and serves to integrate visual perception with the information from the other sensory systems into the unified experience of the world around us. It plays an important role in memory in both its specific and general aspects. It contains systems which help to preserve the record of conscious experience. Finally, it has such an intimate connection with the structures of the limbic system, which itself has far reaching connections, that its functional boundaries as well as its morphological boundaries are ill-defined. It is through this system that the temporal lobes help to provide part of the anatomical substrate for the integration of the emotional and motivational aspects of the organism with informational content coming from all those sensory systems situated behind the central fissure and, through its connections with the frontal lobes, with those systems for plans of action which are formulated in these regions. This anatomical and functional complexity means that one must be cautious of over simplified conceptions based on an examination of lesions in specific parts of the temporal lobes. Williams says of temporal lobe syndromes '...it is more true of this part of the nervous system than of any other that disturbances of the part must include consideration of the whole' (1969, p. 700). Therefore, the division of topics in what follows is an arbitrary one. It is particularly oriented to those disorders the examination of which will prove useful in trying to provide a basis for understanding the complex integrative functions which the temporal lobes serve. In the first section, the main areas deal with the effects of unilateral temporal lobe lesions on auditory perception, visual perception, intellectual changes and modality or material specific memory processes, while the second section deals with the complex disturbances of behaviour and experience caused by temporal lobe epilepsy and the non-specific disorders of memory which are such a prominent feature of interruption to the mesial temporal lobe structures and their connections. For lack of space, some areas, such as the perception of time and the participation of the temporal lobes in alerting mechanisms, will have to be omitted.

ANATOMICAL FEATURES

The temporal lobe lies below the lateral cerebral fissure or fissure of Sylvius. The lateral surface is divided into three convolutions or gyri (superior, middle and inferior gyri) by two sulci. The superior temporal sulcus runs approximately parallel to the lateral cerebral fissure, beginning near the temporal pole in front and running back until, near its end, it turns upward for a short distance into the parietal lobe where it is surrounded by the angular gyrus. On the inner portion of the lateral sulcus the cortex of the superior temporal gyrus dips into the insula in several short horizontal convolutions known as the anterior transverse gyri of Heschl. The middle temporal sulcus, which is often in two disconnected parts, divides the middle from the inferior temporal gyrus, a portion of which lies on the inferior or basal portion of the lobe. The artificial lines of demarcation of the boundaries of the lobe with the parietal and occipital lobes are shown in Figure 5.1. The posterior boundary is formed by an imaginary line joining the parieto-occipital sulcus to the pre-occipital notch, and the superior boundary runs backwards from the upper end of the lateral sulcus to join the posterior boundary at right angles. Thus the temporal lobe merges into the visual cortex behind and the inferior parietal lobule above. The inferior parietal lobule is made up of the supramarginal and angular gyri. The supramarginal gyrus surrounds the ascending branch of the lateral sulcus.

The inferior parietal lobule lies at the confluence of the parietal, temporal and occipital lobes, i.e. with those posterior or retrorolandic portions of the cerebral cortex that are concerned with the various sensory systems of the body. As this area is rich in multisensory connections, it is concerned with the integration of sensory information. Lesions in the lobule, particularly in the dominant hemi-

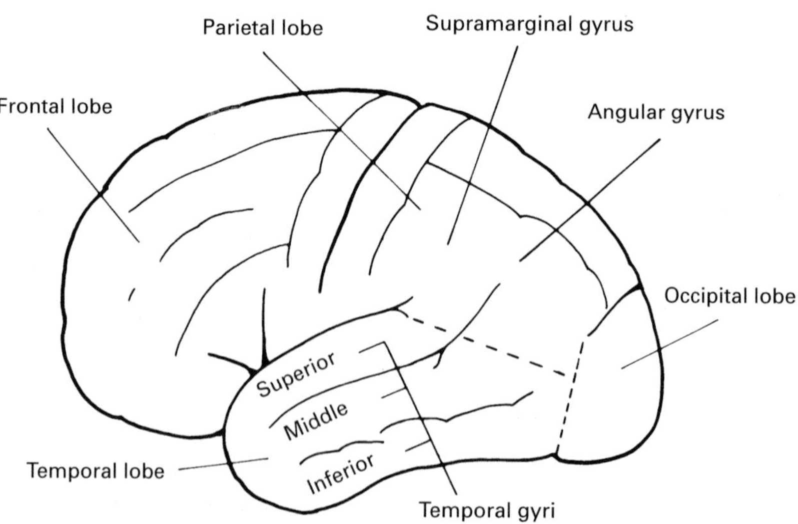

Fig. 5.1 Lateral aspect of the cerebral hemisphere.

sphere, give rise to symptoms which are characteristically different from lesions in other areas. Whereas lesions in the primary projection areas and the association areas which surround them are modality specific, giving deficit in only one sensory system, lesions in the supramarginal and angular gyri disrupt 'the mnemonic constellations that form the basis for understanding and interpreting sensory signals…(which are based on) multisensory perceptions of a higher order' (Carpenter 1972, p. 17). Luria (1973) has also given prominence to this area, considering it as the crowning level of the hierarchically organized systems concerned with gnostic function.

The inferior surface of the temporal lobe (Fig. 2.11) is also divided into three major gyri. Part of the inferior temporal gyrus occupies the lower lateral aspect of the lobe and is separated from the fusiform gyrus by the inferior temporal sulcus. The fusiform gyrus is separated from the hippocampal gyrus by the collateral fissure. The anterior portion of the hippocampal gyrus bends around the hippocampal fissure to form the uncus.

The mesial surface, largely the hippocampal gyrus, slopes downwards to the inferior surface (Fig. 5.2).

The cross-sectional view (Fig. 5.3) relates the three surfaces to each other and should be of value in understanding descriptions of lesions in this area.

FUNCTIONAL ORGANIZATION

The auditory system

The auditory cortex, like the cortex devoted to other sense modalities, may be divided into two zones: (i) the primary projection area for auditory sensation; and (ii) the secondary or auditory association cortex.

Primary auditory projection. The primary projection area is largely buried in

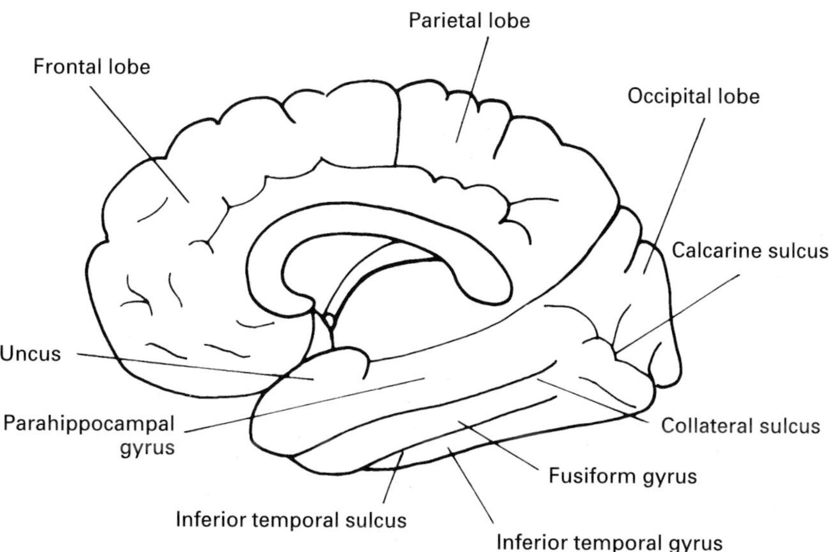

Fig. 5.2 Medial aspect of the cerebral hemisphere.

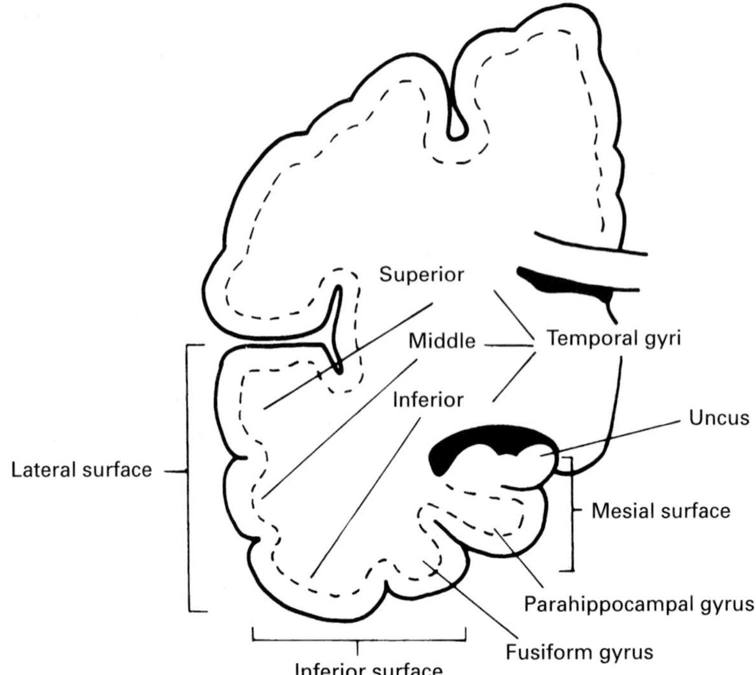

Fig. 5.3 Coronal section through one hemisphere showing the three surfaces of the temporal lobe.

that infolded region of the cortex termed the insula which lies at the junction of the frontal and parietal lobes above the temporal lobes below. This means that a portion of the superior surface of the temporal lobe is hidden from sight when the brain is viewed from its lateral aspect. This insular portion of the superior temporal cortex which serves auditory sensation may contain one, or sometimes two, anterior transverse temporal gyri, or gyri of Heschl (Fig. 5.4).

Auditory information is transmitted from the sense receptors in the cochlea of the inner ear via the auditory pathways. The pathways for auditory information in the brain stem are exceedingly complex and, even now, some of the details appear to be incomplete. The main features of the pathways (Fig. 5.5) are provided principally to demonstrate the fact that information from one ear may travel via a number of different routes to reach the auditory cortex of both hemispheres. After relaying at several points on the way, auditory information reaches its final relay station in the medial geniculate body at the base of the thalamus from which it travels to the primary projection area in Heschl's gyrus.

Damage to the peripheral receptors or acoustic nerve results in deafness on the side of the damage; but damage in the principal auditory pathway in the brain stem (Fig. 5.5) causes a partial deafness since there are both crossed and uncrossed pathways in this tract.

There are certain similarities and also important differences in the transmission of photo- and phono-reception that are important in understanding the effects of lesions in the two sense modalities of vision and audition. Both sys-

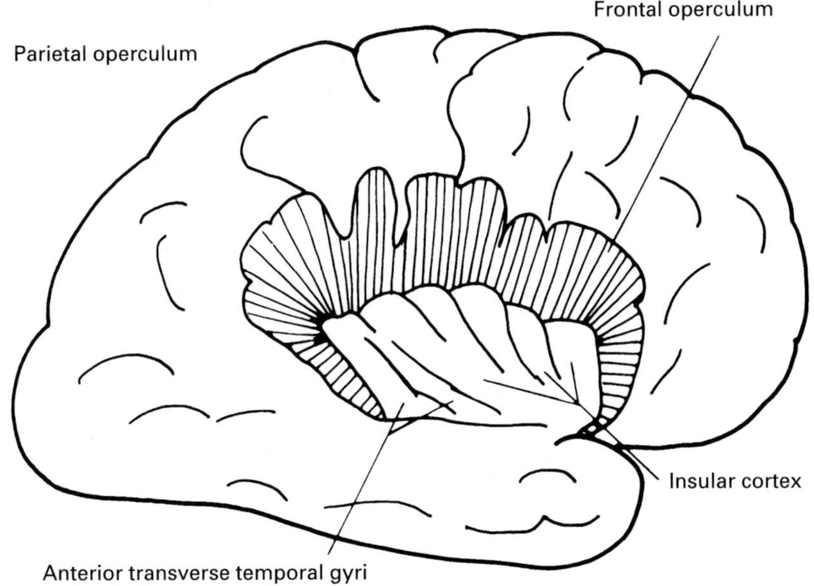

Fig. 5.4 Insular cortex.

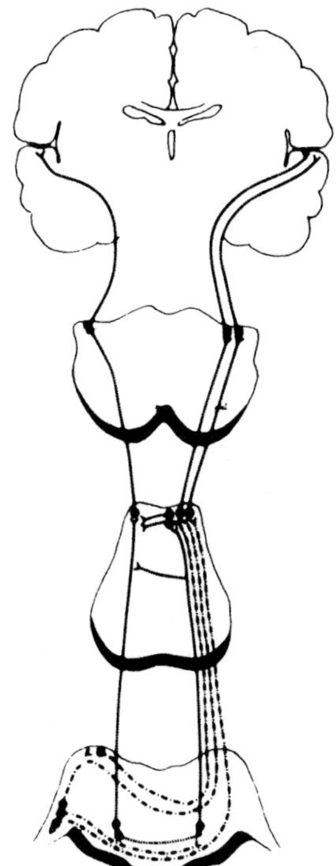

Fig. 5.5 The complex auditory pathways.

tems relay their modality-specific information via specialized thalamic nuclei, and both auditory and visual cortex have a topological structure, i.e. the relationships of the stimuli as they impinge on the organism are preserved from receptor to primary cortex. In the case of audition this is termed tonotopic localization. Fibres carrying impulses produced by high frequency sounds are found in the medial portions of the cortex while the fibres carrying information produced by low frequency sounds terminate in the lateral parts of the auditory cortex.

In the visual system there is a partition of information from each eye, certain fibres from each organ going to one hemisphere and other fibres to the other hemisphere (see Ch. 7 for further detail). In audition the fibres from the receptor organ (the organ of Corti) in each ear are projected to both primary zones of the auditory cortex. This representation is, however, not equal, each ear being represented more strongly in the opposite hemisphere, i.e. the ears are bilaterally but unequally represented in the cortex. Because of this bilateral representation of each organ, complete cortical or cerebral deafness would require lesions affecting the transverse gyri of Heschl bilaterally. Such a situation is exceedingly rare. Unilateral lesions of the primary auditory zones of the cortex do not have a marked effect on auditory acuity, but careful testing reveals an elevation of auditory thresholds in the ear contralateral to the lesion.

Auditory association areas. The secondary or association areas of the auditory cortex give clear cut evidence of lateral specialization, the cortex of the hemisphere which is dominant for speech being particularly concerned with the analysis of speech sounds, while the auditory perception of non-verbal material including music appears to be mediated more by the non-dominant hemisphere. This partition or specialization of function is in accordance with what Luria (1973) termed the law of progressive lateralization and forms an important aspect of the asymmetry of function dealt with in Chapter 8.

Auditory perception

Lesions in the auditory association cortex of the left side produce *sensory aphasia.* The difficulty arises only when the patient has to distinguish speech sounds, and the older term auditory or acoustic agnosia is in some ways to be preferred since it points to the primary difficulty from which a number of other symptoms flow. However, usage is too well established to allow the change, and the term acoustic agnosia is best preserved for the inability to distinguish non-verbal sounds, which is associated with right hemisphere lesions. The disorder of phonemic hearing is produced largely by lesions affecting the superior temporal gyrus in the region adjacent to the primary auditory cortex of the left hemisphere. A phoneme is the smallest distinctive group of sounds in a language, and one of the principal tasks in learning a language is to distinguish readily between phonemes. The nature of phonemic distinction becomes apparent when we endeavour to learn a new language since the distinctive speech sounds are not the same in all languages and the difficulties which a person may have with learning a new language will depend on the phonemic distinctions which are brought to the task. The ease with which we are able to distinguish p and b in words such as peach and beach will be lacking for people whose primary language has but a single phoneme for these sounds.

It follows that a person who has an acquired difficulty in discriminating between similar phonemes will have difficulty in understanding spoken speech. Luria expresses this concisely. 'As words in his own language fail to be differentiated his attitude towards words in his native tongue will begin to resemble that to words in a foreign language' (Luria 1973). Since patients' basic difficulty lies in auditory discrimination, they are deprived of the regulation of their own speech via the monitoring of their own vocal productions. They are therefore unaware of their own defective speech and hence see no necessity for correcting it. Moreover, if they have difficulty in producing the correct word to name an object, prompting is of no avail since they are unable to fit the information into a phonemic system. Structured language disappears and is replaced by very fragmented utterances that have been called a 'word salad'.

The failure to distinguish the vital differences in the acoustic content of words means that patients are unable to write material that is dictated to them, whereas they may be readily able to copy verbal material when it is presented visually. An important exception to the inability to write words from dictation is in the ability to write words which have become so familiar that they no longer require precise analysis of their acoustic content. Prime examples of this conversion of words into motor stereotypes are the patient's signature and the most frequently used words in the person's trade or profession. Luria and colleagues have pointed out that this is an example of how the cerebral organization of a process may change over time (Luria et al 1970). In the process of learning to write words, careful acoustic analysis is needed at first, but the motor aspects of writing become more and more automatic with use and less dependent upon auditory discrimination so that the writing of a familiar word comes to have a different neuronal or cerebral organization from a relatively new word. This means that lesions in different sites will have different effects and, once again, a careful qualitative analysis of the precise form of difficulty which the patient has (in this case with some words and not with others) will point more precisely to the location of the lesion.

As one moves away from the area surrounding the primary projection area for audition there is a decrease in phonological disturbances and, in the region of the middle temporal gyrus, the most prominent defect is one of audioverbal memory, an *auditory amnesic aphasia*. The characteristic feature of these memory disorders is the inability to repeat a series of words which has been presented acoustically despite the fact that the patient may be able to retain and repeat single words. With a series of words the patient may show a primacy effect (the reproduction of the first word given) or a recency effect (the reproduction of the last word given), other members of the series being lost. Luria et al (1967) have analyzed these disturbances of audioverbal memory and suggest that the fault lies in the increased mutual inhibition of the auditory traces. This hypothesis is supported by their finding that increasing the time interval between the presentation of members of the series greatly reduces or eliminates the difficulty. The extension of the time between words is thought to reduce the mutually inhibitory effects which adjacent members of the series have on each other. This type of finding is also relevant to an examination of the amnesic syndrome which follows bilateral mesial temporal lesions discussed below. The major pathology is in the dominant hemisphere with the temporal lobe always affected (e.g. Sakurai et al 1991, Servan et al 1995).

Left-sided posterior temporal lesions sometimes lead to a difficulty in using words to name objects, the so-called *nominal aphasia*. The patient perceives the objects and their significance and can, usually in a round-about fashion known as circumlocution, describe their use or function. It is the association between the visual apprehension of a particular object and a particular word which is lost.

A second effect of lesions which disrupt the coordinated action of vision and audition in this borderland region between the temporal and occipital lobes is an inability to draw objects on verbal request ('please draw a clock'), while retaining the ability to draw the same object when a copy is presented. It might be assumed that, because of disconnection of portions of the auditory and visual regions from each other, words no longer evoke images which would form the basis for executing a drawing of the object named.

So far we have dealt with difficulties which arise with the understanding of speech sounds. Man must also be able to discriminate and attach meaning to other environmental sounds. The finding of impairment in the recognition of these non-verbal sounds was described in the literature for many decades under the term *acoustic agnosia,* though this term is seldom used in the recent literature, having been replaced by the term *auditory agnosia.* Even this term has ambiguities. Used in a general sense it means that the person has a difficulty in recognizing sounds both of speech and non-speech despite adequate hearing on audiometry. With the increasing specificity of the neuropathology of causative lesions, it might be preferable to use more category specific terms such as auditory sound agnosia, auditory verbal agnosia and other categories in the way suggested by Bauer (1993).

Unfortunately, the term auditory agnosia has been used somewhat indiscriminately at times to refer to difficulty with the recognition of any kind of auditory material including speech. In a review of the earlier clinical literature, Vignolo (1969) employed the term in its original sense of 'defective recognition of non-verbal sounds and noises'. This group addressed itself to two major aspects of the problem of auditory agnosia, namely the relationship of auditory agnosia to aphasia, and the relationship of auditory agnosia to hemispheric location of the lesion. The two experiments described by Vignolo (1969) are summarized here in some detail. These experiments demonstrate the value of the clinico-experimental method in neuropsychology for testing hypotheses suggested by clinical findings. They have led to the concept of the double dissociation of auditory functions between the two temporal lobes. The practical diagnostic value of these findings is discussed at the end of this section.

In the first experiment, a test of auditory recognition was given to normal subjects and to patients with unilateral temporal lesions (both right- and left-sided). Left-sided patients were defined as aphasic if their scores fell below a certain point on one of a number of tests of aphasia. These aphasic patients were then further categorized into types and degrees of aphasia.

The auditory test required subjects to select from four pictures on a card the source of a common environmental sound played to them. The sounds were unambiguous, e.g. baby crying, ambulance siren, yapping dog. Four separate pictures were presented with each sound, each having the following categories of sound source: (i) the correct source (e.g. canary whistling); (ii) acoustically similar source (man whistling); (iii) similar class or semantic category (cock crowing); (iv) unrelated sound source (train). Thus the subjects could have three types of misrecognition, acoustic errors, semantic errors and unrelated errors. The findings supported a distinction made by Vignolo between two different types of auditory agnosia. An inability to discriminate accurately the sound pattern produced a *perceptual-discriminative sound agnosia*, while an inability to associate the auditory stimulation with its meaning resulted in an *associative-sound agnosia*. As might have been anticipated, sound recognition defects were more frequently associated with marked sensory aphasia than they were with other types of aphasia. Thus auditory verbal comprehension and the recognition of non-verbal sound sources were closely related.

An examination of the type of error made by the aphasic and non-aphasic groups showed a highly significant difference with regard to the 'semantic' errors but not to the other types, i.e. 'auditory' or 'unrelated'. This suggested that the difficulties in recognition by the aphasic patients were due, not to any inability to discriminate, but to an inability to associate the sound which had been perceived with its usual meaning. On the other hand, two patients with right hemisphere lesions who performed poorly on this test did so because of an increase in acoustic errors, i.e. their difficulty appeared to be discriminative rather than semantic-associative.

The second experiment strengthened and clarified this distinction. Two tests were employed. One, the Meaningful Sounds Identification Test, was similar to the test employed in the first experiment, requiring the subject to select the correct pictorial representation of a well-known environmental sound. The second task, the Meaningless Sounds Discrimination Test, required the subject to discriminate between pairs of complex sounds which had been 'mixed' artificially in a sound studio. Again, groups of left and right brain damaged patients, and normal subjects were used.

Each of the brain damaged groups performed poorly on one of the tests, the deficit varying according to the hemispheric locus of the lesion. Left-sided damage was related to poor performance on the test of semantic association (Meaningful Sounds), while this group's performance on the discrimination test (Meaningless Sounds) was normal. The right hemisphere group reversed the pattern of deficit, having a normal performance on the semantic-associative task and a very poor performance on the perceptual-discriminative test. In keeping with the findings from the first experiment, all patients with an exclusively semantic-associative defect were aphasic. Though there have been very few cases of auditory sound agnosia described in the literature, a case such as that of Fujii et al (1990) lends weight to the Vignolo findings. Their right-handed patient could not recognize the meaning of non-verbal sounds while showing no language comprehension difficulties, and CT scan showed a lesion in the right temporal lobe.

This double dissociation of function of the two temporal lobes with respect to auditory perception further supports the lateral specialization of function shown by the studies of material specific memory defects, dichotic listening studies and cortical stimulation of the temporal regions described elsewhere in this chapter, and the finding of asymmetry of auditory recognition is in keeping with the broader notion of cerebral hemisphere asymmetry of function reviewed in Chapter 8. These findings also have a practical application in diagnosis, since they appear to make an unequivocal distinction between unilateral lesions of the temporal lobes.

Dichotic listening studies. Auditory material is presented simultaneously to the two ears by means of a stereophonic tape-recorder. The material may consist of pairs of digits; when three pairs of these are given in fairly quick succession, the subjects can normally repeat all six digits, usually reporting the three digits which were presented to one ear followed by the three presented to the other. In right-handed subjects (assumed to be left hemisphere language dominant) the digits from the right ear are normally reported first. This may be assumed to be in keeping with the verbal nature of the material and stronger contralateral representation of the auditory input mentioned at the beginning of the chapter. This finding is sometimes referred to as ear asymmetry or interaural rivalry. It might be better to avoid such terms since they focus attention on the periphery rather than on the asymmetry of processing by the two hemispheres.

Attention was directed to this area by the early work of Kimura. In her studies with Milner at Montreal (Milner 1962) it had been found that certain aspects of the Seashore Measures of Musical Talents differentiated between patients who had undergone right or left anterior temporal lobectomy for epilepsy. In particular, right temporal lobectomy produced a marked deficit of tonal memory, while left-sided operations had no effect on this subtest. These deficits appeared to be of a higher order or agnostic type, since hearing as measured by audiometric testing was apparently unaltered. Following these findings, Kimura (1961) employed Broadbent's dichotic technique in the assessment of temporal lobe damage. Patients with temporal lobe epilepsy were examined before and after lobectomy. Patients with temporal lobe seizures performed poorly before operation, but following operation the left temporal group became much worse, while the level of performance of the right temporal group remained the same. These right-sided patients, however, now reported more of the right ear digits than they had before the operation. In more general terms, unilateral temporal lobectomy impaired the recognition of material by the contralateral ear. The fact that the left temporal lobectomy group performed very poorly is related to the verbal nature of the material used, i.e. the deficit is a function of the type of material presented. This point of view was strongly supported when Kimura (1964) developed her dichotic test using short melodic patterns instead of verbal material.

Kimura (1961) assumed that the superiority of the right ear in dichotic listening (verbal) experiments was due to a direct relation between cerebral dominance and the verbal nature of the perception. However, subsequent studies have shown that much of the effect can be accounted for by what has come to be termed the 'ear order effect' (Satz et al 1965, Inglis & Sykes 1967, Schulhoff & Goodglass 1969). This effect represents a greater decay related to material reported from the ear which is reported second. The first ear report is closer in time to immediate apprehension of the stimuli while the second report is subject to decay in short term memory (STM).

Clinical studies of *amusia* reported in the literature have often given equivocal findings with regard to the question of localization. Though many cases implicate the anterior regions of the left hemisphere, some patients clearly have right fronto-temporal lesions (Confavreux et al 1992), and jargon amusia accompanied jargon aphasia in one man with a left parieto-occipital infarction (Hofman et al 1993). One rare case with a lesion in the right insular region showed a receptive musical deficit which was dissociated from a normal appreciation of speech and environmental sounds (Griffiths et al 1997). Since amusia in its various forms almost always accompanies other deficits, particularly aphasia, interpretation of test results has often confounded any loss of musical recognition with verbal aspects of the test situation such as comprehension of verbal instructions and naming difficulties. Kimura devised a test which consisted of the simultaneous presentation to each ear of melodic patterns of four seconds duration. Each pair of melodies was followed by four single melodies and the subject was asked to identify the position of the two dichotically presented patterns in the series, e.g. 'first and third', 'second and third', 'first and fourth'. Kimura's findings of a left ear (right hemisphere) superiority in the perception of melodies (Kimura 1964, 1967) were confirmed by Shankweiler (1966), and other workers demonstrated a dichotic superiority for the perception of the intonational aspects of speech, again for the left ear (Blumstein & Cooper 1974, Zurif 1974). Kimura (1967) pointed out that this auditory asymmetry for words and music provided a new technique for the study of cerebral dominance. Her findings were supplemented by others (Schuloff & Goodglass 1969, Sparks et al 1970) who found a bilateral decrement in auditory recognition with damage to either lobe which varied with the nature of the material presented – left hemisphere lesion cases showed a severe bilateral deficit with words as stimuli, while right hemisphere cases showed a marked bilateral deficit with tonal sequences. In each case there was also a falling off in efficiency of the ear contralateral to the lesion for the other class of material, i.e. with left hemisphere lesions there was a right ear loss for tonal sequences while with right hemisphere lesions there was a left ear loss of efficiency for digits.

A study by Zurif and Ramier (1972) came close to the same distinction made by Vignolo. Using dichotic digits and dichotic sequences of phonemes, they found differences between left- and right-sided lesions, suggesting that the left hemisphere is more concerned with the processing of phonological information, while the right hemisphere is more concerned with the acoustic parameters of speech.

The question of whether primary sensory deficits contribute to the agnosic or so-called higher order defects is one which is frequently raised. In some instances there are those who doubt the existence of certain 'pure' syndromes such as visual object agnosia (Ch. 7) in the absence of a primary sensory deficit. As mentioned earlier, primary sensory deficits of cortical origin in audition are difficult to detect because of the bilateral representation of each ear in the cortex. Oxbury and Oxbury (1969) compared the dichotic findings with digits in groups of cases in each hemisphere where the cortex of Heschl's gyrus was either completely removed or completely spared. Before operation, the order of reporting the digits favoured the right ear, i.e. although digits arrived simultaneously, the subjects most frequently reported those from the right ear before they reported those from the left. Left temporal lobectomy including Heschl's gyrus increased right ear errors but did not alter the order of report. Left temporal lobectomy sparing Heschl's gyrus reversed the order of report, i.e. left digits were reported before right; but there was no increase in errors. Right temporal lobectomy including Heschl's gyrus did not increase errors and exaggerated the primacy of reporting right ear digits. Right temporal lobectomy sparing Heschl's gyrus led to no alteration on either measure. These data show clearly the importance of loss of the primary auditory cortex in producing the deficits. A later study of Efron and Crandall (1983) on a small number of temporal lobectomies suggested that operation decreases the perceptual salience of the tone presented to the ear contralateral to the lesion.

Finally, dichotic performance has been studied in a few instances where the interhemispheric fibres were interrupted, either from agenesis of the corpus callosum or operative division of the fibres for the relief of epilepsy. Two studies (Milner et al 1968a, Bryden & Zurif 1970) described failure to report digits presented to the left ear when dichotic stimulation was used on commissurotomy patients. Sparks and Geschwind's patient showed complete extinction of digits received by the left ear. The fact that failure to report from the left ear in this patient was so much greater than any right hemisphere cases suggested the importance of the commissural pathways in dichotic stimulation (Sparks & Geschwind 1968). Two studies of agenesis of the corpus callosum (Saul & Sperry 1968, Bryden & Zurif 1970) report no auditory asymmetry, nor is there any evidence of marked unilateral auditory effects with hemispherectomy (Curry 1968, Bryden & Zurif 1970).

The studies cited above are a small sample of the extensive studies which have been carried out on auditory asymmetry. An extensive review was given by Bradshaw and Nettleton (1983).

Inferring language dominance. It was hoped that dichotic listening results might be used to infer functional asymmetry of the brain in individual cases, without having to resort to the Wada technique of intracarotid sodium amytal injection described below. Knowledge of cerebral dominance is desirable in certain neurosurgical procedures and in the application of unilateral electroconvulsive therapy (ECT). However, numerous studies attest to the fact that not only are the differences small, but the reliability of the usual method of dichotic recall is unacceptably low (Pizzamiglio et al 1974, Blumstein et al 1975, Berlin 1977, Fennell et al 1977, Colbourn 1978), while others question the dubious logic employed in drawing inferences from the test results (Satz 1977, Teng 1981).

A more robust test termed *dichotic monitoring* was developed by Geffen (1976). This requires the subject to make a manual response on detection of the stimulus, rather than using verbal recall. A validation study (Geffen & Caudry 1981) showed considerably larger measures of ear advantage than for the usual dichotic recall method.

While a more robust non-invasive technique may be helpful, even this fails to satisfy requirements in one of the most common situations, namely proposed temporal lobe surgery for intractable epilepsy where amytal ablation remains the preferred technique.

Music and the brain. Apart from dichotic listening studies, the testing of patients with unilateral lesions (particularly in the temporal lobes) lends general support to a hemispheric asymmetry of function with regard to the perception and execution of music, although the evidence as to which particular characteristics relate to the dominant or non-dominant side is still far from clear. Damasio and Damasio (1977), having reviewed the evidence to that time, felt the evidence supported a major role for the right hemisphere for musical *execution.* As in the case report of McFarland and Fortin (1982), they felt that this could be dissociated from musical training and experience. The unsatisfactory state of our knowledge is shown by the edited collection of Critchley and Henson (1977) and the later review of Henson (1985).

The cocktail party effect. This term refers to the ability of normal individuals to note information, such as one's name, in one of a number of simultaneous auditory channels of information even though that particular channel appears not to be the central focus of attention. This capacity is lowered on the contralateral side for those who have undergone the operation of anterior temporal lobectomy (Efron et al 1983). Details of attentional shifts and subsequent recall in normal subjects have been reported by Wood and Cowan (1995a, b).

Visual perception

The temporal lobes are neither concerned with the primary reception of visual information nor with its elaboration into meaningful wholes. They are concerned however with the integration of visual experience with all forms of sensory information coming from the receptors of the other special senses and from the receptors of the bodily senses. Disturbances of all forms of perception of the individual's internal and external worlds are seen in all their complexity in temporal lobe epilepsy, examples of which are described below.

The temporal lobes contain a portion of the optic radiations which curve forward into the lobe after leaving the lateral geniculate bodies before looping back to their termination in the occipital lobes. Temporal lobe lesions thus produce visual field defects which characteristically affect the upper homonymous quadrants (see Ch. 7) but may sometimes produce a complete hemianopia (Falconer & Wilson 1958). Even in cases where no field loss was apparent to normal examination, changes were detected after temporal lobectomy in the form of raised flicker fusion thresholds for both left- and right-sided cases. Differences between the impact of the lesions according to the side have been demonstrated in a number of studies. Thus, Dorff et al (1965) found that, using the method of presenting two stimuli simultaneously one to each of the visual fields, the left temporal group was impaired in the right (contralateral) visual field, while the right temporal lobe group was impaired in both left and right fields.

Other studies have suggested that lesions of the right temporal lobe might produce disruptions of visual perception that are not shown by comparable lesions on the left side. Milner (1958) found that patients with right temporal lobe lesions had difficulty in recognizing objects from an incomplete pictorial representation of them, a difficulty which was not shown by patients with left-sided lesions. Milner also described an impairment in right-sided cases in the ability to recognize anomalies in pictures, e.g. a picture in which a painting is shown hanging on the wall inside a monkey house. However, using the same test – the McGill Picture Anomalies Test – Shalman (1961) failed to confirm this finding in a small highly selected sample. McFie (1960) described defects in the Picture Arrangement subtest of the Wechsler Scale, again restricted to right hemisphere cases. Kimura (1963), using tachistoscopic presentation, found that lesions on the right side impaired subjects' recognition when the material was unfamiliar, while left temporal subjects were more impaired when familiar material was being presented.

Warrington and James (1967b) failed to confirm Kimura's general finding of impaired number estimation on tachistoscopically presented material with right temporal damage, but did find significantly raised recognition thresholds in the contralateral left visual fields. Rubino (1970) found that right temporal lobe removal rendered the patient less able to identify meaningless visual patterns than did left-sided removals.

Further support to the association of special defects with right temporal lesions was given by Lansdell (1962a) who found right temporal lobectomy patients to be poorer on a design preference test than left lobectomy patients. In a later study, Lansdell (1968) reported that right-sided operations led to poorer performance also on a visuospatial abstract reasoning task that was relatively unaffected by left-sided operations. The more extensive the removals were on the right side the greater were these deficits.

Though both temporal lobes are intimately concerned with perceptual processing, it appears that the lateral specialization shown in auditory perception extends also to the visual modality in this area. From the sample of evidence cited, the relationship between the side of the lesion and the nature of the perceptual deficit, however, is still far from clear.

Olfactory function

The olfactory receptive area is located in the uncus and adjoining parts of the parahippocampal gyrus. Damage to the olfactory pathways or cortex produces *anosmia*. Olfactory hallucinations are often the signal of irritative lesions in the region and are known as *uncinate fits*, sometimes occurring as an epileptic aura.

Following temporal lobectomy, Rausch and Serafetinides (1975a, b) described an elevation in the threshold of detection for the quality or identity of an odour. A further study of lobectomy patients (Rausch et al 1977) showed more errors in odour recall for operated subjects, with right lobectomy patients performing more poorly than left. In another study, right lobectomy patients only were impaired on matching odours (Abraham & Mathai 1983) though discrimination as such was not affected. Finally, Eskenazi et al (1983) found no laterality effects, though all subjects postoperatively had poorer immediate and delayed odour memory than controls and also showed impairment on a wide range of tests of olfactory functioning.

COMPLEX PARTIAL SEIZURES (temporal lobe epilepsy)

Behavioural change

This issue has been the subject of debate for several decades. From the 1950s, epidemiological studies in several countries had suggested that there might be a higher frequency of psychopathology in those with temporal lobe epilepsy, compared with those with other neurological disorders including other forms of epilepsy. There were also some negative studies. A pivotal report was that of Bear and Fedio (1977), who compared patients with unilateral temporal lobe foci with normal subjects and those with neuromuscular disorders on specific aspects of behaviour. The selected traits were examined both by self-report and close observer rating. Bear and Fedio claim to have demonstrated characteristic patterns in the interictal behaviour of their temporal lobe subjects that were different from the other two groups and, moreover, differences which reflected an asymmetry of the expression of affect between those with right- versus left-sided foci. Hermann and Riel (1981) lent partial support to Bear and Fedio's contention by finding characteristic differences between those with temporal lobe seizures and those with generalized epilepsy on a self-report questionnaire. In a further study, Bear et al (1982) obtained quantitative ratings from blind interviews of temporal lobe subjects who had been hospitalized for psychiatric reasons, others with epilepsy, and psychiatric patients with no history of epilepsy. The authors claimed a distinctive profile, which included 'desire for social affiliation, circumstantiality, religious and philosophic interests, and deepened affects, among the temporal lobe epileptics'.

Bear (1979) theorized that the connections between sensory cortex and limbic system form the substrate for 'attributing visceral or emotional significance to perceived stimuli' (p. 358). This could lead to an increased connection as the result of heightened electrical activity in temporal lobe seizures, which might alter the affective experience in this group.

The original article of Bear and Fedio has produced vigorous discussion and at least two negative attempts at replication (Mungas 1982, Brumback 1983). The subsequent debate has highlighted the methodological problems inherent in this complex area (Bear 1983, Mungas 1983, Silberman 1983).

A second area of interest is the relationship between temporal lobe epilepsy and psychotic behaviour. In 1969 Flor-Henry made a retrospective case history evaluation of 50 temporal lobe patients who had been hospitalized with psychotic episodes; he claimed that temporal lobe epilepsy of the dominant hemisphere predisposed to psychosis and that this psychosis was schizophreniform in nature, while psychosis accompanying non-dominant hemisphere epilepsy tended to be manic-depressive in nature.

Both the major areas mentioned in this section have been ably reviewed by Trimble (1983).

Complex partial seizures arising in the temporal region were outlined in Chapter 3. The term 'temporal lobe epilepsy' was introduced by Lennox (1951). Part of the complexity of the syndrome no doubt lies in the spread of excitation from the numerous possible sites of origin of the electrical abnormalities, though some regions such as the mesial temporal areas are more often involved than others. Williams points out that the way in which the term temporal lobe epilepsy has been used 'reflects the difficulty we have in considering disturbance of complex functions in relation to equally complex structures which have a very extensive network of communications throughout the hemisphere. The phrase simply implies that the more evident origins of the disturbances are situated below the sylvian fissure…' (1969, p. 700).

The complex symptomatology of temporal lobe epilepsy has been described in detail in its many guises by Lennox and Lennox (1960) and numerous other authors. The following two cases taken from the previously cited work of Williams are particularly illustrative of the multiform nature of the disorder.

> A woman surgeon developed temporal lobe epilepsy as the result of head injuries caused by being knocked down by a car. The attacks were all heralded by appearance of a human face and shoulders clothed in a red jersey. The figure was intensely and distressingly identified with the patient. The hallucination would then topple sideways and disintegrate into

> discrete fragments like a jigsaw puzzle, the patient meanwhile experiencing extreme fear with an unnatural quality to it, followed by amnesia in which a general convulsion occurred. The patient had total amnesia for the accident, but it is incidentally interesting that long after the traumatic epilepsy became established she learnt that she had been wearing a red jumper when the car struck her. Here then is a visual hallucination identified with the self, compounded with an emotion, and having in it fragments of memory in time. In another case a woman of 30 had epilepsy for 15 years. The attacks only happened when she was applying her eye shadow; then, her face close to the mirror attending fixedly to the eyes, the reflected image would change, becoming more intense and dominating her. She would then seem to see a scene with her grandparents and parents, which seemed to be vividly remembered from a former experience. The scene was visualized but was not seen as an hallucination – 'it was in my mind's eye'. This visual memory was accompanied by unremembered words, the whole event being pleasurable and associated with a general sense of sexual excitement. This then is the experience of visual and auditory hallucination inter-mixed, related to past experience, and having visceral, sensory and emotional components, induced by a highly specific visual precipitant which must be closely identified with the self and also with sexuality. (Williams 1969, p. 709)

Hallucinations and illusions of the temporal lobe

Disordered perception in the form of either illusions or hallucinations has been recognized as part of epileptic symptomatology for a very long time. If the perception refers to a person or object present in the environment we speak of an illusion or false perception. With temporal lobe attacks part or all of the object may be distorted, e.g. everything may appear visually larger or smaller (macropsia, micropsia) or the relative size of parts may appear distorted (metamorphopsia), or sounds louder or softer than usual. These distortions are often accompanied by a feeling that the person is somehow detached from his/her own body (depersonalization) or that things are unreal (derealization). Though these disorders are common in the visual modality they are by no means restricted to this sense. Hughlings Jackson's case with olfactory hallucinations was described in Chapter 3. These olfactory auras appear to be associated with the anterior and inferior portions of the lobe including the uncus. The odours are always described as being disagreeable or offensive, never pleasant (Penfield & Jasper 1954).

Hallucinations refer to perceptual experiences which do not correspond in any way to stimuli in the current environment. The patient is often aware of the 'unreal' nature of the hallucinated objects. The hallucination may be accompanied by emotional experiences which are usually unpleasant, though pleasurable feelings and even short periods of ecstasy have been described infrequently (Lennox & Lennox 1960). Williams (1956) has examined these emotional experiences and related them to specific locations in the temporal lobe. The change in affect at the time of seizure is most commonly that of fear (Williams 1956, Daly 1975), and this fear has been evoked by stimulation through implanted electrodes (Bancaud et al 1994). Some patients experience unprecipitated fear in the interictal period (Hermann & Chhabria 1980). While there is as yet no supporting evidence, these interictal phenomena may be associated with abnormal electrical discharges in structures forming the anatomical substrate of emotional experience.

With temporal lobe disturbances there is a fresh interpretation of current experience. Simpson (1969) suggests that, for learning to take place, or to decide whether an object or situation is 'familiar', one must compare the present sensory input with the neural record of past experience, and he interprets the data of temporal lobe epilepsy as demonstrating the presence in the temporal lobe of 'coincidence detection circuits'. If the comparison of the input with the record of the past produces a coincidence or familiarity response, the present stimulation will appear familiar even if nothing similar had occurred in the subject's prior experience. This is the well known phenomenon of *déjà vu* (seen before), which is experienced at times by normal subjects but more frequently and with greater vividness by some patients with temporal lobe epilepsy. On the other hand, a matching which produces a 'no coincidence' response leads to the experience of *jamais vu* or *jamais entendu* (never seen, never heard), even though the stimulus pattern or one very similar has been frequently encountered in the past. Penfield (1954) referred to these alterations in the perception of the present as 'interpretive illusions'. While déjà vu experiences are associated with pleasant or neutral affect, those of jamais vu may be accompanied by negative affect such as fear (Sengoku et al 1997).

On some occasions the hallucinations can be shown to be quite clearly related to prior experience and the evidence from cortical stimulation outlined below supports Penfield's contention that they are 'a reactivation of a strip of the record of the stream of consciousness'.

ELECTRICAL STIMULATION OF THE TEMPORAL LOBE

Temporal lobe surgery, particularly surgical procedures for the treatment of intractable complex partial seizures, presented an opportunity to study the effects of electrical stimulation from both the temporal cortex and subcortical regions. Several classes of mental phenomena have been elicited: (i) visceral sensation, fear and anxiety (Jasper & Rasmussen 1958, Chapman 1960, Van Buren 1961, Heath 1964, Kim 1971); (ii) complex hallucinations and experiential changes including déjà vu (Mullan & Penfield 1959, Sem-Jacobsen & Torkildsen 1960, Penfield & Perot 1963, Horowitz et al 1968, Weingarten et al 1977); and (iii) changes in memory (Bickford et al 1958, Pampiglione & Falconer 1960, Brazier 1968, Halgren et al 1978). Most of these studies have found a marked inter- and intra-individual variability in response. Only a small proportion of stimulations produce mental phenomena, even where evoked potentials and/or after discharges have been recorded (Chapman 1958, Pampiglione & Falconer 1960, Walker & Marshall 1961, Angeleri et al 1964, Halgren et al 1978), certainly on less than 10% of occasions. It has also proved difficult to obtain similar experiences on repeated stimulation in the same subject. Halgren et al (1983) have reviewed the stimulation studies of the medial temporal lobe and hippocampal formation.

Apart from the well known relation between medial temporal structures and memory, Perrine et al (1993b) point out that their studies and the earlier studies of Ojemann (1981) suggest a role for the *lateral* temporal cortex in memory and suggest mapping prior to resection.

In 1938, Penfield produced for the first time an evocation of experience by stimulating the temporal cortex in a conscious human subject. These experiences were of two kinds: firstly the evocation of an experience which the subject had undergone on a number of previous occasions during epileptic seizures, and, secondly, the production of previous happenings which had not been seen during the attacks but here also clearly related to specific prior experiences.

Penfield used the term *experiential hallucination* when the phenomenon occurred spontaneously, and *experiential response* when it was elicited by stimulation.

Several features stand out clearly in the very large number of cases where stimulation of the brain was employed (Penfield & Perot 1963):

i. Despite the stimulation of practically every accessible spot on the cerebral cortex, experiential responses were evoked only from the temporal lobe (a total of 612 patients in Penfield's series were stimulated in non-temporal areas and produced not a single experiential response).

ii. In almost all cases of evoked experiences, the patients were suffering from temporal lobe epilepsy.

iii. Only about 8% of temporal lobe cases stimulated gave rise to experiential responses.

iv. Responses were evoked from both sides of the brain but there was a marked asymmetry.

Figure 5.6 shows the points in the two cerebral hemispheres where electrical stimulation produced an experiential response. The greatest concentration of the responses was in the superior temporal convolution of both hemispheres, with the frequency on the right side being greater than that on the left. On the right side, too, the points giving rise to experiential responses extended more posteriorly along the superior temporal convolution and the posterior portion of the whole right lobe is productive, while the corresponding regions on the left are almost silent to stimulation.

Auditory responses evoked by stimulation are shown in Figure 5.7. They are concentrated on the superior regions of the lobes with greater frequency on the right. Within this distribution no further finer topographical distribution was discovered, nor did there appear to be any separate effects related to laterality.

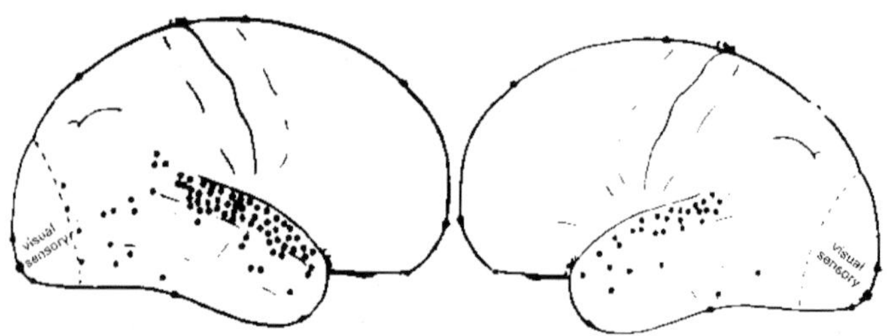

Fig. 5.6 Points on the lateral aspects of the hemispheres where stimulation evoked experiential responses (from Penfield & Perot 1963).

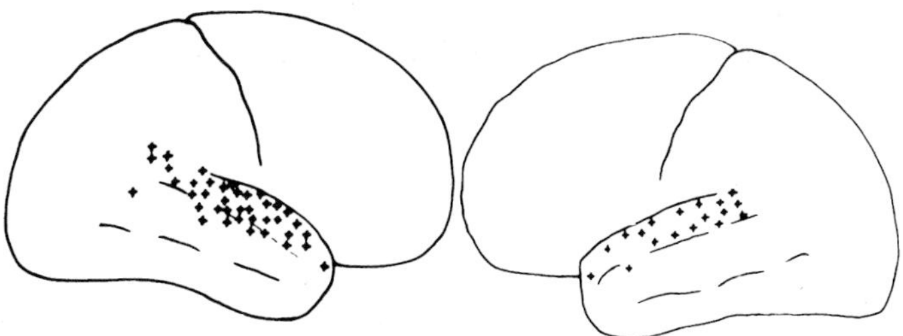

Fig. 5.7 Auditory experiential responses.

The responses were most often a voice or voices, though sometimes meaningful environmental sounds or music were elicited. The following case is condensed from Penfield and Perot (1963, p. 639). The patient's verbatim responses are reported in full.

> A 25-year-old man with six-year history of epileptic seizures which were at first characterised by vertigo and auditory experiential hallucinations and later changed their character to generalized seizures. Stimulation of a number of points on the cortex of the first or superior temporal convolution produced the following responses: STIMULATION 'Just like someone whispering, or something, in my left ear, it sounded something like a crowd.' REPEAT STIMULATION 'Again someone trying to speak to me, a single person…a man's voice. I could not understand what he said.' ANOTHER POINT STIMULATED 'Something brings back a memory, I could see Seven-Up Bottling Company – Harrison Bakery.' ANOTHER POINT 'I am trying to find the name of a song. There was a piano and someone was playing. I could hear the song, you know. It is a song I have sung before but I cannot find out quite what the title of the song is. That is what I was trying to do when you finished stimulating!' REPEAT STIMULATION 'Someone was speaking to another and he mentioned a name but I could not understand it.' REPEAT STIMULATION 'Yes, 'Oh Marie Oh Marie' - someone is singing it.' REPEAT 'Someone telling me in *my left* (*contralateral ear*) (author's italics) Sylvere, Sylvere (the patient's name). It could have been the voice of my brother.' ANOTHER POINT 'It is a woman calling but I cannot make out the name.'

Combined auditory and visual responses were evoked on only very few occasions. Though also few in number, experiences of music were more frequently reported from the right side; this is in keeping with clinical reports of amusia and the experimental findings of the greater importance of the right temporal lobe for the perception of music and the melodic elements of speech mentioned in this chapter and elsewhere in the literature.

Temporal lobe stimulation sometimes evoked visual experiences. There was an even greater preponderance of responses from the right side and the experiences were evoked over a much wider range of points in the right temporal lobe than was the case with auditory responses. A detailed study of stimulation in 16 cases has given further detail on the anatomical origin of several of the phenomena described in this section (Bancaud et al 1994), involving particularly the temporal neocortex, anterior hippocampus and amygdala.

Finally, there is a small amount of evidence that gelastic seizures (those characterized by outbursts of laughter) are dependent upon pathology in the temporal lobes. Three such cases with electrical stimulation of the fusiform and parahippocampal gyri gave bursts of laughter accompanied by a feeling of mirth (Arroyo et al 1993).

An extensive treatment of these phenomena is provided in the recent textbook of Gloor (1997).

TEMPORAL LESIONS AND COGNITIVE CHANGE

Unilateral lesions

Intelligence test differences

There have been frequent assertions that the differential effects of unilateral temporal lobectomy according to the side of the lesion are examples of what Blakemore (1969) calls 'the broad generalization that lesions occurring in the hemisphere of the brain which is dominant for speech produce deficits in performance on tasks which are essentially verbal in nature, while lesions in the non-dominant hemisphere produce performance impairments on essentially non-verbal (visual-spatial and perceptual-motor) tasks'. The question of the hypothesized hemispheric differences, both with regard to the temporal lobes and other areas, is the special theme of Chapter 8. It will be sufficient here to outline a sample of findings from the temporal lobectomy studies.

Left unilateral anterior temporal lobectomy is often followed by aphasia which is, however, transient in nature. Though language disturbance may cease to be clinically apparent, there are numerous studies which show that there are verbal deficits which are apparent for some time after operation when appropriate tests are employed. The early studies of Meyer and Yates (1955) and Meyer and Jones (1957) suggested that the decline in verbal intelligence test scores which was found by studies such as Milner (1954a, b, 1958) and Meyer (1959) after left temporal lobectomy was an aggravation of a deficit which patients with a left-sided lesion had before operation. The three latter studies reported no significant change in the verbal subtests of the Wechsler Scale after operation on the right temporal lobe. Milner's data suggested that there was also no decline on the Wechsler Performance subtests with right-sided operations. However, Miller (1972) reinterpreted Milner's data in the light of the large practice effect from Form I to Form II of the Wechsler-Bellevue Scale which had been demonstrated by Gerboth (1950), and came to the conclusion that the data did in fact demonstrate a decline in Performance Scale score after right temporal operations. Care must be taken in allowing for practice effects in neurological populations since many such groups fail to show such an effect (Shatz 1981). Blakemore and Falconer (1967) also described a lowering of the Performance Intelligence Quotient after right anterior temporal lobectomy. In one of the earliest studies of right temporal lobectomy, Hebb (1939) had noted a lowering of non-language abilities, particularly those associated with visual form perception.

The general relation of verbal deficits with left-, and performance deficits with right-sided lesions was supported by the studies of Lansdell (1962b),

Dennerll (1964) and Blakemore et al (1966). On the other hand the verbal versus non-verbal character of deficits related to the laterality of the lesion was not confirmed by Parsons and Kemp (1960).

A rather different set of findings was reported by Halstead (1958) on 21 cases with epilepsy subjected to small anterior temporal lobe resections. Firstly, the results of operation on the left versus the right side did not support the contention that important differences exist between the dominant and non-dominant temporal lobes. Secondly, of major interest was the fact that a significant difference between patients and control subjects which existed on several intellectual measures before operation actually improved, though impairment in relation to normal performance was still seen on some tasks. Such results may be due to the smaller nature of the operations compared with the larger temporal excisions in Milner's series and possible differences in the patient populations selected for operation. In the printed discussion at the end of Halstead (1958), Cobb remarked concerning the postoperative improvement on test measures – 'it seems extraordinary, and, if it is true, it must be that the operation removes some noxious influence (if I may speak in very vague terms) that was actually impairing function'. Our own experience would support this position, since those with improvement in cognitive measures tend to be those with clinical improvement in their epilepsy. A similar example of 'improvement of function' after removal of cerebral tissue is seen in the discussion of hemispherectomy in Chapter 8.

Several follow-up studies after anterior temporal lobectomy have shown recovery of both the verbal losses which follow left-sided operations (Milner 1958, Meyer 1959) and the non-verbal losses which follow right-sided ones within a year of surgery (Blakemore & Falconer 1967). The latter study covers a period of 10 years and it is difficult to reconcile this with the findings of Meier and French (1966) that, while performance scale scores 1 year after right-sided operations showed no decline over the preoperative level, the scores at 3 years did show such a decline.

Material specific memory loss

The introduction of anterior temporal lobectomy as a standard treatment for intractable complex partial seizures offered a unique opportunity for the study of the role of the mesial temporal structures in memory processes. The resection typically includes the anterior 6 cm or so of the temporal lobe and the underlying structures, the uncus, amygdaloid nucleus, and part of the hippocampus and parahippocampal gyrus. The evidence from this source strongly supports a complementary role for each temporal lobe.

Many studies have reported loss on verbal memory tests postoperatively, although this loss is seldom of clinical significance, i.e. it does not inconvenience the patient in everyday life (Meyer & Yates 1955, Milner 1958, 1967, Blakemore & Falconer 1967, Weingartner 1968, Làdavas et al 1979, Zaidel & Rausch 1981). Support for this relationship comes from other unilateral lesion studies, for example Coughlan and Warrington (1978) found patients with left hemisphere lesions to be generally poorer than those with right hemisphere lesions. Of the left-sided group, those with temporal lesions were more impaired than those with lesions elsewhere in the hemisphere.

Operations and lesions of the right temporal lobe differentially affect visuospatial and non-verbal pictorial material (Kimura 1963, Prisko 1963, Warrington & James 1967a, Milner & Teuber 1968, Taylor 1969, Làdavas et al 1979). Smith and Milner (1981) also implicated the right temporal lobe in the memory for the location of objects.

This evidence is usually interpreted as showing a *material specificity* of memory loss with unilateral temporal lesions. Milner summarized her point of view in the following way. 'It is now well established that a left temporal lobe lesion in the dominant hemisphere for speech impairs the learning and recognition of verbal material whether aurally or visually presented, and regardless of whether retention is measured by recognition, free recall, or rate of associative learning.' She cites her own work (Milner 1958, 1962, Milner & Kimura 1964) and that of Meyer and Yates (1955) in support of this view. Further support came from Weingartner (1968) who tested serial verbal learning after both right-sided and left-sided operations and found a learning deficit with left-sided lesions despite the visual presentation of the material.

Some evidence for the opposite point of view came from Meyer (1959). Following an earlier study (Meyer & Yates 1955) which demonstrated a severe impairment with aurally presented material for left-sided lesions and not right, Meyer specifically tested this proposition employing both visual and auditory (and tactile) modalities in an examination of learning with both verbal and non-verbal materials. Right-sided removals produced no postoperative deficit, while left-sided removals produced a marked impairment of verbal paired associate learning only with auditory presentation and not with visual. Several other studies (Luria et al 1967, Luria & Karasseva 1968, Warrington & Shallice 1969) support the view that, while patients with left temporal or left temporoparietal lesions may have difficulty with verbal memory for all forms of auditory material – words, letters, numbers – they have little or no difficulty with the same material presented via the visual modality. This apparent contradiction over material versus modality specificity still remains to be resolved. There is no doubt of the greater sensitivity of verbal memory to left-sided lesions, the deficit being demonstrable with cerebral tumours (Meyer & Falconer 1960) and after unilateral ECT on the left side but not on the right (see below).

Finally, Blakemore (1969) reported an earlier study in which the rate of presentation of items was varied by altering the time between words and between pairs in paired associate learning. Patients after left temporal lobectomy showed the anticipated deficits at normal and rapid rates of presentation but, when the rate was slowed appreciably, the patients demonstrated that they could learn almost as well as before operation. Blakemore argued that the longer time intervals allow verbal mediation to be effective. Thus the frequent assertion that the deficits after operation should be interpreted as learning deficits as such should be viewed with caution.

While there is a great weight of evidence to support dissociation of function after operative lesions, the evidence for such differences in non-operated subjects with unilateral temporal foci is equivocal. Many comparisons of temporal versus other epileptic groups and with normals have failed to find a significant difference on memory tests (Mirsky et al 1960, Scott et al 1967, Stevens et al 1972, Silverstein et al 1973). Others, while finding memory impairment in the temporal lobe patients, found no relationship between laterality and specificity of memory loss (Schwartz & Dennerll 1969, Glowinski 1973).

Unilateral electroconvulsive therapy has provided further evidence for lateral specificity of memory function. Inglis (1970) pointed to a close resemblance between the effects of temporal lobectomy and ECT. Verbal memory is disrupted by left-sided or bilateral treatment but not by right (Gottlieb & Wilson 1965, Zamora & Kaelbling 1965, Fleminger et al 1970, Pratt et al 1971) while right-sided ECT has a differential effect on non-verbal memory (Halliday et al 1968, Berent et al 1975, d'Elia 1976, d'Elia et al 1976).

The demonstration of detrimental effects of bilateral ECT or dominant side ECT, combined with the demonstration of comparable effectiveness of non-dominant ECT led to fall off in the use of the first two procedures (Squire & Slater 1978). However, earlier studies in which subjects were randomly assigned to the three modes of treatment strongly support the double dissociation of memory (Cohen et al 1968, Halliday et al 1968). With the accumulated evidence to that time, Squire and Slater (1978) chose verbal and non-verbal tests known to be sensitive to left and right temporal lobe dysfunction. Their patients with bilateral ECT showed impairment for both classes of material, while those with right-sided ECT were impaired on non-verbal material only, and this was less than for the bilateral group.

Semantic memory loss

The first clear description of neuropsychological findings in three relatively pure cases of semantic amnesia was given by Warrington (1975). A small number of cases of the selective impairment of semantic memory have appeared since, though some have had accompanying defects. Several of the reports have concerned patients with widespread disorders such as encephalitis but, even here, the critical neuropathology appears to be in the left mesial temporal region. In one such case with encephalitis and a striking dissociation of semantic from episodic (autobiographical memory), MRI showed damage almost completely confined to the left mesial temporal region (De Renzi et al 1987).

A semantic memory disorder appears as the principal feature of the recently described *semantic dementia* (Basso et al 1988, Snowden et al 1989, Hodges et al 1992, Talbot et al 1995). This is clinically a grammatically fluent form of progressive aphasia, in which progressive dissolution of the lexicon occurs as a prominent feature, with preservation of non-verbal new learning, orientation and aspects of everyday memory allowing differentiation from typical Alzheimer's disease. Pronounced dominant inferior temporal lobe atrophy is seen on neuroimaging studies (Hodges et al 1992, Talbot et al 1995), though asymmetrical bilateral lesions are also seen. A recent case of the authors is given in more detail in Chapter 10 (QS).

Amytal ablation – the Wada technique

In 1949 Wada developed the method for determining directly the side of the hemisphere which played the major role in subserving speech functions. A temporary cessation or *functional ablation* was effected by injecting a solution of rapidly acting anaesthetic agent into the internal carotid artery which supplies one side of the brain. This intracarotid sodium amytal injection technique produced the following evidence of functional loss: (i) hemiplegia; (ii) hemianaesthesia; and (iii) half visual field loss (hemianopia) – all on the side opposite the side of the injection. If the hemisphere injected was dominant for language, aphasia was also produced. These effects cleared within about 5 minutes, though subtle changes in language function could be elicited on careful examination for as long as 30 minutes after the injection. Even where amytal injection produces marked difficulty of expressive speech, some patients may preserve the ability to comprehend semantic relations (Hart et al 1991).

In a recent study with a large number of subjects, Wyllie et al (1990) confirmed previous findings that subjects with left hemisphere language dominance shown on Wada testing revealed no language areas in the right hemisphere on cortical stimulation, but two of those with right hemisphere dominance had language areas on the left, arguing for caution in the evaluation of apparently right-dominant subjects proposed for large left or right surgical ablations.

The amytal ablation technique has several advantages. Firstly, it allows the neurosurgeon to determine the lateralization of language function quite unequivocally, and to gauge the probable effect on language of an operation in either hemisphere, since separate injections can be made on either side on two different occasions. The method came to be used extensively to determine the anticipated effects on memory as well as language (Milner et al 1962, 1964, 1966, Kløve et al 1969, 1970), most frequently in anterior temporal lobectomy for the treatment of epilepsy. Verbal and non-verbal tasks were administered during the period of functional ablation. The rationale for Milner's test of memory and similar procedures was based on an assumption derived from the findings stated above, namely that the loss of function in only one temporal lobe does not produce a generalized memory loss. However, if an unsuspected lesion is affecting the hippocampal zone of the opposite hemisphere, then amytal ablation of one temporal lobe should produce transiently the functional effect of a bilateral lesion, namely, the pervasive non-specific amnesic syndrome described in the next section. This generalized memory loss should be apparent for the time of the ablation and clear up as the effect of the anaesthetic agent wears off. This reversible functional ablation greatly diminishes the potential risk of producing a lasting undesirable result from surgery. It should be remembered that a non-functioning (atrophic) hippocampus on the side contralateral to proposed surgery may be silent to electroencephalographic examination. However, since the advent of imaging techniques, these formerly silent lesions are readily demonstrated and appropriate neuropsychological testing reveals a strong material specific memory loss consistent with the laterality of the lesion.

Obviously the short time available, 3–5 minutes, limits the amount of testing possible, and it has been established that prediction is much more accurate the earlier the stimulus presentation occurs after the amytal injection (Loring et al 1994). Also, left/right asymmetry of performance seems reliable in predicting amnesia risk for those with left-sided lesions, but not for those with right-sided lesions (Loring et al 1995), and even the type of stimulus material used has a bearing, e.g. presentation of real objects appears more reliable than the much more commonly used line drawings (Loring et al 1997).

Quite early, Milner (1966) presented strong evidence for the bilateral basis of the general amnesic syndrome, e.g. each of three cases who had already been subjected to anterior temporal lobectomy showed a pronounced memory defect during the injection period when the other hemisphere was chemically ablated. Also, of 216 injections, some 27 cases of anterograde amnesia were produced and, in the 18 cases where the amnesic condition was most clearly produced, all occurred after ablation of the hemisphere contralateral to the side of the temporal lobe lesion. The value of preoperative testing under amytal ablation is one that recommended itself because of the very drastic changes caused by bilateral lesions. 'The fact that there has been no incidence of postoperative memory loss in patients screened by this method, although the series included a number of cases of bilateral EEG abnormality furnishes some evidence of its validity' (Milner 1966). Despite these findings it is difficult to understand the anatomical basis involved. 'Branches of the anterior choroidal artery (which usually arise from the internal carotid) supply the pyriform cortex uncus, posterior medial half of the amygdaloid nucleus, anterior hippocampus and dentate gyrus. We do not yet understand the reasons for memory dysfunction (in cases with contralateral mesial temporal lobe abnormalities) after injection of amobarbital into the internal carotid artery, which perfuses only the anterior part of the hippocampal formation' (Blume et al 1973). Perhaps some form of spreading depression or regional suppression of function takes place for some time after the injection.

Nonetheless, standard amytal testing has continued to show dissociations between test material such as words and pictures of common objects which are related to the two hemispheres in the 'cross over interaction' model described in Chapter 10 (Christianson et al 1990, Perrine et al 1993a). Evidence is emerging that neuronal loss in the hippocampal subfield known as CA3 is the critical lesion (Sass et al 1991).

In recent years technical improvements in catheterization plus dissatisfaction with the confusion sometimes produced by the standard Wada method led to selective injection of the posterior cerebral artery (Jack et al 1988, 1989). Miller and Fedio (1988) comment that this posterior injection 'may be valuable if surgery is limited to a restricted medial resection of the temporal lobe in patients with clinical and neuropsychometric evidence that they are at high risk for postoperative amnesia'. This would be the case in some centres, but the risks of posterior catheterization are significant and such an injection does not clarify the question of language dominance which is central to most investigations, so that traditional methodology is likely to remain.

The carotid amytal ablation technique has also been used in testing for lateralization of functions other than language. Bogen and Gordon (1971) looked at musical ability during depression of activity of the non-dominant (right) hemisphere in six patients. Injection of the right side caused a marked temporary disturbance of singing ability, whereas in five of the six patients 'speech remained unaffected except for slight slowing and slurring of words and the presence of some monotonicity, the intelligibility and rhythmicity of speech were hardly affected'. Such a finding is in keeping with the evidence cited elsewhere of the greater importance of the non-dominant hemisphere in certain musical abilities.

On the negative side Serafetinides (1966) noted that visual recognition of geometrical designs was not affected by ablation of either side though the impairment of verbal recall with amytal ablation of the dominant hemisphere was again confirmed.

Opportunities for studying the neuropsychological effects of amytal ablation with special tests occur in only a few centres. Apart from the restriction of time, the presence of hemianopia and occasional somnolence of the subject together with aphasia and hemiplegia or hemiparesis makes testing difficult. On occasions we have been defeated by the sudden loss of consciousness, especially where both anterior cerebral arteries arise from one side. Furthermore, Rausch et al (1984) found that more sustained disruption occurs with left versus right hemisphere injections and recovery is prolonged if injection is made in the side opposite the seizure focus.

Perhaps the most important contribution to the everyday usefulness of the amytal ablation technique is that of Bouwer et al (1993). They demonstrated that information from implanted electrodes showed that slow waves in the medial temporal region dissipated earlier than the apparent return of function as measured by the frequently employed motor or sensory tests. Thus, measures of hippocampal function based solely on the latter may be somewhat unreliable.

Finally, of great clinical importance is the basing of predictions of postoperative functions, particularly of memory, on 'passing' or 'failing' tests such as the intracarotid amytal test. This is of particular importance where left-sided resection is being proposed since some studies (e.g. Hermann et al 1995, Kneebone et al 1995) indicate that reports from both patients and families demonstrate significantly poorer memory outcome in those patients who have shown no evidence of hippocampal sclerosis preoperatively than in those with evidence of sclerosis. The question of whether transfer of function or some other accommodation has taken place in the latter group, or whether the patients notice no difference from an already lowered premorbid state remains open.

A review of material specific memory deficits following medial or lateral temporal lobe damage, which also covers much of the literature relating to amytal ablation studies, has been given by Smith (1989), while an up-to-date review covering neuropsychological testing, amytal ablation, MRI volumetric analysis of the hippocampus and some postoperative histological data is provided by Baxendale (1995). Another review (Trenerry & Loring 1995) relates the imaging techniques to Wada predictions. The somewhat intrusive Wada method may become redundant as these other methods develop. The changing role of neuropsychological testing in relation to temporal lobe surgery is discussed by Trenerry (1996).

Bilateral lesions and the general amnesic syndrome

Unlike the mild material specific memory losses caused by unilateral lesions, the memory difficulties of patients with bilateral lesions affecting the medial temporal regions are profound, pervasive and generally lasting. Several lines of evidence support this relationship.

The first strong line of evidence came from a prolonged and intensive series of investigations carried out on a patient with bilateral operations that included an extensive amount of medial temporal tissue including the amygdala and much of the hippocampi (Scoville & Milner 1957). This patient, known as HM, developed a stable amnesia almost completely free of other cognitive deficits which has persisted for decades. Many studies of this individual are reported in the various summaries (Milner 1970, Scoville & Correll

1973, Iversen 1977, Ogden 1996) and a similar case was reported by Duyckaerts et al (1985).

Immediately after the operation, HM demonstrated both a retrograde and anterograde amnesia. The retrograde amnesia cleared but the patient was left with some confusion about the chronological order of events, particularly with regard to a period of 1–2 years before the operation. On the other hand, the anterograde amnesia remained severe with an almost total lack of registration for everyday events. He repeatedly re-read the same papers and repeated tasks over and over without giving any evidence of having done them before. He failed to learn the location of his house or the location of objects within it. He was unable to learn the name of visitors even after they had been visiting the house frequently over some years and failed to recognize them.

On the other hand, HM's immediate span of attention was normal. He could, provided there was no distraction, repeat a normal span of six or seven digits. This preservation of immediate memory in the clinical testing of amnesic patients had been reported many years earlier by Zangwill (1946) and has been confirmed frequently since. The preservation of intelligence can be seen in a reported Wechsler Intelligence Quotient of 118 some 9 years after operation.

The marked degree of anterograde amnesia in this syndrome has led to a tendency on the part of some writers to overgeneralize and oversimplify the learning and retention deficit. There is now ample evidence that some learning and retention takes place even in such pronounced cases as HM. Motor skills do not suffer to the degree shown by many other tasks. HM improved his performance with practice on a mirror drawing task even though he was unaware that he had done the task before (Milner 1962). He also showed improvement on a number of manual tracking and coordination tasks (Corkin 1968).

In 1962 Milner reported HM's complete inability to learn a visually guided stylus maze of the type described in Chapter 4. However, when the number of choice points was reduced so that it fell within his immediate memory span, he demonstrated extensive saving in the number of trials to relearn the maze a week after the initial trials and a comparatively rapid relearning after 2 years (Milner et al 1968b). The learning occurred despite HM's denial of previous experience with the tasks. Milner (1970) also demonstrated that HM was able to learn the identity of 20 incomplete outline drawings (Gollin 1960). When retested 1 hour after first exposure to the stimuli he showed even greater savings than a group of normal subjects.

The amnesic syndrome with unilateral lesions. Despite the weight of evidence in favour of the amnesic syndrome being produced only by bilateral lesions, occasional reports suggest that unilateral lesions may produce the loss. Penfield and Milner (1958) reported two cases of the syndrome after unilateral anterior temporal lobectomy in the hemisphere dominant for language. They attributed this effect to the unsuspected presence of a lesion in the hippocampal region of the non-operated side so that what was a unilateral operation in one sense produced a bilateral lesion in another. Their contention was borne out in one case by the finding of a wasted hippocampal region in the non-operated hemisphere at post mortem and by the presumptive evidence of EEG abnormality in the other case in the side opposite the operation. Baldwin (1956) had previously described similar bilateral effects in unilateral left lobectomies only, in cases with bilateral EEG abnormalities. Similarly, less severe amnesia was described by Serafetinides and Falconer (1962) after right lobectomy in cases with added left-sided EEG abnormalities. All these cases appear explicable in terms of the production of a functionally bilateral lesion by a unilateral operation.

In 1964 Dimsdale and colleagues described the occurrence of a case of general amnesia after right lobectomy in which there had been no neurological evidence whatsoever of a lesion on the other side. The authors attributed the memory defect to the extensive nature of the operation. Milner however pointed to the authors' report of a verbal memory defect before operation as presumptive evidence of a left temporal lobe lesion which was then compounded with the right-sided lobectomy to produce the effect. This implied bilaterality of lesion, one preoperative (left hippocampal) and one operative (right temporal lobectomy), was confirmed 28 years later by the finding of left hippocampal sclerosis at autopsy (Warrington & Duchen 1992). In one of our own cases (see Walsh 1991, p. 256) we have had confirmation that in fact clinical, radiological and electrographic evidence may be negative while the hippocampus in the 'silent' temporal lobe may be completely wasted. Our patient, who was a candidate in prospect for left-sided lobectomy, died of a cause unrelated to her epilepsy and the right hemisphere at autopsy showed wasting in the hippocampal region. Earlier psychological testing in this case had pointed to a lowering of function in certain non-verbal functions usually associated with the 'minor' hemisphere. Cases of this type are now being shown up clearly by MRI scanning.

Finally the cases described by Stepien and Sierpinski (1964) are quite contrary to all the above findings. These three cases had a general memory defect before the operation and EEG evidence of abnormality on both sides. Removal of one temporal lobe, rather than aggravating the defect as Milner's hypothesis would suggest, resulted in a disappearance of the amnesia. These findings are difficult to reconcile with the numerous studies cited earlier.

A further landmark in the neurological basis of memory disorders was the report of Rose and Symonds (1960) of four cases of severe amnesia occurring after recovery from what may be assumed to be viral encephalitis. Barbizet (1970) pointed to a similar post-encephalitic case reported by Hillemand and colleagues in 1931, a patient whose memory disorder was essentially unchanged when Barbizet examined him 36 years later. The features of these cases are essentially those of the general amnesic syndrome, namely, a gross defect of recent memory with difficulty in the registration of ongoing events and some retrograde amnesia, with relatively little impairment of other intellectual functions. A constant feature of these hippocampal amnesias is preservation of immediate memory (Drachman and Arbit 1966).

Further reports of post-encephalitic amnesia became almost commonplace (e.g. Adams et al 1962, Drachman & Adams 1962, Beck & Corsellis 1963, Leman et al 1963, Hall 1963, 1965, Zangwill 1966, Barbizet et al 1967, Lhermitte & Signoret 1972). While many of the cases described in the literature have profound, lasting amnesia, a few cases of our own who have had a clear-cut amnesic syndrome after a viral illness have gone on to complete or almost complete recovery.

The most common cause appears to be a necrotic encephalitis of herpetic origin causing bilateral hippocampal damage and sometimes other lesions. The neuropathological evidence is reviewed is some detail in Brierley (1977).

The third major cause of medial temporal amnesia is bilateral compromise of the posterior cerebral arteries. The memory problems may be of a transient or permanent nature. Occasionally, after several transient amnesic episodes the patient may die of a massive cerebrovascular accident, as in the case described by Whitty and Lishman (1966).

Typically, the onset is sudden so that the term 'amnesic stroke' is used. Bilateral infarction is common, since both posterior cerebral arteries arise from the single parent vessel, the basilar artery. For the same reason patients often suffer a cerebral blindness, which may partially remit. A typical report is that of Victor et al (1961). Their patient who had been followed for a period of five years prior to death showed:

> ...a profound defect in recent memory and inability to learn new facts and skills. His general intellectual functions remained at a 'bright normal' level, although certain mild and relatively inconspicuous abnormalities were disclosed by the tests designed to measure concentration, shifting of mental set, and abstract thinking. He also showed an incomplete retrograde amnesia, covering the two-year period prior to the onset of his illness. His memory for remote events was virtually unaffected. (Victor et al 1961, p. 261)

Post-mortem examination of the brain showed old bilateral infarctions in the inferomedial portions of the temporal lobes. Since that time further studies have described the association of serious memory defect in life with post-mortem evidence of bilateral infarction in the territory of the posterior cerebral arteries (Boudin et al 1967, 1968, De Jong et al 1968, 1969). Trillet et al (1980) described 30 cases of vascular origin (17 permanent and 13 transient) with anterograde amnesia as the principal finding. All had cerebral blindness at the outset. These authors reviewed the literature and their own experience and concluded that the typical case closely resembles the original description of the syndrome first described by Dide and Botcazo (1902), viz., cerebral blindness, amnesia and posterior cerebral softening. The latter characteristically includes the fusiform and lingual gyri and cuneus, together with the hippocampus. The thalamus and mamillary bodies may be involved in some cases (Van Buren and Borke 1972).

Benson et al (1974) reported the acute onset of amnesia in 10 patients, associated with unilateral or bilateral visual field defects clearly caused by posterior cerebral artery territory infarction. In our experience there is always CT evidence of infarction in such cases.

A severe amnesia may be produced by infarction in the dominant hemisphere only (Geschwind & Fusillo 1966, Mohr et al 1971). It is possible that, because of the common use of largely verbal or verbally mediated tests of memory, these cases may appear to be instances of the general amnesic syndrome rather than, as we believe, cases of severe verbal specific memory deficits. It is also possible that there may be bilateral but asymmetrical involvement of the posterior regions with pathological emphasis on the dominant side. Once again, modern imaging techniques do much to clarify the nature and extent of the lesions.

Whatever turns out to be the case, severe memory impairment seems more related to the dominant than the non-dominant hemisphere in unilateral cases. The predominant mechanism of production of amnesia may be involvement of the inferomedial parts of the temporal lobes, including the hippocampus. The single case of a severe amnesic syndrome produced by infarction in the area of the left anterior choroidal artery would fit this proposition (Amarenco et al 1988).

Finally, hypoxic injury to the brain following cardiac or respiratory arrest may result in cognitive loss, in which the most prominent feature is a general amnesic syndrome (Muramoto et al 1979, Volpe & Hirst 1983). This may be linked to the known neuronal loss in the hippocampus which accompanies more diffuse cortical damage (Brierley & Cooper 1962, Adams et al 1966, Brierley 1977).

Preserved learning in amnesia

Not all memory functions are lost even in a 'general' amnesia; for example it has been known since the work of Corkin (1965, 1968) that motor learning may be intact in the amnesia which follows some bitemporal lesions. Other tasks without a significant motor component may also be preserved, and much attention has been given to the topic, often termed procedural or *implicit memory*, in recent years. This work is reviewed in Chapter 9.

Transient global amnesia (TGA)

This term was introduced by Fisher and Adams (1958, 1964) for a condition described earlier by Bender (1956) and Guyotat and Courjon (1956). The case histories of Fisher and Adams describe the condition very clearly. The attack is marked by confusion, during which the patient has repetitive queries and shows a total inability to form any new memories. There is retrograde amnesia during the attack for events extending back for days or, in some cases, even years before the present but, as the confusion and anterograde amnesia clear, the retrograde amnesia shrinks to leave amnesia only for the period of the attack itself. Most often there are no accompanying neurological signs and symptoms. The condition, unlike transient ischaemic attacks (Ch. 3), is benign with no added risk of stroke or other vascular problems shown on follow-up (Hinge et al 1986, Frederiks 1993, Zorzon et al 1995). The case reported by Gorelick et al (1988) is an exception. This patient had two characteristic episodes of transient global amnesia before undergoing thalamic infarction (affecting the dorsomedial nucleus), after which his amnesia became fixed.

Transient global amnesia is more often seen in those of middle age or older. The event lasts around 4–8 hours, may be a single event, or may recur a number of times. There is a strong association of TGA with migraine, with dozens of reports of transient amnesic attacks in *migraineurs* (e.g. Olivarius & Jensen 1979, Caplan et al 1981, Crowell et al 1984, Zorzon et al 1995). The amnesic episodes appear to be precipitated by factors which are commonly inducers of classical migraine. In one migraineuse (Damasio et al 1983) the amnesia was largely verbal, the non-verbal memory being relatively spared. Matias-Guiu and Codina (1986) reported a further four cases of *transient partial amnesia* restricted to verbal material and listed the features which should be present for a case to fit this category. This is important since there are numerous cases of transient memory difficulty which do not meet the criteria for either transient global or partial amnesia. Transient topographical amnesia (see Ch. 6) also occurs. One study found 10 such cases in 3 years (Stracciari et al 1994). Transient autobiographic amnesia is reported with ictal bilateral temporal and parietal hypoperfusion on SPECT and no evidence of psychiatric disorder (Venneri & Caffarra 1998).

Despite a strong association with migraine, TGA has been reported with a particularly wide range of factors, such as immersion in cold or hot water, sexual intercourse, or highly emotional experience, and the disorder has also been described with a wide variety of pathological conditions such as mild head trauma (Haas & Ross 1986), hydrocephalus (Giroud et al 1987) and cerebral tumours. There are several reports of TGA after vertebral angiography (Caplan 1985, Brady et al 1993, Schamschula & Soo 1994, Jackson et al 1995). TGA has even been reported in four brothers (Corston & Godwin-Austen 1982). For more extensive reviews see Caplan et al (1981), Fisher (1982a), Caplan (1985) and Hodges (1998).

The most common opinion is that the condition is due to temporary ischaemia in the territory of the posterior cerebral arteries, though a pioneer in the field was strongly opposed to this view (Fisher 1982a). This author believed that the greater part of the evidence was consistent with cerebral seizure. Since then, several studies have failed to find any EEG abnormalities in a substantial number of cases (Miller et al 1987, Jacome 1989, Melo et al 1994); Cole et al (1987) have reported a case of a subject who had a transient amnesic episode while undergoing EEG examination and the trace remained normal. The EEG may also be misleading, since although the case of Venneri and Caffarra (1998) showed ictal frontotemporal slowing, SPECT showed temporoparietal hypoperfusion.

Overwhelming support for a vascular basis has come from cases where it has been possible to carry out SPECT examinations both during and after the event. These have demonstrated temporary hypoperfusion in many different parts of the territory of the posterior cerebral arteries, with return to normal consonant with the return of memory to normal levels (Stillhard et al 1990, Goldenberg et al 1991, Tanabe et al 1991, Evans et al 1993, Lin et al 1993, Hodges 1994, Attarian et al 1995). As expected, the hippocampus is frequently implicated (Onishi et al 1995). The case of Baron et al (1994), where the hypoperfusion was over the entire right lateral frontal cortex, is a marked exception to a posterior vascular hypothesis, as is that of Venneri and Caffarra (1998), though this may account for differences in clinical features. A recent case series reported left or bilateral medial temporal lobe diffusion-weighted abnormalities on MRI in 7 of 10 patients scanned within 40 hours of onset (Strupp et al 1998). The distribution was more consistent with a spreading depression hypothesis than specific vascular territories.

Neuropsychological testing. With the growing interest in TGA, especially as a tool for the understanding of the neural basis of memory functions, there have been a number of reports of test findings both during and after the attacks. Several series have been well documented (Stracciari et al 1987, Kritchevsky et al 1988, Hodges & Ward 1989, Kritchevsky & Squire 1989). One study of two patients has shown the preservation both of semantic memory and frontal executive function assessed by several measures

(Hodges 1994). The case of Evans et al (1993) also showed relative preservation of semantic memory.

In essence the transient condition closely resembles the lasting general amnesic syndrome of central origin following bilateral damage to the medial temporal or medial diencephalic regions. For this reason the present authors would prefer the term *transient general amnesia* for the condition since, unlike the *global* amnesia of late Alzheimer's disease, immediate and long term memory are usually much less affected.

The principal features are:

1. Preservation of immediate memory.
2. A general, i.e. verbal and non-verbal, anterograde amnesia. (On occasions we have noted cases where non-verbal memory does not appear to be as severely affected as verbal memory. Okada et al (1987) describe two such cases whose non-verbal memory also recovered earlier. An interesting feature of two studies carried out during the attacks has been the preservation of semantic memory in the face of severe episodic memory impairment (Evans et al 1993, Hodges 1994)).
3. Some retrograde amnesia. This may be patchy and in the series cited above was highly variable, ranging from a day or two to several years. Following the attack this retrograde amnesia shrinks rapidly, though many are left with a hiatus of a day or two. Pure retrograde amnesia is also reported (Venneri & Caffarra 1998).
4. Other cognitive functions such as language, problem solving and visuospatial functions are generally well preserved, though Kritchevsky et al (1987) reported poor copying of a complex figure and possible difficulty with confrontation naming. Preservation of other functions stands in stark contrast to the amnesia.

Recovery and prognosis. Clinical writers have stressed the rapid recovery of memory, most subjects reporting that they are back to normal within a day. However, it is apparent from follow-up testing that recovery is more gradual than is suggested by the clinical picture, and a residual memory weakness in the form of a new learning deficit may be present in some cases even months after the attack (Mazzucchi et al 1980, Stracciari et al 1987, Gallassi et al 1988). This slow restoration is similar to that shown by a related type of case (KN) detailed in Walsh (1991), though it must be admitted that this is not a typical 'neurologically asymptomatic' case.

The recent large follow-up study of Gallassi et al (1993) shows the generally benign nature of the disorder. Minor deficits may follow multiple attacks, but these may not be of clinical significance. One case whose memory had been tested before the attack showed no deficit following the episode, even showing a normal 'practice effect' on one of the tasks (Stracciari & Morreale 1987).

Few data exist on other psychological functions in TGA patients. Data from Mazzucchi and colleagues (1980) appear to show some cases with a lower verbal than performance IQ, differences in this direction being unusual in subjects of normal or above normal ability. Other studies have not shown this trend consistently and it would be wrong to conclude that there is a hemisphere relationship; certainly there are cases of TGA with right hemisphere lesions (Matias-Guiu & Codina 1985). Inferences from group data must be treated with caution because of the obvious heterogeneity of what is at present spoken of as a single syndrome. Baron and co-workers (1994) suggest that, like permanent amnesia, TGA 'may be a core syndrome with several possible foci of dysfunction along the neuronal networks that subserve explicit memory'.

Finally, though there may be a superficial resemblance between TGA and an hysterical or dissociative amnesia (or fugue), there is little difficulty with differential diagnosis provided the episode has been witnessed and reported by a reliable observer (Merriam 1988). In all cases of transient amnesia care should be taken to abide by the criteria stressed by Caplan (1986).

Whiplash amnesia

A type of transient amnesia with all the features of an episode of transient global amnesia has been described following whiplash injury to the neck, usually in motor vehicle accidents (Fisher 1982b, Hofstad & Gjerde 1985, Matias-Guiu et al 1985). Apparently full recovery may be a function of the type of evaluation, since the detailed examination of a case described by Walsh (1994) revealed major recovery but significant residual memory difficulty.

Vertebrobasilar insufficiency (VBI)

Atherosclerosis in the posterior circulation, viz. vertebral, basilar and posterior cerebral arteries, may cause transient attacks of brain stem vascular insufficiency, the most common symptoms being those of vestibular and cerebellar disturbance. Very little attention was paid to possible disorders of higher cerebral function in these cases. More recently it has been noted that patients showing symptoms of VBI are often forgetful, have poor concentration and occasionally have attacks of transient global amnesia (Rivera & Meyer 1976). Two small studies (Donnan et al 1978, Ponsford et al 1980) suggested that patients with chronic VBI may show evidence of a mild memory problem which has the characteristics of an axial amnesia.

Neuropsychological characteristics of hippocampal amnesia

There is some evidence to suggest that while general amnesias arising from differently located lesions may share a number of common features, such as preserved immediate memory and poor spontaneous recall with relatively better recognition memory, the different locations impress certain characteristics upon the amnesia, so that one might think of different amnesic syndromes or, at least, different discriminable subtypes of the overall amnesic syndrome. This comparison is taken up in Chapter 9.

Amygdala lesions and cognition

Patients with isolated lesions of the amygdala are rare (e.g. Bechara et al 1995, Angrilli et al 1996, Scott et al 1997). The cases available support a role in emotional processing, including the linking of sensory information to emotionally relevant behaviours, particularly responses to fear and anger (Bechara et al 1995, Scott et al 1997). A comparison of the ability to acquire either visual or aural conditioning responses to aural unconditioned stimuli showed a double dissociation between lesions involving the amygdalar and hippocampal regions. The amygdala was implicated in conditioned learning but not episodic memory (Bechara et al 1995). Normal autonomic responses to the unpleasant unconditioned stimulus occurred even when an amygdala lesion was present. Bechara et al (1995) conclude that the amygdala is '…essential for the coupling of sensory stimuli with affect – the establishment of sensory-affective associations' (p. 1117), regardless of modality of presentation, and that the '…amygdala is essential for association of contextual (complex) or discrete (simple) cues with affect, whereas the hippocampus is critical for learning the relations among contextual cues' (p. 1117). Contralateral startle response, recognition of facial emotion and other aspects of facial gesture were reported as deficient with a unilateral right amygdala lesion, leading to the hypothesis that the learning of socially relevant stimuli may be in part mediated through the amygdala (Angrilli et al 1996).

References

Abraham A, Mathai K V 1983 The effect of right temporal lobe lesions on matching of smells. Neuropsychologia 21: 277–281

Adams J H, Brierley J B, Connor R C T, Treip C S 1966 The effects of systemic hypotension upon the human brain. Clinical and neuropathological observations in 11 cases. Brain 89: 235–268

Adams R D, Collins G H, Victor M 1962 Troubles de la mémoire et de l'apprentissage chez l'homme. In: Centre National de la Recherche Scientifique (eds) Physiologie de l'hippocampe. Centre National de la Recherche, Paris, pp 273–291

Amarenco P, Cohen P, Roullet E, Dupuch K, Kurtz A, Marteau R 1988 Amnesic syndrome caused by infarction in the area of the left anterior choroidal artery. Revue Neurologique 144: 36–39

Angeleri F, Ferro-Milone F, Parigi S 1964 Electrical activity and reactivity of the rhinencephalic, pararhinencephalic and thalamic structures: Prolonged implantation of electrodes in man. Electroencephalography and Clinical Neurophysiology 16: 100–129

Angrilli A, Mauri A, Palomba D, Flor H, Birbaumer N, Sartori G, di Paola F 1996 Startle reflex and emotion modulation impairment after a right amygdala lesion. Brain 119: 1991–2000

Arroyo S, Lesser R P, Gordon B et al 1993 Mirth, laughter and gelastic seizures. Brain 116: 757–780

Attarian S, Michel B, Delaforte C et al 1995 A case of transient global amnesia associated with cerebral thrombophlebitis: The contribution of neuroimaging techniques to the study of the pathogenesis of transient amnesias. Revue Neurologique 151: 552–558

Baldwin M 1956 Modifications psychiques survenant après lobectomie temporal subtotale. Neurochirurgie 2: 152–167

Bancaud J, Brunet Bourgin F, Chauvel P, Halgren E 1994 Anatomical origin of déjà vu and vivid 'memories' in human temporal lobe epilepsy. Brain 117: 71–90

Baron J C, Petit-Taboué M C, Le Doze F et al 1994 Right frontal cortex hypometabolism in transient global amnesia. Brain 117: 545–552

Barbizet J 1970 Human memory and its pathology. Freeman, San Francisco

Barbizet J, Devic J M, Duizabo P 1967 Etude d'un cas d'encéphalite amnésiante d'origine hérpetique. Société Médicale des Hôpitaux de Paris 118: 1123–1132

Basso A, Capitani E, Laiacona M 1988 Progressive language impairment without dementia: a case with isolated category specific semantic defect. Journal of Neurology, Neurosurgery and Psychiatry 51: 1201–1207

Bauer R M 1993 Agnosia. Ch. 9 In: Heilman K M, Valenstein E (eds) Clinical neuropsychology, 3rd edn. Oxford University Press, New York

Baxendale S A 1995 The hippocampus: functional and structural correlations. Seizure 4: 105–117

Bear D M 1979 Temporal lobe epilepsy - a syndrome of sensory-limbic hyperconnection. Cortex l: 357–384

Bear D M 1983 Behavioral symptoms in temporal lobe epilepsy (letter). Archives of General Psychiatry 40: 467–468

Bear D M, Fedio P 1977 Quantitative analysis of interictal behavior in temporal lobe epilepsy. Archives of Neurology 34: 454–467

Bear D, Levin K, Blumer D, Chetham D, Ryder J 1982 Interictal behaviour in hospitalised temporal lobe epileptics: relationship to idiopathic psychiatric syndromes. Journal of Neurology, Neurosurgery and Psychiatry 45: 481–488

Bechara A, Tranel D, Damasio H, Adolphs R, Rockland C, Damasio A R 1995 Double dissociation of conditioning and declarative knowledge relative to the amygdala and hippocampus in humans. Science 269: 1115–1118

Beck E, Corsellis J A 1963 Das Fornixsystem des Menschen im Lichte anatomischer und pathologischer Untersuchungen. Zentralblatt für die gesamte Neurologie und Psychiatrie 173: 220–221

Bender M B 1956 Syndrome of isolated episode of confusion with amnesia. Journal of the Hillside Hospital 5: 212–221

Benson D F, Marsden C D, Meadows J C 1974 The amnesic syndrome of posterior cerebral artery occlusion. Acta Neurologica Scandinavica 50: 133–145

Berent S, Cohen B D, Silverman A J 1975 Changes in verbal and non verbal learning following a single left or right unilateral electroconvulsive treatment. Biological Psychiatry 10: 95–100

Berlin C I 1977 Hemispheric asymmetry in auditory tasks. In: Harnad S, Doty R W, Goldstein L, Jaynes J, Krauthamer G (eds) Lateralization in the nervous system. Academic Press, New York, pp 303–323

Bickford R G, Mulder D W, Dodge H W, Svien H J, Rome H P 1958 Changes in memory function produced by electrical stimulation of the temporal lobe in man. Research Publications, Association for Research in Nervous and Mental Disease 36: 227–243

Blakemore C B 1969 Psychological effects of temporal lobe lesions in man. In: Herrington R N (ed) Current problems in neuropsychiatry: schizophrenia, epilepsy, the temporal lobe. British Journal of Psychiatry, Special publication no 4, ch 10, pp 60–69

Blakemore C B, Falconer M A 1967 Long-term effects of anterior temporal lobectomy on certain cognitive functions. Journal of Neurology, Neurosurgery and Psychiatry 30: 364–367

Blakemore C B, Ettlinger G, Falconer M A 1966 Cognitive abilities in relation to frequency of seizures and neuropathology of the temporal lobes in man. Journal of Neurology, Neurosurgery and Psychiatry 29: 268–272

Blume W T, Grabow J D, Darley F L, Aranson A E 1973 Intracarotid amobarbital test of language and memory before temporal lobectomy for seizure control. Neurology 23: 812–819

Blumstein S, Cooper W 1974 Hemispheric processing of information contours. Cortex 10: 146–158

Blumstein S, Goodglass H, Tartter V 1975 The reliability ear advantage in dichotic listening. Brain and Language 2: 226–236

Bogen J E, Gordon H W 1971 Musical test for functional lateralization with intracarotid amobarbital. Nature 230: 524–525

Boudin G, Barbizet J, Derouesné C, Van Amerongen P 1967 Cécité corticale et problème des 'amnésies occipitales'. Revue Neurologique 116: 89–97

Boudin G, Brion S, Pepin B, Barbizet J 1968 Syndrome de Korsakoff d'étiologie artèriopathique. Revue Neurologique 119: 341–348

Bouwer M S, Jones-Gotman M, Gotman J 1993 Duration of sodium amytal effect: Behavioral and EEG measures. Epilepsia 34: 61–68

Bradshaw J L, Nettleton N 1983 Human cerebral asymmetry. Prentice-Hall, Englewood Cliffs, N J

Brady A P, Hough D M, Lo R, Gill G 1993 Transient global amnesia after cerebral angiography with iohexol. Canadian Association of Radiologists Journal 44: 450–452

Brazier M A B 1968 The electrical activity of the nervous system, 3rd edn. Pitman, London

Brierley J 1977 The neuropathology of amnesic states. In: Whitty C W M, Zangwill O L (eds) Amnesia, 2nd edn. Butterworths, London, pp 199–223

Brierley J B, Cooper J E 1962 Cerebral complications of hypotensive anaesthesia in a normal adult. Journal of Neurology, Neurosurgery and Psychiatry 25: 24–30

Brumback R A 1983 Personality analysis of epileptics. Archives of Neurology 40: 68

Bryden M P, Zurif E B 1970 Dichotic listening performance in a case of agenesis of the corpus callosum. Neuropsychologia 8: 371–377

Caplan L R 1985 Transient global amnesia. In: Vinken P J, Bruyn G W, Klawans H L (eds) Handbook of clinical neurology. New series l. Elsevier, Amsterdam, vol 4, pp 205–218
Caplan L R 1986 Transient global amnesia: criteria and classification. Neurology 36: 441
Caplan L, Chedru F, Lhermitte F, Mayman F 1981 Transient global amnesia and migraine. Neurology 31: 1167–1170
Carpenter M B 1972 Core text of neuroanatomy. Williams and Wilkins, Baltimore
Chapman W P 1958 Studies of the periamygdaloid area in relation to human behavior. Research Publications, Association for Research in Nervous and Mental Disease 36: 258–277
Chapman W P 1960 Depth electrode studies in patients with temporal lobe epilepsy. In: Ramey E R, O'Doherty D S (eds) Electrical studies on the unanesthetized brain. Hoeber, New York, pp 344–350
Christianson S A, Saisa J, Silfenius H 1990 Hemisphere memory differences in Sodium Amytal testing of epileptic patients. Journal of Clinical and Experimental Neuropsychology 12: 681–694
Cohen B D, Noblin C D, Silverman A J, Penick S B 1968 Functional asymmetry of the human brain. Science 162: 475
Colbourn C J 1978 Can laterality be measured? Neuropsychologia 16: 283–298
Cole A J, Gloor P, Kaplan R 1987 Transient global amnesia: the electroencephalogram at onset. Annals of Neurology 22: 771–772
Confavreux C, Croisile B, Garussus P, Aimard G, Trillet M 1992 Progressive amusia and aprosody. Archives of Neurology 49: 971–976
Corkin S 1965 Tactually-guided image learning in man. Effect of unilateral cortical excisions and bilateral hippocampal lesions. Neuropsychologia 3: 339–351
Corkin S 1968 Acquisition of motor skill after bilateral medial temporal-lobe excision. Neuropsychologia 6: 255
Corston R N, Godwin-Austen R B 1982 Transient global amnesia in four brothers. Journal of Neurology, Neurosurgery and Psychiatry 45: 375–377
Coughlan A K, Warrington E K 1978 Word-comprehension and word-retrieval in patients with localized cerebral lesions. Brain 101: 163–185
Critchley M, Henson R A 1977 Music and the brain. Studies in the neurology of music. Heinemann, London
Crowell G F, Stump D A, Biller J, McHenry L C, Toole J F 1984 The transient global amnesia – migraine connection. Archives of Neurology 41: 75–79
Curry F K W 1968 A comparison of the performance of a right hemispherectomized subject and 24 normals on four dichotic listening tasks. Cortex 4: 144–153
Daly D D 1975 Ictal clinical manifestations of complex partial seizures. In: Penry J K, Daly D D (eds) Advances in Neurology. Raven, New York, vol 11, pp 75–84
Damasio A R, Damasio H 1977 Musical faculty and cerebral dominance. In: Critchley M, Henson R A (eds) Music and the brain. Heinemann, London, pp 141–155
Damasio A R, Graff-Radford N R, Damasio H 1983 Transient partial amnesia. Archives of Neurology 40: 656–657
De Jong R N, Itabashi H H, Olson J R 1968 'Pure' memory loss with hippocampal lesions: a case report. Transactions of the American Neurological Association 93: 31–34
De Jong R N, Itabashi H H, Olson J R 1969 Memory loss due to hippocampal lesions. Archives of Neurology 20: 339–348
d'Elia G 1976 Memory changes after unilateral electroconvulsive therapy with different electrode positions. Cortex 12: 280–289
d'Elia G, Lorentzson S, Raotma H, Widepalm K 1976 Comparison of unilateral dominant and non-dominant ECT on verbal and non-verbal memory. Acta Psychiatrica Scandinavica 3: 85–94
Dennerll R D 1964 Prediction of unilateral brain dysfunction using Wechsler test scores. Journal of Consulting Psychology 28: 278–284
De Renzi E, Liotti M, Nichelli P 1987 Semantic amnesia with preservatlon of autographic memory. A case report. Cortex 23: 575–597
Dide M, Botcazo M 1902 Amnésie continué, cécité verbale pure, perte du sens topographique, ramollissement double du lobe lingual. Revue Neurologique 10: 676–686
Dimsdale H, Logue V, Piercy M 1964 A case of persisting impairment of recent memory following right temporal lobectomy. Neuropsychologia 1: 287–298

Donnan G A, Walsh K W, Bladin P F 1978 Memory disorder in vertebrobasilar disease. Journal of Clinical and Experimental Neurology 15: 215–220

Dorff J E, Mirsky A F, Mishkin M 1965 Effects of unilateral temporal lobe removals on tachistoscopic recognition in the left and right visual fields. Neuropsychologia 3: 39–51

Drachman D A, Adams R D 1962 Acute herpes simplex and inclusion body encephalitis. Archives of Neurology 7: 45–63

Drachman D A, Arbit J 1966 Memory and the hippocampal complex. Archives of Neurology 15: 52–61

Duyckaerts C, Derouesné C, Signoret J L, Escourolle R, Castaigne P 1985 Bilateral and limited amygdalohippocampal lesions causing a pure amnesic syndrome. Annals of Neurology 18: 314–319

Efron R, Crandall P H 1983 Central auditory processing II. Effects of anterior temporal lobectomy. Brain and Language 19: 237–253

Efron R, Crandall P H, Koss B, Divenyi P L, Yund E W 1983 Central auditory processing. III. The "cocktail party" effect and anterior temporal lobectomy. Brain and Language 19: 254–263

Eskenazi B, Cain W S, Novelly R A, Friend K B 1983 Olfactory functioning in temporal lobectomy patients. Neuropsychologia 21: 365–374

Evans J, Wilson B, Wraight E P, Hodges J R 1993 Neuropsychological and SPECT scan findings during and after transient global amnesia: evidence for the differential impairment of remote episodic memory. Journal of Neurology, Neurosurgery and Psychiatry 56: 1227–1230

Falconer M A, Wilson J L 1958 Visual changes following anterior temporal lobectomy: their significance in relation to 'Meyer's loop' of the optic radiation. Brain 81: 1–14

Fennell E B, Bowers D, Satz P 1977 Within-modal and cross-modal reliabilities of two laterality tests. Brain and Language 4: 63–69

Fisher C M 1982a Transient global amnesia. Precipitating activities and other observations. Archives of Neurology 39: 605–608

Fisher C M 1982b Whiplash amnesia. Neurology 32: 667–668

Fisher C M, Adams R D 1958 Transient global amnesia. Transactions of the American Neurological Association 83: 143–146

Fisher C M, Adams RD 1964 Transient global amnesia. Acta Neurologica Scandinavica 40 (suppl 19): 1–83

Fleminger J J, de Horne D J, Nott P N 1970 Unilateral electroconvulsive therapy and cerebral dominance: effect of right- and left-sided electrode placement on verbal memory. Journal of Neurology, Neurosurgery and Psychiatry 23: 408–411

Flor-Henry P 1969 Schizophrenic-like reactions and affective psychosis associated with temporal lobe epilepsy: etiological factors. American Journal of Psychiatry 126: 400–403

Frederiks J A 1993 Transient global amnesia. Clinical Neurology and Neurosurgery 95: 265–283

Fujii T, Fukatsu R, Watabe S et al 1990 Auditory sound agnosia without aphasia following a right temporal lesion. Cortex 26: 263–268

Gallassi R, Stracciari A, Morreale A, Lorusso S, Ciucci G 1988 Transient global amnesia follow-up: a neuropsychological investigation. Italian Journal of Neurological Science Supplement 9: 33–34

Gallassi R, Stracciari A, Morreale A et al 1993 Transient global amnesia: Neuropsychological test findings after single and multiple attacks. European Neurology 33: 294–298

Geffen G 1976 The development of hemispheric specialization for speech perception. Cortex 2: 337–346

Geffen G, Caudrey D 1981 Reliability and validity of the dichotic monitoring test for language laterality. Neuropsychologia 19: 413–423

Gerboth R 1950 A study of the two forms of the Wechsler-Bellevue Intelligence Scale. Journal of Consulting Psychology 14: 365–370

Geschwind N, Fusillo M 1966 Color naming defects in association with alexia. Archives of Neurology 15: 137–146

Giroud M, Guard D, Dumas R 1987 Transient global amnesia associated with hydrocephalus. Report of two cases. Journal of Neurology 235: 118–119

Gloor P 1997 The temporal lobe and limbic system. Oxford University Press, New York

Glowinski H 1973 Cognitive deficits in temporal lobe epilepsy: an investigation of memory functioning. Journal of Nervous and Mental Disease 17: 129–137

Goldenberg G, Podreka I, Pfaffelmeyer N, Wessely P, Deecke L 1991 Thalamic ischemia in transient global amnesia: a SPECT study. Neurology 41: 1748–1752

Gollin E S 1960 Development studies of visual recognition of incomplete objects. Perceptual and Motor Skills 11: 289–298

Gorelick P B, Amico L L, Ganellan R, Benevento L A 1988 Transient global amnesia and thalamic infarction. Neurology 38: 496–499

Gottlieb G, Wilson I 1965 Cerebral dominance: temporary disruption of verbal memory by unilateral electroconvulsive shock treatment. Journal of Comparative and Physiological Psychology 60: 368–372

Griffiths T D, Rees A, Witton C et al 1997 Spatial and auditory processing deficits following right hemisphere infarction. Brain 120: 785–794

Guyotat J, Courjon J 1956 Les ictus amnésiques. Journal de Médicine de Lyon 37: 697–701

Haas D C, Ross G S 1986 Transient global amnesia triggered by mild head trauma. Brain 109: 251–257

Halgren E, Walter R D, Cherlow D G, Crandall P H 1978 Mental phenomena evoked by electrical stimulation of the human hippocampal formation and amygdala. Brain 101: 83–117

Halgren E, Engel J, Wilson C L, Walter R D, Squires N K, Crandall P H 1983 Dynamics of the hippocampal contribution to memory: Stimulation and recording studies in humans. In: Seifert W (ed) Neurobiology of the hippocampus. Academic Press, New York, pp 29–72

Hall P 1963 Korsakov's syndrome following herpes zoster encephalitis. Lancet 1: 72–73

Hall P 1965 Subacute viral encephalitis amnesia. Lancet 2: 1077

Halliday A M, Davison K, Browne M W, Kreeger L C 1968 A comparison of the effects on depression and memory of bilateral ECT and unilateral ECT to the dominant and non-dominant hemispheres. British Journal of Psychiatry 114: 997–1012

Halstead W C 1958 Some behavioral aspects of partial temporal lobectomy in man. Research Publications, Association for Research in Nervous and Mental Disease 36: 478–490

Hart J, Lesser R P, Fisher R S, Schwerdt P, Bryan R N 1991 Dominant-side intracarotid amobarbital spares comprehension of word meaning. Archives of Neurology 48: 55–58

Heath R G 1964 Pleasure response of human subjects to direct stimulations of the brain. In: Heath R G (ed) The role of pleasure in behavior. Harper and Row, New York, pp 219–243

Hebb D O 1939 Intelligence in man after large removals of cerebral tissue: defects following right temporal lobectomy. Journal of General Psychology 21: 437–446

Henson R A 1985 Amusia. In: Vinken P J, Bruyn G W, Klawans H L (eds) Handbook of clinical neurology. New series l. Elsevier, Amsterdam, vol 4, pp 483–490

Hermann B P, Chhabria S 1980 Interictal psycho-pathology in patients with ictal fear. Archives of Neurology 37: 667–668

Hermann B P, Riel P 1981 Interictal personality and behavioral traits in temporal lobe and generalized epilepsy. Cortex 17: 125–128

Hermann B P, Seidenberg M, Dohan F C, Wyler A R, Haltiner A et al 1995 Reports by patients and their families of memory change after left anterior temporal lobectomy: relationship to degree of hippocampal sclerosis. Neurosurgery 36: 39–45

Hillemand P, Laurent M, Mézard J, Stehelin J 1931 Un cas d'encéphalite accompagnée de paraplegie au décours d'une fiévre typhoï de ostréaire chez une vaccinée. Revue Neurologique 38: 794–801

Hinge H H, Jensen T S, Marquardsen J, de Fine Olivarius B 1986 The prognosis of transient global amnesia. Archives of Neurology 43: 673–676

Hodges J R 1994 Semantic memory and frontal executive function during transient global amnesia. Journal of Neurology, Neurosurgery and Psychiatry 57: 605–608

Hodges J R 1998 Unraveling the enigma of transient global amnesia. Annals of Neurology 43: 151–153

Hodges J R, Ward C D 1989 Observations during transient global amnesia. A behavioural and neuropsychological study of five cases. Brain 112: 595–620

Hodges J R, Patterson K, Oxbury S, Funnell E 1992 Semantic dementia: progressive fluent aphasia with temporal lobe atrophy. Brain 115: 1783–1806

Hofman S, Klein C, Arlazaroff A 1993 Common hemisphericity of language and music in a musician. A case report. Journal of Communication Disorders 26: 73–82

Hofstad H, Gjerde I O 1985 Transient global amnesia after whiplash injury. Journal of Neurology, Neurosurgery and Psychiatry 48: 956–957

Horowitz M J, Adams J E, Rutkin B B 1968 Visual imagery on brain stimulation. Archives of General Psychiatry 19: 469–486
Inglis J 1970 Shock, surgery, and cerebral asymmetry. British Journal of Psychiatry 117: 143–148
Inglis J, Sykes D H 1967 Some sources of variation in dichotic listening in children. Journal of Experimental Child Psychology 5: 480–488
Iversen S D 1977 Temporal lobe amnesia. In: Whitty C W M, Zangwill O L (eds) Amnesia, 2nd edn. Butterworths, London, pp 136–182
Jack C R, Nichols D A, Sharbrough F W, Marsh W R, Petersen R C 1988 Selective posterior cerebral artery Amytal test for evaluating memory function before surgery for temporal lobe seizure. Radiology 168: 787–793
Jack C R, Nichols D A, Sharbrough F W et al 1989 Selective posterior cerebral artery injection of amytal: New method of preoperative memory testing. Mayo Clinic Proceedings 64: 965–975
Jackson A, Stewart G, Wood A, Gillespie J E 1995 Transient global amnesia and cortical blindness after vertebral angiography: further evidence for the role of arterial spasm. Americal Journal of Neuroradiology 16: 955–959
Jacome D E 1989 EEG features in transient global amnesia. Clinical Electroencephalography 20: 183–192
Jasper H H, Rasmussen T 1958 Studies of clinical and electrical responses to deep temporal stimulation in man with some considerations of functional anatomy. Research Publications, Association for Research in Nervous and Mental Disease 36: 316–334
Kim Y K 1971 Effects of basolateral amygdalectomy. In: Umbach W (ed) Special topics in stereotaxis. Hippokrates-Verlag, Stuttgart, pp 69–81
Kimura D 1961 Some effects of temporal lobe damage on auditory perception. Canadian Journal of Psychology 15: 156–165
Kimura D 1963 Right temporal lobe damage: perception of unfamiliar stimuli after damage. Archives of Neurology 8: 264–271
Kimura D 1964 Left-right differences in the perception of melodies. Quarterly Journal of Experimental Psychology 16: 35–38
Kimura D 1967 Functional asymmetry of the brain in dichotic listening. Cortex 3: 163–178
Kløve H, Grabow J D, Trites R L 1969 Evaluation of memory functions with intracarotid sodium amytal. Transactions of the American Neurological Association 94: 76–80
Kløve H, Trites R L, Grabow J D 1970 Intracarotid sodium amytal for evaluating memory function. Electroencephalography and Clinical Neurophysiology 28: 418–419
Kneebone A C, Chelune G J, Dinner D S, Naugle R I, Awad I A 1995 Intracarotid amobarbital procedure as a predictor of material-specific memory change after anterior temporal lobectomy. Epilepsia 36: 857–865
Kritchevsky M, Squire L R 1989 Transient global amnesia: evidence for extensive, temporally graded retrograde amnesia. Neurology 39: 213–218
Kritchevsky M, Graff-Radford N R, Damasio A R 1987 Normal memory after damage to medial thalamus. Archives of Neurology 44: 959–962
Kritchevsky M, Squire L R, Zouzounis J A 1988 Transient global amnesia: characterization of anterograde and retrograde amnesia. Neurology 38: 213–219
Làdavas E, Umiltà C, Provinciali L 1979 Hemisphere-dependent cognitive performances in epileptic patients. Epilepsia 20: 493–502
Lansdell H 1962a A sex difference in effect of temporal lobe neurosurgery on design performance. Nature 194: 82–84
Lansdell H 1962b Laterality of verbal intelligence in the brain. Science 13: 922–923
Lansdell H 1968 The use of factor scores from the Wechsler-Bellevue Scale of Intelligence in assessing patients with temporal lobe removals. Cortex 4: 257–268
Leman P, Loiseau P, Cohadon F 1963 Sur deux cas d'encéphalite rappelant cliniquement les encéphalites nécrosantes temporales mais d'évolution favorable. Revue Neurologique 198: 798–806
Lennox W G 1951 Phenomena and correlates of the psychomotor triad. Neurology 1: 365–371
Lennox W G, Lennox M A 1960 Epilepsy and related disorders. Little Brown, Boston
Lhermitte F, Signoret J L 1972 Analyse neuro-psychologique et différenciation des syndromes amnésiques. Revue Neurologique 126: 161–178

Lin K N, Liu R S, Yeh T P et al 1993 Posterior ischaemia during an attack of transient global amnesia. Stroke 24: 1093–1095
Loring D W, Meador K J, Lee G P, King D W, Gallagher B B 1994 Stimulus timing effects on Wada memory testing. Archives of Neurology 51: 806–810
Loring D W, Meador K J, Lee G P, King D W, Nichols M E et al 1995 Wada memory asymmetries predict verbal memory decline after anterior temporal lobectomy. Neurology 45: 1329–1333
Loring D W, Hermann B P, Perrine K, Lee G P et al 1997 Effect of Wada memory stimulus type in discriminating lateralised temporal lobe impairment. Epilepsia 38: 219–224
Luria A R 1973 The working brain. Allen Lane, The Penguin Press, London
Luria A R, Karasseva T A 1968 Disturbances of auditory speech memory in focal lesions of the deep regions of the left temporal lobe. Neuropsychologia 6: 97–104
Luria A R, Sokolov E N, Klimkovsky M 1967 Towards a neuro-dynamic analysis of memory disturbances with lesions of the left temporal lobe. Neuropsychologia 5: 1–12
Luria A R, Simernitskaya E G, Tubylevich B 1970 The structure of psychological processes in relation to cerebral organization. Neuropsychologia 8: 13–20
Matias-Guiu J, Codina A 1985 Neuropsychological functions in the follow-up of transient global amnesia. Journal of Neurology, Neurosurgery and Psychiatry 48: 713
Matias-Guiu J, Codina A 1986 Transient global amnesia: Criteria and classification. Neurology 36: 441–442
Matias-Guiu J, Buenaventura I, Codina A 1985 Whiplash amnesia. Neurology 35: 1259
Mazzucchi A, Moretti G, Caffarra P, Parma M 1980 Neuropsychological functions in the follow-up of transient global amnesia. Brain 103: 161–178
McFarland H R, Fortin D 1982 Amusia due to right temporoparietal infarct. Archives of Neurology 39: 725–727
McFie J 1960 Psychological testing in clinical neurology. Journal of Nervous and Mental Disease 131: 383–393
Meier M J, French L A 1966 Longitudinal assessment of intellectual functioning following unilateral temporal lobectomy. Journal of Clinical Psychology 22: 22–27
Melo T P, Ferro J M, Paiva T 1994 Are brief or recurrent transient global amnesias of epileptic origin? Journal of Neurology, Neurosurgery and Psychiatry 57: 622–625
Merriam A E 1988 Emotional arousal-induced amnesia. Case report, differentiation from hysterical amnesia, and an etiologic hypothesis. Neuropsychiatry, Neuropsychology, and Behavioral Neurology 1: 73–78
Meyer V 1959 Cognitive changes following temporal lobectomy for temporal lobe epilepsy. Archives of Neurology and Psychiatry 81: 299–309
Meyer V, Falconer A 1960 Defects of learning ability with massive lesions of the temporal lobe. Journal of Mental Science 106: 472–477
Meyer V, Jones H G 1957 Patterns of cognitive test performances as functions of the lateral localization of cerebral abnormalities in the temporal lobe. Journal of Mental Science 103: 758–772
Meyer V, Yates A J 1955 Intellectual changes following temporal lobectomy for psychomotor epilepsy. Journal of Neurology, Neurosurgery and Psychiatry 18: 44–52
Miller D L, Fedio P 1988 Whither the Wada? Radiology 168: 871–872
Miller E 1972 Clinical neuropsychology. Penguin Books, Harmondsworth, Middlesex
Miller J W, Yanagihara T, Petersen R C, Klass D W 1987 Transient global amnesia and epilepsy. Electroencephalographic distinction. Archives of Neurology 44: 629–633
Milner B 1954a Intellectual function of the temporal lobe. Psychological Bulletin 51: 42–64
Milner B 1954b Psychological defects produced by temporal lobe excision. Research Publications, Association for Research in Nervous and Mental Disease 36: 244–257
Milner B 1958 Psychological defects produced by temporal lobe excision. Research Publications, Association for Research in Nervous and Mental Disease 36: 244–257
Milner B 1962 Laterality effects in audition. In: Mountcastle V B (ed) Interhemispheric relations and cerebral dominance. Johns Hopkins Press, Baltimore, ch 9
Milner B 1966 Amnesia following operations on the temporal lobes. In: Whitty C W M, Zangwill O L (eds) Amnesia. Butterworth, London
Milner B 1967 Brain mechanisms suggested by studies of temporal lobes. In: Darley F L (ed) Brain mechanisms underlying speech and language. Grune and Stratton, New York

Milner B 1970 Memory and the medial temporal regions of the brain. In: Pribram K H, Broadbent D E (eds) Biology of memory. Academic Press, New York, pp 29–50

Milner B, Kimura D 1964 Dissociable visual learning defects after temporal lobectomy in man. Paper read at the 35th Annual Meeting of the Eastern Psychological Association, Philadelphia

Milner B, Teuber H L 1968 Alteration of perception and memory in man: reflections on methods. In: Weiskrantz L (ed) Analysis of behavioral change. Harper and Row, New York, ch 11

Milner B, Branch C, Rasmussen T 1962 Study of short term memory after intracarotid injection of sodium amytal. Transactions of the American Neurological Association 87: 224–226

Milner B, Branch C, Rasmussen T 1964 Observations on cerebral dominance. In: de Reuck A V S, O'Connor M (eds) Disorders of language. Churchill, London

Milner B, Branch C, Rasmussen T 1966 Evidence for bilateral speech representation in some non-right handers. Transaction of the American Neurological Association 91: 306–308

Milner B, Taylor L, Sperry R W 1968a Lateralized suppression of dichotically-presented digits after commissural section in man. Science 161: 184–186

Milner B, Corkin S, Teuber H L 1968b Further analysis of the hippocampal amnesic syndrome: 14 year follow-up study of H.M. Neuropsychologia 6: 215

Mirsky A, Primac D, Marsan C, Rosvold H, Stevens J 1960 A comparison of the psychological test performance of patients with focal and non-focal epilepsy. Experimental Neurology 2: 75–89

Mohr J P, Leicester J, Stoddard L T, Sidman M 1971 Right hemianopia with memory and colour deficits in circumscribed left posterior cerebral artery territory infarction. Neurology 21: 1104–1113

Mullan S, Penfield W 1959 Illusions of comparative interpretation and emotion. Archives of Neurology and Psychiatry 81: 269–284

Mungas D 1982 Interictal behavior abnormality in temporal lobe epilepsy. Archives of General Psychiatry 39: 108–111

Mungas D M 1983 Behavioral symptoms in temporal lobe epilepsy (letter). Archives of General Psychiatry 40: 468–469

Muramoto O, Kuru Y, Sugishita M, Toyokura Y 1979 Pure memory loss with hippocampal lesions. Archives of Neurology 36: 54–56

Ogden J A 1996 Marooned in the moment: H.M., a case of global amnesia. In: Ogden J A Fractured minds: a case-study approach to clinical neuropsychology. Oxford University Press, Oxford, ch 3, pp 41–58

Ojemann G 1981 Interrelationship in the localization of language, memory and motor mechanisms in human cortex and thalamus. In: Thompson R (ed) New perspectives in cerebral localization. Raven Press, New York, pp 157–175

Okada F, Ito N, Tsukamoto R 1987 Two cases of transient partial amnesia in the course of transient global amnesia. Journal of Clinical Psychiatry 48: 449–450

Olivarius B de F, Jensen T S 1979 Transient global amnesia in migraine. Headache 19: 335–338

Onishi T, Hoshi H, Nagamachi S et al 1995 High-resolution SPECT to assess hippocampal perfusion in neuropsychiatric diseases. Journal of Nuclear Medicine 36: 1163–1169

Oxbury J M, Oxbury S M 1969 Effects of lobectomy on the report of dichotically presented digits. Cortex 5: 1–4

Pampiglione G, Falconer M A 1960 Electrical stimulation of the hippocampus in man. In: Field J, Magoun H W, Hall V E (eds) Handbook of physiology. Section l, Neurophysiology. American Physiological Society, Washington, vol 2, pp 1391–1394

Parsons O A, Kemp D E 1960 Intellectual functioning in temporal epilepsy. Journal of Consulting Psychology 24: 408–414

Penfield W 1938 The cerebral cortex in man. Archives of Neurology and Psychiatry 40: 417–442

Penfield W 1954 Temporal lobe epilepsy. British Journal of Surgery 41: 337–343

Penfield W, Jasper H 1954 Epilepsy and the functional anatomy of the human brain. Little Brown, Boston

Penfield W, Milner B 1958 Memory deficit produced by bilateral lesions of the hippocampal zone. Archives of Neurology and Psychiatry 79: 475–497

Penfield W, Perot P 1963 The brain's record of auditory and visual experience. Brain 86: 595–697

Perrine K, Gershengorn J, Brown E R et al 1993a Material-specific memory in intracarotid amobarbital procedure. Neurology 43: 706–711
Perrine K, Uysal S, Dogali M, Luciano D J, Devinsky O 1993b Functional mapping of memory and other nonlinguistic cognitive abilities in adults. Advances in Neurology 63: 165–177
Pizzamiglio L, De Pascalis C, Vignati A 1974 Stability of dichotic listening test. Cortex 10: 203–205
Ponsford J L, Donnan G A, Walsh K W 1980 Disorders of memory in vertebrobasilar disease. Journal of Clinical Neuropsychology 2: 267–276
Pratt R T C, Warrington E K, Halliday A M 1971 Unilateral ECT as a test for cerebral dominance, with a strategy for treating left handers. British Journal of Psychiatry 119: 78–83
Prisko L H 1963 Short-term memory in focal cerebral damage. Unpublished doctoral dissertation, McGill University
Rausch R, Serafetinides E A 1975a Specific alterations of olfactory function in humans with temporal lobe lesions. Nature 255: 557–558
Rausch R, Serafetinides E A 1975b Human temporal lobe and olfaction. In: Denton D A, Coghlan J P (eds) Olfaction and taste. Academic Press, New York, pp 321–324
Rausch R, Serafetinides E A, Crandall P H 1977 Olfactory memory in patients with anterior temporal lobectomy. Cortex 13: 445–452
Rausch R, Fedio P, Ary C M, Engel J, Crandall P H 1984 Resumption of behavior following intracarotid sodium amobarbital injection. Annals of Neurology 15: 31–35
Rivera V M, Meyer J S 1976 Dementia and cerebrovascular disease. In: Meyer J S (ed) Modern concepts of cerebrovascular disease. Eighth International Congress, Salzburg. Thieme, Stuttgart
Rose F C, Symonds C P 1960 Persistent memory defect following encephalitis. Brain 83: 195–212
Rubino C A 1970 Hemispheric lateralization of visual perception. Cortex 6: 102–130
Sakurai Y, Momose T, Watanabe T et al 1991 Slowly progressive fluent aphasia: clinical features and an imaging study including MRI, SPECT, and PET. Rinsho Shinkeigaku 31: 505–511
Sass K J, Lencz T, Westerveld M, Novelly R A, Spencer D D, Kim J H 1991 The neural substrate of memory impairment demonstrated by the intracarotid amobarbital procedure. Archives of Neurology 48: 48–52
Satz P 1977 Laterality tests: an inferential problem. Cortex 13: 208–212
Satz P, Aschenbach K, Fennell E 1965 Order of report, ear asymmetry, and handedness in dichotic listening. Cortex 1: 377–396
Saul R, Sperry R W 1968 Absence of commissurotomy symptoms with agenesis of the corpus callosum. Neurology 18: 307
Schamschula R G, Soo M Y 1994 Transient global amnesia following cerebral angiography with non-ionic contrast medium. Australasian Radiology 38: 196–198
Schulhoff C, Goodglass H 1969 Dichotic listening: side of brain injury and cerebral dominance. Neuropsychologia 7: 149–160
Schwartz M, Dennerll R 1969 Immediate visual memory as a function of epileptic seizure type. Cortex 5: 69–74
Scott D, Moffett A, Matthews A, Ettlinger G 1967 Effects of epileptic discharges on learning and memory in patients. Epilepsia 8: 188–194
Scott S K, Young A W, Calder A J, Hellawell D J, Aggleton J P, Johnson M 1997 Impaired auditory recognition of fear and anger following bilateral amygdala lesions. Nature 385: 254–257
Scoville W B, Correll R E 1973 Memory and the temporal lobe. A review for clinicians. Acta Neurochirurgica 28: 21–28
Scoville W B, Milner B 1957 Loss of recent memory after bilateral hippocampal lesions. Journal of Neurology, Neurosurgery and Psychiatry 20: 11–21
Sem-Jacobsen C W, Torkildsen A 1960 Depth recording and electrical stimulation in the human brain. In: Ramey E R, O'Doherty D S (eds) Electrical studies on the unanesthetized brain. Hoeber, New York, pp 275–290
Sengoku A, Toichi M, Murai T 1997 Dreamy states and psychoses in temporal lobe epilepsy: mediating role of affect. Psychiatry and Clinical Neurosciences 51: 23–26

Serafetinides E A 1966 Auditory recall and visual recognition following intracarotid amytal. Cortex 2: 367–372
Serafetinides E A, Falconer M A 1962 Some observations on memory impairment after temporal lobectomy for epilepsy. Journal of Neurology, Neurosurgery and Psychiatry 25: 251–255
Servan J, Verstichel P, Catala M, Yakovleff A, Rancurel G 1995 Aphasia and infarction of the posterior cerebral artery territory. Journal of Neurology 242: 87–92
Shalman D C 1961 The diagnostic use of the McGill Picture Anomalies Test in temporal lobe epilepsy. Journal of Neurology, Neurosurgery and Psychiatry 24: 220–222
Shankweiler D P 1966 Effects of temporal lobe damage on the perception of dichotically presented melodies. Journal of Comparative and Physiological Psychology 62: 115
Shatz M W 1981 WAIS practice effects in clinical neuropsychology. Journal of Clinical Neuropsychology 3: 171–179
Silberman E K 1983 Behavioral symptoms in temporal lobe epilepsy (letter). Archives of General Psychiatry 40: 468
Silverstein M L, Schwartz M, Rennick P 1973 Recall of verbal material in temporal lobe epilepsy and schizophrenia. Diseases of the Nervous System 34: 234–240
Simpson J A 1969 The clinical neurology of temporal disorders. British Journal of Psychiatry. Special publication no 4: 42–48
Smith M L 1989 Memory disorders associated with temporal-lobe lesions. In: Boller F, Grafman J (eds) Handbook of neuropsychology. Elsevier, Amsterdam, vol 3, ch 4
Smith M L, Milner B 1981 The role of the right hippocampus in the recall of spatial location. Neuropsychologia 19: 781–793
Snowden J S, Goulding P J, Neary D 1989 Semantic dementia: a form of circumscribed cerebral atrophy. Behavioural Neurology 2: 167–182
Sparks R, Geschwind N 1968 Dichotic listening in man after section of the neocortical commissures. Cortex 4: 3–16
Sparks R, Goodglass H, Nickel B 1970 Ipsilateral versus contralateral extinction in dichotic listening from hemisphere lesions. Cortex 6: 249–260
Squire L R, Slater P C 1978 Bilateral and unilateral ECT: effects on verbal and nonverbal memory. American Journal of Psychiatry 13: 1316–1320
Stepien L, Sierpinski S 1964 Impairment of recent memory after temporal lesions in man. Neuropsychologia 2: 291–303
Stevens J, Milstein V, Goldstein S 1972 Psychometric test performance in relation to the psychopathology of epilepsy. Archives of General Psychiatry 26: 32–38
Stillhard G, Landis T, Scheiss R et al 1990 Bitemporal hypoperfusion in transient global amnesia: 99m-Tc HM PAO SPECT and neuropsychological findings during and after an attack. Journal of Neurology, Neurosurgery and Psychiatry 53: 339–342
Stracciari A, Morreale A 1987 Memory performances before and after transient global amnesia. Stroke 18: 813–814
Stracciari A, Rebucci G G, Gallassi R 1987 Transient global amnesia: neuropsychological study of a "pure" case. Journal of Neurology 234: 126–127
Stracciari A, Lorusso S, Pazzaglia P 1994 Transient topographical amnesia. Journal of Neurology, Neurosurgery and Psychiatry 57: 1423–1425
Strupp M, Brüning R, Wu R H, Deimling M, Reiser M, Brandt T 1998 Diffusion-weighted MRI in transient global amnesia: elevated signal intensity in the left mesial temporal lobe in 7 of 10 patients. Annals of Neurology 43: 164–170
Talbot P R, Snowden J S, Lloyd J J, Neary D, Testa H J 1995 The contribution of single photon emission tomography to the clinical differentiation of degenerative cortical brain disorders. Journal of Neurology 242: 579–586
Tanabe H, Hashikawa K, Nakagawa Y et al 1991 Memory loss due to transient hypoperfusion in the medial temporal lobes. Acta Neurologica Scandinavica 84: 22–27 (see erratum published in Acta Neurologica Scandinavica 84: 463)
Taylor L 1969 Localization of cerebral lesions by psychological testing. Clinical Neurosurgery 16: 269–287
Teng E L 1981 Dichotic ear difference is a poor index for the functional asymmetry between the cerebral hemispheres. Neuropsychologia 19: 235–240
Trenerry M R 1996 Neuropsychologic assessment in surgical treatment of epilepsy. Mayo Clinic Proceedings 71: 1196–1200

Trenerry M R, Loring D W 1995 Intracarotid amobarbital procedure. The Wada test. Neuroimaging Clinics of North America 5: 721–728
Trillet M, Fischer C, Serclerat D, Schott B 1980 Le syndrome amnésique des ischemies cérébrales posterieures. Cortex 16: 432–434
Trimble M R 1983 Interictal behaviour and temporal lobe epilepsy. In: Pedley T A, Meldrum B S (eds) Recent advances in epilepsy. Number one. Churchill Livingstone, Edinburgh, pp 211–229
Van Buren J M 1961 Sensory, motor and autonomic effects of mesial temporal lobe stimulation in man. Journal of Neurosurgery 18: 273–288
Van Buren J M, Borke R C 1972 The mesial temporal substratum of memory. Anatomical studies in three individuals. Brain 9: 599–632
Venneri A, Caffarra P 1998 Transient autobiographic amnesia: EEG and single-photon emission CT evidence of an organic etiology. Neurology 50: 186–191
Victor M, Angevine J B, Mancall E L, Fisher C M 1961 Memory loss with lesions of the hippocampal formation. Report of a case with some remarks on the anatomical basis of memory. Archives of Neurology 5: 244–263
Vignolo L A 1969 Auditory agnosia. A review and report of recent evidence. In: Benton A L (ed) Contributions to neuropsychology. Aldine, Chicago, ch 7
Volpe B T, Hirst W 1983 The characterization of an amnesic syndrome following hypoxic ischemic injury. Archives of Neurology 40: 436–440
Wada J 1949 A new method for the determination of the side of cerebral speech dominance. A preliminary report on the intracarotid injection of sodium amytal in man. Igaku to Siebutsugaku 14: 221–222
Walker A E, Marshall C 1961 Stimulation and depth recording in man. In: Sheer D E (ed) Electrical stimulation of the brain. University of Texas Press, Austin, pp 514–518
Walsh K W 1991 Understanding brain damage. A primer of neuropsychological evaluation, 2nd edn. Churchill Livingstone, Edinburgh
Walsh K 1994 Neuropsychological assessment of patients with memory disorders. In: Toyuz S, Gilandas A, Byrne D (eds) Neuropsychology in clinical practice. Harcourt Brace Jovanovich, Marrickville, Australia, pp 107–127
Warrington E K 1975 The selective impairment of semantic memory. Quarterly Journal of Experimental Psychology 27: 635–657
Warrington E K, Duchen L W 1992 A re-appraisal of persistent global amnesia following right temporal lobectomy: a clinico-pathological study. Neuropsychologia 30: 437–450
Warrington E K, James M 1967a An experimental investigation of facial recognition in patients with cerebral lesions. Cortex 3: 317–326
Warrington E K, James M 1967b Tachistoscopic number estimation in patients with unilateral cerebral lesions. Journal of Neurology, Neurosurgery and Psychiatry 30: 468–474
Warrington E K, Shallice T 1969 The selective impairment of auditory verbal short-term memory. Brain 92: 885–896
Weingarten S M, Cherlow D G, Halgren E 1977 Relationship of hallucinations to the depth structures of the temporal lobe. In: Sweet W H et al (eds) Neurosurgical treatment in psychiatry, pain, and epilepsy. University Park Press, Baltimore, pp 553–568
Weingartner H 1968 Verbal learning in patients with temporal lobe lesions. Journal of Verbal Learning and Verbal Behavior 7: 520–526
Whitty C W M, Lishman W A 1966 Amnesia in cerebral disease. In Whitty C W M, Zangwill O L (eds) Amnesia. Appleton Century-Crofts, New York
Williams D 1956 The structure of emotions reflected in epileptic experiences. Brain 79: 28–67
Williams D 1969 Temporal lobe syndromes. In: Vinken P J, Bruyn G W (ed) Handbook of clinical neurology. North-Holland, Amsterdam, vol 2, ch 22
Wood N, Cowan N 1995a The cocktail party phenomenon revisited: how frequent are attention shifts to one's name in an irrelevant auditory channel? Journal of Experimental Psychology. Memory, Learning and Cognition 21: 255–260
Wood N, Cowan N 1995b The cocktail party phenomenon revisited: attention and memory in the classic selective listening procedure of Cherry (1953). Journal of Experimental Psychology: General 124: 243–262
Wyllie E, Luders H, Murphy D et al 1990 Intracarotid amobarbital (Wada) test for language: correlation with results of cortical stimulation. Epilepsia 31: 156–161

Zaidel D W, Rausch R 1981 Effects of semantic organization on the recognition of pictures following temporal lobectomy. Neuropsychologia 19: 813–817

Zamora E N, Kaelbling R 1965 Memory and electro-convulsive therapy. American Journal of Psychiatry 122: 546–554

Zangwill O L 1946 Some qualitative observations on verbal memory in cases of cerebral lesions. British Journal of Psychology 37: 8–19

Zangwill O 1966 The amnesic syndrome. In: Whitty C W M, Zangwill O (eds) Amnesia. Butterworths, London, pp 77–91

Zorzon M, Antonutti L, Mase G et al 1995 Transient global amnesia and transient ischemic attack. Natural history, vascular risk factors, and associated conditions. Stroke 26: 1536–1542

Zurif E B 1974 Auditory lateralization: Prosodic and syntactical factors. Brain and Language 1: 391–404

Zurif E B, Ramier A M 1972 Some effects of unilateral brain damage on the presentation of dichotically presented phoneme sequences and digits. Neuropsychologia 10: 103–110

6

The parietal lobes

The middle third of the cerebral hemispheres, strategically situated between the frontal, occipital and temporal lobes, is closely related in function to each of these regions of the brain. Partly as a result of this, a greater variety of clinical manifestations is likely to result from disease of the parietal lobe than from disturbance of any other part of the hemispheres. It must be emphasized, however, that these phenomena require special techniques for their elicitation, otherwise they may be easily overlooked or discounted.

ANATOMICAL FEATURES

The parietal lobe has two main surfaces, one lateral and the other medial. The anterior border of the lateral aspect is formed by the central sulcus, while the posterior border is formed by the parieto-occipital sulcus and a line drawn from the end of this sulcus to the pre-occipital notch on the inferolateral border of the hemisphere (Fig. 6.1). The lower border separates the inferior part of the parietal lobe from the superior portion of the temporal lobe. It is made up of the lateral sulcus and a line continued back from it to reach the posterior line of demarcation.

Two well-marked sulci lie within the parietal lobe. The post-central sulcus delimits the post-central gyrus, which is concerned with somatic sensation. The intraparietal sulcus runs roughly parallel to the lower margin of the lobe about midway in the lobe, separating it into a superior and an inferior parietal lobule. The ends of two (sometimes three) sulci invade the inferior parietal lobule. The anterior of these is the posterior branch of the lateral sulcus, while just posterior to it is the end of the superior temporal sulcus. The cortex of the inferior parietal lobule around the end of the lateral sulcus is the supramarginal gyrus, that around the superior temporal sulcus is the angular gyrus. Not infrequently the sulci of the supramarginal and angular gyri are independent of the lateral and superior temporal gyri.

The anterior border of the medial aspect of the parietal lobe is formed by a line which extends about midway through the paracentral lobule from the point on the superomedial border of the hemisphere reached by the central

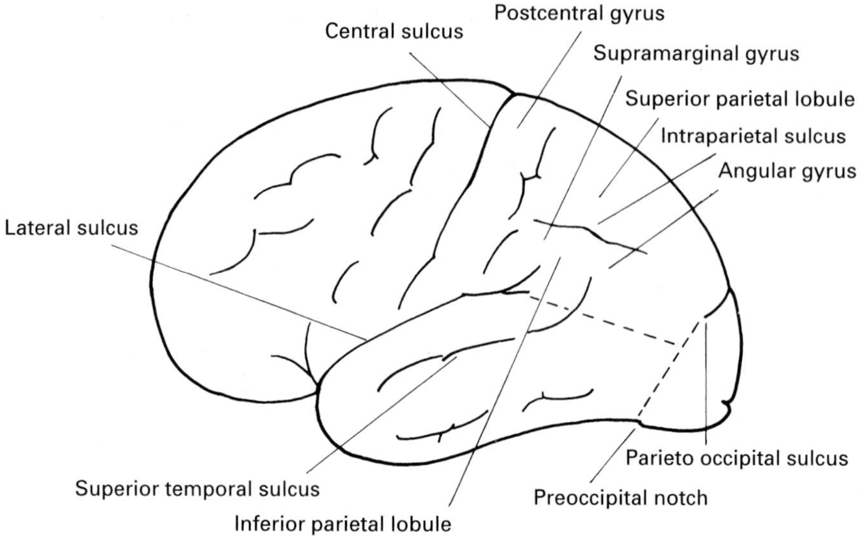

Fig. 6.1 Lateral aspect of the parietal lobe.

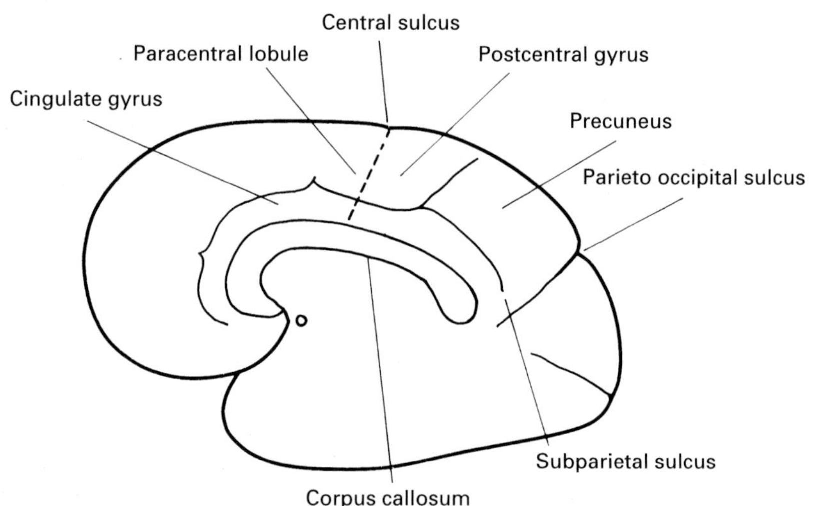

Fig. 6.2 Medial aspect of the parietal lobe.

sulcus, to the top of the corpus callosum (Fig. 6.2). Thus only the posterior half of the paracentral lobule belongs to the parietal lobe. The posterior border is formed by the parieto-occipital sulcus, which is usually very distinct. The region anterior to this sulcus is the precuneus which extends anteriorly to the continuation of the post-central gyrus and is continuous around the subparietal sulcus with the cingulate gyrus. A branch or continuation of the cingulate sulcus, the marginal sulcus, separates the anterior border of the precuneus from the posterior border of the paracentral lobule.

Following this description of the parietal lobe as an empirical convention, it would be wise to repeat the warning of Critchley (1953) in his classic monograph on the parietal lobes.

> More than once it has been emphasized that the parietal lobe cannot be regarded as an autonomous anatomical entity. Its boundaries cannot be drawn with any precision except by adopting conventional and artificial landmarks and frontiers. Later, it will also be seen that it is not possible to equate the parietal lobe with any narrowly defined physiological function. In other words, the parietal lobe represents a topographical convenience pegged out empirically upon the surface of the brain. The name serves a mere descriptive role…
>
> Up to 150 years ago, the cerebrum was not divided into lobes or regions by any established figural patterns. In the early nineteenth century Burdach began to speak of the cerebrum as being made up of lobes. These major subdivisions he spoke of as anterior, upper and lower lobes, the operculum, and the island of Reil. At a still later date (cf. Quain 1837) there were three lobes identified, namely, the anterior, posterior and middle lobes, indicating the various positions of the brain as related to the fossae of the base of the skull. This system was adopted and recapitulated in text-books until 1850. Around that time, there developed a tendency to associate regions of the brain with the overlying cranial bones. Thus the anterior lobe became the frontal lobe, while the cortical territory underlying…(the) os parietalis became known as the parietal lobe…
>
> There is no inherent reason to doubt but that the term parietal lobe…and others…will eventually be replaced by some other nomenclature. The ideal would be a less narrow terminology, and one which would include the whole retro-rolandic complex, or a three-dimensional temporo-occipital territory as a functional domain. (p. 55)

Later, Critchley came to term this region the 'parieto-temporo-occipital crossroads'. This term had been used also by early European neurologists.

These notions have been reiterated a number of times in the ensuing decades, although no satisfactory nomenclature has as yet emerged. In what follows it is difficult to disentangle the contribution of separate parts of the posterior cortical territory, though the division into primary, secondary (association) and tertiary (supra-modal) cortex proposed by Luria (1973) and outlined in brief in Chapter 2 seems of value when considering different degrees of complexity of symptoms in the posterior areas. Many studies employ a heterogeneous collection of variously located lesions, while some attempts have been made to separate parietal from non-parietal cases. Certainly some major differences have emerged which are related to the laterality of the lesion in the territory behind the central sulcus.

SENSORY AND PERCEPTUAL DISTURBANCES

The primary reception area for the numerous forms of somatic sensation has its principal locus in the post-central gyrus. The secondary or association cortex posterior to this is thought to deal with the elaboration of the discrete elements into meaningful wholes so that disorders with damage away from the 'somaesthetic' area tend to be more complex, i.e. tend to be perceptual or cognitive in nature rather than simple disturbances of sensation. Further afield in the region of the 'temporo-parieto-occipital crossroads' the disturbances tend to be those which reflect a disruption of intersensory or cross-modal association and integration. Following this 'anatomical' division of deficits according to type of cortex, three types of deficit have been selected for treatment: (i) somatosensory discrimination; (ii) disorders of tactile perception; and (iii) disorders of intersensory association. They by no means cover the gamut of parietal disorders.

Somatosensory discrimination

What is commonly called somatic sensation is made up of a number of separate modalities. Among these are touch, pain, temperature, body position sense, kinaesthesis and vibration. The detailed organization of each of these is dealt with in texts of physiological psychology, such as Galluscio (1990) and Levinthal (1990), as well as in some texts of physiology and neurology. Some major texts do not treat the topic at all!

The somatosensory system is able to combine information from different modalities in different locations and with different temporal relationships. A treatment of these, however, is outside the scope of the present volume which is largely concerned with lesion studies.

The earliest neuropsychological studies of the cerebral basis of somatic sensation in man came from the examination of missile wounds to the head (Head 1920, Holmes 1927). The value of these studies suffered from the inability to localize accurately the site of the lesion for correlation with the results of their painstaking examination of sensory-perceptual capacities. The introduction and increasing use of cortical ablation for the removal of cerebral scars allowed Penfield's group to make the first serious examination of sensory defects following circumscribed ablation of cortical tissue (Evans 1935) (Fig. 6.3). Employing the detailed examination procedure outlined by Head, Evans examined 17 cases, nine posterior and eight anterior.

Evans concluded from the examination of these cases that damage to the extraparietal areas, the pre- and post-central gyri and the central portion of the parietal lobe led to transient sensory dysfunction, if any, 'while limited excisions in the region of the supramarginal gyrus caused extensive and permanent loss of somesthetic sensation'. Such limited case material, supplemented by other smaller studies, formed the basis for conjecture about the cortical basis of somatosensory function until the studies performed on penetrating missile cases after World War II. Numerous studies on such cases provided increasing evidence that performance on many complex sensory discrimination tasks depended on temporal, posterior parietal or parieto-temporo-occipital areas (Blum et al 1950, Teuber 1950, Battersby 1951, Teuber et al 1951, Teuber & Weinstein 1954).

In 1956 Hécaen et al, in a study of patients with surgical lesions of the minor hemisphere, reported that patients with parietal lesions showed no increase in sensory thresholds unless there was also involvement of the rolandic region. They also noted difficulties with complex sensorimotor tasks, such as using scissors, dressing and making block constructions, as well as some of the

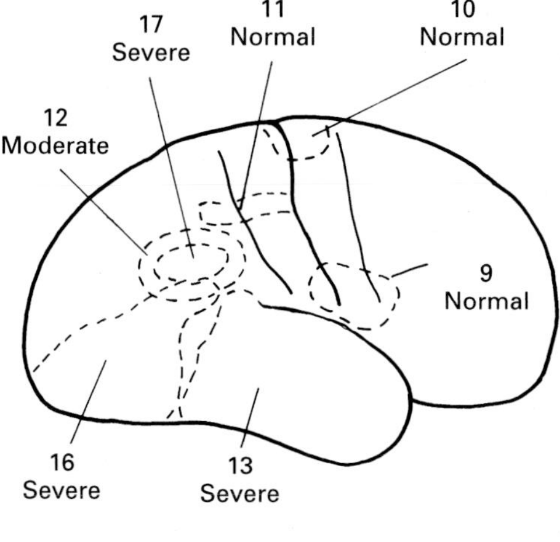

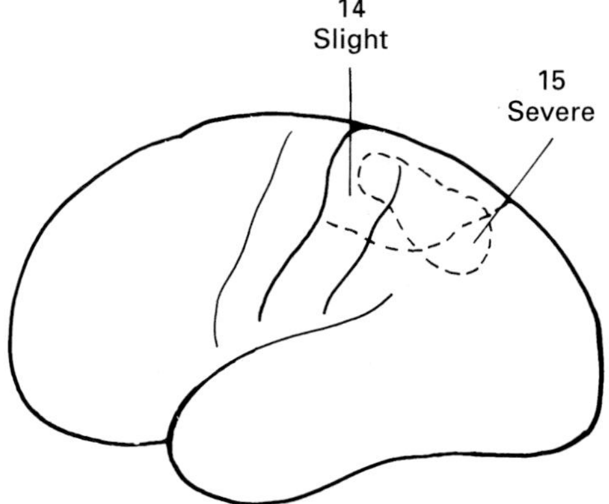

Fig. 6.3 Relation between severity of somatic sensory disturbance and site of lesion (redrawn from Evans 1935. Courtesy of the Association for Research in Nervous and Mental Disease).

visuospatial and body image disturbances described below, in patients with right posterior lesions.

One of the most extensive investigations of somatosensory changes after brain injury was that of Semmes et al (1960). This work summarizes a good deal of the work of this group on the effects of penetrating missile wounds and it is difficult to do justice to it in a brief summary. One major finding worth recording is the fact that this group found bilateral deficits on occasion in patients with left hemisphere lesions but only contralateral deficits after lesions of the right hemisphere. The difference was not statistically significant and to date there has been little or no confirmation of this hemispheric asymmetry. Semmes et al also reported bilateral difficulty in tactually guided learning in patients whose primary sensory deficit seemed restricted to one hand.

Corkin (1964) tested 95 patients who had undergone cortical excision for the relief of epilepsy and compared their performance with that of control subjects on sensory discrimination tasks and tests of tactual learning and problem solving. Her major findings were that sensory deficits and impairment in tactile object recognition were closely related to lesions in the rolandic region of either side. No lasting sensory impairment was seen in patients whose pre- and post-central gyri were spared. The deficits were usually contralateral though some bilateral effects were produced by unilateral excisions. A wide range of measures such as pressure sensitivity, two-point discrimination threshold and point localization were used. More complex functions such as tactually guided learning and problem solving showed deficits with removals in the right hemisphere regardless of location of the lesion within the hemisphere. Generalization from these findings is limited since left parietal lesions were not specifically studied.

An extension of this work was reported by Corkin et al (1970). Tests of pressure sensitivity, two-point discrimination, point localization, position sense and tactual object recognition were given to 127 cases of limited unilateral cortical removal. Preoperative, postoperative and follow-up measurements were taken. This study confirmed the earlier report that lasting sensory loss was highly correlated with lesions of the post-central gyrus and was particularly severe with involvement of the contralateral hand area. Normal scores were reported in patients with pre-central lesions which did not encroach upon the post-central hand area. Lesions of the parietal lobe outside the post-central gyrus produced transient loss or no loss at all. Extraparietal lesions produced little or no sign of somatosensory change. Ipsilateral sensory defects were found in 20 of the 50 parietal lobe patients; unlike the finding of Semmes et al (1960), the defects showed no relation to laterality but did appear to be related to the size of the lesion.

For further detail on sensory disorders, readers should consult texts on physiological psychology and neurology.

Disorders of tactile perception

Judgment of stimulus orientation

The perception of orientation has been studied in detail by Benton and his colleagues for both tactile and visual perception in normal subjects and those with unilateral lesions (see Chs. 7 and 8). Carmon and Bechtoldt (1969) and Fontenot and Benton (1971) tested the perception of the direction of tactile stimulation applied to the palm of the hand. A significant proportion of patients with right hemisphere lesions showed bilateral impairment, whereas patients with left hemisphere lesions showed significant impairment only in the contralateral hand. A test of the detection of three-dimensional orientation was devised by De Renzi et al (1971) for use in both visual and tactile modalities. Using the hand ipsilateral to the lesion, only those with right hemisphere lesions having visual field defects were significantly impaired.

While no sound anatomical data exist on the regions involved, there is presumptive evidence that the right parietal lobe may be crucially involved in this basic spatial function.

Tactile agnosia

The term *astereognosis* has in the past often been used interchangeably with the term *tactile agnosia*. In either case, the patients are unable to recognize objects which they feel. If the disorder is to conform to the general concept of agnosia it should be a higher perceptual disorder in the presence of intact primary sense modalities. Denny-Brown et al (1952) considered the basic disturbance to be a failure to synthesize separate tactile sensations into the perception of form, a process they termed *amorphosynthesis*. Elsewhere they considered the difficulty to be one of inability to carry out a 'summation of spatial impressions' (Denny-Brown & Chambers 1958).

Doubt has been cast on the existence of this, as with other forms of agnosia (Teuber 1965a, b). Several early neuropsychological studies directed themselves in whole or in part to the problem. Corkin (1964) found that impaired tactual recognition was seen only in patients who also had somatosensory deficits. This was confirmed in the 1970 study previously mentioned. 'Impaired tactual recognition of common objects reflected the sensory status of the hand, and, in this series of patients, there were no object-recognition deficits that were disproportionate to the sensory loss' (p. 57).

Semmes (1965) clarified the relation of sensory status to tactile agnosia in a study of left hemisphere, right hemisphere and bilateral lesions. She found that impaired performance on tests of tactual shape discrimination was seen in the absence as well as in the presence of sensory defect. Authors of recent papers (Caselli 1991a, b, Reed & Caselli 1994) also agree that tactile object recognition difficulty can occur in the absence of basic somaesthetic dysfunction, and that relatively normal tactile object recognition can be seen in cases with somatosensory dysfunction. Caselli (1991b) sensibly suggests that the term tactile agnosia, denoting a mild disorder, be reserved for cases where difficulty with tactile object recognition occurs without significant somatosensory loss, i.e. in the general sense of usage of the term agnosia. The term significant somatosensory loss is critical since Maugiere and Isnard (1995), using a method employing evoked potentials, failed to find a case of pure tactile agnosia in their large series. If cases do exist, the lesions responsible are probably in the secondary somatosensory cortex or parietotemporal or insular cortical regions. The term *astereognosis* should be reserved for a 'lower order' somatosensory loss, whether from cortical or spinal or peripheral nerve damage. This form of disorder is a more severe form of deficit. The Caselli opinion, which is supported by imaging information on the distinction, and the editorial by Tranel (1991), greatly clarify the conceptualization and terminology of tactile agnosia.

Semmes' earlier examination of her cases without sensory defect revealed that the impairment was specific to shape, the discrimination of texture, size and roughness being unaffected. The impairment was, however, related to spatial orientation even when this was measured by a visual task. 'It was suggested, therefore, that impaired shape discrimination after brain injury depends on a general spatial factor as well as on the status of somatic sensation' (p. 312). Either of these factors seemed capable of producing impairment of tactile form discrimination, but when both were present the impairment was more severe, suggesting that the factors are independent but additive. Semmes found that they tended to occur together in right hemisphere lesions and she assumed that this was because of the size of the lesion, a large lesion being needed to affect both sensation and orientation. 'Paradoxically although each of the factors is more localizable in the left hemisphere than the right and the parietal region is implicated for both, these factors show no tendency toward association. One must therefore assume separate foci for the two factors within the left parietal region' (p. 312). Both specific testing of tactual recognition (De Renzi & Scotti 1969) as well as the wealth of evidence cited later in this chapter would support the idea that the prime representation of the spatial factor which may contribute to tactile agnosia has its major location in the posterior cerebral areas, particularly of the right hemisphere.

The only standard psychological measure of tactual form perception is the Seguin-Goddard formboard, which has been adapted in the much used Halstead-Reitan battery of tests. Teuber and Weinstein (1954) showed that men with posterior lesions performed significantly poorer on this task than those with anterior lesions, though all brain damaged subjects were significantly inferior to controls. This latter finding has been replicated many times by Reitan and his co-workers (Reitan & Davison 1974). For example, Boll (1974) found that, apart from tactile object recognition, early studies (e.g. Battersby et al 1955) suggested that tactile discrimination learning might not be more impaired with posterior lesions than with lesions in other locations, though Semmes et al (1954) did find that patients with lesions of the parietal lobe, unlike other patients, showed no transfer effect from one modality to another. This may reflect a loss of cross-modal association.

Both Corkin (1965) and Milner (1965) used visually guided and tactually guided maze learning in patients with variously located surgical lesions. Small parietal lesions had little effect upon performance, while right hemisphere lesions, either frontal or temporal, produced a marked impairment. However, the complex nature of the tasks makes interpretation difficult.

A study of De Renzi et al (1970) showed that tactile searching, like visual searching, is poorer for the contralateral field for both left and right hemisphere lesions but that the poorest performances were made by the right posterior group. That the right parietal region specifically is also involved during ipsilateral hemispace exploration was strongly suggested by a recent PET study, using right hand exploration into right hemispace (Gitelman et al 1996).

Finally, visual object recognition also appears to be related more closely to the right parietal regions than anywhere else. Warrington and Rabin (1970) found that a right parietal group was much inferior to others on a series of perceptual matching tasks of simple perceptual attributes, but that this failure was not related to their poor performance on the Gollin incomplete figures test (Gollin 1960), suggesting that failure of recognition of features (which was required in the matching tasks) could not account for impairment on the test of visual recognition. There was, however, a correlation between the performance on matching tasks and more complex tasks of spatial analysis such as Block Designs, suggesting that there was a common spatial element involved in the two types of task but that this differed in complexity. A new test of object recognition was introduced by Warrington and Taylor (1973). This consisted of the recognition of objects photographed from a 'conventional' and an 'unconventional' view. The right posterior group was selectively impaired in this test compared to all other groups, having a very marked deficit, whereas the deficit of other brain damaged groups was much smaller when compared with control subjects. Right posterior subjects were again inferior on the recognition of Gollin's incomplete figures, though not nearly as much as on the new recognition task. Other visuoperceptual tasks such as figure-ground discrimination showed no differences between any of the brain damaged subgroups, though all groups were inferior to controls.

Disorders of intersensory association (cross-modal integration)

Studies on intersensory association or cross-modal integration are of interest because such integration or association between different forms of sense information would appear to be basic to many higher functions. Damage to the region in which such integration is likely to take place, i.e. the area of conjunction of the temporal, parietal and occipital lobes in the dominant hemisphere, has often been said to produce the most marked losses of cognitive functions. Few studies relating cross-modal association problems with locus of lesion have appeared to date.

Butters and Brody (1968) found that patients with neurologically confirmed dominant parietal lobe damage were particularly impaired on cross-modal matching tasks (auditory-visual, tactual-visual, visual-tactual), whereas frontotemporal patients were unimpaired either on intra-modal or cross-modal tasks. Deficits on the auditory-visual matching task were closely associated with reading difficulties, confirming the notion that this cross-modal association is a prerequisite for reading. Many of the parietal patients who were impaired on the visual-tactual and tactual-visual matching tasks were also impaired on copying tests, which are often used to assess constructional praxis, whereas those with mild or no signs of parietal involvement showed little or no copying impairment. 'The possibility that certain kinds of intersensory associations or integrations may underlie some constructional apraxia disorders and other voluntary motor behaviour is intriguing and certainly deserving of further study' (p. 342).

Butters et al (1970a) found some impairment of cross-modal association (auditory-visual matching) in patients with severe parietal signs, but none in those with only mild parietal signs. The care that must be exercised in interpretation of findings was highlighted by the subsequent finding that the impairment of right parietal patients on the auditory-visual task was associated with an auditory decoding problem rather than failure of cross-modal association. The inferred size of the lesions and the propinquity of the auditory association area make it possible that the difficulty arose from disruption of function in this area rather than from parietal damage.

Taking the data from these two studies it does appear that there is some evidence to support the contention that the left parietal area may be dominant for cross-modal associations.

Kotzmann (1972) compared the performance of 10 unilateral left lesion patients with 10 unilateral right and 10 control subjects on a tactile-visual recognition task. Subjects were asked to palpate two classes of objects and to choose the corresponding drawing from a multiple choice visual array. One set of objects was meaningful (pipe, eggcup, bolt, etc.) and the other meaningless (moulded nonsense shapes). The brain damaged groups performed more poorly than control subjects on both tactual recognition tasks. The meaningful/meaningless dichotomy was not related to the laterality of the lesion in any simple way. Left hemisphere subjects had about equal difficulty with the two tactual tasks, while right hemisphere subjects performed more poorly on the meaningless task than on the meaningful. An extension of this work might shed further light on the asymmetry of function with regard to tactual perception in the same way that auditory perceptual studies have done for the different classes of auditory information described in the previous chapter.

Symbolic (quasi-spatial) syntheses

Luria, in a number of publications, pointed to the importance of the 'tertiary zones' of the left hemisphere in relationships which are logical or symbolic in character, arguing that these relationships are 'quasi-spatial' in nature: this conception may provide a basis for understanding what at first appear to be quite separately based disturbances. The first example is acalculia. Although patients with a dominant parietal lesion can understand and remember a problem, and may even think of certain rules which would be appropriate for its solution, they are unable to carry out the necessary operations. As outlined below, if the description of the problem contains a number of symbolic relations the patient will have even further difficulty. The simplest examples may be found in the operations of addition and subtraction. The appropriateness of the term 'quasi-spatial' becomes apparent when it is realized that the significance of a number alters according to its spatial relation to other numbers, e.g. the figure 2 in the number 42 has a different significance from the 2 in 24. Luria provides the following example 'To subtract 7 from 31, as a rule we begin by rounding the first number and obtain the result 30 – 7 = 23. We then add the remaining unit, placing it in the right-hand column, and obtain the result 23 + 1 = 24. The operation is much more complex when we subtract a number of two digits (for example, 51 – 17), when, besides observing the conditions just mentioned, we have to carry over from the tens column and to retain the double system of elements in the operative memory' (1973, pp. 154–155).

If one employs a series of mathematical operations of increasing difficulty (e.g. addition or subtraction of one figure numbers, addition or subtraction of two figure numbers, of three figure numbers, multiplication of two or three figure numbers) patients with lesions in this region will break down well below the level which might be expected of them from their educational or occupational level. For the 'spatial' reason mentioned above, patients who have no difficulty with a problem such as 796 – 342 will fail repeatedly on seemingly similar problems, e.g. 534 – 286, as well as more complex mathematical operations, since the 'spatial' or 'carry-over' element is essential for the solution of the second problem but not the first. The rather different characteristics which frontal patients experience with numerical problem solving have been described in Chapter 4.

The other major area of difficulty for patients with lesions of the dominant inferior parietal region is that involving the abstract logical relations of syntax. The communication of such relationships can be greatly affected by the sequence of words, by the introduction of relational terms such as prepositions of space or time, or by more complex syntactical structures. Note the completely different meaning of 'my wife's brother' from 'my brother's wife', or 'the bridge over the water' and 'the water over the bridge'. Identical words in different situations take on quite different meanings dictated by the structure of the whole. It is this significance of structure that may present difficulties for patients with lesions of the dominant parietal region, though they show clear evidence of understanding the individual elements. The Token Test provides excellent opportunities for demonstrating these difficulties and is one of the reasons why this test is so sensitive to dominant hemisphere impairment. The difficulty with logico-grammatical constructions forms part of 'semantic aphasia'.

DISORDERS OF SPATIAL ORIENTATION

It will become obvious that the concept of spatial disorientation as employed in clinical neurology encompasses a variety of different disorders, and even some of these, about which there is some consensus as to their validity as distinct entities, may well turn out on further investigation to be more complexly determined than is thought at present. The brief description of the commonly reported spatial disabilities which follows obviously overlaps in part with the preceding section on perceptual disorders and that on disorders of personal space or body schema which follows. The disorders in this section are mainly of the appreciation of spatial relationships between and within objects in extrapersonal space. The principal categories are: (i) disorders in the judgment of the location or orientation of stimuli both with respect to each other and to the person; (ii) impairment of memory for location; (iii) topographical disorientation and loss of topographical memory; (iv) route finding difficulties; (v) constructional apraxia; and (vi) spatial alexia and acalculia.

Disorders of location and orientation

Benton (1969b) suggests that a distinction might be made between impairment of localization of a single stimulus, which could be termed a difficulty of 'absolute' localization, and difficulty with the perceived spatial relations between two or more stimuli, which could be termed a difficulty of 'relative' localization. Paterson and Zangwill (1944) referred to 'defective appreciation of spatial relations in the visual field with or without impairment of visual localization in the strict sense' as *visuospatial agnosia*, in other words, a dissociation between 'absolute' and 'relative' localization. They also confirmed earlier reports of a tendency to overestimate the distance of very near objects and to underestimate the distance of far objects.

Absolute localization may be checked by asking the patient to point to a stimulus placed in different parts of the visual field. This test is usually failed only by grossly impaired patients. Localization difficulty has also been inferred from other tests such as the bisection of lines. The performance of 12 patients with parieto-occipital traumatic lesions on this bisection task and other spatial tests was described by Bender and Teuber (1947), with the addition of a further occipital trauma case a year later (Bender & Teuber 1948).

Tests of more complex spatial relations often bring out difficulties when none are apparent on simpler tests. The multiple choice version of the Benton Visual Retention Test (Benton 1950) (Fig. 6.4) would appear sensitive to the subtler changes in perception of spatial relations and has been relatively

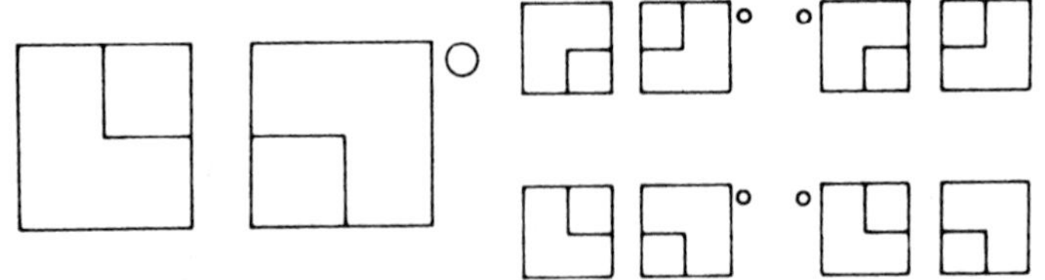

Fig. 6.4 Item 6 from multiple-choice version of the Benton Visual Retention Test (Benton 1950. Courtesy of the American Medical Association).

neglected in the study of parietal lesions since its introduction as a diagnostic aid (Benton 1952), though Alajouanine (1960) employed it in studies of occipital lobe patients. The visuospatial difficulties which many of Alajouanine's occipital patients had on this task remind us of the dangers of dealing rigidly with lobar divisions.

De Renzi et al (1971) have pointed out that spatial perception has been studied very often at a rather complex level, most tests having been derived from tests of intelligence or devised with various neurological symptoms in mind. For this reason they feel that 'it is difficult to disentangle the influence on performance of spatial as compared with praxic, intelligence, and memory factors' (p. 490). They devised a very simple task where two rods jointed together could be placed at various orientations (angles) to each other. The subject's task was to align another pair of rods in the same orientation under the two conditions of visual and tactile assistance. When testing in this way they found that gross impairment was associated almost exclusively with posterior lesions of the non-dominant hemisphere. They contrast this with the less striking asymmetry shown on more complex spatial tasks which are also poorly performed by a proportion of dominant posterior cases. Miller (1972) comments:

> It may well be that the important factor in determining whether an apparently spatial task is affected by left posterior lesions as well as right is the degree of verbal mediation used by the subject. Although a task may be spatial in nature, this does not prevent a subject from using verbal reasoning in its solution and to the extent that this occurs the task will be more liable to disruption by left-sided lesions even though the task may be particularly difficult to verbalize. (p. 86)

Another simple test used by the Milan group was the reproduction of the location of a number of crosses drawn at random on paper, the measure of performance being taken from the sum of the distances by which the subjects' copies deviated from the originals (De Renzi & Faglioni 1967). A right hemisphere group was inferior to a left hemisphere group on this task.

The significance of the right hemisphere for localization was again demonstrated by Faglioni et al (1971). Right posterior lesion patients were most impaired on a visual localization task. The fact that two separate versions of the task, one visual and the other tactile, were both poorly performed supports the notion that many deficits produced by parietal lesions are not modality specific.

Perhaps a separate factor in dealing with spatial relations is the ability to carry out reversible operations in space. Two studies (Butters & Barton 1970, Butters et al 1970a) have employed a number of measures of this type.

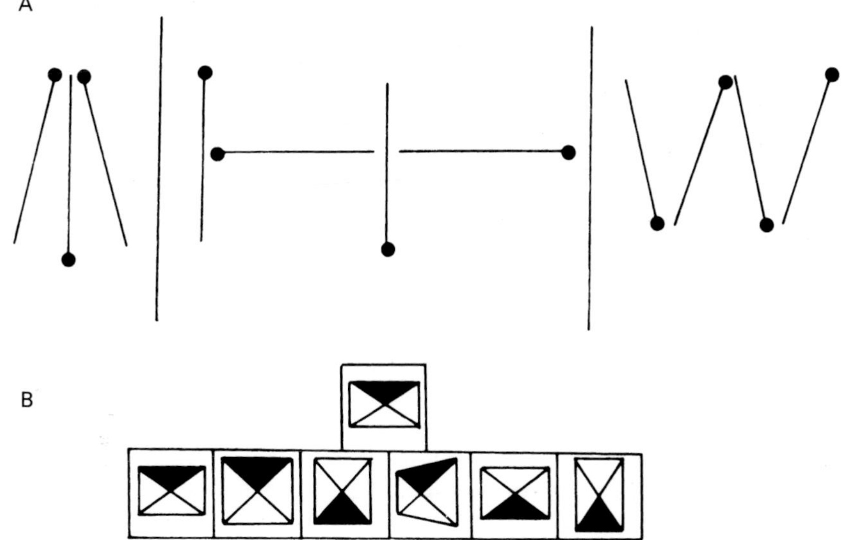

Fig. 6.5 A, Sample designs, Stick Test (from Benson & Barton 1970); B, Pool reflection item (from Butters et al 1970a).

The Stick Test. The patient is shown a simple arrangement of sticks and asked to copy them under the two conditions of sitting alongside or opposite the examiner.

The Pools Reflections Test, which is modelled after one of the subtests of Cattell's *A Culture Free Test* (Cattell 1944). From a number of alternatives, the subject must select the one which represents the reflection which the sample would present to the viewer (see Fig. 6.5).

The Village Scene Test. Here the subject is shown the model of a village and is asked to choose the correct photograph representing the scene from six photographs, one of which is correct, the others being similar views in which the spatial relationships of features of the scene have been altered before being photographed.

Both these studies produced data which suggest that this type of task is performed poorly by patients with either left or right parietal lesions. Patients with lesions in other areas showed little or no difficulty with these spatial reversible operations.

There also appears to be a little evidence that a dissociation may exist between localization disorders and the topographical disorders of orientation and memory (Hécaen et al 1951, Gilliatt & Pratt 1952), each type of disorder being seen in isolation in some individuals. Marie and his co-workers (1924) described a right prefrontal tumour which produced marked spatial disorientation in the patient but 'l'absence de troubles dans les fonctions en quelque sort primaires de l'appréciation spatiale, chez ce malade' (p. 217).

Impaired memory for location

Very little systematic work has been done in this area. Impaired memory for location may form part of a general amnesic disorder or it may be seen in association with other spatial difficulties. However, an occasional patient is seen who performs adequately on the usual spatial tasks but who may encounter difficulty when asked to recall spatial relationships even after a short delay. Such difficulties have been described in occipital cases and right parietal cases by Alajouanine (1960), who used the multiple choice version of the Benton Visual Retention Test as a recognition memory task.

Loosely related to this area was the experiment of De Renzi and colleagues (1969a), who tested a large group of unilateral lesion patients on a simple memory for position task under visual guidance or tactual guidance. Though all brain damaged subjects performed more poorly than controls, there was no significant difference between the right and left hemisphere groups. The impairment was greater in those with visual field defects than those without. 'However, the finding that this impairment was significantly more marked on the tactile than on the visual memory tests suggests that it is related to the concomitant injury of posterior areas of the brain rather than to the effect of the visual deficit' (p. 283).

Patients are seen frequently who have a disproportionate difficulty on the memory-for-location aspect of the Tactual Performance Test (TPT) of the Reitan Neuropsychological Test Battery. Though a large number of studies have been reported in which the TPT is demonstrated to be generally sensitive to cerebral impairment (Reitan & Davison 1974), there is little or no available information on any differential effect of location of lesion on the memory aspect of the task. Since patients are not advised in advance that they will be asked to recall the location as well as the shapes of the objects which are to be placed in the formboard (using only tactile information), inferences about any individual patient's performances must be limited. It is a striking fact, nevertheless, that after the prolonged experience which this test gives, many patients with cerebral impairment will fail to recall correctly the location of even one of the shapes.

A comparison of differences between the recall and copying versions of the Rey Figure (Rey 1941, Osterrieth 1944, Rey 1959) might also prove valuable in this regard.

Topographical disorientation and loss of topographical memory

Several different difficulties may be encompassed under this heading: (i) the inability to recall the spatial arrangement of familiar surroundings, such as the disposition of rooms within the patient's house or the disposition of furniture within a room; and (ii) the inability to recall and describe well-known geographical relationships with which the patient was formerly familiar.

Benton (1969b) considered the basic defect to be difficulty in calling up visual images – 'We deal here with an impairment in 'revisualization', a failure to retrieve long-established visual memories' (p. 219). This is similar to the 'visual irreminiscence' of Critchley (1953), which is mentioned in the next chapter in relation to lesions of the occipital lobes.

Compared with other aspects of spatial ability, topographical orientation has received comparatively little attention. Ratcliff and Newcombe (1973) noted that most studies had been concerned with situations in which patients could

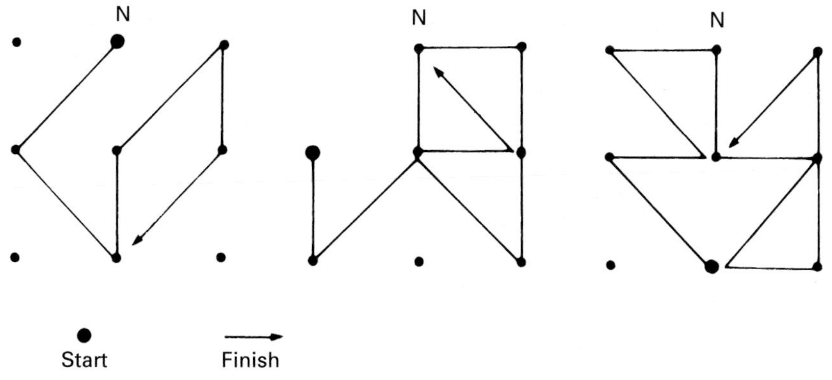

Fig. 6.6 Three items from a locomotor map following test (after Semmes et al 1955, courtesy of Dr Josephine Semmes).

explore spatial relationships without gross changes in their own position, i.e. they have been more concerned with spatial agnosia.

In 1955 Semmes and her co-workers described an objective test of spatial orientation. This consisted of 15 diagrams of the type shown in Figure 6.6. The nine dots on each map represented nine circles on the floor of a room, the circles being some 137 cm apart. One wall of the room was designated as North, and North was marked on the maps. With the map maintained in constant orientation to the body, the subject was required to walk around each designated path. In this way the orientation of the person to the room was constantly changing. Both visual maps and 'tactile-only' versions were provided. The performance of parietal lobe cases was significantly inferior to that of non-parietal patients and control subjects. There was no difference between non-parietal cases and controls. Furthermore, as the disorder proved to be unrelated to perceptual modality (visual or tactile), Semmes and her colleagues felt that it was incorrect to label the difficulty as part of visuospatial agnosia. A second study (Weinstein et al 1956) confirmed the poor performance of parietal subjects on the route finding task but, in this study, poor performance was also shown by frontal subjects though to a lesser degree. These frontal subjects also performed poorly on a test of personal orientation.

A later study (Semmes et al 1963) extended these findings and compared the results on this test of extra-personal orientation with a test of personal space, in which subjects were asked to touch parts of their own bodies in the order indicated by numbers on diagrams of the human body. Brain impairment affected both tasks to an approximately equal degree. Statistical analysis showed that, though the two tasks were significantly related in the brain-injured group studied, there were also independent elements.

With regard to the locus of the lesion 'both personal and extra-personal orientation were impaired by lesions of the posterior part of the left hemisphere. Anterior lesions (particularly those of the left hemisphere) tended to impair personal but not extra-personal orientation, whereas the converse was the case for right posterior lesions' (Semmes et al 1963, p. 769).

Two studies cited in the previous section (Butters & Barton 1970, Butters et al 1970a) have shown that parietal patients have difficulty with reversible mental spatial operations, while other patients do not. Butters, Soeldner and Fedio

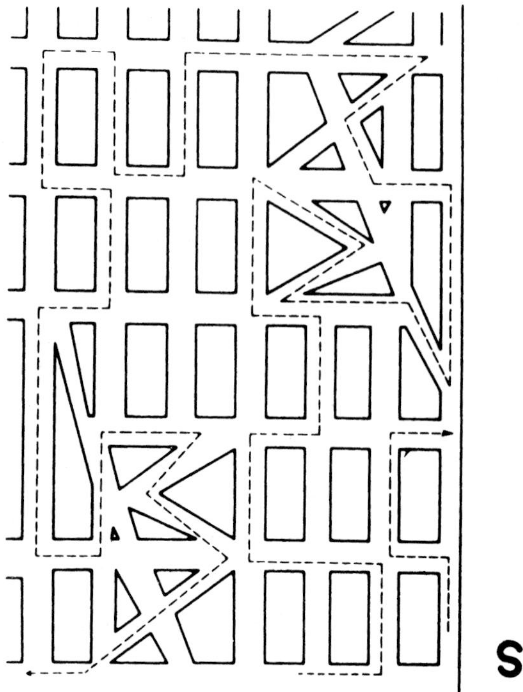

Fig. 6.7 Money's Standardized Road-Map Test of Direction Sense.

(1972) extended these findings by including a test which cannot be performed by rotating an external object either at the concrete or the abstract level. In the test, Money's Standardized Road-Map Test of Direction (Fig. 6.7), patients need the ability to rotate themselves in imagery or on an abstract level. With the road map in a fixed stationary relationship they are required to describe the right or left turns which would need to be made while following the route.

A comparison of left frontal and right parietal patients on this task allowed a test of Teuber's hypothesis that the frontal and parietal regions mediate qualitatively different spatial abilities: (i) spatial orientation to external objects mediated by the parietal regions, particularly the right; and (ii) spatial discrimination involving the subject's own body mediated particularly by the left frontal region. The study demonstrated a partial double dissociation between the two groups on the test of personal or egocentric space (Money's Test) and a test of extra-personal space (the Stick Test described above). While the authors mention a number of clinical, statistical and methodological restrictions, there appears to be tentative support for Teuber's hypothesis. This difference could, of course, represent the general difficulty frontal patients have with hypothetical ('as if') situations.

Two early studies of Pierre Marie reported disorientation in space with major lesions of the frontal lobe, comprising a traumatic left frontal case, a case of right frontal trauma and a right frontal tumour (Marie & Behague 1919, Marie et al 1924).

In testing for difficulties in spatial orientation, care should be taken in excluding topographical difficulties on the basis of verbal tests only.

‘Longstanding associations of a purely verbal character may enter into the verbal descriptions and give an impression of the appreciation of topographic relationships which in fact the patient no longer possesses’ (Benton 1969b, p. 221). Benton reports a case of De Renzi and Faglioni (1962) who was ‘completely unable to make localizations on a map of Milan, nevertheless could name the streets and public buildings associated with a given locality as well as all the gates of the city. However he could not specify the spatial relationships among the gates and his descriptions of routes were schematic and imperfect’ (pp. 220–221).

Benton and others (1974) later made a more systematic study of this distinction. Geographic orientation was assessed in patients with unilateral cerebral disease using two types of task. The first required the localization of states and cities on a map of the United States while the second was a verbal test of the directional relations between places. Two subtests in this second (verbal) category failed to discriminate between left and right hemisphere cases or brain impaired subjects from controls on the map localization test. A ‘vector’ score was calculated showing a tendency of the subject to shift localization either toward the right or left part of the map. This score differentiated between the two hemisphere groups and suggested neglect of the visual field contralateral to the side of the lesion in some of the patients. These findings demonstrate the interaction of defects in producing impaired performance on complex tasks.

It has become evident that the relation between locus of lesion and topographical loss is less clear than with some other ‘spatial’ disorders, probably because of the complexity of the notion. The most frequent reports have been after posterior lesions – right, left or bilateral (Kleist 1934, Brain 1941, Paterson & Zangwill 1945, Cogan 1960, De Renzi & Faglioni 1962, Hécaen 1969, Obi et al 1992) – though ‘pure’ cases are probably more common with right parietal or right parahippocampal lesions (Hublet & Demeurisse 1992). Topographical disorientation is particularly associated with infarcts of the right posterior cerebral artery producing lesions in the medial aspect of the temporo-occipital cortex (Landis et al 1986, Habib & Sirigu 1987). The latter authors suggest that appropriate testing of patients with these infarctions would probably show the defect to be more common than reported. The role of the frontal lobes in contributing to functions which take part in this complex area has been mentioned many times in the preceding sections. The study of Maguire et al (1996), which compared unilateral temporal lobectomy cases with controls, shows a clear role for both temporal and parietal lobes in route finding.

A prime difficulty in studying topographical disorientation is the fact that it is most often seen in association with other difficulties (e.g. Ishii et al 1992, Zarranz et al 1995), and there is often an admixture of perceptual and memory based components. Dissociation between these components may occur with callosal lesions, such as in the case of Bottini et al (1992) where a patient with a splenial lesion had topographical memory impairment but performed normally on perceptual topographic tests.

Methods of coping with the disability may remain hidden unless specific exploration is made of the strategies used in individual cases; some of these may be left hemisphere dependent (Clarke et al 1993).

Route finding difficulties

The neurological literature has occasionally reported cases where the principal deficit lies in the patients' inability to find their way about in long familiar surroundings or in locations frequently encountered in the recent past. Such patients may be well able to give adequate verbal descriptions of familiar routes but are unable to execute them either by drawing or by taking them in real life situations. They become lost in the hospital environs or en route to the hospital.

Perhaps for lack of a more appropriate term, such a disorder is often termed *topographical amnesia*. An extensive review is provided by De Renzi (1982). It is impossible to tell in most reported cases just how much of the route finding difficulty is due to memory disturbance because of inadequate examination. Brain (1941) pointed to at least four basic disorders which might lead to route finding difficulties: (i) perceptual disorders of the location and relative position of objects; (ii) failure of recognition of environmental features through object agnosia; (iii) topographical amnesia; and (iv) unilateral spatial neglect. This latter cause may result in the patient failing to take appropriate left-hand turns, with a resulting preponderance of right-hand turns (Gloning 1965).

If one excludes perceptual and attentional defects, there remain two basic difficulties to be disentangled, namely *topographical agnosia* and *topographical amnesia*, a distinction first put forward in the classical paper of Paterson and Zangwill (1945).

Topographical agnosia

While some reports suggest that inability to recognize objects that serve as landmarks might be the predominant topographical difficulty in a small number of cases, even these have shown associated perceptual or agnosic difficulties (Pallis 1955, De Renzi & Faglioni 1962). It is obvious that, even if a separate category of topographical agnosia were to be established, it would fail to account for the majority of cases of route finding difficulties produced by brain lesions especially if, as Byrne (1982) suggests, such schemata may be developed by different individuals in different ways. As long ago as 1948 Tolman conceived of the notion of a cognitive map to account for the spatial maze learning of the white rat. 'The alternative possibility (to S-R theory) is that the learner is following signs to a goal, is learning his way about, is following a sort of map – in other words, is learning not movements but meanings. The organism learns sign-significant relations, it learns a behaviour route, not a movement pattern' (Hilgard 1956, p. 191). Experimental investigation of the development of such 'maps' or schemata might pave the way for more life-related clinical tests of topographical ability.

Topographical amnesia

Cases where amnesia for topography forms the sole or major complaint are likewise rare. The amnesia may include long stored topographical information as well as material more recently acquired, e.g. Paterson and Zangwill's patient (1945) displayed an inability to describe previously experienced topographical relationships and could not recall whether to turn right or left when leaving the ward doorway to visit the toilet. Both patients described by

De Renzi & Faglioni (1962) and Scotti (1968) had a very short forgetting period for spatial information.

However, it is noteworthy that one of these cases (Scotti 1968) showed a dissociation between recent and long term topographical memory, since he was quite competent in finding his way in previously familiar locations but not in recent ones, such as the hospital. On the other hand the patient of De Renzi et al (1977), who had a right temporo-parietal softening, showed both topographical amnesia and an inability to learn a visually-guided stylus maze problem over 275 trials although she was free from spatial perceptual disorder and had no apparent verbal or visual memory deficit. Other cases with topographical amnesia as a major feature have been described by Whitty and Newcombe (1973), Whiteley and Warrington (1978) and Hécaen and colleagues (1980). Even migraine has been cited as a possible cause for a transient form of topographical amnesia (Mazzoni et al 1993).

A very recent study of a case with topographical disorientation as an isolated disorder was reported by Incisa della Rocchetta et al (1996). Extensive neuropsychological testing showed preservation of intellectual, language and basic perceptual and spatial skills. However, both episodic and semantic memory of topographical items and routes were poor; other aspects of both forms of memory were unaffected. Of particular note is the fact that this patient had experienced a similar episode 30 years earlier which resolved.

Clinico-experimental study in this area is hampered by our paucity of knowledge of how geographical knowledge is developed in the normal subject. The review by Byrne (1982) makes a number of important distinctions. Prime among these is the difference between spatial information, which can be gained from a single viewpoint (visuospatial perception), and the topographical schema of large scale space which is typically acquired by personal locomotor experience. Many of the tasks used in the laboratory and clinic fail to come to grips with the ways in which the dynamically evolved cognitive representation of large scale space is disrupted.

CONSTRUCTIONAL APRAXIA

The first modern description of constructional difficulties in patients with cerebral impairment is usually attributed to Kleist (Strauss 1924, Kleist 1934). After first considering certain drawing disabilities of neurological patients to be a form of 'optic apraxia', Kleist later introduced the term 'constructional apraxia'. Moreover, Benton (1969a) pointed out that Kleist insisted that this particular disorder was to be distinguished from others that were obviously rooted in visuoperceptual disorders and thought that the basis of the disorder lay in a disruption between visual and kinesthetic processes. This would accord well with what we would call today the general conception of a 'disconnection syndrome', alluded to in earlier chapters.

Many early investigators had felt that the failure of patients on certain tasks such as drawing and route finding reflected a visuospatial disturbance. While many patients with constructional difficulties did have visuospatial problems there were also those who had, for example, severe difficulties with drawing without showing a spatial deficit (Kroll & Stolbun 1933, Lhermitte & Trelles

1933, Mayer-Gross 1935). Strauss (1924) defined a pure case of constructional apraxia as one with adequate form perception, perceptual discrimination and perceptual localization, and absence of ideomotor apraxia or motor disability.

Later definitions include those of Critchley (1953), 'an executive defect within a visuospatial domain', and Benton (1967) 'an impairment in combinatory or organizing activity in which details must be clearly perceived and in which the relationships among the component parts of the entity must be apprehended if the desired synthesis of them is to be achieved'.

Constructional apraxia is often said to be the apraxia of the psychologist since it is more often revealed on neuropsychological examination than clinically exhibited. The present summary builds on earlier reviews such as those of Benton (1969a) and Warrington (1969).

Status of the concept

One of the most frequently asked questions is the following. Is constructional apraxia a single entity or are there separate, distinct types of disorder under this heading? In 1957 Ettlinger and his co-workers reported 10 cases with right posterior cerebral lesions who showed disturbances in spatial perception and manipulation. An investigation of individual performances suggested the possibility of different varieties of constructional difficulty. Benton and Fogel (1962) pointed to the possible relation with the type of test employed or the activity under examination.

> Constructional praxis is a broad concept which has been applied to a number of rather different types of activities. These activities have in common the characteristic that they require the patient to assemble, join or articulate parts to form a single unitary structure. However, they may differ from each other in many respects, e.g. in complexity, in the type of movement and the degree of motor dexterity required in achieving the task, in the demands made on the higher intellectual functions, and in whether they involve construction in two or three spatial dimensions.

Critchley (1953) had pointed out that three-dimensional construction tasks appeared to be necessary, since some patients with parietal lesions who had no difficulty on the commonly employed two-dimensional tests displayed gross abnormalities of construction when the test moved into the third dimension. Such abnormalities could not be elicited by the usual clinical examination. Benton and Fogel (1962) confirmed this by demonstrating only a weak positive correlation between the performance of brain damaged subjects on a drawing test (Benton Visual Retention Test) and their newly constructed Three Dimensional Constructional Praxis task (Fig. 6.8). 14 patients were adequate on the copying task but defective on the three-dimensional task, whereas another eight were adequate on the three-dimensional task but showed defective copying.

In a later study, Benton (1967) addressed himself specifically to the question and, since it appears to be the only such study, it is worth referring to in a little detail. Benton employed four apparently dissimilar tests – Benton Visual Retention Test, Stick-construction, Block Designs, Three Dimensional Constructional Praxis – and measured the concordance between various com-

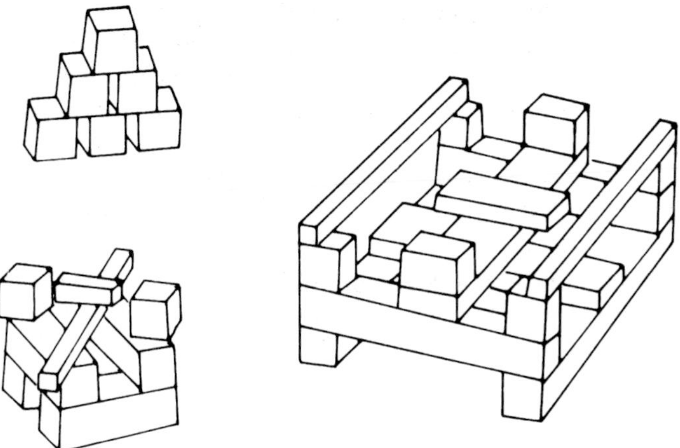

Fig. 6.8 Three Dimensional Constructional Praxis Test (drawn from Benton & Fogel 1962, courtesy of the American Medical Association).

binations of tests. The concurrence of failure varied from chance level upward for different pairs of tests, but even the highest degree of concurrence fell well below perfect agreement. There was also considerable intra-individual variation in performance level on these tests. However, there did seem to be more relation between the last three tests than there was between any of these and the drawing test (VRT). Benton concluded that there may be at least two types of tests, namely graphic tasks and assembly tasks, and that empirical study may well reveal others.

The variety of tests which have been used to elicit constructional apraxia is great:

1. spontaneous or free drawing – for a careful and detailed description with illustration of the common errors seen with drawing tasks the reader is referred to Warrington (1969)
2. drawing from a model, e.g. Benton Visual Retention Test (Benton 1962) as well as simpler clinical versions
3. stick pattern constructions, e.g. Stick Test (Goldstein & Scheerer 1941)
4. block designs, usually modelled on the Kohs test (Goldstein & Scheerer 1941, Wechsler 1958)
5. test of spatial analysis (mentioned above)
6. three-dimensional constructions (Critchley 1953, Benton & Fogel 1962)
7. reconstruction of puzzles, e.g. Benson and Barton (1970) and the Object Assembly subtest of the Wechsler Adult Intelligence Scale (WAIS).

In view of the fact that many brain damaged patients fail on some of these and pass on others, it is obviously unsatisfactory to use failure on any one as an operational definition of constructional apraxia as some writers have done. Since the WAIS is about the most widely used test in the assessment of higher functions it provides the most frequent opportunity to observe the dissociation which so often occurs between performance on the Block Design and Object Assembly subtests. Obviously many tests, particularly Block Design, are multifactorial in nature; failure on such a test may arise from a number of causes which need to be explored if the significance of the failure is to be seen. The failure may rest on inability to analyze the model visually, or be made difficult by disruption of the patient's spatial schemata or, as outlined below, be impossible because the patient is unable to initiate, monitor and execute a plan for the solution of the task.

Some of the factors which need to be taken into consideration in interpreting a patient's failure on constructional tasks have been mentioned in the study by Benson and Barton (1970) and are further discussed in relation to clinical assessment in Chapter 10. Benson and Barton suggest that the more general term 'constructional disability' would be more appropriate for most findings, reserving the term 'constructional apraxia' for the case having the features outlined by Kleist. Their study with a variety of tests showed that right hemisphere lesions produced more consistent disturbance than left, while posterior lesions of either hemisphere produced more consistent disturbances than anterior ones.

Laterality and constructional apraxia

Most early cases described as showing constructional apraxia had bilateral posterior lesions. Later, cases were described where constructional apraxia was seen together with one or more symptoms of the Gerstmann syndrome (see below), which suggested that the left or dominant parietal area was of importance as part of the substratum of constructional abilities. Still later, attention began to be paid to the role of the minor hemisphere when it was clearly demonstrated that unilateral right hemisphere lesions could produce the symptom (Paterson & Zangwill 1944, Ajuriaguerra & Hécaen 1960).

The first large systematic survey of laterality of lesion and constructional apraxia was that of Piercy et al (1960). Of 403 consecutive cases with unilateral cerebral lesions, 67 cases showed constructional apraxia. Of these, 42 had lesions on the right and 25 on the left. This represented 22.3% of the right hemisphere cases and 11.6% of the left. The disproportion between right and left cases was even greater for retrorolandic cases, some 37.8% of the right posterior cases showing apraxia against 16.1% of the left. Since that time, numerous studies have confirmed the much higher incidence of constructional apraxia with non-dominant hemisphere lesions (e.g. Benton 1962, Benton & Fogel 1962, Costa & Vaughan 1962, Piercy & Smyth 1962, Arrigoni & De Renzi 1964, Newcombe 1969, Black & Strub 1976).

Many studies have reported that constructional apraxia is not only more frequent with right hemisphere lesions but that it also tends to be more severe, i.e. patients show more grossly defective performances (Benton & Fogel 1962, Benton 1967, Gainotti et al 1972a). However, other well controlled studies have not shown hemispheric differences, particularly where the severity of general psychological deficit has been taken into account (Warrington et al 1966, De Renzi & Faglioni 1967, Benson & Barton 1970, Dee 1970, Gainotti et al 1977).

The assumption of a true relationship between lesions of the non-dominant hemisphere and constructional apraxia has been seriously challenged by the study of Arrigoni and De Renzi (1964). While they also found a higher incidence of difficulties in right-sided lesions on each of three constructive tests in an unselected sample of hospitalized patients, they felt that at least part of the

Table 6.1 Constructional apraxia and side of lesion		
	Present	**Absent**
Right hemisphere	27	17
Left hemisphere	17	27

difference might lie in the possibility that the lesions of the right hemisphere group were consistently larger. This possibility has also been alluded to by Costa and Vaughan (1962) and Benton (1965). Wolff (1962) had suggested that one reason for this might be the earlier presentation of dominant lesions because of language disturbances.

From their larger group, Arrigoni and De Renzi matched left and right cases for severity of impairment using a reaction time measure which their earlier work had suggested was an index of cerebral impairment that was not affected by the location of lesion. The two groups of 44 patients produced the findings listed in Table 6.1.

The difference was in the 'predicted' direction but was no longer significant (when tested by *chi square*). 'This result should make us extremely cautious in attributing a dominance (even if relative) to the right hemisphere with regard to constructive capacities' (p. 190). Benton (1969a), in a summary of evidence to that time, pointed out that 'defective performance on the part of patients with left hemisphere disease is not at all rare. Thus, if right hemisphere 'dominance' for visuoconstructive performance does exist, it does not appear comparable to the 'dominance' for language performance exercised by the left hemisphere'. This does not mean that there are no qualitative differences between the two sides. In fact Arrigoni and De Renzi describe such differences.

Qualitative differences and laterality

Relation between visuoperceptive and visuoconstructive deficits

Qualitative differences between the two hemispheres are dealt with in Chapter 8, but numerous studies, including that of Arrigoni and De Renzi (1964), show characteristic differences in quality of performance on constructional tasks between left and right hemisphere cases (McFie & Zangwill 1960, Piercy et al 1960, Warrington et al 1966, Gainotti et al 1972a, Collignon & Rondeaux 1974). The study of Warrington and her colleagues was directed to an examination of specially designed drawing tests which were rated by independent judges. Though there was no significant difference in degree of disability between the two groups, they showed a dissociation of predominant types of error. 'The type of error made by patients with right hemisphere lesions suggest that these patients have difficulty in incorporating spatial information into their drawing performance, leading to disproportion and faulty articulation of parts of the drawing, while the patients with left hemisphere lesions seemed to experience difficulty in planning the drawing process, leading to simplified drawings of the model' (p. 82). Similar findings were described by Gainotti and his colleagues (1972a), who found that left hemisphere cases produced simplified drawings which were helped by the presentation of a model for copying, while

Table 6.2 Laterality of lesion and characteristics of drawing

Right hemisphere	Left hemisphere
Scattered and fragmented	Coherent but simplified
Loss of spatial relations	Preservation of spatial relations
Faulty orientation	Correct orientation
Energetic drawing	Slow and laborious
Addition of lines to try to make drawing correct	Gross lack of detail

the visuospatial disturbances of the right hemisphere cases were not helped to any degree by a model. Table 6.2, drawn largely from Warrington (1969), summarizes the main differences.

Both Warrington (1969) and Benson and Barton (1970) have put forward hypotheses about the relative contributions of the left and right hemispheres to visuoconstructive tasks: '...right hemisphere lesions produce disorders of visuo-spatial perception while left-sided lesions disturb motor function (apraxia)' (Benson & Barton, p. 21); '...the suggestion that right hemisphere supplies a perceptual and the left hemisphere an executive component to the task' (Warrington 1969, p. 80). Earlier studies had already suggested this hypothesis (Hécaen et al 1951, Duensing 1954, Ettlinger et al 1957, Ajuriaguerra & Hécaen 1960, McFie & Zangwill 1960, Piercy et al 1960). Several of these studies are cited by both authors. The argument that the right hemisphere contributes a perceptual element is supported indirectly by studies showing that purely perceptual tasks (without a constructional component) are more poorly performed by patients with right hemisphere lesions (Ch. 8).

Despite the strong clinical evidence of laterality differences, experimental studies have given conflicting results. One group of studies supports the contention that a perceptual difficulty usually lies at the root of the trouble. Kleist himself postulated that the left hemisphere was the one mainly implicated in patients with constructional difficulties which were not on the basis of visuoperceptive defects (Piercy & Smyth 1962, De Renzi & Faglioni 1967, Dee 1970, Gainotti & Tiacci 1970). Dee (1970) found that 42 out of 46 patients with constructional apraxia had significant visuoperceptive defects and was unable to demonstrate any hemispheric differences apart from the finding that three of the four patients with apraxia and no perceptual deficit had lesions in the left hemisphere. Dee concluded that most constructional apraxia is due to a disorder of visual perception irrespective of the side of the lesion though allowing that other explanations must be sought for the minority of cases. Further study of the cases in the 1970 study by Dee and Benton showed that the patients with constructional apraxia also failed on a haptic-spatial task, supporting the contention of Semmes (1965, 1968) that many spatial disorders extend beyond a single modality and are not determined by primary sensory, perceptual defect, i.e. they are multimodal in character. Other studies, e.g. De Renzi and Scotti (1969), show that posterior lesions may produce spatial difficulties embracing more than one sense modality.

On the other hand, there are studies claiming evidence that the correlation between perceptual and constructional difficulties is higher in right than left hemisphere lesion patients (Costa & Vaughan 1962, Warrington et al 1966).

Results of constructional tests in a small number of patients who had undergone cerebral commissurotomy have been cited as additional evidence of the greater role of the non-dominant hemisphere in constructional performance (Gazzaniga et al 1965, Gazzaniga 1970). Though commissurotomy subjects may perform better when using the left hand (right hemisphere) than the right hand, the fact that performance was below par with either hand suggests bilateral but unequal representation of constructional abilities.

Constructional apraxia and locus of lesion

There seems little doubt that, if one can consider frontal constructional difficulties as forming a separate entity, the parietal lobe, particularly on the non-dominant side, is most closely related with constructional disabilities which have the characteristics of the Kleist-Strauss formulation. Writers not wishing to be limited by the artificial lobar boundaries often relate constructional apraxia to the ill-defined area at the junction of the parietal, temporal and occipital lobes – Luria's zone of overlapping. In a study of 105 cases with tumours of the temporal lobe, Petrovici (1972) found a complete absence of constructional apraxia in the 77 cases which were completely restricted to the temporal lobe, or in 4 frontotemporal cases. On the other hand, the remaining 24 cases with added involvement of the parietal lobe or the parietal and occipital lobes had 11 cases of constructional apraxia (4 left and 7 right).

A factorial study could be conducted to see whether the parietal, overlapping and occipital areas contribute separate factors to the 'posterior type' of constructional disability. There are, however, anatomical and pathological reasons why this is difficult if not impossible.

Bilateral parietal or diffuse cerebral lesions lead to very marked disturbances both of constructional praxis and spatial orientation, though they are often masked by accompanying organic dementia (Allison 1962).

Resolving the confusion

This confusing state of affairs can be attributed to the interaction of two factors, viz. the over-inclusive nature of the concept of constructional apraxia together with the great variety of clinical and experimental measures, often of some complexity, which have been used to elicit constructional difficulties. It might be better to abandon the concept or term constructional apraxia in favour of an examination of the seemingly separate component functions and their relation to tests as factorially simple as possible. The warning given earlier about the multiple determination of responses on most tests applies particularly here, since even apparently simple perceptual tasks may allow different strategies to be brought into play (Bryden 1977, Birkett 1978).

There have been studies which have aimed at clarifying the issue by separating out perceptual and executive functions. Arena and Gainotti (1978) employed two relatively pure measures of perceptual and constructional ability, the multiple choice version of the Benton Visual Retention Test and the usual graphomotor version of the same test. No differences were found between right and left hemisphere damaged subjects on these measures with respect to either incidence or severity of deficient performance. On the other

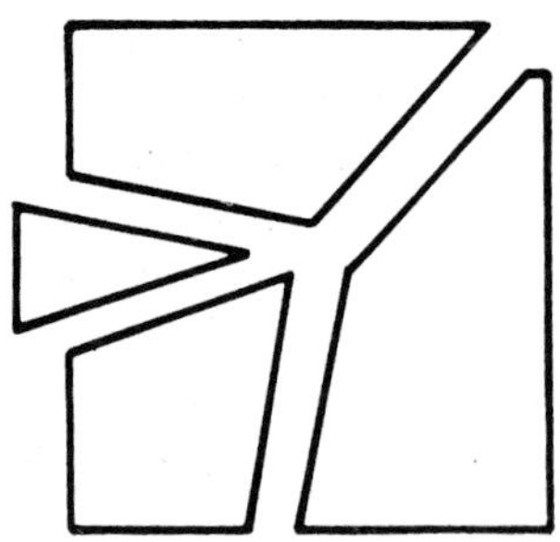
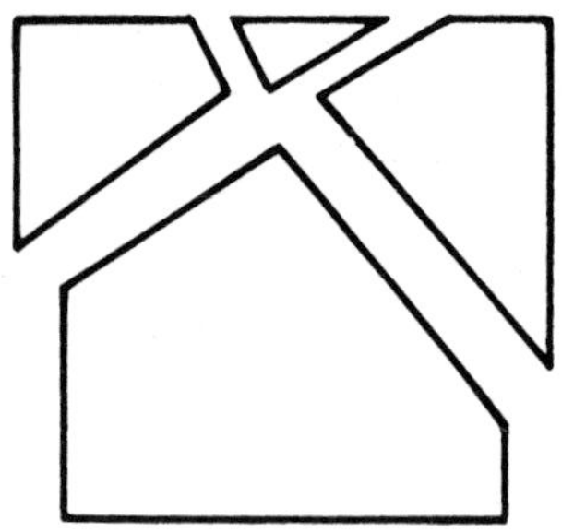

Fig. 6.9 Form assembly task (from Mack & Levine 1981).

hand, Mack and Levine (1981) devised a visuoconstructive task, termed the Form Assembly Task, which required the subjects to assemble geometrical pieces with different lengths of lines and different angles, to form a square (Fig. 6.9). This test was given, together with two visual discrimination tasks, to patients with unilateral lesions. All but one of the right hemisphere subjects failed on the Form Assembly Task but only 7 out of 19 of the left hemisphere subjects failed, and the degree of impairment was greater in the former group. Comparison of the relationship between performance on the three tests was consistent with the hypothesis already mentioned above that perceptual deficits may underlie constructional difficulties among those with right but not left hemisphere damage. Further studies of this kind are clearly necessary.

A discussion of the relative contributions of visuo-perceptual versus executive disorders is given by Carlesimo et al (1993).

Associated disabilities

The most widely quoted study of disabilities associated with constructional difficulties is that of McFie and Zangwill (1960). They compared the visual-constructive impairment of 8 left hemisphere cases (all in the posterior parietal region) with that of right-sided cases from earlier studies of the Cambridge group. Table 6.3 gives the quantitative features of the study.

It is clear that there is a strong association between the first five symptoms and right-sided lesions, while the last two symptoms are seen almost exclu-

Table 6.3 Comparison between left and right sided lesions (McFie & Zangwill 1960)

	Left		Right	
	No. examined	No. with disability	No. examined	No. with disability
Unilateral neglect	8	1	21	14
Dressing disability	8	1	15	10
Cube counting	6	1	7	6
Paper cutting	4	0	10	9
Topographical loss	8	1	18	9
Right-left discrimination	8	5	21	0
Weigl's sorting test	6	5	16	1

sively with left-sided lesions. McFie and Zangwill felt that their left-sided cases corresponded more closely to the classical description of constructional apraxia, whereas the difficulties encountered by the right hemisphere patients were more closely associated with visuospatial agnosia. As well as the difference in associated symptoms, there also appeared to be qualitative differences in the constructional disabilities of left and right cases. Failure of a high proportion of left-sided cases on Weigl's sorting test appeared to be part of a general intellectual impairment which was not seen with right-sided cases. Gainotti and colleagues (1972a) confirmed this relationship. In right-sided cases there was no relation between constructional apraxia and mental impairment, while with left-sided cases there was a significant relationship between constructional apraxia, mental impairment and ideomotor apraxia. A number of studies by Benton (Benton 1962, Benton & Fogel 1962, Benton 1967) have shown a generally higher incidence of mental impairment in brain damaged patients with constructional apraxia than those without such apraxia. Despite this general relationship, there were both patients with severe mental impairment who showed no defective praxis and patients with severe constructional impairment whose intelligence levels were around the level expected from their educational background. The impairment level was based on the work of Fogel (1962, 1964) using the difference between obtained and expected intelligence scores.

The problems which arise in the interpretation of the significance of associated disabilities are discussed by Warrington (1969).

Frontal apraxia

Constructional difficulties with anterior lesions have been reported sporadically since the early finding of Pollack (1938) that frontal lesions may occasionally disturb constructional praxis. Luria and Tsvetkova (1964) summarized the difference between anterior and posterior lesions:

> In lesions of the parieto-occipital part of the brain the general factor underlying constructive disturbances is a loss of spatial organization of the elements…In lesions of the frontal lobes the general factor underlying constructive disturbances is a loss of programming and regulating of sequential behaviour…instability of the primary intention or program and to the inability to compare the results with the preliminary intention… (p. 95)

This type of disruption has been considered in Chapter 4.

Constructional apraxia as a disconnection syndrome

In a largely neglected paper, Nielsen (1975) drew attention to the marked similarity in the drawing errors of patients with right and left hemisphere lesions and the errors made by the left and right hands of commissurotomy patients. This led to the postulation that the observed constructional difficulties in patients with unilateral lesions might be explained at least partially by a disconnection effect. This thesis is supported by such cases as that of Boldrini et al (1992).

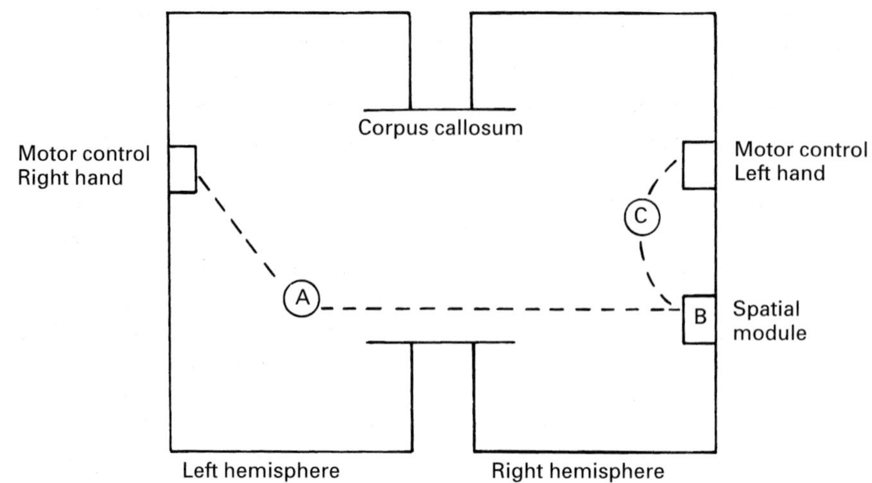

Fig. 6.10 Constructional apraxia as a disconnection syndrome.

Independently, Le Doux and his colleagues (1978) put forward the same argument based on observation of a patient with complete commissurotomy. This patient, while showing equal perceptual ability of either hemisphere for block design matching (Le Doux et al 1977) showed a clear inferiority of the right hand (left hemisphere) in executing the block design problems compared with the left hand (right hemisphere).

According to such a model, left-sided lesions may produce constructional difficulties in the right hand (but not the left) since they disconnect the vital right posterior region from the left motor cortex controlling the right hand. It could be postulated that the right posterior cortex contains the basic module for spatial integration (Fig. 6.10), a plausible position in view of accumulated neuropsychological evidence. It would thus be possible to have three situations: (i) a lesion at A would produce only right-handed constructional problems; (ii) a lesion at B would result in constructional difficulty for either hand; while (iii) a lesion at C would produce left-handed difficulties only.

The situation is obviously more complex than this: for example, constructional apraxia is never seen alone, always in association with other difficulties. Much has obviously been overlooked however in the failure to examine systematically the performance of each hand, and the disconnection notion is open to experimental verification.

SPATIAL ALEXIA AND ACALCULIA

Spatial alexia

This form of alexia may be clearly distinguishable at times from alexia of a symbolic nature. The patient can recognize letters and words but may be unable to read. At least part of this difficulty is attributable to difficulty with the continuous scanning movements necessary for reading. The disorganization in the directional control of eye movements varies a good deal from patient to patient, but in severely disabled patients the fixations appear to be made at random, so that fixation may jump from one part of a line to another and from part of one line to another line some distance away. Obviously a patient with this difficulty cannot make sense of printed material. Less severely affected patients may skip only occasional words so that they are able to fill in the sense of what they are reading.

Some patients' reading difficulties appear to depend largely upon unilateral spatial neglect. For this reason spatial alexia is seen rather more frequently with right hemisphere lesions. Benton (1969a) explains the effect in the following way: 'The patient initially fixates on a point which is at some distance to the right of the beginning of the line, reads to the end of the line and then returns to a point on the next line which is somewhat to the right of the beginning of the line. The result is, of course, that he cannot make any sense of what he reads and he soon becomes confused' (p. 219). This explanation is very similar to that usually employed in the explanation of reading difficulty of the hemianopic patient (especially those with a left half-field loss), which is described in the next chapter.

Spatial acalculia

Hécaen and his collaborators divided calculation difficulties into three types, each the product of a different mechanism (Hécaen et al 1961, Hécaen 1969). These are: (i) acalculia based on an alexia of figures and numerals; (ii) inability to do arithmetical sums (anarithmia); and (iii) acalculia of the spatial type. Hécaen and Angelergues (1961) found a predominance of left hemisphere lesions with the first two types and a predominance of right hemisphere lesions with the third. Approximately 24% of 148 right hemisphere cases had this disorder compared with only 2% of 195 left hemisphere cases.

Grafman et al (1982) studied 76 subjects with unilateral damage resulting from focal haemorrhage, having first established the subjects' competence to read and write numbers. They were then given a written calculation test, together with neuropsychological tests covering perception, construction and intelligence. Both right and left hemisphere subjects were poorer than controls, but those with left posterior lesions were particularly impaired even after the calculation test score had been corrected for the results on the other tests. This would seem to confirm the presence of the type 2 acalculia and relate it to the left posterior region. Three similar cases of Takayama et al (1994) implicate the region of the left intraparietal sulcus.

SPATIAL DISORDERS: GENERAL COMMENTS

The hemispheric asymmetry of function with regard to spatial disorders is summarized in Chapter 8. Bender and Diamond (1970) remind us of the

> ...extensive interrelationships among the various sensory-motor systems that characterize normal perceptual function...cerebellar, oculomotor and vestibular influences are prominent factors in visual function besides the visual projection system itself and the subject's state of alertness. It is not

possible therefore to ascribe disturbances in perception of space to disease of the parietal lobe or, more specifically, to disease of the right parietal lobe. (p. 184)

While one might agree with this statement if it means only to disease of the parietal lobe, there is little doubt that the accumulated evidence indicts the right parietal lobe most strongly in certain disorders. There is some evidence, too, that the presence of residual perceptual and spatial deficits may be the principal reason why recovery after right hemisphere strokes is more difficult to achieve than after seemingly comparable lesions in the left hemisphere (Marquardsen 1969, Hurwitz & Adams 1972).

Finally, it is obvious that the concept of 'spatial disorientation' or even 'spatial difficulty' is a very gross one. Dee and Benton (1970) comment: 'Assuming that spatial perception may be analyzed into 'partial' functions, it would not be surprising to find hemispheric differences in the representations of such functions' (p. 270). It would also be surprising if these partial functions were not closely related to the specific outlying association areas of the different modalities.

UNILATERAL SPATIAL NEGLECT (USN)

As early as 1876 Jackson described a patient who neglected the left side of the page when reading. As with so many later reports, the lesion was in the right posterior region. A more complete description of visual inattention came from Holmes (1918) and the phenomenon was confirmed by Poppelreuter (1923) and Riddoch (1935), but it was not until the detailed description by Brain (1941) of inattention for the left half of space in three patients with large right-sided parietal lesions that the condition attracted much attention. It has been variously defined, but the essential features are expressed in the following definition of Gainotti and his colleagues (1972b, p. 545). The 'syndrome consists of a tendency to neglect one half of extrapersonal space in such tasks as drawing and reading which require a good and symmetrical exploration of space'.

In everyday activities patients may neglect food on one side of their plates, may fail to use cutlery on one side, may collide with a wall along a corridor and, when asked to read, may read only portions of the page and even fractions of words. The most striking examples are seen in those with left-sided neglect.

Testing for neglect

Simple clinical tasks include asking the patient to copy a simple symmetrical drawing such as a daisy. The patient will often be satisfied with drawing half the figure, usually the right. Asked to bisect a line drawn on a paper placed directly in front, the patient will place the mark towards the normal side. This test was first devised by Axenfeld in 1894 (De Renzi 1982). However, care must be taken in reporting results of such tests to provide specific procedural details, since the degree of neglect shown on such a task as line bisection can be affected by factors like spatial motor cues, such as the starting position of the hand (Halligan et al 1991). Body or trunk orientation has likewise been shown to affect certain neglect tasks (Karnath et al 1991).

Other 'experimental' measures have been employed, e.g. the omission of items on the neglected side of space with the Poppelreuter overlapping figures test (Critchley 1953, Hécaen & Angelergues 1963). Costa et al (1969) devised an empirical position preference score from Raven's Coloured Progressive Matrices. Specially constructed tasks have been produced, e.g. that of De Renzi and Faglioni (1967); the most favoured has been that of Albert (1973). The importance of using several measures in the one patient is shown by the study of Ogden (1985), where some patients showed clear visual hemineglect on some tasks but not on others. A study by Seki and Ishiai (1996) of 69 neglect subjects demonstrates that different performances by subjects may arise from different levels rather than different types of neglect.

Laterality of lesion and USN

The first clear statement on a relation between laterality and neglect also came from Brain (1945), who considered that the deficit was very largely restricted to right hemisphere or non-dominant lesions. This point of view has received very wide support, though Brain was aware that the apparently low incidence of report of USN in left hemisphere or dominant lesions might be caused by the masking effects of other symptoms such as severe aphasia. A direct attempt to test this proposition was made by Battersby et al (1956) during a study of 75 cases with unilateral space occupying lesions. The authors suggest that the apparently high association found between neglect phenomena and the non-dominant hemisphere might be a spurious one. There are a number of factors which make comparison studies exceedingly difficult if not impossible. Chief among these are the characteristics of the groups under study: e.g. (i) the presence and degree of sensory deficits; (ii) the presence and degree of aphasia; (iii) the presence of intellectual deterioration; and (iv) the relative size of the lesion. The sobering effect of the findings of Arrigoni and De Renzi (1964) with regard to laterality and another disorder (constructional praxis) has already been mentioned.

A brief review of studies since 1960 does lend weight to Brain's original hypothesis. In a study of other symptoms associated with constructional apraxia occurring in unilateral cases, McFie and Zangwill (1960) found that only one of their 8 left hemisphere cases showed neglect compared with 14 out of 21 right hemisphere cases from previous studies from Zangwill's laboratory (Paterson & Zangwill 1944, 1945, McFie et al 1950, Ettlinger et al 1957). The right-sided predominance was also reported by Piercy and co-workers (1960). Hécaen (1962) reviewed a large number of retrorolandic cases which showed that only 4 out of 206 left hemisphere cases had the deficit as against 52 out of 154 right hemisphere cases. A much higher incidence of qualitative errors suggesting left hemi-inattention was found for right hemisphere cases than left hemisphere cases in Arrigoni and De Renzi's (1964) study of constructional apraxia. A specific test of the laterality hypothesis by Gainotti (1968) using a battery of simple tests showed that unilateral neglect is both significantly more frequent and more severe in patients with lesions of the right hemisphere than of the left. This finding was strongly confirmed in a later study (Gainotti & Tiacci 1971), and other studies have continued to add to the consensus. Oxbury et al (1974), for example, found no cases of neglect in their patients with either left hemisphere or brain stem strokes, while 7 of their 17 right hemisphere stroke cases showed the symptom. In an extensive review of studies relating unilateral neglect to laterality, Hécaen (1962) concludes that prevalence of neglect in right-sided lesions appears established even after factors such as sampling bias have been considered. Not only has evidence of a quantitative difference between the two hemispheres gained support, but the hypothesis has been advanced that qualitative differences also exist. Gainotti and co-workers (1972a) compared patients with unilateral lesions on various tasks of copying drawings. They described for the first time what appears to be a unique feature in the performance of some right hemisphere cases, namely, 'the tendency to neglect one half of a figure (on the side opposite to the hemispheric locus of lesion), while reproducing designs that are placed even more laterally on the neglected side' (p. 546). Examples of this qualitatively different sign are shown in Figure 6.11.

The majority of earlier references to neglect phenomena were concerned with visuospatial neglect. It can also occur in other modalities. The finding of unilateral neglect in the tactile modality by De Renzi and colleagues (1970) suggested to those authors 'that hemi-inattention does not depend so much on perceptual and motor factors as on a mutilated representation of space' (p. 202). Heilman and Valenstein (1972a) found 17 cases of auditory unilateral neglect in a 10 month survey. Of 10 cases with positive brain scans, 9 lesions were in the right inferior parietal lobule and one in the left frontal region. Though the defect became most apparent in test situations employing simultaneous stimulation, it was not restricted to these, being apparent as an abnormal responsiveness when the patients were addressed from the neglected side. There was no loss of auditory acuity in these patients. There may also be an interaction between the nature of the task employed and the laterality of the

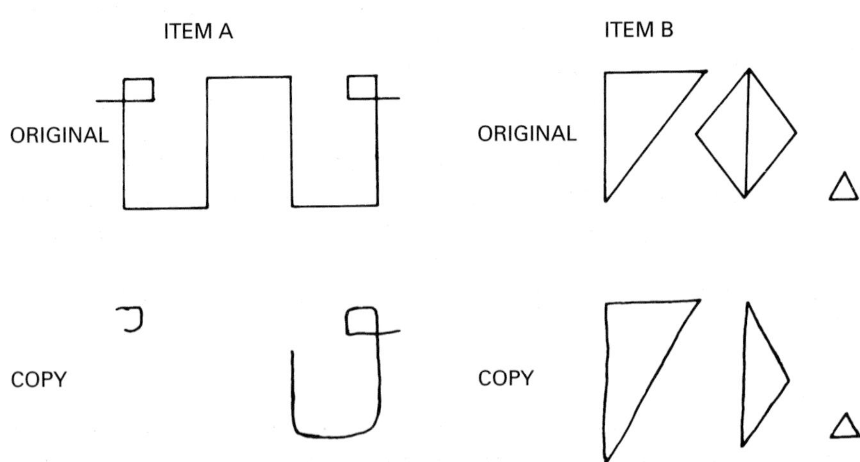

Fig. 6.11 Examples of copying defects in right hemisphere patients (after Gainotti et al 1972b, courtesy of the authors and editors).

lesions. Leicester et al (1969) found that not only did neglect appear with lesions of either hemisphere but also that, with particular tasks, neglect occurred predominantly or exclusively with lesions of one hemisphere, e.g. a language related task of matching letters to an auditory sample showed neglect only on the right with dominant left hemisphere lesions. This study also revealed that neglect appeared not 'on every test, but only on those which, for some reason they could not do correctly' (p. 586).

Locus of lesions causing neglect

Although most studies of USN implicate posterior parts of the brain (e.g. Fujii et al 1995), with particular emphasis on the non-dominant parietal lobe, neglect phenomena may be seen with lesions in other locations, both cortical and subcortical.

Parietal lobe

Apart from a large number of case reports, two sources of evidence for a preponderant role for the parietal lobe come from neurosurgical reports and localization studies using computed tomography (CT scan).

In patients who had undergone surgery for epilepsy, Hécaen et al (1956) found the critical area to be the supramarginal and angular gyri (the inferior parietal lobule) and part of the adjacent superior temporal gyrus. This was confirmed by the study of Heilman and Watson (1977), which showed radionucleotide uptake to be maximal in this region in 14 out of 19 cases with neglect. Similarly, the CT scan study of Bisiach et al (1979) implicated the multimodal cortex at the junction of the parietal, temporal and occipital lobes with heavy emphasis on the inferior parietal lobule. However, caution should be used in inferring the predominant importance of a particular region in view of the studies which follow.

Frontal lobe

The first description of frontal lobe neglect was by Heilman and Valenstein (1972b). All 6 patients were right-handed and had right-sided lesions, 3 dorsolateral and 3 medial. More recently, Damasio and his associates (1980) described 5 cases of neglect with lesions in the frontal lobe or basal ganglia. In this study, 4 of the 5 cases were in the left hemisphere. That frontal neglect is not uncommon was confirmed by Ogden (1985). While contralateral neglect was more severe with right-sided posterior lesions, some neglect was also seen with about half her patients with left-sided lesions, being more common with a frontal locus. Two further cases of right frontal lesions with neglect and confirmation of lesion site by PET have been described by Maeshima et al (1994).

Subcortical lesions

A number of reports of neglect and extinction phenomena have been reported with subcortical lesions in the thalamus or basal ganglia (Hier et al 1977, Watson & Heilman 1979, Damasio et al 1980, Valenstein & Heilman 1981). With one exception all cases have affected the right hemisphere.

Unilateral neglect and perceptual disorders

The higher incidence of impairment of patients with right hemisphere lesions on tasks of complex visual perception (described in Ch. 8), together with the higher incidence of neglect with right-sided lesions, has suggested the hypothesis that the two are causally related. Two experiments by Gainotti and Tiacci (1971) add weight to the hypothesis that some perceptual difficulties are caused, at least in part, by unilateral spatial neglect. On an overlapping figures test, right hemisphere patients made more total errors as well as more errors and omissions for figures lying to one side (left) of the midline than the left hemisphere group, while there was no significant difference between the two groups for errors on figures lying to the right of the midline. Furthermore the right hemisphere group with neglect tended to overvalue drawings on the right half of the midline when asked to compare the size of two figures, one to the left and one to the right. The authors suggest that the overvaluation may result from a tendency to gaze to the right (non-neglected) side invoking Piaget's theory of the 'fixation effect' (Piaget 1969) '...the space of visual perception is not homogeneous, but the elements on which the gaze is mostly fixed are systematically overvalued' (Gainotti & Tiacci 1971, p. 456).

A much higher incidence of visual field defects has been found in right hemisphere groups, with a higher incidence of visual spatial neglect (Battersby et al 1956, McFie & Zangwill 1960, Hécaen 1962). There is also a generally poorer performance on visual perceptual tasks by patients with right hemisphere lesions and neglect than by those with right hemisphere lesions without neglect (Oxbury et al 1974). These authors employed a wide range of tests of visual perception and spatial analysis, all of which showed a greater deficit in patients with neglect. However, the fact that some patients with clearly marked perceptual and spatial disorders showed no evidence of neglect suggested that, while visuospatial neglect may be an important factor in producing impairments of perception and spatial analysis in patients with non-dominant retrorolandic lesions, it certainly cannot be the whole answer.

The role of visual field defects in the disorders of visual perception which are so often associated with unilateral neglect has been the subject of frequent study. The Milan group has produced many studies showing that the perceptual deficits of non-dominant lesions are almost always associated with visual field defects (De Renzi & Spinnler 1967, De Renzi et al 1969a, b, 1970, Faglioni et al 1969). Ratcliff & Newcombe (1973) likewise found greatest impairment on a perceptual task for posterior right hemisphere lesions with visual field defects. Costa et al (1969) inferred that the strong right position preference shown by their right hemisphere cases on Raven's Progressive Matrices was indicative of visual spatial neglect and this was strongly associated in their material with visual field defects.

The relation between field defects and neglect is far from simple; Vallar et al (1991) have shown by the use of evoked brain potentials that early sensory processing of material from the 'neglected' side does take place in some subjects at least, though this information is not accessible to consciousness.

Nature of the defect

Theories of neglect phenomena are many and no single conception appears adequate to explain fully the findings. There is also overlap between what appear at first to be separate theories. Four classes of explanation cover most of the opinions.

Sensory synthesis

Denny-Brown and his colleagues (1952) considered that a disruption of sensory transmission and synthesis in one hemisphere was the causative process. Battersby et al (1956) felt that mental deterioration needed to be superadded; this was far from universally present in the studies of Hécaen and Angelergues (1963) and Gainotti (1968), though a half to three quarters of subjects did have such impairment.

Attentional deficit

Critchley (1949) in a discussion of tactile inattention argued strongly for an attentional deficit as the basis of the disorder. Heilman and associates have been the most enthusiastic proponents of this view (Heilman & Watson 1977, Heilman & Valenstein 1979, Heilman et al 1983). They pointed out that all the anatomical structures described as producing neglect have been shown to be involved in arousal or activation and attention, and supported their argument with experimental studies in animals (Heilman et al 1983). More recently this group (Meador et al 1988) trained subjects who were being investigated for the possibility of epilepsy surgery on a non-verbal tactile attention task and retested them after either left or right hemisphere sodium amytal ablation. Subjects with right hemisphere ablation showed more extinction responses and greater inattention than those with left hemisphere ablation. Again these authors argue that this result arises from a greater dominance by the right hemisphere for attentional mechanisms for scanning the environment.

If attentional mechanisms are at the basis of neglect, it is apparent from the complex patterns of dissociation between different aspects of so-called neglect seen in individual patients that the mechanisms must operate at various levels (Gentilini et al 1989, Cubelli et al 1991). Recently Ishiai et al (1997) showed that, when given a verbal instruction, patients with left-sided neglect could perform a copying task normally, whereas unaided they omitted the content of the left side of the given design.

Internal representation of space

Neither of the above explanations accounts for the difficulties which some neglect patients appear to have with the internal representation of space. 'This behaviour is suggestive of a deficit not restricted to perception but one also involving also a mutilated mental representation of space.' (De Renzi 1982, p. 110). This latter expression had also been used earlier by De Renzi, Faglioni and Scotti (1970), who were impressed by the fact that neglect was not restricted to the visual modality only, but affected the tactile modality as well. Some of their subjects confined their tactile exploration to the right (ipsilateral) side as though the left side of space did not exist for them.

Bisiach and Luzzatti (1978) asked two patients with left-sided neglect to describe imagined perspectives (the buildings on either side of the well known piazza outside the Milan cathedral). The subjects failed to allude to buildings on their left as they tried to imagine themselves facing the cathedral. A most impressive fact was that, when asked to imagine themselves now faced about, the subjects now omitted buildings on their *imagined left*, buildings which they had only recently reported. In a recent rare case with a right parietal lesion, neglect was limited to mental representation, visual perception being unaffected (Beschin et al 1997).

Similar support for an inability to deal with the left side of spatial representation came from an experimental study using laboratory apparatus which precluded perceptual scanning as a contributing factor (Bisiach et al 1981). The study employed only right-lesioned patients, and a replication with the same test using also left-lesioned subjects demonstrated the same difficulty in both groups. The fact that left-sided lesions showing neglect tend to be anterior conforms with the evidence of the role of this region (as well as the right posterior cortex) in spatial representation, cited earlier in the chapter.

The question of whether there is separate (modality specific) or supramodal representation of space in the right parietal region is still being explored (Villardita 1987, Farah et al 1989, Fujii et al 1991).

Neuronal network asymmetry

In a number of publications, Heilman and his colleagues (Heilman & Valenstein 1979, Heilman & Van Den Abell 1980, Heilman et al 1985) have suggested the hypothesis that the attentional neurons of the right parietal region may have bilateral receptive fields whereas those of the corresponding left hemisphere have only contralateral fields.

Such an explanation might account for the asymmetry of contralateral neglect supported by the literature, but also suggests that ipsilateral neglect might also be found with right-sided lesions. This latter finding received support from a study by Weintraub and Mesulam (1987, 1988), but a study by Gainotti et al (1990) using large groups failed to support the hypothesis and suggests that there are probably different mechanisms for ipsilateral versus contralateral neglect. PET studies in volunteers, however, tend to support bilateral right and contralateral left hemisphere attentional responsibilities (Corbetta et al 1993, Gitelman et al 1996).

Unilateral neglect and recovery of function

The more striking features of hemineglect after cerebrovascular lesions tend to ameliorate in the first few weeks, but may remain relatively stable thereafter (Gainotti 1968, Campbell & Oxbury 1976). Follow-up studies suggest that persistence of neglect may be a key factor in the lesser degree of improvement in independence and social adjustment shown by left hemiplegics compared with right (Denes et al 1982).

Despite this poor prognosis, there are those who feel that neglect may be amenable to rehabilitation (Lawson 1962), and rehabilitative techniques have shown some promise of transferring improved scanning, for example, from training to everyday situations (Diller & Weinberg 1977).

Motor neglect

Many patients with unilateral (sensory) neglect also may fail to use their contralateral arm, although they are able to do so when pressed and show no obvious motor defect when they do. However, Laplane and Degos (1983) have described 20 cases of 'pure' motor neglect, i.e. without sensory neglect. The motor neglect was always contralateral. 15 cases were frontally located, 4 were in the parietal region and 1 was thalamic. In another series, all directional motor neglect patients had frontal lesions while, in those with perceptual neglect, the frontal lobes were spared (Ladavas et al 1993). A novel use of a cancellation test using an interposed mirror also found dissociable frontal and parietal groups (Tegnér & Levander 1991). Another recent case of pure neglect had MRI evidence of a discrete left parietal infarct with sparing of the sensorimotor cortex (Triggs et al 1994). An interesting case with sequential infarctions in right frontal then parietal regions showed initial motor or exploratory neglect, with additional sensory neglect only after the second infarction (Daffner et al 1990).

Umilta (1995) points out in his review that not only may there be a dissociation between perceptual and motor neglect, but also that sensory neglect may show a dissociation between modalities such as visual and tactile. Even motor neglect itself may be further subdivided. Heilman et al (1993) prefer the term 'action-intentional disorders', and outline a number of subtypes which include motor impersistence, motor extinction, akinesia and hypokinesia, while Simon et al (1995) recommend a division based on the hemispace in which the required task is to be performed.

DISORDERS OF THE BODY SCHEMA

Disorders of the body schema are usually attributed to impairment of parietal lobe function. Some observations would suggest that these disorders are more prominent with right parietal lesions than with left. Absence of the disorders of communication seen with left hemisphere lesions at least make the body schema disorders caused by right hemisphere damage appear more apparent and striking. There are often associated motor and sensory deficits from spread of the lesions to somaesthetic, visual and motor pathways. The first systematic studies of disorders of 'the body image' were published by Lhermitte (1942, 1952). Only a sample of the most frequently seen syndromes will be outlined; these are (i) anosognosia, (ii) bodily agnosia, and (iii) right-left discrimination, together with a consideration of the Gerstmann syndrome. The related area of unilateral neglect for external space has been treated separately above. Body schema disorders were dealt with extensively by Frederiks (1969).

Anosognosia

This term means a failure to perceive illness. Observations of single cases were described late in the 19th century, but the coining of the term by Babinski in 1914 to describe lack of awareness of, or unconcern about, (left) hemiplegia stimulated systematic study. The normal clinical usage implies a failure to perceive a defect or the denial of a defect. This association between denial or imperception of hemiplegia is a very common finding and in the majority of cases the paralysis is on the left side. While the lesion is usually centred in the right parietal lobe, it is seldom restricted to this site, the lesions with anosognosia being invariably large (Hier et al 1983a). Nathanson and his co-workers (1952) observed that some 70% of patients with denial of unilateral paralysis had damage to the right hemisphere, and this accent on right hemisphere lesions continues to be reported (Stone et al 1993). Patients with this disorder may rationalize about their failure to use the paralyzed limbs and sometimes even have the delusion that the limbs do not belong to them, i.e. they are seen as being outside the patient's own body image. Anosognosia is seen in the acute stages of a disorder, being quite uncommon in chronic hemiplegics (Cutting 1978, Hier et al 1983b), and may be so elaborated as to appear delusional (Halligan et al 1995). Amelioration has also been reported with various vestibular stimulations (Rubens 1985, Vallar et al 1993).

Some writers have suggested that the asymmetrical reporting of anosognosia may be in part a relative absence of reports from patients with left hemisphere lesions and associated aphasia. Eight subjects who underwent consecutive Wada ablations of each hemisphere were tested by Gilmore et al (1992). The results were compelling. All subjects recalled their hemiplegia and aphasia after recovery from the left hemisphere injection, but none recalled their hemiplegia after recovery from the right hemisphere injection. In a recent study, patients with both aphasia and left-sided neglect from left hemisphere lesions showed dissociated transient improvement in the USN with vestibular stimulation but no change in language disorder (Vallar et al 1995).

The term anosognosia has also been extended by some writers to the denial or imperception of other deficits, so that qualifying terms need to be added. It is interesting to note that these phenomena may sometimes be dissociated, with unawareness or denial of one deficit but not another (e.g. Kotler Cope & Camp 1995). Recent studies of Alzheimer patients, where lack of recognition of cognitive defects is very common, strongly suggest that dysfunction of the *right* frontal lobe may be the key determining factor (Reed et al 1993, Lopez et al 1994, Michon et al 1994, Starkstein 1995). The non-recognition of a defect ranges from minimization, through apparent lack of concern, to frank denial. Numerous reviews have appeared, e.g. Hécaen and Ajuriaguerra (1952), Critchley (1953), Alajouanine and Lhermitte (1957) and Frederiks (1969).

Anosognosia for hemiplegia (Babinski's syndrome) is almost always associated with acute, massive vascular lesions affecting the retrorolandic area, with accompanying hemiplegia, hemianopia and hemianaesthesia. The middle cerebral artery is most often implicated as the seat of the trouble.

Related, but somewhat less striking, is the symptom of relative inattention to one side of the body. Once again this deficit is mostly for the left half of the body. It is also related in many patients to the neglect of one half of external space, as already described. It should be stressed that in these cases there is no weakness or paralysis, though patients may fail to move their limbs spontaneously such as not swinging the affected arm when walking. They may neglect the left half of the body when bathing, dressing or combing the hair. Hécaen et al (1956) found that patients with surgical lesions in the right posterior parieto-temporal area had marked difficulties with complex sensorimotor activities including dressing. One patient could dress store dummies at his work, but had difficulty in dressing himself, which may suggest that one of the fundamental deficits in dressing apraxia is unawareness of the position of the limbs. This may be part of the general unawareness of body parts. The so-called 'dressing apraxia' would appear to have a number of determinants, only one of which is bodily inattention.

Lack of awareness of body parts

This disturbance of the body image declares itself in the patients' inability to name and localize parts of their own bodies. Methods of examination have been described in detail by Benton (1959). Common clinical tests include the following: (i) asking the patient to identify parts of the body named by the examiner or to move the named parts; (ii) asking the patient to identify body parts on a diagram or on the examiner; (iii) asking the patient to move parts shortly after the examiner has touched them; (iv) asking the patient to touch one part of the body with another, e.g. 'place your (right) hand on your (left) ear'. This latter task is often known as Head's 'hand-eye-ear' test (Head 1920) and forms part of many routine screening devices for higher function disorders, such as the Halstead-Wepman Aphasia Screening Test (Russell et al 1970). Head's test is also commonly used for determining difficulties with right-left orientation.

One of the most commonly described disorders in this category is finger agnosia, first described by Gerstmann in 1924 (see Gerstmann 1930). It was defined in a later publication in the following way – 'It consists in a *primary* disturbance or loss of ability to recognize, identify, differentiate, name, select, indicate and orient as to the individual fingers of either hand, the patient's own, as well as those of other persons' (Gerstmann, 1957, p. 886). Some writers would prefer a term like 'faulty finger localization'.

Finger agnosia has been studied experimentally by Kinsbourne and Warrington (1962). They examined 12 patients with this symptom using a number of specially constructed tests, most of which require only minimal verbal response. Two of these tests are as follows:

The In-Between Test. Two fingers are simultaneously touched. The patient is asked to state the number of fingers between the ones touched. Thus the answer may be 0, 1, 2 or 3 (Fig. 6.12A).

Two-Point Finger Test. The fingers are touched in two places. The patient judges whether the two touches are both on the same finger or on different fingers (Fig. 6.12B.).

Warrington (1973) considers Test 1 to be the most clinically useful. Unlike the three studies cited below, Kinsbourne and Warrington maintained that the conjunction of the other Gerstmann symptoms with finger agnosia was more than coincidental.

Warrington cites Lunn's 1948 review of the published cases of finger agnosia '...after excluding cases with widespread lesions and subjects with mixed handedness (they) found no case of finger agnosia with a right hemisphere lesion' (p. 273). There seems little doubt from the accrued evidence that finger agnosia is a sign par excellence of a dominant hemisphere posterior lesion.

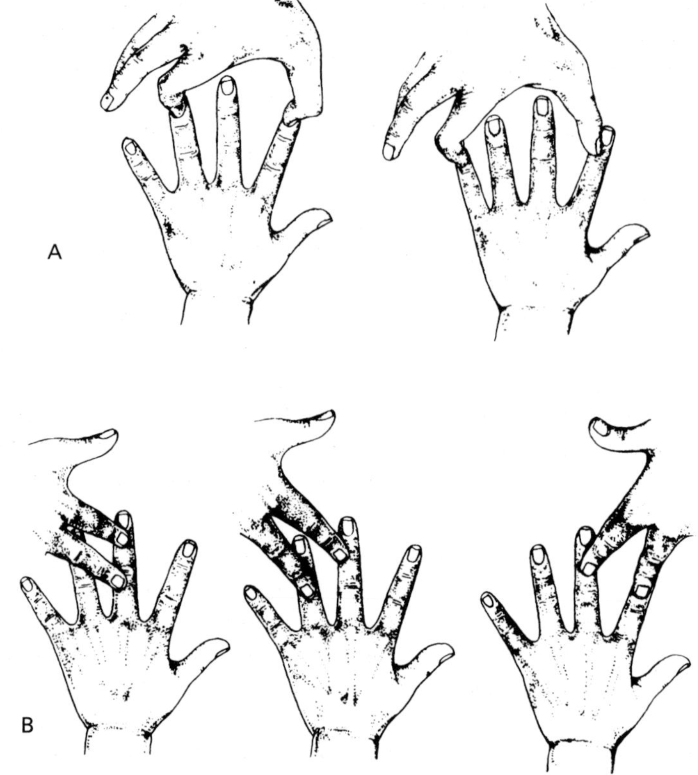

Fig. 6.12 A, The In-Between Test of Finger Agnosia; B, Two-Point Finger Test (from Kinsbourne & Warrington 1962).

Right-left disorientation

This disorientation reflects itself in confusion between left and right for all parts of the body. It is a complex disorder or set of disorders and its significance is still not yet fully understood. Many factors may be involved, apraxic, aphasic and agnosic. Poeck and Orgass (1966) stressed the role of aphasia though the deficit may be seen in the absence of clinically demonstrable aphasia. The complexity was brought out clearly in a factorial study of Poeck and Orgass (1967). Benton (1959), in a developmental study of lateral orientation in normal children, has stressed the dependency of this type of ability on language. Like the other symptoms under discussion of right-left hemisphere malfunction, minor degrees of the disorder are difficult to establish since many normal individuals continue to have lateral confusion in adult life without any apparent signs of cerebral impairment.

THE GERSTMANN SYNDROME

In 1924 Gerstmann described finger agnosia and, in the ensuing 6 years, studied 4 such cases, all of whom had associated deficits. This experience suggested that four of the features formed a unique constellation to which others gave the title of Gerstmann's syndrome. To the two symptoms mentioned above (finger agnosia and right-left disorientation) must be added agraphia and acalculia. These four deficits formed for Gerstmann a unique constellation reflecting disturbance of the person's knowledge of his or her hand and its use. Such a constellation appeared to result from dominant hemisphere lesions affecting the region of the angular gyrus and adjacent part of the occipital lobe (Gerstmann 1930). Many neurologists readily accepted the syndrome as having significant localizing value. However, with the passage of time doubt arose over the validity of the syndrome and the 1960s produced several direct attempts at verification. Critchley, in the William Gowers lecture for 1965, commented elegantly upon the evidence to that time (Critchley 1966).

The first major objective study to find against the validity of the Gerstmann syndrome was that of Benton (1961), whose designation of the syndrome as a 'fiction' attracted wide support. Benton studied the concordance between a number of deficits in a group of patients with cerebral disease, arguing that the strength of concordance should be a measure of the viability of the concept of a syndrome. His summary is well worth quoting:

> Systematic, objective analysis of the performance of patients with cerebral disease on seven 'parietal' tasks (right-left orientation, finger localization, writing, calculation, constructional praxis, reading, visual memory) indicates that many combinations of deficits, including those known as the 'Gerstmann syndrome', may be observed. The syndrome appears to be no different from the other combinations in respect to either the strength of mutual interrelationships among its elements or the strength of the relationships between its elements and performances not belonging to it. These results hold both for patients with diverse cerebral conditions and for those with focal lesions of the dominant parietal lobe.
>
> The findings are interpreted as indicating that the Gerstmann syndrome is an artifact of defective and biased observation. Further, a review of the pertinent clinical literature offers little support for its alleged focal diagnostic significance. (p. 181)

Benton's analysis was soon followed by another large study (Heimburger et al 1964). Of 456 patients with cerebral disease, some 111 showed one or more Gerstmann symptoms. 33 cases showed one symptom, 32 two symptoms, 23 three symptoms and 23 showed all four. These four groups were then related to the nature and extent of pathology. Group I (one symptom only) tended to have small static lesions. An increase in the number of symptoms was paralleled by an increase in the extent and destructiveness of lesions up to Group IV (having all four Gerstmann symptoms). An analysis of Group IV also showed that the angular gyrus does not need to be involved, as earlier writers, particularly Gerstmann himself, believed. At least 3 of the 23 cases had autopsy confirmation of absence of a lesion affecting the angular gyrus. With regard to the localizing value of the Gerstmann symptoms, Heimburger et al found that the probability of a dominant hemisphere lesion increased with the number of symptoms but that they were of no value for localizing within the hemisphere. They concluded 'As to localizing significance, Gerstmann's syndrome has approximately the same degree of cogency as dysphasia' (p. 57).

The results of Poeck and Orgass (1966) supported the contention of the two previous studies that the syndrome does not occur in isolated form. They noted that the complete syndrome was rarely observed without aphasia which they believed was the 'common denominator of the four symptoms'. 'The performances which are disturbed in the so-called Gerstmann syndrome are closely related to language. However, aphasia also produces other behavioural deficits, appearing as 'concurrent' symptoms. It is therefore not justified to regard the four symptoms as a natural syndrome. They are an arbitrary partial grouping of the numerous neuropsychological disturbances resulting from lesion of the leading hemisphere' (p. 436). This association of aphasia with Gerstmann symptoms following infarction of the left parietal lobe continues to be reported (e.g. Kumar & Mollison 1993).

Against this apparently impressive accumulation of negative evidence are those rare cases with all four classical features with no associated deficits, following infarction to the left angular gyrus (Roeltgen et al 1983, Sukumar & Ferguson 1996). Roeltgen and colleagues commented 'Perhaps the pure Gerstmann syndrome is a rare disorder because the lesions are rarely restricted to the area critical to this syndrome' (p. 47). A CT scan in Sukumar and Ferguson's case showed the lesion confined to the angular gyrus. In a review of the syndrome Benton (1992) agreed that imaging has now confirmed the presence of pure cases, albeit rare. Cortical stimulation appears to have further clarified the situation, with pure deficits being elicited in discrete cortical areas between angular and supramarginal gyri (Morris et al 1984).

Moreover, Strub and Geschwind (1983) point out that most of the contrary evidence is based on a misunderstanding by the opponents of the syndrome of the traditional usage of the term 'syndrome' in clinical medicine; the fact that patients may show other associated neurobehavioural disorders 'in no way negates the utility and certainly not the existence of the syndrome' (p. 315). Certainly the presence of several (not necessarily all) of the four classical features has powerful localizing significance suggesting pathology in the left parietal lobe. Discussion of the different uses of the term 'syndrome' has been presented in Chapter 1.

The review of Strub and Geschwind cited above not only provides an appraisal of evidence but also describes methods of examination of the component deficits.

THE PARIETAL LOBE AND SHORT TERM MEMORY (STM)

To date there is only a small amount of evidence about the localization of anatomical systems concerned with short term memory dysfunction. Much of the work has been carried out by Warrington and her colleagues and reviewed by her in several articles (Warrington 1971, Warrington & Weiskrantz 1972, Warrington & Baddeley 1974). The first report concerned one patient (KF) who had many years earlier received an injury to the left parietal region (Warrington & Shallice 1969). This patient had a marked impairment of the ability to repeat auditory verbal stimuli, which contrasted with much less difficulty with comparable visual verbal stimuli. This case suggested the possibility of modality specific short term memory defects. KF's difficulty could not be accounted for by faulty auditory perception or speech defect. A further study of the same patient (Shallice & Warrington 1970) confirmed the presence of a modality specific STM defect. Later Warrington and her colleagues (1971) added two further patients with lesions in the left parietal regions, this time employing 'psychological tests differentially loaded with short-term and long term memory components'. Results showed that: (i) long term memory functions in audition were relatively intact while auditory STM was impaired; and (ii) the disability was specific to the auditory modality, visual STM (as measured by relatively normal decay function) being little affected. Peterson and Peterson techniques were used in all instances. Further testing of KF in 1972 confirmed his rapid forgetting in auditory STM compared with relatively normal visual STM (Warrington & Shallice 1972).

Additional differentiation of the STM defect came with a study of KF and one other patient (Shallice & Warrington 1974). Within the auditory modality two tests were employed, one verbal (letters) and one non-verbal (meaningful sounds). The two patients exhibited a dissociation between these two tasks showing impairment on the verbal task but not on the non-verbal.

Against these studies supporting modal specificity is the study of Butters et al (1970b). These authors compared the performance of frontal and parietal cases, both left and right, on a variety of short term visual and auditory tasks, again employing the distractor technique. The right hemisphere group showed more severe impairment on visual STM tasks compared with auditory, while the two left-sided groups (frontal and parietal) showed separate characteristics. Left frontal patients had predominantly registration but not memory deficits. Left parietal patients had memory deficits. However, neither of the left groups showed modal specificity; visual and auditory material both being affected. Butters et al (1970b) consider that their results can be interpreted 'as supporting the notion that the right hemisphere, especially the parietal region, is involved in the processing of visual information both verbal and patterned, while the left hemisphere is concerned with verbal material irrespective of sensory modality' (p. 458). Further studies are needed to resolve this early apparent difference of findings.

Since a disproportionate impairment in the repetition of verbal stimuli is the most prominent symptom of 'conduction aphasia', Warrington considers that the results in her three patients with left parietal lesions add weight to the anatomical basis of this syndrome, which has been variously centred in the inferior parietal or temporo-parietal region. Many of the studies referring to the anatomical basis of repetition difficulty on conduction aphasia are given in Warrington, Logue and Pratt (1971). Certainly, the obvious clinical feature on which these cases were selected was their marked impairment for repetition of digits on the Digit Span subtest of the WAIS.

POSTURAL ARM DRIFT

A common clinical test used in neurological examination requires the patient to maintain a static position of the outstretched arms in a horizontal position with the eyes closed. In some brain damaged patients there may be considerable drift, usually, but not always, towards the midline. Since this drift is so frequently seen with parietal lesions it has come to be called by some clinicians 'parietal drift'. Only one experimental study relating postural arm drift to localization and lateralization appears to have been made (Wyke 1966). The findings of this study suggest that the more general term 'postural arm drift' should be used since it is by no means uncommon with extraparietal lesions. All Wyke's patients with lesions of the parietal region showed significant drift compared with two thirds of frontal and half of temporal patients. Left hemisphere cases showed some ipsilateral drift plus a more severe drift in the contralateral arm, while right hemisphere cases showed only a contralateral drift effect.

References

Ajuriaguerra J de, Hécaen H 1960 Le cortex cerebral. Masson, Paris
Alajouanine T 1960 Les grandes activités du lobe occipital. Masson, Paris
Alajouanine T, Lhermitte F 1957 Des agnosognosies électives. Encéphale 4: 509–519
Albert M L 1973 A simple test of visual neglect. Neurology 23: 58–64
Allison R S 1962 The senile brain: a clinical study. Arnold, London
Arena R, Gainotti G 1978 Constructional apraxia and visuoperceptive disabilities in relation to laterality of cerebral lesions. Cortex 14: 463–473
Arrigoni G, De Renzi E 1964 Constructional apraxia and hemispheric locus of lesion. Cortex l: 170–197
Babinski J 1914 Contribution a l'étude des troubles mentaux dans l'hémiplégie organique cérébrale. Revue Neurologique 1: 845–848
Battersby W S 1951 The regional gradient of critical flicker frequency after frontal or occipital injury. Journal of Experimental Psychology 42: 59–68
Battersby W S, Krieger H P, Bender M B 1955 Visual and tactile discriminative learning in patients with cerebral tumors. American Journal of Psychiatry 70: 703–712
Battersby W S, Bender M B, Pollack M, Kahn R L 1956 Unilateral 'spatial agnosia' ('inattention') in patients with cerebral lesions. Brain 79: 68–93
Bender M B, Diamond S P 1970 Disorders in perception of space due to lesions of the nervous system. Research Publications, Association for Research in Nervous and Mental Disease 48: 176–185
Bender M B, Teuber H L 1947 Spatial organization of visual perception following injury to the brain. Archives of Neurology and Psychiatry 58: 721–738
Bender M B, Teuber H L 1948 Spatial organization of visual perception following injury to the brain. Archives of Neurology and Psychiatry 59: 39–62
Benson D F, Barton M I 1970 Disturbances in constructional ability. Cortex 6: 19–46
Benton A L 1950 A multiple choice type of the Visual Retention Test. Archives of Neurology and Psychiatry 4: 699–707
Benton A 1952 La signification des tests du rétention visuelle dans le diagnostic clinique. Revue de Psychologie Appliquée 2: 151–179
Benton A L 1959 Right-left discrimination and finger localization. Hoeber, New York
Benton A L 1961 The fiction of the 'Gerstmann syndrome'. Journal of Neurology, Neurosurgery and Psychiatry 24: 176–181
Benton A L 1962 The visual retention test as a constructional praxis task. Confinia Neurologica 22: 141–155
Benton A L 1965 The problem of cerebral dominance. Canadian Psychologist 6: 332–348
Benton A L 1967 Constructional apraxia and the minor hemisphere. Confinia Neurologica 29: 1–16
Benton A L 1969a Constructional apraxia, some unanswered questions. In: Benton A L (ed) Contributions to clinical neuropsychology. Aldine, Chicago, ch 5
Benton A L (ed) 1969b Contributions to clinical neuropsychology. Aldine, Chicago
Benton A L 1992 Gerstmann's syndrome. Archives of Neurology 49: 445–447
Benton A L, Fogel M L 1962 Three dimensional constructional praxis. Archives of Neurology 7: 347–354
Benton A L, Levin H S, Van Allen M W 1974 Geographic orientation in patients with unilateral cerebral disease. Neuropsychologia 12: 183–191

Beschin N, Cocchini G, Della Sala S, Logie R H 1997 What the eyes perceive, the brain ignores: a case of pure representational neglect. Cortex 33: 3–26
Birkett P 1978 Hemispheric differences in the recognition of nonsense shapes. Cortex 14: 245–249
Bisiach E, Luzzatti C 1978 Unilateral neglect of representational space. Cortex 14: 129–133
Bisiach E, Luzzatti C, Perani D 1979 Unilateral neglect nonrepresentational schema and consciousness. Brain 102: 609
Bisiach E, Capitani E, Luzzatti C, Perani D 1981 Brain and conscious representation of outside reality. Neuropsychologia 19: 543–551
Black F W, Strub R L 1976 Constructional apraxia in patients with discrete missile wounds of the brain. Cortex 12: 212–220
Blum J S, Chow K L, Pribram K H 1950 A behavioral analysis of the organization of the parieto-temporo-preoccipital cortex. Journal of Comparative Neurology 93: 53–100
Boldrini P, Zanella R, Cantagallo A, Basaglia N 1992 Partial hemisphere disconnection syndrome of traumatic origin. Cortex 28: 135–143
Boll T J 1974 Right and left cerebral hemisphere damage and tactile perception: Performance of the ipsilateral and contralateral sides of the body. Neuropsychologia 12: 235–238
Bottini G, Cappa S, Geminiani G, Sterzi R 1992 Topographic disorientation – a case report. Neuropsychologia 28: 309–312
Brain R 1941 Visual disorientation with special reference to lesions of the right hemisphere. Brain 64: 244–272
Brain W R 1945 Speech and handedness. Lancet 2 : 837–842
Bryden M P 1977 Strategy effects in the presence of hemispheric asymmetry. In: Underwood G (ed) Strategies of information processing. Academic Press, London
Butters N, Barton M 1970 Effect of parietal lobe damage on the performance of reversible operations in space. Neuropsychologia 8: 205–214
Butters N, Brody B A 1968 The role of the left parietal lobe in the mediation of intra and cross-modal associations. Cortex 4: 328–343
Butters N, Barton M, Brody B A 1970a Role of the right parietal lobe in the mediation of cross-modal associations and reversible operations in space. Cortex 6: 174–190
Butters N, Samuels I, Goodglass H, Brody B 1970b Short term visual and auditory memory disorders after parietal and frontal lobe damage. Cortex 6: 440–459
Butters N, Soeldner C, Fedio P 1972 Comparison of parietal and frontal lobe spatial deficits in man: extra-personal vs personal (egocentric) space. Perceptual and Motor Skills 34: 27–34
Byrne R W 1982 Geographical knowledge and orientation. In: Ellis A W (ed) Normality and pathology in cognitive functions. Academic Press, London, pp 239–264
Campbell D C, Oxbury J M 1976 Recovery from unilateral visual-spatial neglect. Cortex 12: 303–312
Carlesimo G A, Fadda L, Caltagirone C 1993 Basic mechanisms of constructional apraxia in unilateral brain-damaged patients: role of visuo-perceptual and executive disorders. Journal of Clinical and Experimental Neuropsychology 15: 342–358
Carmon A, Bechtoldt H P 1969 Dominance of the right cerebral hemisphere for stereopsis. Neuropsychologia 7: 29–39
Caselli R J 1991a Bilateral impairment of somesthetically mediated object recognition in humans. Mayo Clinic Proceedings 66: 357–364
Caselli R J 1991b Rediscovering tactile agnosia. Mayo Clinic Proceedings 66: 129–142
Cattell R B 1944 A culture-free test. The Psychological Corporation, New York
Clarke S, Assal G, de Tribolet N 1993 Left hemisphere strategies in visual recognition, topographical orientation and time planning. Neuropsychologia 31: 99–113
Cogan D G 1960 Hemianopia and associated symptoms due to parieto-temporal lobe lesions. American Journal of Ophthalmology 50: 1058–1066
Collignon R, Rondeaux J 1974 Approche clinique des modalités de l'apraxie constructive secondaire aux lésions corticales hémisphèriques gauches et droites. Acta Neurologica Belgica 74: 137–146
Corbetta M, Miezin F M, Shulman G L, Petersen S E 1993 A PET study of visuospatial attention. Journal of Neuroscience 13: 1202–1226
Corkin S H 1964 Somesthetic function after cerebral damage in man. Unpublished doctoral dissertation, McGill University

Corkin S 1965 Tactually-guided image learning in man. Effect of unilateral cortical excisions and bilateral hippocampal lesions. Neuropsychologia 3: 339–351
Corkin S, Milner B, Rasmussen T 1970 Somatosensory thresholds – contrasting effects of postcentral-gyrus and posterior parietal lobe excisions. Archives of Neurology 23: 41–58
Costa L, Vaughan H 1962 Performance of patients with lateralized cerebral lesions. 1: Verbal and perceptual tests. Journal of Nervous and Mental Disease 134: 162–168
Costa L D, Vaughan H G Jr, Horwitz M, Ritter W 1969 Patterns of behavioral deficit associated with visual spatial neglect. Cortex 5: 242–263
Critchley M 1949 The phenomenon of tactile inattention with special reference to parietal lesions. Brain 72: 538–561
Critchley M 1953 The parietal lobes. Arnold, London
Critchley M 1966 The enigma of Gerstmann's syndrome. Brain 89: 183–198
Cubelli R, Nichelli P, Bonito V, Inzaghi M G 1991 Different patterns of dissociation in unilateral spatial neglect. Brain and Cognition 15: 139–159
Cutting J 1978 Study of anosognosia. Journal of Neurology, Neurosurgery and Psychiatry 41: 548–555
Daffner K R, Ahern G L, Weintraub S, Mesulam M-M 1990 Dissociated neglect behavior following sequential strokes in the right hemisphere. Annals of Neurology 28: 97–101
Damasio A R, Damasio H, Chang Chui H 1980 Neglect following damage to frontal lobe and basal ganglia. Neuropsychologia 18: 123–132
Dee H L 1970 Visuoconstructive and visuoperceptive deficit in patients with unilateral cerebral lesions. Neuropsychologia 8: 305–314
Dee H L, Benton A L 1970 A cross-modal investigation of spatial performances in patients with unilateral cerebral disease. Cortex 6: 261–277
Denes G, Semenza C, Stoppa E, Lis A 1982 Unilateral spatial neglect and recovery from hemiplegia. A follow-up study. Brain 105: 543–552
Denny-Brown D, Chambers R A 1958 The parietal lobe and behavior. Research Publications, Association for Research in Nervous and Mental Disease 3: 35–117
Denny-Brown D, Meyer J S, Horenstein S 1952 The significance of perceptual rivalry resulting from parietal lesions. Brain 75: 433–471
De Renzi E 1982 Disorders of space exploration and cognition. Wiley, New York
De Renzi E, Faglioni P 1962 Il disorientamento spatiale da lesione cerebrale. Sistema Nervoso 14: 409–436
De Renzi E, Faglioni P 1967 The relationship between visuo-spatial impairment and constructional apraxia. Cortex 3: 327–342
De Renzi E, Scotti G 1969 The influence of spatial disorders in impairing tactile recognition of shapes. Cortex 5: 53–62
De Renzi E, Spinnler H 1967 Impaired performance on color tasks in patients with hemispheric damage. Cortex 3: 194–217
De Renzi E, Faglioni P, Scotti G 1969a Impairment of memory for position following brain damage. Cortex 5: 274–284
De Renzi E, Scotti G, Spinnler H 1969b Perceptual and associative disorders of visual recognition. Neurology 19: 634–642
De Renzi E, Faglioni P, Scotti G 1970 Hemispheric contribution to exploration of space through the visual and tactile modality. Cortex 6: 191–203
De Renzi E, Faglioni P, Scotti G 1971 Judgment of spatial orientation in patients with focal brain damage. Journal of Neurology, Neurosurgery and Psychiatry 34: 489–495
De Renzi E, Faglioni P, Villa P 1977 Topographical amnesia. Journal of Neurology, Neurosurgery and Psychiatry 40: 498–505
Diller L, Weinberg J 1977 Hemi-inattention in rehabilitation: the evolution of a rational remediation program. Advances in Neurology 18: 63–82
Duensing F 1954 Raumagnostische und ideatorischapraktische Störung des gestaltenden Handelns. Deutsche Zeitschrift für Nervenheilkunde 170: 72–94
Ettlinger G, Warrington E, Zangwill O L 1957 A further study of visual-spatial agnosia. Brain 80: 335–361
Evans J P 1935 A study of the sensory defects resulting from excision of the cerebral substance in humans. Research Publications, Association for Research in Nervous and Mental Disease 15: 331–370
Faglioni P, Spinnler H, Vignolo LA 1969 Contrasting behavior of right and left hemisphere

damaged patients on a discriminative and a semantic task of auditory recognition. Cortex 5: 366–389
Faglioni P, Scotti G, Spinnler H 1971 The performance of brain-damaged patients in spatial localization of visual and tactile stimuli. Brain 94: 443–454
Farah M J, Wong A B, Monheit M A, Morrow L A 1989 Parietal lobe mechanisms of spatial attention: modality specific or supramodal? Neuropsychologia 27: 461–470
Fogel M L 1962 Intelligence Quotient as an index of brain damage. American Journal of Orthopsychiatry 32: 338–339
Fogel M L 1964 The Intelligence Quotient as an index of brain damage. American Journal of Orthopsychiatry 34: 555–562
Fontenot D J, Benton A L 1971 Tactile perception of direction in relation to hemispheric locus of lesion. Neuropsychologia 9: 83–88
Frederiks J A M 1969 Disorders of the body schema. In: Vinken P J, Bruyn G W (eds) Handbook of clinical neurology. North-Holland, Amsterdam, vol 4, ch 11
Fujii T, Fukatsu R, Kimura I, Saso S, Kogure K 1991 Unilateral spatial neglect in visual and tactile modalities. Cortex 27: 339–343
Fujii T, Fukatsu R, Ayumu O, Kimura I, Yamadori A 1995 Left unilateral spatial neglect and its relation to testing methods, neurological manifestations and lesion site. No To Shinkei 47: 255–259
Gainotti G 1968 Les manifestations de négligence et d'inattention pour l'hémispace. Cortex 4: 64–91
Gainotti G, Tiacci C 1970 Patterns of drawing disability in right and left hemispheric patients. Neuropsychologia 8: 379–384
Gainotti G, Tiacci C 1971 The relation between disorders of visual perception and unilateral spatial neglect. Neuropsychologia 9: 451–458
Gainotti G, Messerli P, Tissot R 1972a Troubles du dessin et lésions hémisphèriques rétrorolandiques unilaterales gauches et droites. Encephale 1: 245–264
Gainotti G, Messerli P, Tissot R 1972b Qualitative analysis of unilateral spatial neglect in relation to laterality of cerebral lesions. Journal of Neurology, Neurosurgery and Psychiatry 35: 545–550
Gainotti G, Miceli G, Caltagirone G 1977 Constructional apraxia in left brain damaged patients: a planning disorder? Cortex 13: 109–118
Gainotti G, Giustolisi L, Nocentini U 1990 Contralateral and ipsilateral disorders of visual attention in patients with unilateral brain damage. Journal of Neurology, Neurosurgery and Psychiatry 53: 422–426
Galluscio E H 1990 Biological psychology. Macmillan, New York
Gazzaniga M S 1970 The bisected brain. Appleton-Century-Crofts, New York
Gazzaniga M S, Bogen J E, Sperry R W 1965 Observations on visual perception after disconnexion of the cerebral hemispheres in man. Brain 88: 221–230
Gentilini M, Barbieri C, De Renzi E, Faglioni P 1989 Space exploration with and without the aid of vision in hemisphere-damaged patients. Cortex 25: 643–651
Gerstmann J 1924 Fingeragnosie: Ein unschriebene Störung der Orientierung am eigenen Korper. Wiener Klinische Wochenschrift 37: 1010–1012
Gerstmann J 1930 Zur Symptomatologie der Hirnlasionen im Uebergangsgebeit der unteren Parietal und mittleren Occipitalwindung. Nervenarzt 3: 91–95
Gerstmann J 1957 Some notes on the Gerstmann syndrome. Neurology 7: 866–869
Gilliatt R W, Pratt R T C 1952 Disorders of perception in a case of right-sided cerebral thrombosis. Journal of Neurology, Neurosurgery and Psychiatry 15: 264–271
Gilmore R L, Heilman K M, Schmidt R P, Fennell E M, Quisling R 1992 Anosognosia during Wada testing. Neurology 42: 925–927
Gitelman D R, Alpert N M, Kosslyn S, Daffner K, Scinto L, Thompson W, Mesulam M M 1996 Functional imaging of human right hemispheric activation for exploratory movements. Annals of Neurology 39: 174–179
Gloning K 1965 Die zerebral bedingten Storungen des Raumlichen Schens und des Raumerlebens. Maudrich, Wien
Goldstein K, Scheerer M 1941 Abstract and concrete behavior: An experimental study with special tests. Psychological Monographs 43: 1–151
Gollin E S 1960 Development studies of visual recognition of incomplete objects. Perceptual and Motor Skills 11: 289–298

Grafman J, Passafiume D, Faglioni P, Boller F 1982 Calculation disturbances in adults with focal hemispheric damage. Cortex 18: 37–50
Habib M, Sirigu A 1987 Pure topographical disorientation: a definition and anatomical basis. Cortex 23: 73–85
Halligan P W, Manning L, Marshall J C 1991 Hemispheric activation vs spatio-motor cueing in visual neglect: a case study. Neuropsychologia 29: 165–176
Halligan P W, Marshall J C, Wade D T 1995 Unilateral somatoparaphrenia after right hemisphere stroke: a case description Cortex 31: 173–182
Head H 1920 Studies in neurology. Oxford University Press, Oxford
Hécaen H 1962 Clinical symptomatology in right and left hemispheric lesions. In: Mountcastle V B (ed) Interhemispheric relations and cerebral dominance. Johns Hopkins Press, Baltimore, ch 10
Hécaen H 1969 Aphasic, apraxic and agnosic syndromes in right and left hemisphere lesions. In: Vinken P J, Bruyn G W (eds) Handbook of clinical neurology. North-Holland, Amsterdam, vol 4, ch 15
Hécaen H, Ajuriaguerra J de 1952 Méconnaissances et hallucinations corporelles. Masson, Paris
Hécaen H, Angelergues R 1961 Etude anatomo-clinique de 280 cas de lésions rétro-rolandiques unilatérales des hémisphères cérébraux. Encephale 6: 533–562
Hécaen H, Angelergues R 1963 La cécité psychique. Masson, Paris
Hécaen H, Ajuriaguerra J de, Massonet J 1951 Les troubles visuo-constructifs par lésion pariéto-occipitale droite. Encephale 40: 122–179
Hécaen H, Penfield W, Bertrand C, Malmo R 1956 The syndrome of apractognosia due to lesions of the minor cerebral hemisphere. Archives of Neurology and Psychiatry 75: 400–434
Hécaen H, Angelergues R, Houillier S 1961 Les variétés cliniques des acalculies au cours des lésions rétrorolandiques: aproche statistique du problème. Revue Neurologique 105: 85–103
Hécaen H, Tzortzis C, Rondot P 1980 Loss of topographic memory with learning deficits. Cortex 16: 525–542
Heilman K M, Valenstein E 1972a Auditory neglect in man. Archives of Neurology 26: 32–35
Heilman K M, Valenstein E 1972b Frontal lobe neglect in man. Neurology 22: 660–664
Heilman K M, Valenstein E 1979 Mechanisms underlying hemispatial neglect. Annals of Neurology 5: 166–170
Heilman K M, Van Den Abell T 1980 Right hemispheric dominance for attention: the mechanism underlying hemispheric asymmetries of inattention (neglect). Neurology 30: 327–330
Heilman K M, Watson R T 1977 The neglect syndrome – a unilateral defect of the orienting response. In: Harnad S et al (eds) Lateralization in the nervous system. Academic Press, New York, pp 285–302
Heilman K M, Watson R T, Valenstein E, Damasio A R 1983 Localization of lesions in neglect. In: Kertesz A (ed) Localization in neuropsychology. Academic Press, New York, pp 471–492
Heilman K M, Valenstein E, Watson A T 1985 The neglect syndrome. In: Vinken P J, Bruyn G V, Klawans H L (eds) Handbook of clinical neurology. Elsevier, Amsterdam
Heilman K M, Watson R T, Valenstein E 1993 Neglect and related disorders. In: Heilman K M, Valenstein E (eds) Clinical neuropsychology, 3rd edn. Oxford University Press, New York, ch 10
Heimburger R F, Demeyer W, Reitan R M 1964 Implication of Gerstmann's syndrome. Journal of Neurology, Neurosurgery and Psychiatry 27: 52–57
Hier D B, Davis K R, Richardson E P 1977 Hypertensive putaminal haemorrhage. Annals of Neurology 1: 152–159
Hier D B, Mondlock J, Caplan L R 1983a Behavioral abnormalities after right hemisphere stroke. Neurology 33: 337–340
Hier D B, Mondlock J, Caplan L R 1983b Recovery of behavioral abnormalities after right hemisphere stroke. Neurology 33: 345–350
Hilgard E R 1956 Theories of learning, 2nd edn. Appleton-Century-Crofts, New York, pp 185–222
Holmes G 1918 Disturbances of visual orientation. British Journal of Ophthalmology 2: 449–469

Holmes G 1927 Disorders of sensation produced by cortical lesions. Brain 49: 413–428
Hublet C, Demeurisse G 1992 Pure topographical disorientation due to a deep seated lesion with cortical remote effects. Cortex 28: 123–128
Hurwitz L J, Adams G F 1972 Rehabilitation of hemiplegia: indices of assessment and prognosis. British Medical Journal 1: 94–98
Incisa della Rocchetta A, Cipolotti L, Warrington E K 1996 Topographical disorientation: selective impairment of locomotor space? Cortex 32: 727–735
Ishiai S, Seki K, Koyama Y, Izumi Y 1997 Disappearance of unilateral spatial neglect following a simple instruction. Journal of Neurology, Neurosurgery and Psychiatry 63: 23–27
Ishii K, Kita Y, Nagura H, Bandoh M, Yamanouchi H 1992 A case report of cerebral achromatopsia with bilateral occipital lesion. Rinsho Shinkeigaku 32: 293–298
Jackson J H 1864, 1874, 1876 See Taylor J (ed) Selected writings of John Hughlings Jackson. Basic Books, New York, 1958
Karnath H O, Schenkel P, Fischer B 1991 Trunk orientation as the determining factor of the 'contralateral' deficit in the neglect syndrome and as the physical anchor of the internal representation of body orientation in space. Brain 114: 1997–2014
Kinsbourne M, Warrington E K 1962 A study of finger agnosia. Brain 85: 47–66
Kleist K 1934 Gehirnpathologie. Barth, Leipzig
Kotler Cope S, Camp C J 1995 Anosognosia in Alzheimer disease. Alzheimer Disease and Associated Disorders 9: 52–56
Kotzmann M 1972 Tactile discrimination of three-dimensional form in brain-damaged patients. Unpublished Masters thesis, University of Melbourne.
Kroll M B, Stolbun D 1933 Was ist konstructive Apraxie. Zeitschrift für die gesamte Neurologie und Psychiatrie 148: 142–158
Kumar A, Mollison L 1993 Cerebral infarction following thoracic herpes zoster. Australasian Journal of Dermatology 34: 113–114
Ladavas E, Umilta C, Ziani P, Brogi A, Minarini M 1993 The role of right side objects in left side neglect: a dissociation between perceptual and directional motor neglect. Neuropsychologia 31: 761–773
Landis T, Cummings J L, Benson D F, Palmer P E 1986 Loss of topographic familiarity. Archives of Neurology 43: 132–136
Laplane D, Degos J D 1983 Motor neglect. Journal of Neurology, Neurosurgery and Psychiatry 46: 152–158
Lawson I R 1962 Visual-spatial neglect in lesions of the right cerebral hemisphere: a study in recovery. Neurology 12: 23–33
Le Doux J E, Wilson D H, Gazzaniga M S 1977 Manipulo-spatial aspects of cerebral lateralization: Clues to the origin of lateralization. Neuropsychologia 15: 743–750
Le Doux J E, Wilson D H, Gazzaniga M S 1978 Block design performance following callosal sectioning. Archives of Neurology 35: 506–508
Leicester J, Sidman M, Stoddard L T, Mohr J P 1969 Some determinants of visual neglect. Journal of Neurology, Neurosurgery, and Psychiatry 32: 580–587
Levinthal C F 1990 Introduction to physiology, 3rd edn. Prentice-Hall, Englewood Cliffs, New Jersey
Lhermitte J 1942 De l'image corporelle. Revue Neurologique 74: 20–38
Lhermitte J 1952 L'image corporelle en neurologie. Schweizer Archiv für Neurologie und Psychiatrie 9: 213–223
Lhermitte J, Trelles J O 1933 Sur l'apraxie pure constructive. Encephale 28: 413–444
Lopez O L, Becker J T, Somsak D, Dew M A, DeKosky S T 1994 Awareness of cognitive deficits and anosognosia in probable Alzheimer's disease. European Neurology 34: 277–282
Luria A R 1973 The working brain. Allen Lane, The Penguin Press, London
Luria A R, Tsvetkova L D 1964 The programming of constructive activity in local brain injuries. Neuropsychologia 2: 95–108
Mack J L, Levine R N 1981 The basis of visual constructional disability in patients with unilateral cerebral lesions. Cortex 17: 515–532
Maeshima S, Funahashi K, Ogura M, Iyakura T, Komai N 1994 Unilateral spatial neglect due to right frontal haematoma. Journal of Neurology, Neurosurgery and Psychiatry 57: 89–93
Maguire E A, Burke T, Phillips J, Staunton H 1996 Topographical disorientation following unilateral temporal lobe lesions in man. Neuropsychologia 34: 993–1001

Marie P, Behague P 1919 Syndrome de désorientation dans l'espace consécutif aux plaies profondes du lobe frontal. Revue Neurologique 26: 1–14

Marie P, Bouttier H, van Bogaert L 1924 Sur un cas de tumeur préfrontale droite. Troubles de l'orientation dans l'espace. Revue Neurologique 31: 209–221

Marquardsen J 1969 The natural history of acute cerebrovascular disease: a retrospective study of 79 patients. Acta Neurologica Scandinavica 38: 1–192

Maugiere F, Isnard J 1995 Tactile agnosia and dysfunction of the primary somatosensory area. Data of the study by somatosensory evoked potentials in patients with deficits of tactile object recognition. Revue Neurologique 151: 518–527

Mayer-Gross W 1935 The question of visual impairment in constructional apraxia. Proceedings of the Royal Society of Medicine 29: 1396–1400

Mazzoni M, Del Torto E, Vista M, Moretti P 1993 Transient topographical amnesia: a case report. Italian Journal of Neurological Sciences 14: 633–636

McFie J, Zangwill O L 1960 Visual-constructive disabilities associated with lesions of the left cerebral hemisphere. Brain 83: 243–260

McFie J, Piercy M F, Zangwill O L 1950 Visual spatial agnosia associated with lesions of the right cerebral hemisphere. Brain 73: 167–190

Meador K J, Loring D W, Lee G P et al 1988 Right cerebral specialization for tactile attention as evidenced by intracarotid sodium amytal. Neurology 38: 1763–1766

Michon A, Deweer B, Pillon B, Agid Y, Dubois B 1994 Relation of anosognosia to frontal lobe dysfunction in Alzheimer's disease. Journal of Neurology, Neurosurgery and Psychiatry 57: 805–809

Miller E 1972 Clinical neuropsychology. Penguin Books, Harmondsworth, Middlesex

Milner B 1965 Visually-guided maze learning in man: effects of bilateral hippocampal, bilateral frontal and unilateral cerebral lesions. Neuropsychologia 3: 317–338

Morris H H, Lüders H, Lesser R P, Dinner D S, Hahn J 1984 Transient neuropsychological abnormalities (including Gerstmann's syndrome) during cortical stimulation. Neurology 34: 877–883

Nathanson M, Bergman P S, Gordon G G 1952 Denial of illness. Archives of Neurology and Psychiatry 68: 380–387

Newcombe F 1969 Missile wounds of the brain. Oxford University Press, Oxford

Nielsen H 1975 Is constructional apraxia primarily an interhemisphere disconnection syndrome? Scandinavian Journal of Psychology 16: 113–124

Obi T, Bando M, Takeda K, Sakuta M 1992 A case of topographical disturbance following a left medial parieto-occipital infarction. Rinsho Shinkeigaku 32: 426–429

Ogden J A 1985 Anterior-posterior interhemispheric differences in the loci of lesions producing visual hemineglect. Brain and Cognition 4: 59–75

Osterrieth P A 1944 Le test de copie d'une figure complexe. Archives de Psychologie 30: 206–353

Oxbury J M, Campbell D C, Oxbury S M 1974 Unilateral spatial neglect and impairments of spatial analysis and visual perception. Brain 97: 551–564

Pallis CA 1955 Impaired identification for faces and places with agnosia for colours. Journal of Neurology, Neurosurgery and Psychiatry 18: 218–224

Paterson A, Zangwill O L 1944 Disorders of visual space perception associated with lesions of the right cerebral hemisphere. Brain 67: 331–358

Paterson A, Zangwill O L 1945 A case of topographical disorientation associated with a unilateral cerebral lesion. Brain 68: 188–212

Petrovici I N 1972 Schlafenlappen und Apraxie. Fortschritte der Neurologie und Psychiatrie 40: 656–672

Piaget J 1969 The mechanisms of perception. Routledge and Kegan Paul, London

Piercy M F, Smyth V 1962 Right hemisphere dominance for certain non-verbal intellectual skills. Brain 85: 775–790

Piercy M, Hécaen H, Ajuriaguerra J de 1960 Constructional apraxia associated with unilateral cerebral lesions – left and right sided cases compared. Brain 83: 225–242

Poeck K, Orgass B 1966 Gerstmann's syndrome and aphasia. Cortex 2: 421–437

Poeck K, Orgass B 1967 Uber Störungen der Recht-links Orientierung. Nervenarzt 38: 285–291

Pollack F 1938 Zur Pathologie und Klinik der Orientierung. Schweizer Archiv für Neurologie und Psychiatrie 42: 141–164

Poppelreuter W 1923 Zur Psychologie und Pathologie der optischen Wahrnemung. Zeitschrift für die gesamte Neurologie und Psychiatrie 83: 26–152
Ratcliff G, Newcombe F 1973 Spatial orientation in man: effects of left, right, and bilateral posterior lesions. Journal of Neurology, Neurosurgery and Psychiatry 3: 448–454
Reed B R, Jagust W J, Coulter L 1993 Anosognosia in Alzheimer's disease: relation to depression, cognitive function, and cerebral perfusion. Journal of Clinical and Experimental Neuropsychology 15: 231–244
Reed C L, Caselli R J 1994 The nature of tactile agnosia: a case study. Neuropsychologia 32: 527–539
Reitan R M, Davison L A (eds) 1974 Clinical neuropsychology: current status and applications. Wiley, New York
Rey A 1941 L'examen psychologique. Archives de Psychologie 28: 112–164
Rey A 1959 Le test de copie de figure complexe. Editions Centre de Psychologie Appliquée, Paris
Riddoch G 1935 Visual disorientation in homonymous half-fields. Brain 58: 376–382
Roeltgen D P, Sevush S, Heilman K M 1983 Pure Gerstmann's syndrome from a focal lesion. Archives of Neurology 40: 46–47
Rubens A B 1985 Caloric stimulation and unilateral visual neglect. Neurology 35: 1019–1024
Russell E W, Neuringer C, Goldstein G 1970 Assessment of brain damage: a neuropsychological key approach. Wiley, New York
Scotti G 1968 La perdita della memoria topografica: descrizione di un caso. Sistema Nervoso 20: 352–361
Seki K, Ishiai S 1996 Diverse patterns of performance in copying and severity of spatial neglect. Journal of Neurology 243: 1–8
Semmes J 1965 A non-tactual factor in astereognosis. Neuropsychologia 3: 295–315
Semmes J 1968 Hemispheric specialization: a possible clue to mechanism. Neuropsychologia 6: 11–26
Semmes J, Weinstein S, Ghent L, Teuber H L 1954 Performance on complex tactual tasks after brain injury to man: analyses by locus of lesion. American Journal of Psychology 7: 220–240
Semmes J, Weinstein S, Ghent L, Teuber H L 1955 Spatial orientation in man after cerebral injury – 1: Analysis by locus of lesion. Journal of Psychology 39: 227–244
Semmes J, Weinstein S, Ghent L, Teuber H L 1960 Somatosensory changes after penetrating brain wounds in man. Harvard University Press, Cambridge, Massachusetts
Semmes J, Weinstein S, Ghent L, Teuber H L 1963 Correlate of impaired orientation in personal and extra-personal space. Brain 86: 747–772
Shallice T, Warrington E K 1970 Independent functioning of verbal memory stores: a neuropsychological study. Quarterly Journal of Experimental Psychology 22: 261–273
Shallice T, Warrington E K 1974 The dissociation between short-term retention of meaningful sounds and verbal material. Neuropsychologia 12: 553–555
Simon E S, Hegarty A M, Mehler M F 1995 Hemispatial and directional performance biases in motor neglect. Neurology 45: 525–531
Starkstein S E, Vazquez S, Migliorelli R, Teson A, Sabe L, Leiguarda R 1995 A single-photon emission computed tomographic study of anosognosia in Alzheimer's disease. Archives of Neurology 52: 415–420
Stone S P, Halligan P W, Greenwood R J 1993 The incidence of neglect phenomena and related disorders in patients with an acute right or left hemisphere stroke. Age and Ageing 22: 46–52
Strauss H 1924 Uber Konstruktive Apraxie. Monatsschrift für Psychiatrie und Neurologie 63: 739–748
Strub R L, Geschwind N 1983 Localization in Gerstmann syndrome. In: Kertesz A (ed) Localization in neuropsychology. Academic Press, New York, pp 295–321
Sukumar S, Ferguson G C 1996 Gerstmann's syndrome. Postgraduate Medical Journal 72: 314
Takayama Y, Sugishita M, Akiguchi I, Kimura A 1994 Isolated acalculia due to left parietal lesion. Archives of Neurology 51: 286–291
Tegnér R, Levander M 1991 Through a looking glass: a new technique to demonstrate directional hypokinesia in unilateral neglect. Brain 114: 1943–1951
Teuber H L 1950 Neuropsychology. In: Harrower M R (ed) Recent advances in diagnostic psychological testing. Thomas, Springfield, Illinois, ch 2

Teuber H-L 1965a Preface: disorders of higher tactile and visual functions. Neuropsychologia. 3: 287–294
Teuber H-L 1965b Postscript: some needed revisions of the clinical views of agnosia. Neuropsychologia 3: 371–378
Teuber H-L, Weinstein S 1954 Performance on a formboard task after penetrating brain injury. Journal of Psychology 38: 177–190
Teuber H-L, Battersby W S, Bender M B 1951 Performance of complex visual tasks after cerebral lesions. Journal of Nervous and Mental Disease 114: 413–429
Tolman E C 1948 Cognitive maps in rats and men. Psychological Review 55: 189–208
Tranel D 1991 What has been rediscovered in "rediscovering tactile agnosia"? Mayo Clinic Proceedings 66: 210–214
Triggs W J, Gold M, Gerstle G, Heilman K M 1994 Motor neglect associated with a discrete parietal lesion. Neurology 44: 1164–1166
Umilta C 1995 Domain-specific forms of neglect. Journal of Clinical and Experimental Neuropsychology 17: 209–219
Valenstein E, Heilman K M 1981 Unilateral hypokinesia and motor extinction. Neurology 31: 445–448
Vallar G, Sandroni P, Rusconi M L, Barbieri S 1991 Hemianopia, hemianesthesia, and spatial neglect: a study with evoked potentials. Neurology 41: 1918–1922
Vallar G, Antonucci G, Guariglia C, Pizzamiglio L 1993 Deficit of position sense, unilateral neglect, and optokinetic stimulation. Neuropsychologia 31: 1191–1200
Vallar G, Papagno C, Rusconi M L, Bisiach E 1995 Vestibular stimulation, spatial hemineglect and dysphasia. Selective effects? Cortex 31: 589–593
Villardita C 1987 Tactile exploration of space and visual neglect in brain-damaged patients. Journal of Neurology 234: 292–297
Warrington E 1969 Constructional apraxia. In: Vinken P J, Bruyn G W (eds) Handbook of clinical neurology. North-Holland, Amsterdam, vol 4, ch 4
Warrington E K 1971 Neurological disorders of memory. British Medical Bulletin 3: 243–247
Warrington E K 1973 Neurological deficits. In: Mittler P (ed) The psychological assessment of mental and physical handicaps. Tavistock Publications, London, ch 9
Warrington E K, Baddeley A D 1974 Amnesia and memory for visual location. Neuropsychologia 12: 257–263
Warrington E K, Rabin P 1970 Perceptual matching in patients with cerebral lesions. Neuropsychologia 8: 475–487
Warrington E K, Shallice T 1969 The selective impairment of auditory verbal short-term memory. Brain 92: 885–896
Warrington E K, Shallice T 1972 Neuropsychological evidence of visual storage in short-term memory tasks. Quarterly Journal of Experimental Psychology 24: 30–40
Warrington E K, Taylor A M 1973 The contribution of the right parietal lobe to object recognition. Cortex 9: 152–164
Warrington E K, Weiskrantz L 1972 An analysis of short-term and long-term memory defects in man. In: Deutsch J A (ed) The physiological basis of memory. Academic Press, New York, pp 365–395
Warrington E K, James M, Kinsbourne M 1966 Drawing disability in relation to laterality of cerebral lesion. Brain 89: 53–82
Warrington E K, Logue V, Pratt R T C 1971 The anatomical localization of selective impairment of auditory short-term memory. Neuropsychologia 9: 377–387
Watson R T, Heilman K M 1979 Thalamic neglect. Neurology 29: 90–94
Wechsler D 1958 The measurement and appraisal of adult intelligence, 4th edn. Williams and Wilkins, New York
Weinstein S, Semmes J, Ghent L, Teuber H L 1956 Spatial orientation in man after cerebral injury. 11. Analysis according to concomitant defects. Journal of Psychology 42: 249–263
Weintraub B, Mesulam M-M 1987 Right cerebral dominance in spatial attention. Archives of Neurology 44: 621–625
Weintraub B, Mesulam M-M 1988 Visual hemispatial inattention: stimulus parameters and exploratory strategies. Journal of Neurology, Neurosurgery and Psychiatry 51: 1481–1488
Whiteley A M, Warrington E K 1978 Selective impairment of topographical memory. Journal of Neurology, Neurosurgery and Psychiatry 41: 575–578
Whitty C W M, Newcombe F 1973 R C Oldfield's study of visual and topographic

disturbances in a right occipito-parietal lesion of 30 years duration. Neuropsychologia 11: 471–475

Wolff H G 1962 Discussion of Teuber's paper. In: Mountcastle V B (ed) Interhemispheric relations and cerebral dominance. Johns Hopkins Press, Baltimore

Wyke M 1966 Postural arm-drift associated with brain lesions in man. Archives of Neurology 15: 329–334

Zarranz J J, Lasa A, Fernandez M et al 1995 Posterior cortical atrophy with progressive visual agnosia. Neurologia 10: 119–126

7

The occipital lobes

ANATOMICAL FEATURES

The occipital lobes form the most posterior portions of the cerebral hemispheres. On the inner or medial aspects there is a natural line of demarcation, called the parieto-occipital fissure. On the lateral or convex surfaces there are no such gross landmarks and the occipital lobe merges into the parietal lobe above and the temporal lobe below (Figs 7.1 and 7.2).

Following the discovery of the fact that the cerebral cortex varied in the cellular composition of its layers from place to place in the hemisphere, numerous attempts were made to map out regions of the cortex having similar distinctive structure. Such studies are termed *cytoarchitecture*, literally the architecture of the cells. One of the best known of such maps is that of Brodmann (1909) (Fig. 7.3). This difference in structure suggested difference in function and, while such a relationship has not been fully established for all areas, it appears to be largely true in the occipital region.

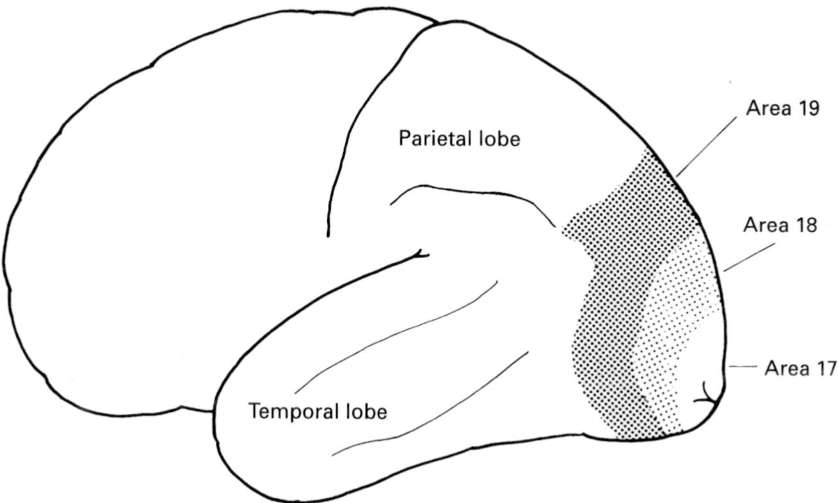

Fig. 7.1 Occipital lobe. Lateral view.

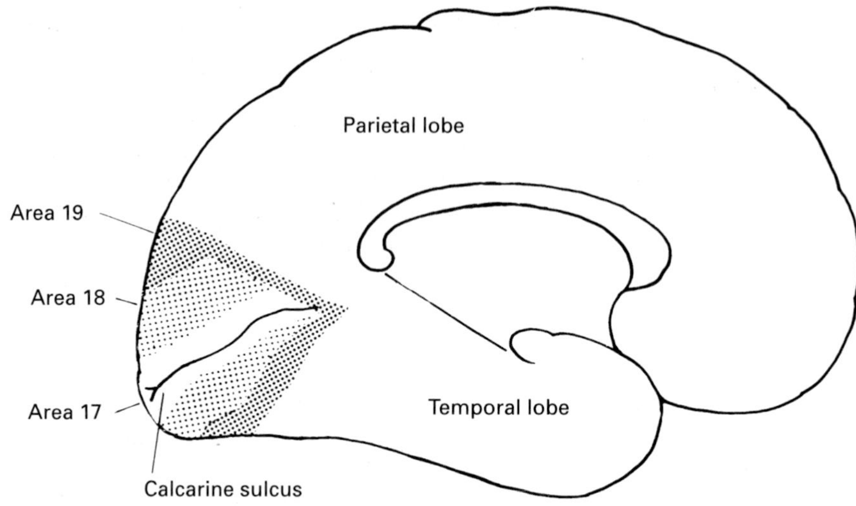

Fig. 7.2 Occipital lobe. Medial view.

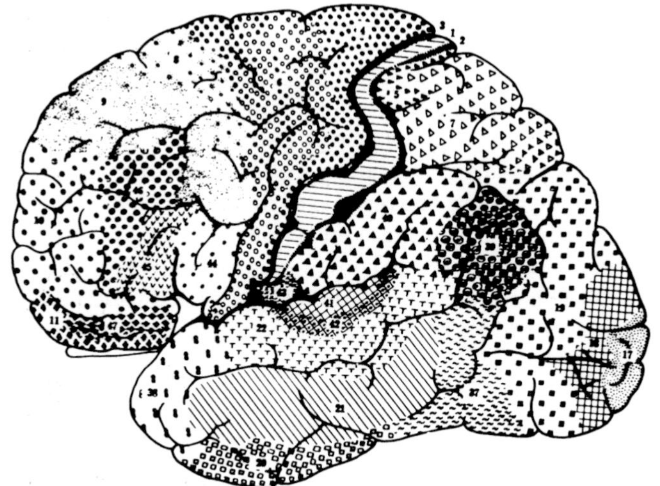

Fig. 7.3 Brodmann's cytoarchitectural map.

Brodmann's method divided each occipital lobe into three areas having different cellular composition (areas 17, 18 and 19). Area 17 borders on the calcarine fissure, which is largely on the medial aspect of the hemisphere, and also covers the posterior pole of the hemisphere. This area is known as the striate area because of the striped appearance when it is sectioned. It is in this area that the neural fibres relaying information from the visual receptors in the retina reach their termination. Area 17 is the primary visual cortex. It is surrounded by area 18, the parastriate region, which in turn is surrounded by area 19, the peristriate region which borders on the parietal and temporal lobes (Figs 7.1 and 7.2).

Area 18 is a secondary sensory area believed to be concerned with the elaboration and synthesis of visual information. This area has numerous interhemispheric or commissural fibre connections with the corresponding area in the other hemisphere.

Area 19 possesses abundant connections with other regions of the hemispheres so that it appears to be chiefly involved in the integration of visual information with the information gathered by the auditory and other sense systems, and it unites visual information with the brain systems subserving speech and other executive functions. It is also concerned, along with areas in the temporal lobes already discussed, with visual memory.

Visual pathways

Knowledge of the basic anatomy of the visual pathways allows an understanding of the diagnostic significance of certain common defects of vision brought about by lesions along the pathways from the eye to the visual cortex. Such lesions will cause the patient to have difficulties with a number of psychological test measures, and an awareness of the nature of the visual defect will help in making correct inferences about the patient's performance on visuoperceptive tasks.

The lens of each eye focuses the stimulation from the outer part of each eye's visual field on to the inner half of each retina, while stimulation arising in the inner half of the visual fields goes to the outer half of each retina. The terms 'temporal' and 'nasal' have often been used to refer to this division of the half-fields of each eye and are included in Figure 7.4 so that the reader may understand texts where these terms occur, but, in what follows, the terms 'left (or

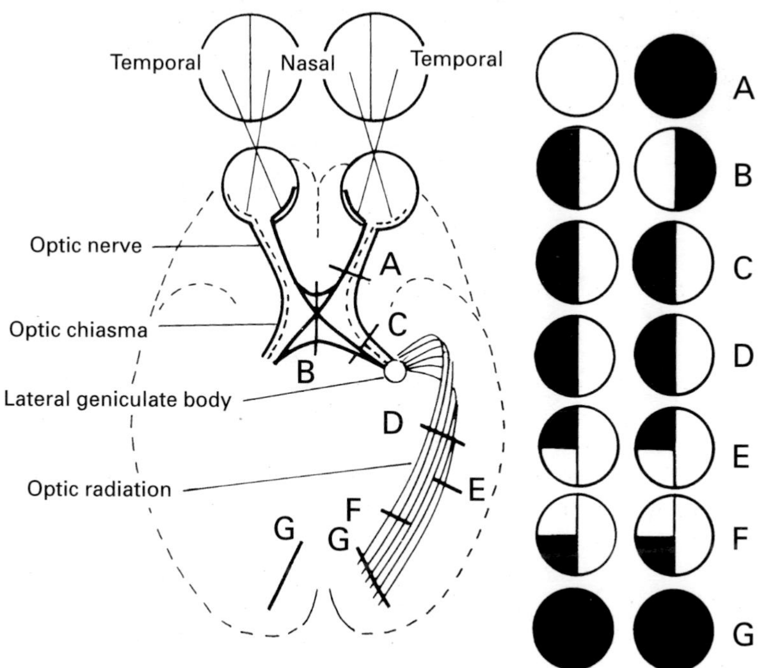

Fig. 7.4 The visual pathways with related field defects.

right) halves of the visual field' will be used since they are less ambiguous in their reference than the terms 'temporal' and 'nasal'.

The fibres which relay information from the retina are gathered together in the optic nerve which travels back to join its partner in the optic chiasma. Here the fibres from the inner half of each retina cross over the midline and go on to enter the contralateral hemisphere while the fibres from the outer halves of each retina enter the hemisphere on the same side as the eye receiving the information. This means that each eye projects visual information to each hemisphere. Furthermore, there is a good deal of overlap between the visual fields of the two eyes so that most of the information (i.e. that seen by the two eyes in common) is analysed by both hemispheres (Fig. 7.5).

From the optic chiasma the visual pathways extend backward to the lateral geniculate bodies. These bodies can be considered as special subdivisions of the thalamus. They relay the visual information to the visual cortex, while the neighbouring structures, the medial geniculate bodies, relay auditory information to the primary projection area for audition situated in the temporal lobes.

The final part of the optic pathway is known as the optic radiation or geniculocalcarine tract. From the geniculate bodies the pathway passes through an area called the temporal isthmus; then its fibres fan out to cover the upper and outer portions of the lateral ventricles before passing to the calcarine cortex.

A lesion in the temporal isthmus forms a good example of the widespread effects that a small lesion may have if it is strategically placed (Ch. 1). Not only does a small lesion in this location lead to an interruption of the visual pathways and hence to a visual field defect, but it also leads to somatosensory and motor changes since fibre pathways related to these functional systems are in close contiguity in this region (Nielsen & Friedman 1942). Moreover, because of the asymmetry of function between the two hemispheres of the brain (see Ch. 8), two clinical syndromes are recognizable according to whether the left or

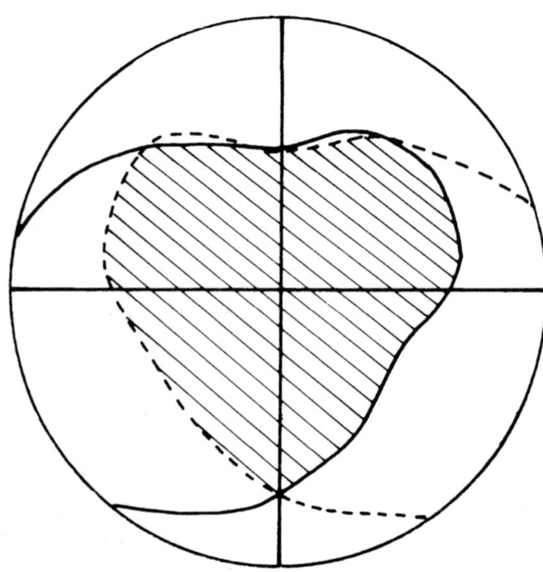

Fig. 7.5 Visual fields with areas of overlap.

right isthmus is damaged. With involvement of the left (dominant) side severe aphasia may accompany the above symptoms, while damage to the right (non-dominant) side may produce anosognosia or delusions of the body schema as well as the visual, motor and sensory disturbances.

Visual field defects. Figure 7.4 represents the effect of lesions interrupting the visual pathways at various points. At A, a lesion produces blindness in the right eye. At B, a lesion will produce a loss in the left half of the left visual field and the right half of the right visual field (a bitemporal hemianopia). At C, a lesion in the right optic tract will produce a loss in the left half of the visual field of each eye (an homonymous hemianopia). At D in the optic radiation, complete lesions also give rise to homonymous hemianopia, while smaller lesions in the radiation, for example at E in the temporal lobe, may cause loss only in the upper homonymous quadrants (quandrantanopia), while lesions in the parietal lobe (at F) may cause visual defects only in the lower quadrants. Bilateral lesions of the occipital lobe (G1 and G2) produce bilateral homonymous hemianopia or cerebral blindness.

Since it is possible that visual field defects may not be readily apparent due to the capacity for adjustment to the defect which many patients show, they may sometimes be overlooked. Patients with homonymous hemianopia affecting the right halves of their visual fields characteristically have difficulty when asked to read normal print since the habitual scanning pattern is from left to right, while those with left-sided hemianopia have difficulty with reading for a different reason. Here patients have difficulty in picking up the correct line as their eyes return to the left to begin scanning the next line. They may begin on a line above or below the appropriate one.

Homonymous hemianopia is an unequivocal sign of a unilateral hemispheric lesion. Some would regard hemianopia as the *only* reliable sign of occipital lobe disease (Cogan 1966, Gloning et al 1968), since more subtle disturbances of visual perception tend to be associated with lesions spreading into neighbouring regions.

Less regular field defects result from partial lesions of the visual cortex or optic radiation, such as those produced by penetrating missile wounds in wartime. The blind area in these cases is known as a scotoma and, particularly if small, may even pass unnoticed by the patient in much the same way as the normal or physiological blind spot in each eye becomes apparent only when the eye is fixated and visual targets are arranged so that they project into the retinal region of the head of the optic nerve where visual receptors are absent.

These traumatically produced lesions of the visual regions have been extensively studied by Teuber and his colleagues (Teuber et al 1960).

The borders of scotomata are usually ill-defined and vary with the attitude and attention of the patient and with the particular methods employed in testing.

Examination of the visual fields. The visual fields are routinely checked in the standard neurological examination. The commonly used method of clinical examination is termed confrontation. The patient faces the examiner and, with one eye shielded, fixates directly into the examiner's eye while the latter checks various parts of the visual field by asking the subject to detect the presence or movement of the visual target, usually the examiner's fingers. This method readily picks out the more obvious field defects. More careful systematic examination is made with a tangent screen or retinal perimeter. These methods are described in standard textbooks of medicine and experimental psychology. Two further procedures may be of value.

1. Since it appears that, in cases of tumour, field defects for coloured test objects invariably appear before those for black and white objects (Bender & Kanzer 1941), Walsh and Hoyt (1969) have suggested that coloured targets be routinely employed. Such an examination is simple enough to be included in a small group of 'neurological' tests employed by the neuropsychologist, and may detect some lesions early in their development.
2. Flicker perimetry may also be sensitive to early lowering of visual efficiency, though such testing is time consuming and needs special facilities not normally available in neuropsychological clinics. The method and its implications for localizing the site of brain damage were described by Parsons and Huse (1958).

CEREBRAL BLINDNESS

One of the most common causes of hemianopic defects is cerebral ischaemia produced by narrowing or occlusion of the posterior cerebral artery. The loss of vision for the contralateral half-field is a prominent symptom of a failure of the vertebrobasilar artery system to provide an adequate blood supply to the posterior regions of one cerebrum (Siekert & Millikan 1955). Where the occipital lobes are affected on both sides a bilateral homonymous hemianopia or complete blindness results.

This blindness has often been termed cortical blindness but the term 'cerebral' is to be preferred since the underlying white matter is usually involved as well as the cortex. The blindness is often accompanied by other neurological signs and, even when the disorder appears to be clinically pure, careful examination will often reveal associated disorders. Since it is most often vascular in origin, the blindness may follow a period of confusion or even unconsciousness because of the 'vascular accident', and testing of the patient may be rendered difficult because of residual confusion. On occasion, there may be an interval of days or weeks between the onset of delirium and visual and neurological symptoms (Verslegers et al 1991). In patients with signs of vertebrobasilar insufficiency even the diagnostic procedure of arteriography may precipitate cerebral blindness (Silverman et al 1961). In our experience this is accompanied on occasions by an amnesic syndrome of marked severity, probably because of bilateral ischaemia of the medial temporal regions supplied by the posterior cerebral arteries.

In patients who survive the precipitating vascular episode, recovery of at least some visual function appears to be the rule (Silverman et al 1961, Gloning et al 1968). This recovery is so frequent that it has led some workers to doubt the validity of earlier reports of lasting cerebral blindness. Of the 32 surviving cases of cerebral blindness in Gloning, Gloning and Hoff's very large series of occipital lobe cases, all recovered some visual function though many stopped short of full recovery. Recovery of the various components of visual experience shows marked variation from case to case. Warrington (1984) described five patients recovered from the acute stage of cerebral blindness who showed differing patterns of dissociation between the fundamental attributes of visual acuity, spatial location, colour and form perception. Such dissociations had been reported in the early literature (e.g. Holmes 1918).

Restitution of visual function appears to take place in a typical order. Firstly, the sensation of darkness becomes punctuated with elementary visual sensations or photisms. Next, the visual field becomes light but no form perception is possible. This is followed by the appreciation of primitive movement, i.e. the appreciation that the object is moving, or has moved, but not the direction or speed. Contours gradually emerge but are vague and unstable. Colour experience is the last to return. Even at this stage the visual processes may readily fatigue so that the percept appears to blur after some time (*asthenopia*). Some patients go on to recover their normal vision but others remain fixed at a stage of partial recovery.

'Blindsight'

Formerly it was believed that destruction of the optic radiation resulted in a total loss of vision in the related parts (or all) of the visual field. This is true if the measure used is the subject's report of the presence or absence of a target in the affected region. However, as early as 1917 Riddoch noted that some patients retained some residual visual function, especially for movement, in the 'blind' area and later work confirmed the capacity of some individuals to detect and localize stimuli within the blind field (Pöppel et al 1973, Weiskrantz et al 1974, Perenin & Jeannerod 1978, Ross Russell & Bharucha 1984). Thus, blindsight 'refers to those subjects who state that they are unaware of the visual stimuli, even when performing discriminations at high levels of proficiency' (Weiskrantz 1990). Such residual visual capacity may be improved by experience or practice (Zihl 1980), suggesting a possible role for rehabilitation. Individuals have also shown the capacity in a forced choice situation to discriminate between wavelengths, i.e. to show colour discrimination, although, once again, the process takes place without awareness (Stoerig & Cowey 1992, Brent et al 1994). As in many areas of function, the detection of deficits may vary with the different task paradigms employed (Corbetta et al 1990). Some writers have assumed that the detection processes are mediated by retinal connections with the brain stem which have been shown to subserve perceptual as well as ocular reflexes in mammals. The anatomical sources of 'blindsight' are still being debated (Barinaga 1992, Stoerig 1993, Weiskrantz 1990, 1993).

The fact that blindsight phenomena also occur in normal subjects as well as the brain damaged (Meeres & Graves 1990, Kolb & Braun 1995) raises fundamental neuropsychological questions about the basis of implicit versus explicit knowledge, and study of such dissociations is of importance for neuropsychological theories of consciousness (Schacter 1992, Farah 1994, Natsoulas 1997). Weiskrantz et al (1995) suggest that it may be possible by brain imaging to determine whether there are structures specifically devoted to conscious perception by comparing performances in the same subject on the same task where the subject does or does not show awareness. The topic is reviewed by Weiskrantz (1996).

Denial of blindness (Anton's syndrome)

It is characteristic of many, though not all, cases of cerebral blindness that the patient appears indifferent to, fails to recognize or even denies the existence of the defect. Post-mortem findings in Anton's case of 1899 showed bilateral softening of the brain in the parieto-occipital regions and this pioneer considered the disconnection of the visual system from other parts of the brain to be the cause of the denial. While there is often evidence of posterior damage, cases showing damage to primary visual cortex alone are rare. One such case (Goldenberg et al 1995) had preserved visual imagery which the authors argue might be aroused by perceptions in other senses thus helping to explain her 'pretended visual experiences'. Denial may also occur for incomplete blindness such as hemianopic defects and it is possible that one explanation may serve to explain both phenomena. There is a strong association between Anton's syndrome and the tendency to confabulate. Even the patient recovering from cerebral blindness who has not explicitly denied the defect may admit to visual difficulties 'but does so almost casually, or lightheartedly, as though it were something not very important' (Critchley 1979, p. 157). Some of these patients may be readily coerced into describing objects they have failed to identify, a condition termed 'confabulatory pseudo-recognition' by Critchley (1979). One of our own patients confidently described my appearance (K.W.) while facing me but was incorrect about every feature.

Many patients with Anton's syndrome also have severe memory disorders because of the effect of the lesion on inferomedial temporal lobe structures. Occasionally, Anton's syndrome is seen with blindness caused by lesions in the anterior visual system, usually in association with confusion and widespread cognitive dysfunction. One recent anterior case without such changes, though with distinctive frontal features, showed a marked tendency to confabulate together with a generalized anosognosia (McDaniel & McDaniel 1991). The mechanism of denial may differ according to the location of the lesion.

While denial may be verbally explicit, some of the patients examined by Gloning and his colleagues admitted their blindness while they were actually under examination, but shortly after again denied visual loss. This meant that patients might invent fictions such as 'It is night now and there is no light in this room' or 'I am in a dark cellar' (Gloning et al 1968, p. 13). Though there was a tendency for all patients to confabulate, a true Korsakoff's syndrome was rare.

Denial occurs with other disorders such as hemiplegia (*Babinski's syndrome*) and we have also noted it on occasions after prefrontal lobotomy where the patient confabulates or rationalizes about the presence of the operative scars. Numerous psychological explanations have been put forward to explain this denial of illness or disability.

Nathanson, Bergman and Gordon (1952) reported 28 cases of denial of hemiplegia in a series of 100 cases. The denial occurred with lesions in either hemisphere, though more frequently with right hemisphere involvement. These authors considered that the denial of illness closely resembled the mechanism of rationalization, or explaining away a defect, found in normal subjects. The difference appeared to be one of degree. In a similar vein, Guthrie and Grossman (1952) pointed to the prior use of denial as a defence mechanism in their two neurological subjects, while the denial of operation was considered by Paganini and Zlotlow (1960) to be a continuation of the use of this defence by their schizophrenic subjects. A low level of intellectual function also seems to be related to the production of denial (Fryer & Rich 1960).

One difficulty in using these explanations for Anton's syndrome lies in the fact that, in some cases where blindness and hemiplegia co-exist, there may be denial of one disability with acceptance of the other. Such a dissociation of the denial of one defect and not another needs to be taken into consideration in a theory which endeavours to explain all forms of denial of illness or disability.

Finally, there has been at least one case of an inverse of Anton's syndrome. An individual with a diagnosis of cerebral blindness with the preservation of only a small portion of the visual fields denied perception despite being able to perform above chance on a variety of tasks (Hartmann et al 1991).

Adaptation to visual field defects

At first sight it is a remarkable thing that persons with quite extensive field defects behave in everyday situations as though their vision was close to normal. The fact that patients are little incommoded by homonymous hemianopia has been commented on by numerous authors, and was the subject of a study by Gassel and Williams (1963) who found that 'the visual function was little impaired, impaired transiently or defective on few occasions in most patients; and the ability to compensate for the visual field defect was remarkable' (Gassel 1969, p. 672).

Since the time of World War I when many patients with traumatic damage to the posterior regions of the brain were examined, cases have been described where patients demonstrate the phenomenon which has been termed *completion*. If those with a hemianopic defect are asked to fixate a point and a card is introduced with, say, half an object depicted on it until the border between the 'half drawing' and the blank portion of the card coincides with the division between the patient's visual field and the visual defect, they may 'see' the whole object (Fig. 7.6). Similarly they may 'see' the whole of the examiner's face despite the fact a portion of it had been covered with a card. Examination of this completion phenomenon has produced both different findings in different studies and different types of explanation to explain the findings (Fuchs 1938, Lashley 1941, Pollack et al 1957, Warrington 1962). Gassel and Williams (1963) suggest that the hemianopic field loss functions as an extensive blind spot. 'The hemianopic field is an area of absence which is discovered rather than sensed, its presence is judged from some specific failure in function rather than directly perceived' (1963, p. 258). For this reason the deficit may not be discovered by the patient, who is often vague about the nature of the impairment.

Gassel further believes that the completion phenomenon is an illusion which is a function of a number of factors, including the patient's expectation and attitude, as well as the testing conditions. In discussing the nature of visual field defects, King (1967) pointed out that incomplete figures (Fig. 7.6) have been as effective as complete figures in eliciting completion (Pollack et al 1957), thus disproving the hypothesis that the phenomenon may be accounted for by remaining visual function in the affected area.

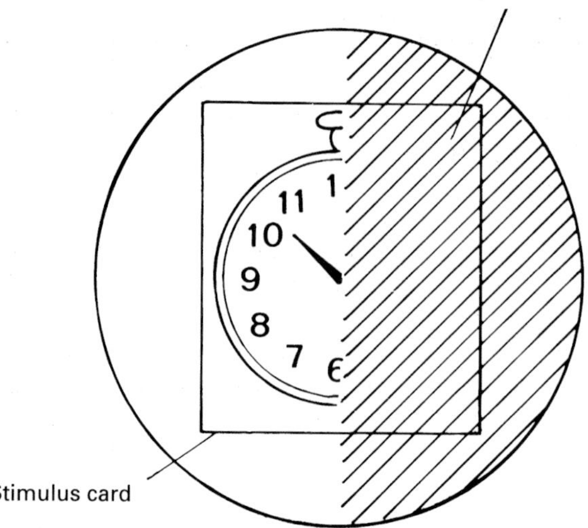

Fig. 7.6 Completion phenomenon.

With regard to the locus of the lesion, Warrington (1962) has observed that completion occurs more commonly, though not exclusively, in patients with parietal lobe lesions.

Apart from being found on routine neurological examination, visual field defects may be discovered on occasion for the first time when a patient has to deal with visual analysis and synthesis of configurations required for successful performance on some psychological tests, e.g. the patient may find difficulty with the Block Design or Object Assembly subtests of the Wechsler Adult Intelligence Scale, one of the most frequently employed tests in neuropsychological assessment. The difficulty with the seemingly easy material of these tests may surprise the patient who has adjusted well to everyday situations in which eye movements and other strategies may have minimized the defect or even rendered the patient unaware of it.

Gassel (1969) argues that the way in which the hemianopic patient adapts to his defect is similar to the operations of visual perception in the normal subject where the imperfections of the eye as an optical instrument do not interfere with the perception of the external world because of rapid eye movements and shifts in attention, both of which are usually carried out without the conscious awareness of the perceiver. 'Thus, in both normal vision and that of patients with homonymous hemianopia what is "seen" is really a conflation of a series of events in space and time, which also involves memory and expectation' (Gassel 1969, p. 674). In other words, the eye-brain analyser is able under normal circumstances to convert a less than perfect set of data into a picture of what is 'out there' in the world and has the ability to continue doing so when the information is further reduced or degraded by visual field defects.

HYSTERICAL BLINDNESS

Hysteria or malingering may form a possible problem in differential diagnosis.

True cerebral blindness shows a lack of both the menace and optokinetic reflexes where the other conditions do not.

The menace reflex is an eyeblink response produced by rapidly approaching the corner of the eye with a menacing object, while the optokinetic reflex consists of jerky eye movements when the patient gazes at a rapidly moving series of objects such as a rotating striped drum.

The electroencephalogram has also proved of use in diagnosis in this situation (Bergman 1957). Most normal subjects show the characteristic 9–13 cycles per second alpha rhythm in the posterior regions of the brain with the subject relaxed with eyes closed, and this alpha activity disappears from the record when visual stimulation is received. The posterior alpha rhythm is absent in cases of cerebral blindness, being replaced by slow waves, and there is no response in the record to opening and closing the eyes. The presence of a normal, reactive alpha rhythm should contradict a diagnosis of cerebral blindness.

Sundry other electrophysiological tests form a ready way of distinguishing functional blindness, two of the most reliable being the suppression of nystagmus (Toglia 1986) and the correlation or otherwise of the pattern electroretinogram (PERG) with the visual evoked potential (VEP) (Röver & Bach 1987).

A simple and readily available test, the Ishihara pseudo-isochromatic colour plates, proved useful in four cases described by Bourke & Gole (1994). A review of functional vision loss (FVL) with case reports is provided by Hoffman & Wilson (1994).

The detection of hysterical and related disorders using neuropsychological assessment is discussed by Walsh (1991).

VISUAL PERCEPTION

Description of sensory disorders such as those of visual location, orientation, stereopsis and colour perception should be sought in texts of experimental neuropsychology.

VISUAL AGNOSIA

Visual agnosia refers to a failure to recognize objects through the visual sense where there is neither a primary sensory loss nor mental deterioration. It is a relatively rare clinical occurrence. The essence of the disorder, as outlined by Freud in 1891 when introducing the term 'agnosia', was a disruption of the relationship between things themselves and the person's concepts of these things ('object concepts') (see Freud 1953). This notion distinguished the disorder from the group of aphasias where there was a disruption in the relationship between the concept of the object and the word used to signify it. The essence of these agnosic defects as Williams points out is 'not so much in non-awareness of the stimuli as in misrecognition of their meaning' (Williams 1970, p. 58). However, these disorders were known before Freud coined the term 'agnosia', and in 1890 Lissauer had distinguished between two classes of such recognition disorders, namely the apperceptive and associative forms. Apperceptive agnosia occurs at the stage of processing of the stimuli into an integrated percept, while in the associative type the percept is formed but does not evoke the memory traces which give the percept its meaning. Some cases may, however, lie between these classical divisions (De Renzi & Lucchelli 1993).

A number of separate forms of visual agnosia have been described as occurring in a pure form, i.e. in isolation from other defects. The validity of these claims is examined at the end of this section. The forms which have attracted most attention, particularly in recent years, are: (i) visual object agnosia; (ii) simultaneous agnosia, or simultanagnosia; (iii) visuospatial agnosia; (iv) agnosia for faces, or prosopagnosia; (v) colour agnosia; and (vi) pure word blindness, or agnosic alexia.

Whatever the status of these separate forms of visual agnosia or even of the validity of the concept of visual agnosia itself, the deficits described are important indicators of lesions in the occipital lobes, and hence it is necessary to understand the manner in which these forms of recognition disorder may present themselves and the tests which might elicit them.

The impaired recognition of spatial relationships – sometimes called spatial or visuospatial agnosia – has been described in Chapter 6.

Visual object agnosia

This is a failure to recognize objects when presented via the visual perceptual modality, with preservation of recognition by other modalities such as touch. Gassel (1969) notes that there is often some difficulty in drawing objects from memory or in describing them so that defective visualization may play a part in these patients' symptoms.

Adequate perceptual function can be demonstrated however by drawing the object (Rubens & Benson 1971) or copying a picture of it (Mack & Boller 1977) or matching objects (Albert et al 1975). Some objects may be recognized, but not others; two-dimensional representations, e.g. photographs, present more difficulty than real objects, and complex pictures present marked problems (Lhermitte et al 1972, Rubens & Benson 1971).

Sometimes patients with visual object agnosia are able to use objects which they have failed to recognize but are unable to state the function of the object when shown it. This clearly distinguishes the condition from a similar deficit seen in amnesic aphasia where the patient, while unable to find the correct name for a thing, is well able to describe its use. Again, this demonstrates that an examination of the qualitative details of a patient's deficit may prove useful in localizing the causative lesion.

Most authors indict the lateral aspect of the dominant occipital lobe as the source of the difficulty. Kleist (1934) pointed to the importance of area 19 on the left side, while Nielsen (1937) felt that, while left-sided lesions were more often the cause, visual agnosia for objects (or mind blindness as it was called earlier) could also occur with lesions of the right occipital region if the lesion lay in the 'cortex of the second and third convolutions'. Nielsen later considered that visual agnosia resulted from interruption of fibre connections between both striate areas and the area of the left occipital region depicted. This hypothesis is supported by the fact that cases with lesions of the left occipital lobe and the posterior portions of the corpus callosum – the splenium – do show agnosia.

Some patients with a lesion confined mainly to the splenium of the corpus callosum have been found to have a marked visual agnosia for objects which fall in the half-fields contralateral to the so-called minor or non-dominant hemisphere, e.g. right-handed patients with left hemisphere dominance for language have difficulty only in their left visual fields (Trescher & Ford 1937, Akelaitis 1942, Gazzaniga et al 1965). Improved experimental techniques of testing since the advent of cerebral commissurotomy in man have clarified and extended the earlier findings (see Ch. 8).

Several well studied cases of visual agnosia have reported post-mortem findings (Lhermitte et al 1972, Benson et al 1974, Albert et al 1979) or CT scan (Mack & Boller 1977). Alexander and Albert (1983), in analysing the anatomical evidence, consider the crucial lesions to be in the fibre pathways beneath the inferior temporo-occipital junction, in particular the inferior longitudinal fasciculus connecting the occipital association cortex with the medial temporal lobe. They hypothesize that this visual-limbic disconnection is the basis of the various forms of visual agnosia. The lesions are usually bilateral infarcts in the territories of the posterior cerebral arteries.

One of the requirements for a diagnosis of visual agnosia would be the absence of primary sensory defects, such as loss of acuity, since, in the sense of Freud's definition, the diagnosis depends on a dissociation between levels of visual function, higher order functions being compromised while primary sensory functions remain intact. A review of the literature shows that, while obvious defects of visual acuity may be present, various perceptual disorders are very frequently present in the case of visual object agnosia. In the extensive report of Gloning and his co-workers (1968) which studied 241 cases of occipital lobe disorder, two findings are pertinent here. Firstly, only three cases of visual agnosia for objects were encountered in the entire series and, secondly, each of these cases suffered also from a number of other perceptual disorders. Despite the relative rarity of visual object agnosia, individual case studies are important for testing neuropsychological theories, for example normal mental imagery has been shown in a case of object agnosia (Behrmann et al 1992), while one case of largely recovered agnosia continues to have difficulty with visual imagery (Wilson & Davidoff 1993).

Simultanagnosia

This form of visual agnosia consists of an inability to appreciate more than one aspect of a stimulus configuration at a time. Single aspects can be identified and pointed out from a stimulus array when it is presented again, suggesting clearly that the subject can identify and remember single features or objects, even quite complex ones. Wolpert (1924) first used the term *simultanagnosia* for one of a number of defects in his stroke victim. This patient, while usually able to name correctly objects or drawings, was unable to grasp the meaning of a complex thematic picture nor could he recognize the significance of playing card combinations such as a 'hand' at poker though he recognized the value of each card separately. There is obvious overlap in the description of cases with simultanagnosia and the relatively rare instances of Balint's syndrome (Balint 1909, Hécaen & Ajuriaguerra 1954). Balint's patient showed defective visual scanning and attention. He seemed unable to carry out voluntary search and, when an object was at the centre of his attention, he failed to notice other stimuli and, unless pressed, was unable to look to the periphery, the so-called *psychic paralysis of gaze*. If he attempted to attend to the details, he lost the whole. He was also unable to carry out visually guided hand and arm movements (*optic ataxia*) and had displacement of visual attention to the right, and left hemineglect. Balint's case and others like it showed bilateral parieto-occipital softenings, both cortical and subcortical.

Luria (1973) described a case of difficulty in grasping the whole while perceiving the parts. His patient was shown a picture of a pair of spectacles. 'He is confused and does not know what the picture represents. He starts to guess 'There is a circle...and another circle...and a stick...and a cross bar...why, it must be a bicycle"' (p. 116). Luria points out that these patients have particular difficulty if drawings are overruled with lines or presented against 'optically complex backgrounds'. Such findings suggest that tests of visual figure-ground discrimination such as the Gottschaldt Hidden Figures Test might prove useful in a diagnostic battery. However, Teuber and Weinstein (1956) demonstrated clearly that impairment on hidden figure tasks followed lesions in any lobe of the brain. They concluded from their very extensive studies that the test deficits were a non-specific sequel of the penetrating brain lesions they were studying. Moreover, impairment on the test was significantly related to aphasia, since aphasic patients performed more poorly than non-aphasic brain damaged subjects. This latter finding was confirmed by Russo and Vignolo (1967) who found that, while visual field defects did not appreciably affect scores on the Gottschaldt Test, the presence and severity of aphasia did so to a marked degree. Furthermore, patients with right hemisphere lesions performed at a poorer level than patients with left hemisphere lesions who were not aphasic. They concluded that the type of ability needed on this test may be impaired by lesions affecting at least two separate abilities, one a factor associated with language and the other a visuospatial factor related to the non-dominant hemisphere. This second aspect is in keeping with the accumulation of recent evidence supporting a major role for the non-dominant hemisphere in subserving visuospatial and visuoconstructive abilities.

Kinsbourne and Warrington (1962, 1963) examined several cases with difficulty in simultaneous form perception with the difficulty of complex figure perception. They recorded the recognition threshold for single and paired stimuli. While the thresholds for single stimuli were close to those of normals, there was invariably a long delay before the second stimulus was perceived. They hypothesized that this slowness in perceiving more than one stimulus at a time might render visual scanning of the whole less efficient, thus lessening the full appreciation of the whole. While there was a delay in recognition, the dual stimuli did appear to be adequately apprehended and one would have expected such patients to be even slower with more complex thematic material, but not to have the total inability that patients with simultanagnosia have, no matter how long they are allowed to attend to the stimuli. The difficulty with 'attention-requiring visual search' has been described in other cases (Coslett & Saffran 1991).

It is obvious that the task of analysing and integrating the information from thematic material is complex indeed, involving as it does the collaboration of visual, perceptual, oculomotor, attentional and cognitive factors. Any number of these in combination may cause a deficit. If one considers that such complex perceptuo-cognitive acts depend on occipito-frontal connections, it is not surprising that both frontal as well as occipital lesions may disrupt the process. The neuropsychologist needs to determine which of the component processes is affected with lesions in different locations in order to determine the boundaries and connections of this occipito-frontal system.

Prosopagnosia (agnosia for faces)

While patients with this disorder are able to recognize that a face is a face and may be able to identify the individual features, they are unable to recognize familiar faces as belonging to a particular friend, acquaintance or family member. In some cases, there is even difficulty with recognition of the patient's own face in the mirror. The first case appears to be that of Quaglino and Borelli in 1867 (see Benton's review of 1990). Charcot described a case in which a patient held out his hand in excuse to another person for having bumped into him when it was, in fact, his own reflection in the mirror (De Romanis & Benfatto 1973). Hoff and Poetzl reawakened interest in the condition in 1937 under the title 'amnesia for faces'. The term 'prosopagnosia' was introduced by Bodamer 10 years later (Bodamer 1947).

Prosopagnosia rarely, if ever, occurs as an isolated defect; it is frequently associated with other disorders, particularly achromatopsia and visual object agnosia. However, unlike patients with visual agnosia, who fail to recognize the nature of objects, i.e. the categories to which they belong, patients with prosopagnosia have difficulty with identification within a category they clearly recognize. This may occur not only for faces but also for other perceptual categories such as chairs (Faust 1955) or cars (Gloning et al 1966, Lhermitte & Pillon 1975) or even farm animals (Assal 1969, Bornstein et al 1969, Assal et al 1984). Some patients show a lack of awareness of impaired facial recognition, while accepting the presence of other deficits (Young et al 1990).

Some patients have difficulties within two or more categories (Alexander & Albert 1983). The report of Assal et al (1984) described the case of a farmer who was no longer able to recognize the identity of his individual cows. Prosopagnosia for human faces was present at the start of his troubles but recovered completely, i.e. there was a dissociation between classes of objects. CT scan showed bilateral temporo-occipital and occipital lesions on the medial surface of both hemispheres. This location corresponds precisely to the critical lesions postulated on the basis of other autopsy and CT findings (see below). Thus, prosopagnosia sits uneasily under the rubric of the agnosias. The rarity of the condition is shown in the numerous reviews, e.g. only one case occurred in several hundred occipital lesions reported by Gloning's group (1968). However, some degree of deficit in the recognition of human faces is much more common when tests of this ability are introduced in the examination of patients with posterior lesions. Where facial recognition is poor, visual defects are almost always present in the form of hemianopia or left upper quadrantanopia, but prosopagnosia can occur without visual field defect (Levin & Peters 1976).

The failure to distinguish between the clinical syndrome of prosopagnosia and relative difficulty with tests of facial perception and recognition has led to some confusion in the neurological and neuropsychological literature.

Location of the lesions

In most studies, there has been direct (post-mortem) or presumptive evidence of *bilateral* lesions in the occipital lobes. Gloning et al (1970), reviewing six cases, concluded that either a bilateral lesion was present or a unilateral lesion was accompanied by involvement of the corpus callosum. They reported post-mortem evidence of bilateral softenings of the brain in the region of the lingual and fusiform gyri in a case which had shown prosopagnosia and other marked signs of visual agnosia, but normal visual acuity. More recently, Damasio and Damasio (1983a) reviewed the eight cases in the literature (1892–1976), where adequate autopsy reports were available. All had bilateral infarctions in the territories of both posterior cerebral arteries affecting the lingual and fusiform gyri or their connections. Likewise, they report three cases of prosopagnosia, where the CT scan showed bilateral lesions in these areas. *They could find no case with autopsy evidence of prosopagnosia caused by a unilateral lesion*. This position continued to find support in sequential lesion cases such as that of Ettlin et al (1992). Damasio and Damasio (op cit pp. 426–427) felt that the strongest possible argument for the necessity of bilateral lesions in the production of prosopagnosia was 'the normal ability to recognize faces exhibited by patients with either left or right hemispherectomy (Damasio et al 1975) and by patients with hemispheres isolated by callosal section (Levy et al 1972)'.

Nevertheless, other reviewers had suggested the possibility of prosopagnosia without bilateral lesions. De Romanis and Benfatto (1973) reviewed 112 cases described in the literature to that time. Of these, 42 appeared to have lesions in the non-dominant hemisphere, 41 were bilateral, and 29 had dominant hemisphere lesions. Some have argued for the adequacy of a right parieto-occipital lesion combined with a left-sided lesion elsewhere in the hemisphere (Rondot & Tzavaras 1969, Lhermitte et al 1972, Meadows 1974) and there is even one report of prosopagnosia with abscess of the left frontal lobe (Cole & Perez-Cruet 1964). One would agree with Bornstein, however, that clinical findings alone are insufficient for the purposes of localization (Bornstein & Kidron 1959, Bornstein 1963, 1965), even though certain reports of prosopagnosia with right occipital lesions have specifically mentioned the absence of evidence of left hemisphere disease (Lhermitte & Pillon 1975, Whiteley & Warrington 1977). Benton's 1990 review, which suggested that the disorder may at times be produced by a right hemisphere lesion alone, has received strong recent support aided by evidence derived from MRI and PET imaging (De Renzi et al 1994, Toghi et al 1994, Carlesimo & Caltagirone 1995, Takahashi et al 1995).

False recognition. This may follow massive damage to the right hemisphere. Rapcsak et al (1994) suggest that, while the left hemisphere may still be able to employ a feature-based analytic strategy, this is prone to error where the complex perceptual analysis, such as that in facial recognition, is largely configural in nature. A further study of focal cases by the same group (Rapcsak et al 1996) suggests that false recognition together with prosopagnosia occurs in right posterior cases while false recognition without prosopagnosia tends to occur in right frontal cases and may be related to confabulation.

Nature of the defect

Benton (1980) pointed out that the most obvious explanation to suggest itself was that of a general perceptual impairment, i.e. the patient suffered from an 'impairment in the analysis and synthesis of complex visual stimulus configurations that is most clearly manifested in defective facial recognition, because individual faces present such a formidable discriminative task' (p. 179). Against this, perhaps the strongest piece of evidence is Benton's own study (Benton & Van Allen 1972), supported by others (Assal 1969, Tzavaras et al 1970, 1971, Malone et al 1982), that some patients with prosopagnosia (familiar faces) have no difficulty with the perceptual discrimination of *unfamiliar* faces, which must be considered equally complex perceptually.

Conversely, although rare, facial recognition may be preserved in the presence of severe visuoperceptive difficulties, as attested by reports, and the rarity of the condition (Meier & French 1965, Russo & Vignolo 1967, Warrington & James 1967, Tzavaras et al 1970, Orgass et al 1972).

Visual fixation difficulties have been considered important by Gloning and colleagues (Gloning et al 1966, 1967), who felt that the prime difficulty lay in identifying the 'eye region', but they later described a case of severe prosopagnosia who had no such difficulty (Gloning et al 1970).

Failure to find a simple unitary cause has led to a close examination of the performance of patients with unilateral lesions, particularly posterior lesions, on tasks requiring the matching of unfamiliar faces and related tests. Such tasks appear to be performed more poorly by those with right hemisphere damage (De Renzi & Spinnler 1966, Warrington & James 1967, Benton & Van Allen 1968, De Renzi et al 1968, Milner 1968, Tzavaras et al 1970, Yin 1970). Benton (1980) points out that the preponderance of right hemisphere lesions on these tasks holds only if it refers to patients without significant language comprehension difficulty. The group of left hemisphere patients with comprehension difficulties contains a significant number with difficulties on unfamiliar face matching tasks, and once again there is a tendency for the posterior lesion cases to have difficulty more frequently than those with anterior lesions (Hamsher et al 1979). It seems as though the two hemispheres may contribute different factors to the total process of facial recognition, in line with the special properties possessed by each hemisphere discussed in Chapter 8. One would thus expect the findings with unilateral lesions to vary somewhat according to the demands of the tasks used and hence the strategies employed (Galper & Costa 1980). In summary, unilateral lesions may render the process of facial recognition inefficient, but only bilateral lesions seem to lead to the clinical condition of prosopagnosia.

Finally, with the advent of imaging techniques the functional anatomy of face and object processing is beginning to be studied in normal subjects as well as in clinical cases. Investigations to date tend to underline the complexity of processes involved in facial recognition tasks, much depending on the requirements of the situation (Sergent & Signoret 1992a–c, Sergent et al 1992, Farah et al 1995a, b). Functional imaging has revealed a large number of discrete cortical regions and pathways in widely dispersed parts of the brain underlying complex perceptual functions such as face recognition (Haxby et al 1993, 1994, Ungerleider & Haxby 1994).

Prosopagnosia – a disconnection syndrome?

At least some cases of prosopagnosia would fit a disconnection model. Bauer and Trobe (1984) described such a case whose other cognitive functions were intact.

If presented with faces simultaneously, the patient could report correctly whether they were the same or different, but could not recognize faces that had been presented to him 90 seconds earlier. He could read and he could name objects correctly, but he could not recognize any previously viewed object among members of its own class. He could copy complex figures, but had trouble synthesizing incomplete visual information. These authors suggest that in this case, and probably in many others, prosopagnosia 'is part of a more general inability to distinguish among objects within a visual semantic class. It results from impaired visual memory and perception caused by visual association cortex damage and interruption of the inferior longitudinal fasciculus connecting visual association cortex and (the) temporal lobe'. The site of the lesion in this case corresponded with that thought to be crucial in the production of prosopagnosia, namely the junction between the medial occipital region and the parahippocampal gyrus (Fig. 7.7) (Damasio et al 1982). Such a lesion could dissociate perceptual analysis from memory processes so that the patient would know that a face is a face but fail to establish the identity of a particular individual within the category. For this reason a term such as *amnesia for identity* might be preferable to prosopagnosia, at least in those cases where perceptual processes are sufficiently intact for the person to be able to identify the class of object and to be able to discriminate between different examples within the class. Careful study of recent cases makes it clear that there are subtypes of facial recognition disorder, e.g. some patients show covert recognition of faces or implicit learning while others do not (Greve & Bauer 1990, Sergent & Poncet 1990, Bruyer 1991, McNeil & Warrington 1991, Diamond et al 1994). Some cases would fit a disconnection model, while others seem more explicable in terms of damage to perceptual units (McNeil & Warrington 1991). Even disconnection cases may differ according to whether the dorsal or occipital pathway to the parietal association cortex or the ventral pathway to the inferior temporal region is affected (Iwata 1990). Recent evidence and the adequacy of various theoretical models is reviewed by Bruyer (1991). De Renzi et al (1991) remind us that the very early division by Lissauer of agnosia into apperceptive and associative types can still be applied to prosopagnosia.

Colour agnosia

Acquired disturbances of colour perception are an important sign of occipital lobe involvement. The basis of the various disturbances of colour sense is still poorly understood but several distinctions are clinically useful. Colour 'agnosia' seems to comprise at least two separate entities, namely visual agnosia for colours and a defect of colour naming.

Patients with agnosia for colours have difficulty in identifying colours in practice. They are unable to match colours or order them in series as in Holmgren's colour sorting test with skeins of wool (Goldstein & Scheerer 1941) or, if they can manage the task, find it a good deal more difficult than normal subjects. In keeping with the general philosophy of the term agnosia no primary sense disability is apparent, e.g. on testing with a pseudo-isochromatic chart such as that of Ishihara (Lhermitte et al 1965). As with other visuognostic

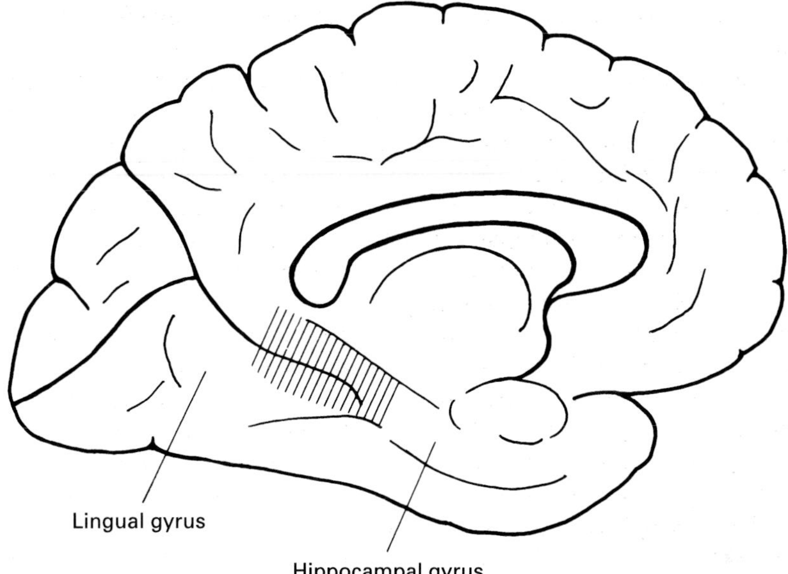

Fig. 7.7 Suggested lesion site for the production of prosopagnosia.

disorders, colour agnosia is often associated with visual field defects, particularly right homonymous hemianopia. Disorders of colour recognition have been reported more frequently with lesions of the dominant hemisphere (Kinsbourne & Warrington 1964).

The colour naming defect is believed by some to be a specific defect (Nielsen 1962). The patient, who performs normally on the Ishihara and Holmgren tests, is unable to name the colour of an object or to recognize it when it is given to him. Though this defect may occur as part of a more general aphasia, it does occur with no observable language difficulty. The failure to recognize the name when given distinguishes it from the amnesic aphasia described earlier. Critchley (1965) has described in detail the features of colour agnosia which distinguish it from other forms of colour blindness.

The relation of colour agnosia to aphasia is one which has to be examined in each case, but there is so far little direct support for Geschwind's hypothesis (Geschwind 1965a, b) that difficulty with colour naming is secondary to language defect. If they understand the instructions, most aphasic patients usually do not show abnormalities on tests of colour vision (Alajouanine et al 1960a).

The nature of the deficit seems to depend to some degree on the type of test administered. The Milan group developed a test in which the patient is required to colour outline drawings of objects having a definite colour, such as cherries, the national flag, and so on (De Renzi & Spinnler 1967). They found that difficulty with this task was particularly associated with lesions of the left hemisphere. Their finding was confirmed by Faglioni et al (1970) and Spinnler (1971), both studies showing that the main defect related to this test was sensory aphasia, and in both studies there was a positive relationship with the

Weigl test of conceptual thinking. They concluded that this reduced ability to associate a drawing with its colour can be viewed as an aspect of the aphasic's impairment in mastering concepts (Spinnler 1971). As Gassel (1969) remarked '*colours*, separate from *coloured objects*, involve a degree of intellectual abstraction' so that the relationship with Weigl's test is not surprising. A greater difficulty with this task for patients with left hemisphere lesions was not found by Tzavaras and Hécaen (1970), though these workers did find a correlation between the degree of deficit in left hemisphere patients and the presence of sensory aphasia.

In 1974, Meadows sought to distinguish three acquired disorders of colour sense. Firstly, *achromatopsia*, as described above, is associated with 'bilateral, inferiorly placed, posterior lesions'. There is a strong association with prosopagnosia. The second disorder, *disconnection colour anomia*, results from disconnection of colour perception from left hemisphere language function (Geschwind & Fusillo 1966). Thirdly, in *aphasic colour anomia* as exemplified in the paper of Kinsbourne and Warrington (1964) colour perception is preserved but the patient has what Meadows terms 'an aphasia related to colour names'. This term was used since the patient may have difficulty not only with naming colours and colouring drawings appropriately, but may also fail on verbal tests where the characteristic colour of a class of object is sought. Since this description demonstrates clearly that the patient has a disorder of knowing the nature and significance of colour in relation to objects, it would be preferable to retain the term visual agnosia for this type of disorder. Analysis of individual cases (e.g. De Vreese 1991) supports the notion of at least two major types of colour naming defect, namely a colour imagery disorder and one caused by disconnection between language and imagery. Defective imagery for colour may be dissociated from other forms of imagery such as that for faces (Goldenberg 1992). Of possible relevance is a recent PET study in subjects who 'see' colours during auditory word discrimination, in whom classical language areas in the left hemisphere were activated (Paulescu et al 1995).

Status of the concept of visual agnosia

There has been a movement in recent times away from the acceptance of visual agnosia in its early accepted sense as a clinical entity, to the position that there are patients with varying degrees of difficulty with visual recognition, not all of which can be accounted for by a single deficiency. The definition of agnosia as a higher order loss without evidence of disturbance of primary visual functions depends on what is accepted as 'primary visual function'. Bay, in a series of papers (e.g. Bay 1953), put forward the notion that visual agnosia results from a combination of faulty visual clues because of lowering of visual function plus an ineffective interpretation by patients of the visual information they have. Bay claimed that the lowering of visual function can be demonstrated by refined means of testing, where normal tests such as retinal perimetry may show the fields to be normal. His theory has received some support (Critchley 1964, Bender & Feldman 1965), though there are also a number of objections. Gassel (1969) pointed out that the findings such as those of Bergman (1957) and Williams and Gassel (1962) demonstrated that many patients with marked visual field constriction do not have disturbances of visual recognition.

Gloning, Gloning and Hoff (1968) do not believe that dissociation of primary and secondary visual functions exists at all in the sense that Freud first suggested. Their own series of cases gives strong support to this view, with only three cases with visual recognition difficulties occurring in 241 cases when those with severe visual disturbances or mental deterioration were excluded. As Critchley remarks 'cases of visual agnosia though a commonplace in medical textbooks, represent – let us admit – an extreme rarity in clinical practice' (Critchley 1964, p. 281).

The rarity of the pure 'syndrome' of visual agnosia should not prevent neuropsychologists from examining the fundamental difficulties which give rise to all forms of visual recognition disorder.

ALEXIA WITHOUT AGRAPHIA

This disorder has been given a number of labels, e.g. *pure alexia, pure word blindness, agnosic alexia,* and recently *word form alexia.* In essence, this form of reading difficulty consists of the failure to recognize words without evidence of aphasia such as speech and writing disorders. Reading difficulties which form part of a written language disturbance are designated *aphasic alexia.* Though the condition is uncommon (Milandre et al 1994), it has received much attention.

Agnosic alexia has been termed alexia *without* agraphia since, unlike the aphasic patient, the patient can write either spontaneously or to dictation. The visual basis of the difficulty becomes apparent when the patient is unable to copy printed material and is unable to read a sentence from a card in front of him which the examiner has just read and the patient has clearly understood. Where the disorder is not very gross the patient may have difficulty only with longer words and a careful search in these cases may reveal elements of simultaneous agnosia. Sometimes the patient can recognize single letters and may even be able to spell words without understanding them, the so-called 'spelling alexia'.

Alexia without agraphia provides a further example of the explanation of neuropsychological symptoms in terms of a disconnection syndrome. Such an explanation has been used to account for the first case of alexia without agraphia described by Déjérine in 1892 as well as later cases (Geschwind 1965b, Walsh & Hoyt 1969). Several findings make such an explanation more easily understood: (i) there is a highly significant correlation between pure word blindness and colour anomia (Gloning et al 1968) – these authors point out that this relationship has been reported frequently since it was first noted by Poetzl in 1928 and suggest the term 'Poetzl's syndrome' for the association; (ii) in some cases (37% of the cases of Gloning et al) the reading of numbers is not disturbed; and (iii) a right homonymous hemianopia is almost always present.

The concurrence of symptoms is explained by a lesion which damages the left occipital region and the splenium (or posterior portion of the corpus callosum) which connects both occipital lobes (Fig. 7.8). Both these regions are supplied by the posterior cerebral artery, and infarction in the distribution of this vessel is almost the sole cause of the syndrome since other lesions are most

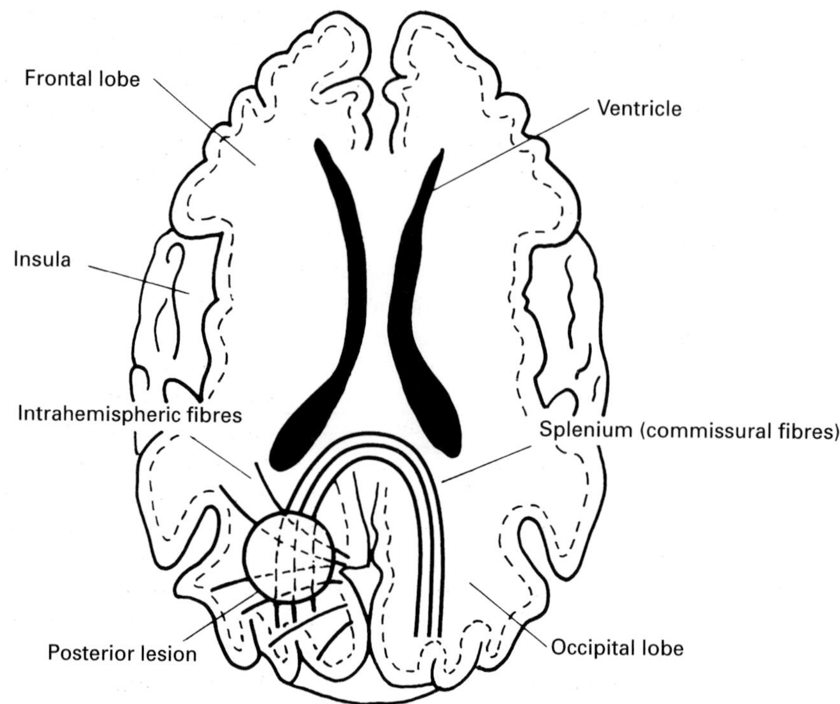

Fig. 7.8 Horizontal section with lesion in the left occipital lobe producing alexia without agraphia.

unlikely to affect both areas so completely and exclusively (Walsh & Hoyt 1969). Since the regions concerned with the non-visual aspects of language are supplied by the other main arteries these latter functions remain unaffected. Careful imaging with respect to the inferior portion of the left side of the splenium of the corpus callosum is recommended by Quint and Gilmore (1992) for patients suspected of having this disorder.

Visual information received by the right occipital lobe cannot reach the language hemisphere (left) because of the interruption to the interhemispheric fibres in the splenium. Thus, while they can see, these patients are unable to interpret or speak about what they see. The preservation of the patient's ability to write spontaneously is accounted for by the fact that non-visual stimuli from both hemispheres can reach appropriate language centres over intra- and interhemispheric connections. The patient is, however, unable to transcribe printed material.

The importance of the splenium of the corpus callosum in the production of this syndrome has been emphasized by numerous authors (Kleist 1934, Alajouanine et al 1960b) and is shown by cases where the callosum has been divided in the removal of cysts of the third ventricle (Trescher & Ford 1937, Maspes 1948) or in cerebral commissurotomy for the relief of epilepsy (Gazzaniga et al 1962, 1965, Geschwind 1962, 1965b, c). These latter patients showed alexia only in the left visual field since this information is transmitted to the right occipital lobe and cannot reach the language centres in the dominant hemisphere over the severed commissural fibres. For a similar reason, removal of the occipital lobe of the language dominant hemisphere has been shown to produce lasting word blindness (Ajuriaguerra & Hécaen 1951).

The anatomic basis of pure alexia has been clarified by Damasio and Damasio (1983b). In their study of 23 cases, the crucial area of involvement was the paraventricular matter of the left occipital lobe that would disrupt both inter- and intrahemispheric visual pathways. Several studies have reported alexia without either agraphia or hemianopia (Iragui & Kritchevsky 1991). In each instance the lesion was in the parietal or parieto-occipital white matter, sparing the optic radiation. Confirmation of the location of causative lesions has come directly from CT scans (e.g. Caffarra 1987, Delreux et al 1987, Weisberg & Wall 1987).

The sparing of the reading of numbers in pure alexia may be accounted for by the preservation of associations such as those developed by counting on the fingers. These associations of somatic with visual information could still reach the language hemisphere over the intact interhemispheric pathways anterior to the splenium. By contrast, the naming of colours is not spared since it involves no associations beside the visuo-auditory ones. 'A colour has no feel, smell, or taste and has no fixed associations but its name' (Geschwind 1965a, p. 99).

A further refinement in the study of disconnection mechanisms underlying alexia comes from a case of Greenblatt (1973). In this case, and a similar one reported by Ajax (1967), the focal lesion involved only the ventro-medial aspect of the left occipital lobe and the splenium of the corpus callosum. The patient had alexia without agraphia but no hemianopia, and colour naming was preserved. Greenblatt put forward the hypothesis that '...within each occipital lobe, the inferior association tracts and the ventro-medial (lingual and fusiform) gyri are necessary for reading. Visual-verbal colour naming, on the other hand, apparently may be served either by the dorsal or by the ventral outflow paths from the calcarine cortex'.

This parcellation of the syndrome has been supported by anatomical evidence from other cases (Ajax et al 1977, Vincent et al 1977, Johansson & Fahlgren 1979).

Finally, Greenblatt (1983) in his comprehensive examination of the pathological basis of all the alexias has further divided alexia without agraphia into a number of subtypes on the basis of functional anatomy. All his evidence fits the disconnection model and provides one of the finest of such arguments in behavioural neurology.

Similarly, the careful symptomatic analysis of a case of agnosic alexia, colour agnosia and severe naming difficulties in a patient with left posterior cerebral artery ischaemia by Lhermitte and Beauvois (1973) has further emphasized the importance of intrahemispheric as well as commissural connections in the production of symptoms in such cases.

Likewise, Albert et al (1973) propose a functional disconnection between the visual, auditory and motor systems used in the understanding of written language as a possible basis for their patient's symptoms. This patient, who had a tumour removed from the left temporo-occipital region, showed alexia without agraphia but was able to spell words presented to him orally and was able to recognize words from their letters spelled out to him, though he was unable to spell words presented in written form and was unable to carry out written commands. It seems important, as in this case, to establish whether the patient has preservation of capacities which are intramodal (within the auditory-oral system) or intermodal (visual-auditory), or both.

Despite the common acceptance of the disconnection theory the advent of neuroimaging may require revision of this approach. Benito-León et al (1997) recently presented MRI and SPECT evidence in a patient with pure alexia, but no right homonymous hemianopia, that damage to the extrastriate visual cortex in the left ventral occipital region may be the critical lesion.

The fact that left hemisphere lesions are paramount in the production of acquired reading disabilities does not imply that the right hemisphere plays no important part in reading. Faglioni, Scotti and Spinnler (1968) have shown that there is a clear dissociation between the effects of left and right hemisphere damage on the subject's performance on visual recognition of verbal material.

Again, as shown for the temporal lobes with regard to auditory material, the dissociation is between the semantic-associative capacities of the left hemisphere and the perceptual-discriminative capacities of the right. An integration of both sets of functions is necessary for effective reading.

Pure alexia has been reported rarely in patients with left homonymous hemianopia, and of these only two cases occurred in clearly right-handed patients (Hirose et al 1977, Mochizuki et al 1980). The former case showed an appropriately sited calloso-occipital lesion on CT scan, while the latter displayed blockage of the right posterior cerebral artery at arteriography.

A detailed and scholarly appraisal of the evidence presented by Déjérine and a critique of his theory in relation to recent hypotheses has been given by Bub et al (1993).

Reversible alexia

Reversible alexia without agraphia caused by migraine was described by Bigley and Sharp (1983). Blood flow studies (SPECT) in a second patient with intermittent alexia showed differences between those taken during the attacks and at normal times, suggesting a vascular (migrainous) basis (Parker et al 1990). Another patient, who had previously suffered an attack of basilar artery migraine, became alexic during the performance of vertebral arteriography (Laurent et al 1984). In this case the alexia coincided with the demonstration of spasm in the left posterior cerebral artery. The alexia lasted up to 1 hour and then resolved. Colour naming was spared during the event but the patient was unable to name well known people from photographs.

VISUAL HALLUCINATIONS

Visual hallucinations are described frequently in conditions affecting the occipital lobes (Allen 1930, Paillas et al 1965, Gloning et al 1968, Anderson & Rizzo 1994). The essential characteristic of these hallucinations is their elementary nature. More organized visual hallucinations of people, objects and scenes usually indicate that the excitation is arising in or has spread to neighbouring regions, particularly the temporal lobes. Complex hallucinations have also been described with frontal pathology (Nakajima 1991).

Elementary hallucinations or photisms have been described by a number of authors (Lhermitte 1951, Ajuriaguerra & Hécaen 1960, Gloning et al 1968). The latter authors found 55 cases of elementary hallucinations in their series. These were almost exclusively projected to the half-field contralateral to the lesion and consisted of points, stars, flames, flashes, wheels, circles and triangles. A few cases of photisms with lesions outside the occipital lobes were reported and each of these seemed to be caused by irritation of the visual pathways.

Elementary hallucinations have been well documented with focal epileptic seizures originating in the occipital lobes (Lhermitte 1951, Penfield & Jasper 1954, Russell & Whitty 1955, Williamson et al 1992). Again, the sensations are referred to the contralateral half-field.

Charles Bonnet hallucinations

The term 'Charles Bonnet syndrome' was coined by De Morsier (1967) to refer to *complex* visual hallucinations in elderly persons without evidence of mental deterioration. Charles Bonnet had described such a situation with his grandfather in 1760. There is characteristically preservation of insight, and cognition is generally intact even on formal testing (Schultz & Melzack 1993), though there may be some exceptions to this latter finding (Cole 1992). Hallucinations do not appear in other sense modalities.

The condition is most frequently seen in the elderly, but an analysis of the literature reveals that it can appear at any age (Schultz & Melzack 1991). The aging subjects almost always have poor vision (e.g. Shedlack et al 1994) and a large prospective review of elderly patients with poor vision found 11% to have the Bonnet phenomenon (Teunisse et al 1995). Most of the 14 patients studied by Teunisse et al (1994) showed evidence of social isolation.

Though the condition is dealt with in this chapter, there is no suggestion that the occipital lobes are the site of origin – this is at present unknown. Also the implication that the condition is not associated with pathology should be regarded with caution since there are two recent reports of patients with the Bonnet syndrome who many months later went on to develop Alzheimer's disease (Crystal et al 1988, Haddad & Benbow 1992).

ELECTRICAL STIMULATION

The findings of studies of spontaneously occurring hallucinations in posterior cerebral lesions have been very strongly confirmed by the results of stimulation, in that complex visual experiences, most frequently of a person or group of persons, are produced from the temporal, temporo-occipital or parieto-occipital regions but not from the visual cortex itself. Gloning, Gloning and Hoff (1968) reported no hemispheric difference in the incidence of complex visual hallucinations in their lesion cases. This is in marked contrast to the stimulation findings reported by Penfield and Perot (1963) where visual hallucinations of prior experience were elicited overwhelmingly from the right hemisphere (Fig. 7.9).

The content of the hallucinations, when complex, may be determined by prior experience. A male patient of Gloning and his colleagues who had been a philatelist saw postage stamps in the hemianopic parts of his visual field while

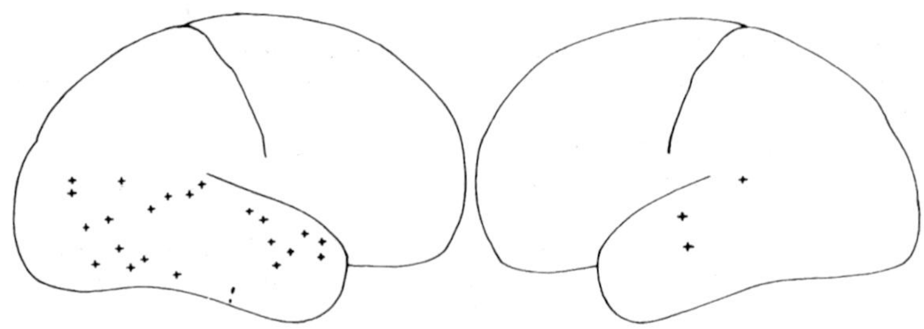

Fig. 7.9 Visual experiential responses evoked by stimulation (from Penfield & Perot 1963).

one of our patients who had been a forestry officer saw predominantly scenes with trees. As is often the case, the hallucinations were vividly coloured, the patient describing them as colours he had not seen before 'colours such as they bring out for new cars each year'. They were so vivid that they prevented the patient getting off to sleep.

Sometimes the experiential hallucination elicited by stimulation is very similar to that experienced by the patient during an epileptic seizure. The following case is condensed from Penfield and Perot (1963).

> Case 3 – a 12-year-old boy with a three year history of seizures. The pattern of his attacks was:
> 1. visual sensation (coloured triangles);
> 2. experiential hallucination – visual;
> 3. automatism...after the visual sensation usually he would see a robber, or a man with a gun, moving towards him. The man was someone he had seen in the movies or the comic strips...(stimulation of several points on the right temporo-occipital cortex produced the following responses). 'Oh gee, gosh, robbers are coming at me with guns!...Pain in my forehead, and there was a robber. He wasn't in front, he was off to the left side'...'Yes, the robbers, they are coming after me'...'Oh gosh! Here they are, my brother is there. He is aiming an air rifle at me.'

The very wide experience of Penfield and his colleagues with brain stimulation (Penfield & Rasmussen 1950, Penfield & Jasper 1954, Penfield & Perot 1963) shows that lights, shadows, colours, movements and other elementary visual sensations occur on stimulation of the occipital lobe (areas 17, 18, 19) and never complex figures or scenes. The fact that Foerster (1936) described the evocation of figures or scenes on stimulation of area 19 might be accounted for by the spread of excitation to regions in front of the occipital lobes. In recent times, three patients receiving stimulation in the medial parieto-occipital region each reported visual motor phenomena (Richer et al 1991).

References

Ajax E T 1967 Dyslexia without agraphia. Archives of Neurology 17: 645–652

Ajax E T, Schenkenberg T, Kosteljanetz M 1977 Alexia without agraphia and the inferior splenium. Neurology 27: 685–688

Ajuriaguerra J de, Hécaen H 1951 La restauration fonctionelle après lobectomie occipitale. Journal de Psychologie Normale et Pathologique 44: 510–546

Ajuriaguerra J de, Hécaen H 1960 Le cortex cerebral. Masson, Paris
Akelaitis A J 1942 Studies on the corpus callosum. V. Archives of Neurology and Psychiatry 47: 971–1008
Alajouanine T, Castaigne P, DeRibaucourt-Ducarne B 1960a Valeur clinique de certains tests perceptifs et perceptivo-moteurs. In: Alajouanine T (ed) Les grandes activités du lobe occipital. Masson, Paris
Alajouanine T, Lhermitte F, De Ribaucourt-Ducarne B 1960b Les alexies agnosiques et aphasiques. In: Alajouanine T (ed) Les grandes activités du lobe occipital. Masson, Paris
Albert M L, Yamadori A, Gardner H, Howes D 1973 Comprehension in alexia. Brain 96: 317–328
Albert M L, Reches A, Silverberg R 1975 Associative visual agnosia without alexia. Neurology 25: 322–326
Albert M L, Soffer D, Silverberg R, Reches A 1979 The anatomic basis of visual agnosia. 29: 86–89
Alexander M P, Albert M L 1983 The anatomical basis of visual agnosia. In: Kertesz A (ed) Localization in neuropsychology. Academic Press, New York, pp 393–415
Allen J M 1930 Clinical study of tumours involving the occipital lobes. Brain 53: 194–243
Anderson S W, Rizzo 1994 M Hallucinations following occipital lobe damage: the pathological activation of visual representations. Journal of Clinical and Experimental Neuropsychology 16: 651–663
Assal G 1969 Régression des troubles de la reconnaisance des physionomies et de la mémoire topographique chez un malade opéré d'un hématome intracérébral pariéto-temporal droite. Revue Neurologique 121: 184–185
Assal G, Favre C, Anderes J P 1984 Non-reconnaissance d'animaux familiers chez un paysan. Zoo-agnosie ou prosopagnosie pour les animaux. Revue Neurologique 140: 580–584
Balint R 1909 Seelenlähmung des 'Schauens', optische Ataxie, raümliche Störung der Aufmerksamkeit. Monatsschrift für Psychiatrie und Neurologie 25: 51–81
Barinaga M 1992 Unraveling the dark paradox of 'blindsight'. Science 258: 1438–1439
Bauer R M, Trobe J D 1984 Visual memory and perceptual impairment in prosopagnosia. Journal of Clinical Neuro-Ophthalmology 4: 39–46
Bay E 1953 Disturbances of visual perception and their examination. Brain 6: 515–550
Behrmann M, Winocur G, Moscovitch M 1992 Dissociation between mental imagery and object recognition in a brain-damaged patient. Nature 359: 636–637
Bender M B, Feldman M 1965 The so-called 'visual agnosias'. Proceedings 8th International Congress of Neurology (Vienna) 3: 153–156
Bender M B, Kanzer M M 1941 Dynamics of homonymous hemianopsias and preservation of central vision. Archives of Neurology and Psychiatry 45: 481–485
Benito-León J, Sánchez-Suárez C, Díaz-Guzmán J, Martínez-Salio A 1997 Pure alexia could not be a disconnection syndrome. Neurology 49: 305–306
Benson D F, Segarra J, Albert M L 1974 Visual agnosia-prosopagnosia. Archives of Neurology 30: 307–310
Benton A L 1980 The neuropsychology of facial recognition. American Psychologist 35: 176–186
Benton A L 1990 Facial recognition 1990. Cortex 26: 491–499
Benton A L, Van Allen M W 1968 Impairment in facial recognition in patients with cerebral disease. Cortex 4: 344–358
Benton A L, Van Allen M W 1972 Prosopagnosia and facial discrimination. Journal of Neurological Science 15: 167–172
Bergman P S 1957 Cerebral blindness. Archives of Neurology and Psychiatry 8: 568–584
Bigley G K, Sharp F R 1983 Reversible alexia without agraphia due to migraine. Archives of Neurology 40: 114–115
Bodamer J 1947 Die Prosop-Agnosie. Archiv für Psychiatrie und Nervenkrankheiten 179: 6–53
Bornstein B 1963 Prosopagnosia. In: Halpern L (ed) Problems in dynamic neurology. Hadassah Medical Organization, Jerusalem
Bornstein B 1965 Prosopagnosia. Proceedings of the 8th International Congress of Neurology (Vienna) 3: 157–160
Bornstein B, Kidron D P 1959 Prosopagnosia. Journal of Neurology, Neurosurgery and Psychiatry 22: 124–131

Bornstein B, Sroka H, Munitz H 1969 Prosopagnosia with animal face agnosia. Cortex 5: 164–169
Bourke R D, Gole G A 1994 Detection of functional vision loss using the Ishihara plates. Australian and New Zealand Journal of Ophthalmology 22: 115–118
Brent P J, Kennard C, Ruddock K H 1994 Residual colour vision in a human hemianope: spectral responses and colour discrimination. Proceedings of the Royal Society of London Series B: Biological Sciences 256: 219–225
Brodmann K 1909 Vergleichende Lokalisationslehre der Grosshirnrinde. Barth, Leipzig
Bruyer R 1991 Covert face recognition in prosopagnosia: a review. Brain and Cognition 15: 223–235
Bub D N, Arguin M, Lecours A R 1993 Jules Déjérine and his interpretation of pure alexia. Brain and Language 45: 531–559
Caffarra P 1987 Alexia without agraphia or hemianopia. European Neurology 27: 65–71
Carlesimo G A, Caltagirone C 1995 Components in the visual processing of known and unknown faces. Journal of Clinical and Experimental Neuropsychology 17: 691–705
Cogan D G 1966 Neurology of the visual system. Thomas, Springfield, Illinois
Cole M G 1992 Charles Bonnet hallucinations: a case series. Canadian Journal of Psychiatry 37: 267–270
Cole M, Perez-Cruet J 1964 Proposognosia. Neuropsychologia 16: 283–289
Corbetta M, Marzi C A, Tassinari G, Aglioti S 1990 Effectiveness of different task paradigms in revealing blindsight. Brain 113: 603–616
Coslett H B, Saffran E 1991 Simultanagnosia. To see but not two see. Brain 114: 1523–1545
Critchley M 1964 The problem of visual agnosia. Journal of Neurological Science 1: 274–290
Critchley M 1965 Acquired anomalies of colour. Brain 88: 711–724
Critchley M 1979 The divine banquet of the brain and other essays. Raven, New York
Crystal H, Wolfson L, Ewing S 1988 Visual hallucinations as the first symptom of Alzheimer's disease. American Journal of Psychiatry 145: 1318
Damasio A R, Damasio H 1983a Localization of lesions in achromotopsia and prosopagnosia. In: Kertesz A (ed) Localisation in neuropsychology. Academic Press, New York, pp 417–428
Damasio A R, Damasio H 1983b The anatomic basis of pure alexia. Neurology 33: 1573–1583
Damasio A R, Lima P A, Damasio H 1975 Nervous function after right hemispherectomy. Neurology 24: 89–93
Damasio A R, Damasio H, Van Hoesen G W 1982 Prosopagnosia: anatomic basis and behavioral mechanisms. Neurology 32: 331–341
Déjerine J 1892 Contribution a l'étude anatomo-pathologique et clinique des différents variétés de cécité verbale. Comptes Rendus, Société de Biologie 4: 61–90
Delreux V, Kevers L, Callewaert A 1987 Alexia without agraphia. Anatomical basis and physiopathological mechanisms. Acta Neurologica Belgica 87: 267–272
De Morsier G 1967 Le syndrome de Charles Bonnet: hallucinations visuelles des viellards sans déficience mentale. Annales Medico-Psychologiques 125: 677–702
De Renzi E, Lucchelli F 1993 The fuzzy boundaries of apperceptive agnosia. Cortex 29: 187–215
De Renzi E, Spinnler H 1966 Facial recognition in brain-damaged patients. Neurology 16: 145–152
De Renzi E, Spinnler H 1967 Impaired performance on color tasks in patients with hemispheric damage. Cortex 3: 194–210
De Renzi E, Faglioni P, Spinnler H 1968 The performance of patients with unilateral brain damage on face recognition tasks. Cortex 4: 1–34
De Renzi E, Faglioni P, Grossi D, Nichelli P 1991 Apperceptive and associative forms of prosopagnosia. Cortex 27: 213–221
De Renzi E, Perani D, Carlesimo G A, Silveri M C, Fazio F 1994 Prosopagnosia can be associated with damage confined to the right hemisphere – an MRI and PET study and a review of the literature. Neuropsychologia 32: 893–902
De Romanis F, Benfatto B 1973 Presentazione e discussione di quattro casi di prosopagnosia. Rivista di Neurologia 43: 111–132
De Vreese L F 1991 Two systems for colour naming defects: verbal disconnection vs colour imagery disorder. Neuropsychologia 29: 1–18
Diamond B J, Valentine T, Mayes A R, Sandel M E 1994 Evidence of covert recognition in a prosopagnosic patient. Cortex 30: 377–393

Ettlin T M, Beckson M, Benson D F et al 1992 Prosopagnosia: a bihemispheric disorder. Cortex 28: 129–134
Faglioni P, Scotti G, Spinnler H 1968 Impaired recognition of written letters following unilateral hemispheric damage. Cortex 5: 120–133
Faglioni P, Scotti G, Spinnler H 1970 Colouring drawings impairment following unilateral brain damage. Brain Research 24: 546
Farah M J 1994 Perception and awareness after brain damage. Current Opinion in Neurobiology 4: 252–255
Farah M J, Levinson K L, Klein K L 1995a Face perception and within-category discrimination in prosopagnosia. Neuropsychologia 33: 661–674
Farah M J, Wilson K D, Drain H M, Tanaka J R 1995b The inverted face inversion effect in prosopagnosia: evidence for mandatory, face-specific perceptual mechanisms. Vision Research 35: 2089–2093
Faust C 1955 Die zerebralen Herderscheinungen bei Hinterhauptsverletzungen und ihre Beurteilung. Thieme Verlag, Stuttgart
Foerster O 1936 Cited in Gloning et al 1968, p 34
Freud S 1953 Zur Auffassung der Aphasien. 1891. International Universities Press, New York
Fryer D G, Rich M P 1960 Denial of illness in relation to intellectual functions. Journal of Nervous and Mental Disease 131: 523–527
Fuchs W 1938 Pseudo-fovea. In: Ellis W D (ed) A source book of Gestalt psychology. Kegan Paul, London
Galper R E, Costa L 1980 Hemispheric superiority for recognizing faces depends upon how they are learned. Cortex 16: 21–38
Gassel M M 1969 Occipital lobe syndromes (excluding hemianopia). In: Vinken P J, Bruyn G W (eds) Handbook of neurology. North-Holland, Amsterdam, vol 2, ch 20
Gassel M M, Williams D 1963 Visual function in patients with homonymous hemianopia. Part III. The completion phenomenon; insight and attitude to the defect; and visual functional efficiency. Brain 86: 229–260
Gazzaniga M S, Bogen J E, Sperry R W 1962 Some functional effects of severing the cerebral commissures in man. Proceedings of the National Academy of Science 48: 165–169
Gazzaniga M S, Bogen J E, Sperry R W 1965 Observations on visual perception after disconnexion of the cerebral hemispheres in man. Brain 88: 221–236
Geschwind N 1962 The anatomy of acquired disorders of reading. In: Money J (ed) Reading disability. Johns Hopkins Press, Baltimore.
Geschwind N 1965a Alexia and colour-naming disturbance. In: Ettlinger G (ed) Functions of the corpus callosum. Churchill, London, pp 95–101
Geschwind N 1965b Disconnection syndromes in animals and man. Part I. Brain 88: 237–294
Geschwind N 1965c Disconnection syndromes in animals and man. Part II. Brain 88: 585–644
Geschwind N, Fusillo M 1966 Color naming defects in association with alexia. Archives of Neurology 15: 137–146
Gloning I, Gloning K, Hoff H, Tschabitscher H 1966 Zur Prosopagnosie. Neuropsychologia 4: 113–132
Gloning I, Gloning K, Hoff H 1968 Neuropsychological symptoms in lesions of the occipital lobes and adjacent areas. Gauthier-Villars, Paris
Gloning I, Gloning K, Jellinger K, Quatember R 1970 A case of 'prosopagnosia' with necropsy findings. Neuropsychologia 8: 199–204
Gloning K, Haub G, Quatember R 1967 Standardisierung einer Untersuchungsmethode der sogenannten Prosopagnosie. Neuropsychologia 5: 99–101
Goldenberg G 1992 Loss of visual imagery and loss of visual knowledge – a case study. Neuropsychologia 30: 1081–1099
Goldenberg G, Mullbacher W, Nowak A 1995 Imagery without perception – a case study of anosognosia for cortical blindness. Neuropsychologia 33: 1373–1382
Goldstein K, Scheerer M 1941 Abstract and concrete behavior: An experimental study with special tests. Psychological Monographs 43: 1–151
Greenblatt S H 1973 Alexia without agraphia or hemianopsia. Anatomical analysis of an autopsied case. Brain 96: 307–316
Greenblatt S H 1983 Localization of lesions in alexia. In: Kertesz A (ed) Localization in neuropsychology. Academic Press, New York, pp 323–356
Greve K W, Bauer RM 1990 Implicit learning of new faces. Neuropsychologia 28: 1035–1041

Guthrie T C, Grossman E M 1952 A study of the syndrome of denial. Archives of Neurology and Psychiatry 68: 362–371

Haddad P M, Benbow S M 1992 Visual hallucinations as the presenting symptom of senile dementia. British Journal of Psychiatry 161: 263–265

Hamsher K de S, Levin H S, Benton A L 1979 Facial recognition in patients with focal brain lesions. Archives of Neurology 36: 837–839

Hartmann J A, Woltz W A, Roeltgen D F, Loverso F L 1991 Denial of visual perception. Brain and Cognition 16: 29–40

Haxby J V, Grady C L, Horwitz B et al 1993 Dissociation of object and spatial visual processing pathways in human extrastriate cortex. In: Gulyás B, Ottoson D, Roland P E (eds) Functional organisation of the human visual cortex. Pergamon, New York, pp 329–340

Haxby J V, Horwitz B, Ungerleider L G et al 1994 The functional organization of human extrastriate cortex: a PET-rCBF study of selective attention to faces and locations. Journal of Neuroscience 11: 636–653

Hécaen H, Ajuriaguerra J de 1954 Balint's syndrome (psychic paralysis of visual fixation) and its minor forms. Brain 77: 373–400

Hirose G, Kin T, Murakami E 1977 Alexia without agraphia associated with right occipital lesion. Journal of Neurology, Neurosurgery and Psychiatry 40: 225–227

Hoff H, Poetzl O 1937 Uber eine optisch-agnostische Störung des 'Physiognomie-Gedachtnisses'. Zeitschrift für die gesamte Neurologie und Psychiatrie 159: 367–395

Hoffman D J, Wilson R 1994 Functional vision loss. Journal of the American Optometric Association 65: 835–844

Holmes G 1918 Disturbances of visual orientation. British Journal of Ophthalmology 2: 449–469

Iragui V J, Kritchevsky M 1991 Alexia without agraphia or hemianopia in parietal infarction. Journal of Neurology, Neurosurgery and Psychiatry 54: 841–846

Iwata M 1990 Visual association pathways in the human brain. Tohoku Journal of Experimental Medicine 161: 61–78

Johansson T, Fahlgren H 1979 Alexia without agraphia: Lateral and medial infarction of the left occipital lobe. Neurology 29: 390–393

King E 1967 The nature of visual field defects. Brain 90: 647–668

Kinsbourne M, Warrington E K 1962 A disorder of simultaneous form perception. Brain 85: 461–486

Kinsbourne M, Warrington E K 1963 The localizing significance of limited simultaneous visual form perception. Brain 86: 697–702

Kinsbourne M, Warrington E K 1964 Observations on colour agnosia. Journal of Neurology, Neurosurgery, and Psychiatry 27: 296–299

Kleist K 1934 Gehirnpathologie. Barth, Leipzig

Kolb F C, Braun J 1995 Blindsight in normal observers. Nature 377: 336–338

Lashley K S 1941 Patterns of cerebral integration indicated by the scotomas of migraine. Archives of Neurology and Psychiatry 46: 331–339

Laurent B, Michel D, Antoine J C, Montagnon D 1984 Migraine basilaire avec alexie sans agraphie: spasme artériel a l'artériographie et l'effet de la naloxone. Revue Neurologique 140: 663–665

Levin H S, Peters B H 1976 Neuropsychological testing following head injuries: Prosopagnosia without field defect. Diseases of the Nervous System 37: 68–71

Levy J, Trevarthen C B, Sperry R W 1972 Perception of bilateral chimeric figures following hemispheric deconnection. Brain 95: 61–78

Lhermitte F 1951 Les hallucinations. Doin, Paris

Lhermitte F, Beauvois M F 1973 A visual-speech disconnexion syndrome. Brain 96: 695–714

Lhermitte F, Pillon B 1975 La prosopagnosie: Rôle de l'hémisphère droit dans la perception visuelle. Revue Neurologique 131: 791–812

Lhermitte F, Chain F, Aron D 1965 10 cas d'agnosie des couleurs. Proceedings of the 8th International Congress of Neurology, Vienna 3: 217–221

Lhermitte F, Chain F, Escourolle R, Ducarne B, Pillon B 1972 Etude anatomo-clinique d'un cas de prosopagnosie. Revue Neurologique 126: 329–346

Lissauer H 1890 Ein Fall von Seelenblindheiten nebst einen Beitrage zur Theorie derselben. Archiv für Psychiatrie und Nervenkrankenheiten 21: 222–270

Luria A R 1973 The working brain. Allen Lane, The Penguin Press, Harmondsworth, Middlesex
Mack J L, Boller F 1977 Associative visual agnosia and its related deficits. The role of the minor hemisphere in assigning meaning to visual perceptions. Neuropsychologia 15: 345–349
Malone D R, Morris H H, Kay M C, Levin H S 1982 Prosopagnosia: a double dissociation between the recognition of familiar and unfamiliar faces. Journal of Neurology, Neurosurgery and Psychiatry 45: 820–822
Maspes P E 1948 Le syndrome expérimental chez l'homme de la section du splenium du corps calleux. Revue Neurologique 80: 100–113
McDaniel K D, McDaniel L D 1991 Anton's syndrome in a patient with posttraumatic optic neuropathy and bifrontal contusions. Archives of Neurology 48: 101–105
McNeil J E, Warrington E K 1991 Prosopagnosia: a reclassification. Quarterly Journal of Experimental Psychology 43: 267–287
Meadows J C 1974 The anatomical basis of prosopagnosia. Journal of Neurology, Neurosurgery and Psychiatry 37: 489–501
Meeres S L, Graves R E 1990 Localization of unseen visual stimuli by humans with normal vision. Neuropsychologia 28: 1231–1237
Meier M J, French L A 1965 Lateralized deficits in complex visual discrimination and bilateral transfer of reminiscence following unilateral temporal lobectomy. Neuropsychologia 3: 261–272
Milandre L, Brosset C, Botti G, Khalil R 1994 A study of 82 cerebral infarctions of the posterior cerebral arteries. Revue Neurologique 150: 133–141
Milner B 1968 Visual recognition and recall after right temporal lobe excision in man. Neuropsychologia 6: 191–209
Mochizuki H, Sugishita M, Tohgi H, Satoh Y 1980 Alexia without agraphia associated with right occipital lobe lesion in a right-hander. Rinsho Shinkeigaku 20: 50–56
Nakajima K 1991 Visual hallucination associated with anterior cerebral artery occlusion. No To Shinkei 43: 71–76
Nathanson M, Bergman P S, Gordon G G 1952 Denial of illness. Archives of Neurology and Psychiatry 68: 380–387
Natsoulas T 1997 Blindsight and consciousness. American Journal of Psychology 110: 1–33
Nielsen J M 1937 Unilateral cerebral dominance as related to mind-blindness. Minimal lesion causing visual agnosia for objects. Archives of Neurology and Psychiatry 38: 108–115
Nielsen J M 1962 Agnosia, apraxia, aphasia. Their value in cerebral localization. Harper, New York
Nielsen J M, Friedman A P 1942 The temporal isthmus and its clinical syndromes. Bulletin of the Los Angeles Neurological Societies 7: 1–11
Orgass B, Poeck K, Kerschensteiner M, Hartje W 1972 Visuo-cognitive performances in patients with unilateral hemispheric lesions. Zeitschrift für Neurologie 202: 177–195
Paganini A E, Zlotlow M 1960 Denial of lobotomy as a continuation of the defense mechanism of denial in schizophrenia. Psychiatric Quarterly 34: 260–268
Paillas J E, Cossa P, Darcourt G, Naquet R 1965 Etude sur l'epilepsie occipital. Eighth International Congress of Neurology, Vienna, vol 3, pp 193–196
Parker D M, Besson J A, McFadyen M 1990 Intermittent alexia. Cortex 26: 657–660
Parsons O A, Huse M M 1958 Impairment of flicker discrimination in brain-damaged patients. Neurology 8: 50–55
Paulescu E, Harrison J, Baron-Cohen S et al 1995 The physiology of coloured hearing. A PET activation study of colour-word synaesthesia. Brain 118: 661–676
Penfield W, Jasper H 1954 Epilepsy and the functional anatomy of the human brain. Little Brown, Boston
Penfield W, Perot P 1963 The brain's record of auditory and visual experience. Brain 86: 595–697
Penfield W, Rasmussen AT 1950 The cerebral cortex of man. Macmillan, New York
Perenin M T, Jeannerod M 1978 Visual function within the hemianopic field following early cerebral decortication in man – l. Spatial localization. Neuropsychologia 16: 1–13
Pollack M, Battersby W S, Bender M B 1957 Tachistoscopic identification of contour in patients with brain damage. Journal of Comparative and Physiological Psychology 50: 220–227

Pöppel E, Held R, Frost D 1973 Residual visual function after brain wounds involving the central visual pathways. Nature 243: 295–296

Quint D J, Gilmore J L 1992 Alexia without agraphia. Neuroradiology 34: 210–214

Rapcsak S Z, Polster M R, Comer J F, Rubens A B 1994 False recognition and misidentification following right hemisphere damage. Cortex 30: 565–583

Rapcsak S Z, Polster M R, Glisky M L, Comer J F 1996 False recognition of unfamiliar faces following right hemisphere damage: neuropsychological and anatomical observations. Cortex 32: 593–611

Richer F, Martinez M, Cohen H, Saint-Hilaire J M 1991 Visual motion perception from stimulation of the human medial parieto-occipital cortex. Experimental Brain Research 87: 649–652

Riddoch G 1917 Dissociation of visual perception due to occipital injuries with special reference to appreciation of movement. Brain 40: 15–57

Rondot P A, Tzavaras A 1969 La prosopagnosie après vingt années d'études cliniques et neuropsychologiques. Journal de Psychologie Normale et Pathologique 66: 133–166

Ross Russell R W, Bharucha N 1984 Visual localisation in patients with occipital infarction. Journal of Neurology, Neurosurgery and Psychiatry 47: 153–158

Röver J, Bach M 1987 Pattern electroretinogram plus visual evoked potential: a decisive test in patients suspected of malingering. Documenta Ophthalmologica 66: 245–251

Rubens A B, Benson D F 1971 Associative visual agnosia. Archives of Neurology 24: 305–316

Russell W R, Whitty C W M 1955 Studies in traumatic epilepsy. 3. Visual fits. Journal of Neurology, Neurosurgery and Psychiatry 18: 79–96

Russo M, Vignolo L A 1967 Visual figure-ground discrimination in patients with unilateral cerebral disease. Cortex 3: 113–127

Schacter D L 1992 Implicit knowledge: new perspectives on unconscious processes. Proceedings of the National Academy of Science 89: 1113–1117

Schultz G, Melzack R 1991 The Charles Bonnet syndrome: 'phantom visual images'. Perception 20: 809–825

Schultz G, Melzack R 1993 Visual hallucinations and mental state. A study of 14 Charles Bonnet syndrome hallucinators. Journal of Nervous and Mental Disease 181: 639–643

Sergent J, Poncet M 1990 From covert to overt recognition of faces in a prosopagnosic patient. Brain 113: 989–1004

Sergent J, Signoret J I 1992a Functional and anatomical decompensation of face processing: evidence from prosopagnosia and PET study of normal subjects. Philosophical Transactions of the Royal Society of London Series B: Biology 335: 55–61

Sergent J, Signoret J I 1992b Varieties of functional deficits in prosopagnosia. Cerebral Cortex 2: 375–388

Sergent J, Signoret J I 1992c Implicit access to knowledge derived from unrecognized faces in prosopagnosia. Cerebral Cortex 2: 389–400

Sergent J, Ohta S, MacDonald B 1992 Functional neuroanatomy of face and object processing. Brain 115: 15–36

Shedlack K J, McDonald W M, Laskowitz D T, Krishnan K R 1994 Geniculocalcarine hyperintensities on brain magnetic resonance with visual hallucinations in the elderly. Psychiatry Research 54: 283–293

Siekert R G, Millikan C H 1955 Syndrome of intermittent inefficiency of the basilar arterial system. Neurology 5: 625–630

Silverman S M, Bergman P S, Bender M B 1961 The dynamics of transient cerebral blindness. Report of nine episodes following vertebral angiography. Archives of Neurology 4: 333–348

Spinnler H 1971 Deficit in associating figures and colours in brain damaged patients. Brain Research 31: 30–31

Stoerig P 1993 Sources of blindsight. Science 261: 493–495

Stoerig P, Cowey A 1992 Wavelength discrimination in blindsight. Brain 115: 425–444

Takahashi N, Kawamura M, Hirayama K, Shiota J, Isono O 1995 Prosopagnosia: a clinical and anatomical study of four patients. Cortex 31: 317–329

Teuber H L, Weinstein S 1956 Ability to discover hidden figures after cerebral lesions. Archives of Neurology and Psychiatry 76: 369–379

Teuber H L, Battersby W S, Bender M B 1960 Visual field defects after penetrating missile wounds of the brain. Harvard University Press, Cambridge, Massachusetts

Teunisse R J, Zitman F G, Raes D C 1994 Clinical evaluation of 14 patients with the Charles Bonnet syndrome (isolated visual hallucinations). Comprehensive Psychiatry 35: 70–75
Teunisse R J, Cruysberg J R, Verbeek A, Zitman F G 1995 The Charles Bonnet syndrome: a large prospective study in the Netherlands. British Journal of Psychiatry 166: 254–257
Toghi H, Watanabe K, Takahashi H 1994 Prosopagnosia without topographagnosia and object agnosia associated with a lesion confined to the right occipitotemporal region. Journal of Neurology 241: 470–474
Toglia J U 1986 Functional amaurosis: diagnostic value of electronystagmography. Neurophysiology 49: 25–35
Trescher J H, Ford F R 1937 Colloid cyst of the third ventricle. Archives of Neurology and Psychiatry 37: 959–973
Tzavaras A, Hécaen H 1970 Color vision disturbances in subjects with unilateral cortical lesions. Brain Research 24: 546–547
Tzavaras A, Hécaen H, Le Bras H 1970 The problem of specificity of deficit of human face recognition in unilateral hemispheric lesions. Neuropsychologia 8: 403–416
Tzavaras A, Hécaen H, Le Bras 1971 Disorders of color vision after unilateral cortical lesions. Revue Neurologique 124: 396–402
Ungerleider L G, Haxby J V 1994 "What" and "where" in the human brain. Current Opinion in Neurobiology 4: 157–165
Verslegers W, De Deyn P P, Saerens J et al 1991 Slow progressive bilateral posterior artery infarction presenting as agitated delirium, complicated with Anton's syndrome. European Neurology 31: 216–219
Vincent F M, Sadowsky C H, Saunders R L, Reeves A G 1977 Alexia without agraphia, hemianopia, or color-naming defect: a disconnection syndrome. Neurology 27: 689–691
Walsh F B, Hoyt W F 1969 The visual sensory system: anatomy, physiology, and topographic diagnosis. In: Vinken P J, Bruyn G W (eds) Handbook of clinical neurology. North-Holland, Amsterdam, vol 2, ch 19
Walsh K W 1991 Understanding brain damage. A primer of neuropsychological evaluation, 2nd edn. Churchill Livingstone, Edinburgh
Warrington E K 1962 The completion of visual forms across hemianopic field defects. Journal of Neurology, Neurosurgery, and Psychiatry 25: 208–217
Warrington E K 1984 Visual deficits associated with occipital lobe lesions. Paper presented to advanced course in neuropsychology, British Postgraduate Medical Federation, Institute of Neurology, London, 10–13 July
Warrington E K, James M 1967 An experimental investigation of facial recognition in patients with cerebral lesions. Cortex 3: 317–326
Weisberg L A, Wall M 1987 Alexia without agraphia: clinical-computed tomographic correlations. Neuroradiology 29: 283–286
Weiskrantz L 1990 Outlooks for blindsight: explicit methodologies for implicit processes. Proceedings of the Royal Society of London B: Biological Sciences 239 (1296): 247–278
Weiskrantz L 1993 Sources of blindsight. Science 26: 493–495
Weiskrantz L 1996 Blindsight revisited. Current Opinions in Neurobiology 6: 215–220
Weiskrantz L, Warrington E K, Sanders M D, Marshall J 1974 Visual capacity in the hemianopic field following a restricted occipital ablation. Brain 97: 709–728
Weiskrantz L, Barbur J L, Sahraie A 1995 Parameters affecting conscious versus unconscious discrimination with damage to the visual cortex (VI). Proceedings of the National Academy of Sciences of the United States of America 92: 6122–6126
Whiteley A M, Warrington E K 1977 Prosopagnosia: A clinical, psychological and anatomical study of three patients. Journal of Neurology, Neurosurgery and Psychiatry 40: 395–403
Williams D, Gassel M M 1962 Visual function in patients with homonymous hemianopia. Part 1. The visual fields. Brain 85: 175–250
Williams M 1970 Brain damage and the mind. Penguin, Harmondsworth, Middlesex
Williamson P D, Thadani V M, Darcey T M et al 1992 Occipital lobe epilepsy: clinical characteristics, seizure spread patterns, and results of surgery. Annals of Neurology 31: 3–13
Wilson B A, Davidoff J 1993 Partial recovery from visual object agnosia: a 10 year follow-up study. Cortex 29: 529–542

Wolpert I 1924 Die Simultanagnosie. Störung der Gesamtauffassung. Zeitschrift für die Gesamte Neurologie und Psychiatrie 93: 397–415

Yin R K 1970 Face recognition by brain-injured patients: dissociable ability. Neuropsychologia 8: 395–402

Young A W, de Haan E H, Newcombe F 1990 Unawareness of impaired face recognition. Brain and Cognition 14: 1–18

Zihl J 1980 'Blindsight': Improvement of visually guided eye movements by systematic practice in patients with cerebral blindness. Neuropsychologia 18: 71–77

8

Hemispheric asymmetry

THE CONCEPT OF CEREBRAL DOMINANCE

The most significant discovery leading to the notion of cerebral dominance was the finding by Dax, Broca and others of a strong relationship between lesions of the left hemisphere and disorders of language, namely disorders of expression, comprehension, reading and writing. For many people the concept of cerebral dominance remained confined to the lateral specialization for language, at least until recent times. However, there were notable exceptions. One of these was the great English neurologist Hughlings Jackson. In 1864, i.e. not long after Broca's first report, Jackson commented 'If, then it should be proved by wider evidence that the faculty of expression resides in one hemisphere, there is no absurdity in raising the question as to whether perception – its corresponding opposite – may not be seated in the other'.

Benton (1965) pointed out that extension of the concept of dominance beyond the sphere of language seemed to be required by the findings of Liepmann and Gerstmann in the early part of the present century. Liepmann had first described apraxia as 'the inability to perform a skilled act or series of movements, this disability occurring within the setting of preserved comprehension and adequate sensory and neuromuscular capacity' (Benton 1965, p. 334). A particular form of this disorder, termed ideomotor apraxia, Liepmann found to be associated with lesions of the left hemisphere. In this disorder the patient was unable to carry out a skilled act on verbal command. Subsequent reviews have supported Liepmann's notion that ideomotor apraxia is associated exclusively with lesions of the left hemisphere. Gerstmann's 'syndrome' has been discussed in Chapter 6 and, despite the doubtful status of the syndrome itself, there is no doubt about the strong association of each of the component symptoms or signs with disorders of the left hemisphere – and their almost complete absence in right hemisphere disease.

While these findings enriched the range of disorders associated with lesions of the left hemisphere, it has been argued that both ideomotor apraxia and the Gerstmann symptoms may be conceptualized as due to a language deficit (Poeck & Orgass 1966, Brewer 1969). Brewer reminds us of the evidence showing that many 'ostensibly non-verbal tasks' are verbally encoded by the subject, so that failure on such a task is only enlightening when we are sure how the subject normally goes about the task. 'Thus, given the current state of knowledge, it is possible to hold the extreme hypothesis, that all tasks showing left-hemispheric dominance are due to an underlying linguistic deficit' (Brewer 1969).

For a long time many neurologists, while accepting the evidence for lateralization of language, were unwilling to admit that the other hemisphere, often termed 'minor' or non-dominant, might also have areas of specialization in which it excelled. Several converging lines of evidence have made it clear that the right hemisphere does, indeed, have such distinctive functions. Zangwill (1961) was one of the first to assemble evidence on the functions of the minor hemisphere and defined the principle of cerebral dominance as follows:

> As ordinarily understood, this principle states that certain higher functions, in particular speech, are differentially represented in the two hemispheres – and are liable to be disturbed, predominantly if not exclusively, by damage to one alone. Further, it has long been accepted that the dominant hemisphere is typically that contralateral to the preferred hand – though many exceptions to this rule are known, particularly among the left handed. (p. 51)

This question of the relationship between lateral hand preference and hemispheric dominance for language has only recently become clarified and will be considered first. This will be followed by the principal lines of evidence which have led to a clearer understanding of the functioning of the two hemispheres. These include the evidence from: (i) naturally occurring cerebral lesions including agenesis or absence of the corpus callosum; (ii) commissurotomy studies; and (iii) hemispherectomy. The chapter concludes with a brief consideration of the concept of cerebral dominance in the light of this knowledge.

Many of the areas of function have been the subject of experimental studies contained in books and journals in the growing specialty of cognitive neuropsychology.

Hand preference and cerebral dominance

Very soon after the introduction of the concept of dominance with the classic formulation that the left hemisphere was dominant in right-handed individuals and vice versa, numerous exceptions were found to the second half of the formula. Study of right-handed aphasics revealed well over 90% to have lesions in the left hemisphere. On the other hand, numerous studies of left-handed aphasics, while varying somewhat in their findings, have tended to show a much lower proportion of left hemisphere lesions and a higher proportion of right hemisphere lesions than in the right-handed groups. Even in groups of left-handed individuals, the left hemisphere appears to be the site of the lesion in 60% or more of the cases. There is also evidence to show that often (but certainly not always) aphasia tends to be less severe and prolonged in left-handed cases (Chesher 1936, Conrad 1949).

Such facts have been thought by some to reflect a bilateral representation of speech in left-handers (Subirana 1958, Zangwill 1960). Support for such a contention comes from the examination of left-handers using the Wada technique (see below).

Benton (1965) points out that the category of left-handedness poses a number of problems if one is to utilize such a category for correlation with pathology. Some 'left-handers' are indeed more skilful with their left hand than with the right and employ it for preference. Other 'left-handers' in fact both employ the right hand more and are more skilled with it. A third and much larger category is much closer to ambidexterity. This fact is in keeping with studies such as that of Hellige et al (1994) which show that non-right-handers show fewer performance asymmetries on a variety of auditory and visual processing tasks. Moreover, even in right-handers, performance asymmetry varied from task to task and between individuals suggesting the need for care when using simple classifications of individuals' asymmetry of function.

The Wada technique

The introduction of the intracarotid sodium amytal test by Wada (1949) has allowed a more definitive statement to be made on the lateral representation of speech. This technique has been extensively employed at the Montreal Neurological Institute where several hundred cases have been studied, the injections on the right and left sides being carried out on separate days. Most of the subjects have been under consideration for surgery and the greater number were left-handed or ambidextrous patients together with a smaller number of right-handed patients for whom the lateralization of language was in doubt (Branch et al 1964, Milner et al 1966, Milner 1974).

In the first report there was a marked difference between the findings for right-handed and non-right-handed patients (Table 8.1).

Several points emerge clearly from these findings. Firstly, there is an absence of bilateral representation in right-handed subjects. Secondly, there is a difference in lateralization between the two non-right-handed groups. The left-handed group has a high percentage of right hemisphere representation and a small percentage of bilateral representation, while the ambidextrous group has by far the highest percentage of bilateral representation and a much smaller percentage of right hemisphere speech representation. Grouped together, the total non-right-handers showed 48% of left, 38% of right and 14% of bilateral representation.

A closer examination showed a further difference when the non-right-handed group was divided into those having clinical evidence of early left hemisphere damage (within the first 5 years of life) and those without.

Table 8.1 Relationship of handedness to speech lateralization (from Branch et al 1964)

Handedness	No. of cases	Speech representation		
		Left	**Bilateral**	**Right**
Left	51	22 (43%)	4 (8%)	25 (49%)
Ambidextrous	20	12 (60%)	6 (30%)	2 (10%)
Right	48	43 (90%)	0 —	5 (10%)

Table 8.2 Handedness and carotid-amytal speech lateralization (from Milner 1974)

Handedness	No. of cases	Speech representation		
		Left	Bilateral	Right
Right	95	87 (92%)	1 (1%)	7 (7%)
Left or ambidextrous				
Without early left hemisphere damage	74	51 (69%)	10 (13%)	13 (18%)
With early left hemisphere damage	43	13 (30%)	7 (16%)	23 (54%)

The difference between the two non-right-handed groups seems to imply that in some cases at least the left-handedness is a reflection of early left hemisphere damage. Milner (1974) also drew attention to the 'impressive tendency for speech to become organized in the left hemisphere'; some two thirds of normal left-handers have speech representation in the left hemisphere and even 30% of those left-handers with gross early damage to the left hemisphere still have the major representation of language on the left side (Table 8.2).

Despite the transfer of language to the right hemisphere after early brain damage the language ability in such patients remains restricted (Helmstaedter et al 1994).

Warrington and Pratt (1973), in examining transient aphasia following electroconvulsive therapy applied unilaterally, found strong confirmation for predominant language representation in the left hemisphere in about 70% of left-handers (Lansdell 1962). Hécaen and Sauguet (1972) have examined the differential characteristics of aphasia in left-handers according to the side of the lesion. Left-handers with left hemisphere lesions tend to have aphasic disturbances as happens with right-handers. However, they have a lower frequency for comprehension and writing defects and a higher frequency for reading difficulties. Disturbances of other functions from left hemisphere lesions, e.g. disorders of calculation, perception and praxis, are similar in the two groups. With right hemisphere lesions, left-handed patients, unlike right-handed, have a high frequency of disturbance of language both oral and written, while the disorders of calculation, perception and praxis are again similar in the two groups.

These authors also found a difference between left-handers according to the presence or absence of left-handedness in the family history. In those with a positive familial history of sinistrality, language disturbances occurred with similar frequency with either left or right hemisphere lesions, whereas language disturbances were almost absent with right hemisphere lesions where there was no familial history of left-handedness.

The importance of a family history of sinistrality in relation to laterality differences in both right- and left-handers has been reported for both auditory and visual perception (Zurif & Bryden 1969, Hines & Satz 1971).

Lansdell (1962) found that not only did the right hemisphere become dominant for speech in some cases of early left hemisphere damage, but that this right hemisphere also became involved with the verbal factor in intelligence.

These few facts merely serve to introduce the general question of hand preference and cerebral asymmetry. More extensive treatments have been provided by Subirana (1969) and Levy (1974a).

Morphological asymmetry

Morphological asymmetry of the human brain had been observed for nearly a century but with the publication of Geschwind and Levitsky's paper in 1968, demonstrating that the superior surface of the temporal lobe (planum temporale) was usually greater on the left side, there was a sudden growth of studies of morphological asymmetry involving sundry anatomical methods as well as a variety of the newly developing imaging techniques which could be employed without risk in the living subject (e.g. Musolino & Dellatolas 1991, Schlaug et al 1995).

No doubt the interest in asymmetry was fuelled by the rapidly growing interest in neuropsychology, since the brain area in question was closely allied to Wernicke's area related to language comprehension. Confirmation of the temporal planum finding has been strong (e.g. Galaburda et al 1978a, b) and other evidence supporting the notion of a language dominant hemisphere soon emerged (Le May & Culebras 1972, Rubens et al 1976, Falzi et al 1982) together with the description of numerous structural differences, such as the greater length of the left hemisphere, which were outlined in the early paper of Le May (1976) and confirmed with CT methodology (Le May & Kido 1978). These asymmetries are evident in the later weeks of gestation (Wada et al 1975), as well as in the newborn (Witelson & Pallie 1973). For a concise summary see Bradshaw and Nettleton (1983).

Several theories linking asymmetry of structure and function have been put forward but no single explanation is adequate at present. Certainly, morphological asymmetry alone seems inadequate to explain the major fact, namely that some 96% of right-handed individuals have language control in their left hemisphere. Moreover, despite anatomic differences, physiological studies of brain activity concurrent with complex psychological functions show increased activity in several areas of each hemisphere, and this is as true for speech as it is for other functions. In recent times, a study of cerebral asymmetry using MRI in cases where the Wada test has given direct evidence of language lateralization, has shown the complexity of the relationships (Charles et al 1994).

The remainder of the chapter is devoted to a sample of some of the main areas that have extended our knowledge of functional asymmetry between the hemispheres. Attempts at replication have not always been successful or have occasionally produced findings which are opposed to any simple theory which would attempt to cover all cases (see Fischer et al 1991), and serious methodological flaws have been highlighted by such analytical papers as that of Soper et al (1988).

UNILATERAL LESION STUDIES

No attempt has been made to present an exhaustive coverage of lesion studies related to asymmetry of hemispheric function. However, most of the principal areas are outlined and these may be supplemented by reviews such as those of

Mountcastle (1962), Hécaen (1969), Subirana (1969), Milner (1971), Benton (1972), Dimond and Beaumont (1974), Kinsbourne and Smith (1974), Schmitt and Worden (1974) and Joynt and Goldstein (1975), and numerous textbooks of neuropsychology.

In reviewing lesion studies there is a tendency to concentrate on lateral differences rather than similarities in function. This often leads to a devaluation of the role of one of the hemispheres in the particular function under scrutiny. Before beginning our review of the evidence for separate functions attributed to each hemisphere, it would be wise to remember that there is no convincing evidence for absolute control of any complex psychological process by either hemisphere. 'The idea of cerebral dominance for a function must be revised, since it appears that there may only be a hemispheric preponderance rather than dominance for a certain behaviour. Thus there are relative rather than absolute contributions from the two hemispheres. This makes it more imminent that we categorise behaviour in its component operations if we wish to make sense out of localisation studies on brain behavior correlations' (Joynt & Goldstein 1975, p. 172).

Visual perception and asymmetry

The following is a sample of the very large amount of information which has accumulated since the 1960s about the asymmetry of function of the hemispheres with relation to visual perception. A good deal of it tends to support the hypothesis of a special role for the minor hemisphere which is the complement of the left hemisphere's specialization in verbal symbolic processes, though both hemispheres carry a role in most functions.

Figure-ground discrimination

While studying perceptual deficits after penetrating missile wounds, Poppelreuter (1917) developed the overlapping figures test. The subject is required to demonstrate the ability to name or outline a number of figures in overlapping drawings (Fig. 8.1) or to select from a number of alternatives the complex figure in which a simpler figure has been 'embedded' (Fig. 8.2).

A number of studies of soldiers with penetrating missile wounds (Poppelreuter 1917, Goldstein 1927, Teuber et al 1951), as well as patients with cerebral tumours (Battersby et al 1953), have shown that difficulty with tasks like the Gottschaldt Hidden Figure Test is a common accompaniment of cerebral lesions. Subsequently, Teuber and Weinstein (1956) and Russo and Vignolo (1967) demonstrated an association of this defect with the presence of aphasia. The latter study compared patients with unilateral right and left lesions with each other and with controls. The presence of aphasia and of visual field defects was checked in each case. While there was a significant association with both the presence and severity of language disorders, visual field defects did not affect scores significantly. Furthermore, considered as single groups, the left and right hemisphere cases did not appear to differ. However, right brain damaged patients did significantly worse than non-aphasic left brain damaged patients, these latter performing very much like the control subjects. Russo and Vignolo suggest that poor performance may be related to the impairment of at least two specific abilities, namely a language

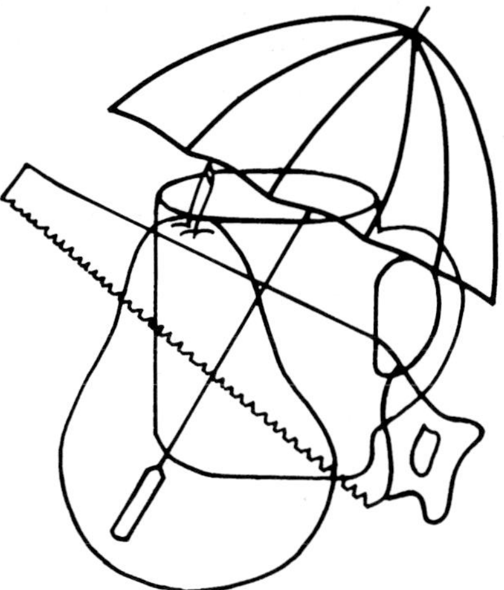

Fig. 8.1 Overlapping drawings test (after Poppelreuter 1917).

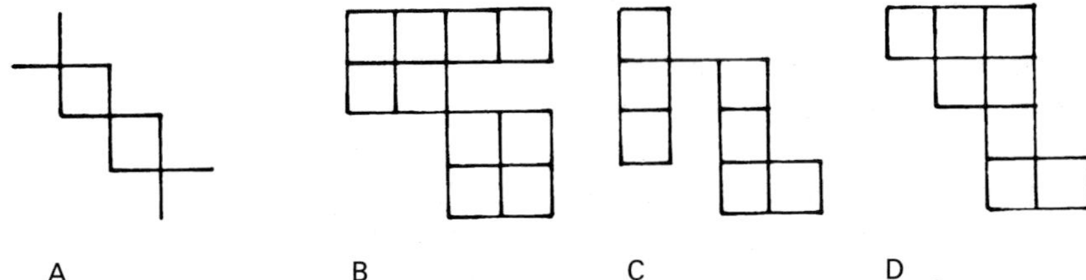

Fig. 8.2 Typical item in embedded figures test. Figure A is embedded in B and D but not in C.

ability and a perceptual factor, the latter being 'preferentially subserved' by the right hemisphere. Poeck et al (1973) confirmed the finding of a disturbance on the Gottschaldt test with lesions of either hemisphere. They suggest that there is a 'common underlying functional disturbance of the visuospatial type associated with the retrorolandic part of both hemispheres'. They point to the evidence from both normal and commissurotomy subjects (see below) which shows that different forms of information processing are utilized by the two hemispheres, i.e. 'non-verbal strategy predominates in visual information processing, unless there is a specific requirement for inner verbalization'. Such complex determination of performance on what appears at first to be a relatively simple perceptual task highlights the care which must be taken in interpreting the findings of lesion studies.

Rubino (1970) extended the knowledge of lateralization in visual perception by greatly reducing the meaningfulness of both 'verbal' and figural material and comparing the performance of left temporal, right temporal and normal control subjects. The verbal material consisted of consonant-vowel-consonant trigrams (CVC), while the non-verbal visual material consisted of randomly generated figures, both sets of stimuli having low association value (meaning). The left temporal group showed a deficit in identification of the nonsense syllables, while the right showed a deficit with the unfamiliar figures. Thus, there appears to be a relation between efficiency of visual recognition, the nature of the visual material and laterality of the lesion.

Facial recognition

Numerous clinical studies have supported the poorer performance of patients with right posterior lesions on tests of facial recognition. These are cited in Chapter 7 in relation to prosopagnosia. It is worth repeating that this latter disorder is seen only with bilateral lesions.

Visuospatial perception

Over the past 50 years a very large number of studies have produced evidence for the relatively greater importance of the right than the left hemisphere for the perception of spatial relationships. The following is a representative sample of earlier significant papers: Paterson and Zangwill (1944); McFie et al (1950); Ettlinger et al (1957); Piercy et al (1960); Milner (1965); Whitty and Newcombe (1965); Warrington and James (1967); Newcombe (1969) and Warrington and Rabin (1970); while summaries are provided by Benton (1982), De Renzi (1982), Young (1983) and Ratcliff (1987). Much of the relevant material has been reviewed in Chapter 6. A few further points might be made.

In order to establish the exact nature of the visuospatial defect which appears to be associated with right posterior lesions it is necessary to show dissociation of the defect from others, e.g. the study of Taylor and Warrington (1973) demonstrates that while patients with right posterior lesions are inferior to other groups on a spatial task of position discrimination they are not inferior on other discrimination tasks such as size and shape. Such studies will help to specify more precisely the nature of the defect.

A second factor which clouds the issue of what is lateralized is the degree of complexity of the task, hence the degree to which sundry factors dependent on different sites (and hemispheres) may enter into the performance. Many of the tasks mentioned in Chapter 6 involve space perception at a rather complex level. De Renzi et al (1971) pointed out that this makes it difficult 'to disentangle the influence on performance of spatial as compared with praxic, intelligence and memory factors'. These authors found that with a very simple test, such as visual (or tactile) judgment of the orientation of a single rod in space, only the right posterior group performed poorly, other brain damaged groups performing very much like controls. Also the fact that there was no significant difference in effect for the different sense modalities stresses the truly 'spatial' nature of the defect. 'It appears, therefore, that when a spatial perception is tested at a very basic and simple level…there is almost a complete dominance of the posterior region of the so-called minor hemisphere. These results must be contrasted with the less striking asymmetry of function shown in more complex spatial tasks – for example, route finding, copying drawings, block designs – that are failed also by patients with damage to the left posterior area' (p. 489). Other studies (Warrington & Rabin 1970, Benton et al 1975) support the importance of the right posterior region in the judgment of orientation and a simple standardized test is now available (Benton et al 1978, 1983).

Miller (1972) reminds us that 'it may well be that the important factor in determining whether an apparently spatial task is affected by left posterior lesions as well as right is the degree of verbal mediation used by the subject. Although a task may be spatial in nature, this does not prevent a subject from using verbal reasoning in its solution and to the extent that this occurs the task will be more liable to disruption by left-sided lesions even though the task may be particularly difficult to verbalize' (pp. 86–87).

The issue of task complexity has been handled by Orgass et al (1972) in a different manner. They began by looking at factor analytic studies of visual cognitive processes in normal subjects and then selected tests related to the three most consistently found factors. The three factors were: (i) speed of visual closure (Street's Figure Completion Test); (ii) flexibility of visual closure (Gottschaldt Embedded Figures Test); and (iii) perceptual speed (form recognition test). Performance on these tests was then related to the lobar and hemispheric locations of lesions, and the presence of aphasia and visual field defects (VFD). The presence of field defects can be taken to indicate the presence of a posterior hemispheric lesion. In keeping with other studies cited above, aphasia was related to factor (ii) (Gottschaldt's Test), while there was no significant relation to laterality, location or presence of field defects. However, the combination of a right-sided lesion with the presence of a visual field defect gave significant impairment of the other two factors, namely speed of closure and speed of recognition. Since neither laterality nor presence of VFD was alone significant, the authors concluded that 'the presence of VFD in the patient with right sided lesions does not act on test performance as a defect in visual function but stands for a critical localization of lesion'.

Finally, Ratcliff and Newcombe (1973) pointed out that a distinction should be made between visuospatial tasks such as those cited above, where subjects can explore spatial relations without any major changes in their position, and tests such as Semmes' locomotor map-reading task (Ch. 6) which measure subjects' topographical orientation ability in a dynamic situation. Using a 'static' task of the first kind they confirmed the expected inferior performance of those with right posterior lesions. However, on the 'dynamic' map-reading task those with unilateral posterior lesions and bilateral frontal lesions were unimpaired, only patients with bilateral posterior lesions showing a lowered performance. They suggest that while the right hemisphere obviously plays an important role in spatial perception 'it does not bear exclusive responsibility for the maintenance of spatial orientation'. The locus of the lesion related to topographical orientation is unclear and may be clarified by the specification of task variables as well as clarification of concepts of personal or egocentric versus extra-personal space along the lines of the study by Butters and colleagues (1972). Certainly disorder of topographical orientation has been described after both left and right frontal lesions (Marie & Behague 1919, Marie et al 1924) as well as with right, left and bilateral posterior lesions (Kleist 1934, Brain 1941, Paterson & Zangwill 1945, Cogan 1960, De Renzi & Faglioni 1962, Hécaen 1969).

The precise factors which the left hemisphere contributes to various forms of spatial processing continue to be elaborated by the Oxford group with their stable population of patients with lateral lesions (Mehta et al 1987, Newcombe et al 1987, 1989, Mehta & Newcombe 1991).

Tactile perception

Somatosensory changes

The most extensive study of somatosensory changes after lesions in various parts of the cerebrum is that of Semmes and her colleagues (1960). These workers examined a large number of patients with brain injuries caused by penetrating missiles in wartime and employed a wide range of measures such as two-point threshold, point localization and pressure sensitivity. One of their findings has relevance to the question of asymmetry of function, namely that they described some bilateral somatosensory deficits after lesions of the left hemisphere but only contralateral deficits after lesions of the right hemisphere. Since this finding has been reported in a number of places it should be pointed out that the differences found were small and did not reach statistical significance and that subsequent workers have not confirmed it, though there has been only a small amount of work done in this field.

Sensory dominance

In the study of Semmes et al (1960), right-handed subjects tended to show a differential sensitivity to pressure stimulation, being more sensitive to pressure on the contralateral (left) hand than on the right. In a subsequent study, Weinstein and Sersen (1961) showed that this 'sensory dominance' varied in a complex manner with the patient's familial history of handedness. Thus lateral hand preference and 'sensory dominance' are not inextricably related. The situation is analogous to crossed aphasia occurring with right hemisphere lesions in some right-handed subjects. It is important to state the nature of the function being affected when employing the term dominance since the present evidence shows that cerebral dominance cannot be a unitary function.

Size discrimination

Tactual size discrimination was found by Teuber and Rudel (1962) to be affected by lesions in either hemisphere, but more frequently with right-sided lesions. The deficit appeared to be independent of sensory loss, but was more severe if this was present.

The information from penetrating missile wounds needs to be interpreted with caution because of the somewhat uncertain nature and extent of the lesions. Another major source has been the study of patients undergoing restricted resection of cortical tissue for epilepsy (Corkin 1964, Corkin et al 1964). Sensory defects appeared to be strictly related to damage to the pre- and postcentral gyri and were mostly for the contralateral side of the body. However localization by the patient of a point on the patient's body touched by the examiner (point localization) showed bilateral effects with unilateral lesions.

Astereognosis

This defect is the inability to appreciate the identity of three-dimensional objects by touch. As with other forms of agnosia this disorder should by definition occur in the absence of sensory loss. The existence of pure astereognosis must be seriously in question in view of Corkin's finding that impairment of tactile object recognition occurred only in those cases with sensory deficits caused by lesions in the vicinity of the central sulcus. Semmes' findings on patients with missile wounds were less clear (Semmes 1965), though she agreed that astereognosis was probably not a clinical entity. She employed tests of roughness, texture and size, together with tests of tactile shape discrimination, in examining patients with right hemisphere, left hemisphere and bilateral lesions. Deficits of shape discrimination were noted with and without the presence of sensory defect. These deficits were related to spatial orientation 'even when this was assessed by a purely visual task'. This finding suggested that shape discrimination may depend on a general spatial factor as well as on the integrity of somatic sensation. Where both factors are affected the disorder is likely to be severe. Semmes' evidence suggested that the factors were organized in a different way in the two hemispheres, though this has not been clarified in the ensuing period.

In contrast to the apparently greater impact of left hemisphere lesions on the sensory system than right hemisphere lesions, Weinstein (1965) found the reverse to be true of the motor system. Using a test of finger movement ('finger oscillation'), he found that lesions of the right hemisphere near the central sulcus tended to produce bilateral slowing with a more marked contralateral effect, whereas left central lesions resulted in contralateral slowing only.

Other studies have lent weight to the greater importance of the right hemisphere in tactile perception.

Auditory perception

Asymmetry effects in auditory perception were treated in Chapter 5. The principal thrust of the evidence demonstrates the superior processing of speech sounds by the left hemisphere and of non-linguistic stimuli by the right. Research with the dichotic listening task proliferated so rapidly that two issues of the journal (1, No. 4 and 2, No. 5) were devoted to this topic. An extensive review of the literature and critical review of theories relating hemisphere specialization for speech and ear advantages was provided by Geffen and Quinn (1984).

Temporal order

The perception of temporal order has been the subject of only few studies in brain impaired individuals (Efron, 1963a, b, Carmon 1971) and even in these studies, perceptual and amnesic processes were possibly confounded. One study (Carmon & Nachson 1971) seems to have shown a clear-cut difference between lateralized lesion groups. Those with left hemisphere lesions were significantly impaired in the identification of the order of both visual and auditory stimuli as compared with normal controls and those with right hemisphere lesions. Efron speculated that speech might be mediated by the left hemisphere because of its serial rather than its linguistic nature. As Poeck (1985) comments: 'The role of temporal analysis in the aphasic language disturbance is still an open question, as is the clinical significance of the fact that the temporal lobe is the "temporal" lobe' (p. 47).

The left hemisphere, particularly the frontal lobe, also plays a major role in judging the relative recency of two events and in programming the order of things (see Ch. 4).

The right hemisphere and communication

Discussion of the role of the right hemisphere in language often turns around evidence derived from the capacities of the isolated non-dominant hemisphere following commissurotomy or hemispherectomy. However, a growing source of interest is the disruption of language or language related skills occasioned by lesions of the right hemisphere itself. Occasionally, cases show clinical evidence of a clear aphasia (Primavera & Bandini 1993, Bakar et al 1996), even a classical Broca's aphasia (Rey et al 1994), with functional imaging showing restriction of the lesion to the right hemisphere.

Apart from the rare cases of *crossed aphasia*, language deficits with right-sided lesions have been described for over 30 years (Critchley 1962, Eisenson 1962), but more recently experimental studies (e.g. Wapner et al 1981) have begun to specify the difficulties such patients have with complex linguistic or ideational materials. While perfectly adequate on traditional tests of aphasia, patients with right hemisphere lesions may have trouble with processing the extra-linguistic aspects of language. Many of our right hemisphere stroke victims would share some of the features mentioned by Wapner and her colleagues (1981, p. 17):

> Superficially, these patients seem to retain the basics of language. However, while their speech may be literally unexceptionable, clinical inspection reveals that such patients often seem to lack a full understanding of the context of an utterance, the presuppositions entailed or the tone of a conversational exchange ...difficulty...in dealing with abstract sentences, logical reasoning, and a coherent stream of thought... In addition, the language of such patients is often excessive and rambling; their comments are often off-color and their humor frequently inappropriate, they tend to focus on insignificant details or make tangential remarks; and the usual range of intonation is frequently lacking.

Such features may present a serious though ill-understood impediment to rehabilitation.

Earlier reviews of the language capabilities of the right hemisphere were published by Searleman (1977, 1983), Bradshaw and Nettleton (1983) and Ardila (1984). A recent review is that of Weekes (1995).

Memory and learning

Reference has already been made to the effects of unilateral temporal lobectomy on memory and learning in Chapter 5. Dominant temporal lobectomy leads to difficulty in the learning and retention of verbal material, whether apprehended via visual or auditory perception and whether tested by recall or recognition (Meyer & Yates 1955, Milner 1958, Blakemore & Falconer 1967, Milner 1967, Milner & Teuber 1968). Resection of the non-dominant temporal lobe leads to difficulties with non-verbal material both visual and auditory. 'Non-verbal' in this sense can be taken to mean those stimuli which are difficult to encode verbally (Kimura 1963, Milner 1968). Milner has also shown that patients with right temporal removals have difficulty with visually or proprioceptively guided maze learning (Corkin 1965, Milner 1965).

Apart from the temporal lobectomy material, only a few studies have concerned themselves directly with laterality and memory. De Renzi and Spinnler (1966) tested patients with lateralized lesions on two tasks of the recognition of familiar figures, one immediate and the other delayed. The registration of familiar visual patterns in this study did appear to be related to the left hemisphere. In the delayed memory test, poor performance was related to the presence of aphasia.

Boller and De Renzi (1967) compared 60 patients with left hemisphere damage with 40 patients with right hemisphere damage on two visual tasks, one easily verbalized (meaningful) and one not easily verbalized (meaningless). The left hemisphere patients were inferior on both tasks, though when the scores were adjusted for the scores obtained on two language tasks, the difference between the left and right groups decreased. The importance of aphasia in lowering the scores appeared to be about as great for the meaningless task as for the meaningful. The authors interpret this as showing 'that, whenever possible, patients try to transform meaningless figures into meaningful ones'.

Warrington and Rabin (1971) used a recognition task of recurring figures similar to that devised by Kimura (1963) and found no significant difference between left and right hemisphere groups, though there was a trend in the predicted direction, right hemisphere patients tending to perform more poorly than left. A consideration of other factors tended to suggest that while temporal and right parietal patients were equally impaired on the recognition memory task the deficit had an amnesic basis in the temporal group and a perceptual basis in the parietal group.

Emotional functions

Two forms of emotional reaction have been described with lateralized lesions. These are particularly evident during certain examinations when the patient is confronted with failure. The first type of emotional response was termed 'the catastrophic reaction' by Goldstein (1939) who noted that it was particularly associated with dominant hemisphere lesions. Goldstein noted that these reactions were 'not only "inadequate" but also disordered, inconstant, inconsistent and embedded in physical and mental shock'. The patient appears not only emotionally distressed but develops signs of incipient physical collapse such as pallor and sweating. It is important to recognize the onset of this catastrophic reaction since, apart from the patient's comfort, performances may be further reduced for some time afterwards and a true picture of the patient's present capacities may not be elicited. '...after a catastrophic reaction his reactivity is likely to be impeded for a longer or shorter interval. He becomes more or less unresponsive and fails even in those tasks which he could easily meet under other circumstances. The disturbing after-effect of catastrophic reactions is long enduring' (Goldstein 1939, p. 37).

The second type of emotional response was originally noted by Babinski (1914) who reported the lack of awareness, indifference, or denial of hemiplegia, particularly of the left side (see *anosognosia*, Ch. 6). The reaction is seen more frequently with right-sided lesions though not exclusively (Hécaen et al 1951, Denny-Brown et al 1952). Gainotti (1972) systematically studied a large series of cases with right and left hemisphere lesions and listed the following symptoms with their association to laterality: symptoms more frequently seen with left-sided lesions were 'anxiety reactions, bursts of tears, vocative utterances, depressed renouncements, or sharp refusals to go on with the examination'. With right-sided lesions the following were more common: 'anosognosia, minimization, indifference reactions and tendency to joke, and expressions of hate towards the paralysed limb'. Gainotti strongly reinforced what had been said by Goldstein and others, namely that catastrophic reactions were found most often in aphasic subjects after repeated failure of their attempts to communicate. 'They seemed due, as Goldstein argues, to the desperate reaction of the organism, confronted with a task it cannot face.'

Further evidence for a dissociation of emotional functions between the two hemispheres comes from lesion studies and this is supported by evidence in normal subjects.

Using the MMPI, Gasparrini et al (1978) found an elevated Depression scale in 7 out of 16 patients with left hemisphere lesions but none of the 8 patients with right hemisphere lesions.

The evaluation of emotional expression appears poorer for those with right than left hemisphere lesions whether perceived visually (Benowitz et al 1983) or auditorily (Heilman et al 1975, Denes et al 1984, Darby 1993). Emotional prosodic deficits are the basis of a putative classification of right hemisphere emotional language disorders proposed by Ross, which he termed the *aprosodias* (Ross 1981, Gorelick & Ross 1987), but whose lateralizing significance is still not clear (Heilman et al 1984, Cancelliere & Kertesz 1990, Darby 1993). A retrospective evaluation of the literature by Sackeim et al (1982) revealed that pathological laughter was predominantly associated with right-sided lesions and pathological crying with left-sided lesions. Gelastic epilepsy (laughing outbursts) was more commonly associated with left-sided foci than with right. One of three patients reported by Arroyo et al (1993) had laughing outbursts with no feeling of mirth. The lesion was in the left medial frontal region with the seizure origin in the left anterior cingulate gyrus as shown by a subdural electrode. The two other cases, who suffered from complex partial seizures, had outbursts of laughter with an accompanying feeling of mirth on stimulation of the fusiform and parahippocampal gyri.

The isolated right hemisphere is more efficient than the left in evaluating visually projected emotional expression (Benowitz et al 1983).

Thus there is a variety of evidence to support a right hemisphere dominance for certain emotional functions. A more complete review was given by Gainotti (1984), who also surveyed the methodological issues. Bear (1982) felt that the fundamental deficit for the right hemisphere patient was 'a failure in emotional surveillance' and considered that it was linked with morphological asymmetries in the brain, particularly cortical-limbic connections, and the work on personality difference in epileptic patients with unilateral temporal lobe foci (see Ch. 5). Bear's theory converges with the attentional asymmetry theory of Heilman outlined earlier.

Hemispheric asymmetry in the perception of affect continues to be studied and continues to produce conflicting results. A sample of studies in the last decade reveals the complexity.

Auditory asymmetry in processing the emotional valence of music received monaurally has been shown by normal subjects (McFarland & Kennison 1989), but this asymmetry was qualified by the handedness of the subject.

EEG recordings taken from the parietal region while emotional stimuli were presented under cognitive or emotional instructional sets to normal subjects showed that the highest level of activation for the emotional condition was in the left hemisphere but the greater differentiation between the cognitive and emotional sets occurred in the right hemisphere (Smith et al 1987). The same investigators showed that the differential processing of affect was less marked in left-handed subjects (Smith et al 1990).

Studies of patients with hemisphere lesions have sometimes failed to support frequently expressed opinions about asymmetry of emotional expression. Mammucari et al (1988) demonstrated that both left and right hemisphere damaged patients showed less spontaneous facial expression to different classes of filmed material than normal subjects, but found no difference between the hemisphere groups. The same workers (Caltagirone et al 1989) found no difference between patients and controls or between hemisphere groups in the ability to pose emotional expressions.

Motor impersistence

In 1956, Fisher described a syndrome 'akin to apraxia', the central features of which were the inability to maintain the eyes closed and the tongue protruded, though these actions could be carried out adequately for a short period. The disorder was strongly associated with left hemiplegia, i.e. with lesions of the minor hemisphere and, though sometimes transient, persisted in some cases for years. This is in sharp contrast to anosognosia, with which it is frequently associated and which tends to clear relatively quickly. Some degree of mental impairment was always present. Fisher was aware that the grouping of several manifestations as a 'syndrome' needed substantiation and suggested hypotheses which might explain the several signs, e.g. failure to maintain a motor set, interference with the persistent control of a motor act, or distractibility. More recently, it has been suggested that impersistence may be associated with lowering of vigilance and sustained concentration but the question of mechanism remains open.

Though of theoretical interest, the value of impersistence as a clinical observation is minimal since it appears to be seen only in the presence of unequivocal lateralizing signs. While some studies (e.g. Hier et al 1983) have found a strong correlation between right-sided lesions and marked impersistence, others (e.g. Joynt et al 1964, Levin 1973) have not found this clear hemisphere difference. The disorder was reviewed by Joynt and Goldstein (1975).

Bilateral effects from unilateral lesions

Apart from the effects caused by permanent damage to functional systems, cerebral lesions may often bring about effects from alteration in neighbouring or remote areas. These effects may alter with time, particularly in areas adjacent to the damaged tissue, because of resolution of oedema and other reversible changes. The term diaschisis was used by von Monakow (1911) to denote functional disturbances in situations anatomically remote from the lesion. Smith (1974) stressed that the consideration of diaschisis may help to resolve some of the apparently conflicting results described in the literature, pointing to many studies of patients with unilateral vascular lesions which reveal bilateral dysfunction.

Observations such as those of Smith are not rare, for example 16 of 18 patients with left hemiplegia in a study by Belmont et al (1971) showed disruption of movement of the intact side when bilateral function was called for, but not when the movement was required only from the intact side.

Bilateral effects from unilateral lesions may involve at least three classes of effect. Firstly, there is the effect of disconnecting an association area of one hemisphere from the association cortex of the opposite side. Many examples of interhemispheric disconnection effects are provided in the later sections of this chapter. Secondly, the possibility of interference or inhibitory influences is suggested by the improvement in function following removal of pathological tissue (as mentioned in the section on hemispherectomy). Such an argument was repeated recently by Bogousslavsky (1994). Thirdly, studies have demonstrated that reduction in cerebral function may follow alteration in hemispheric blood flow. A reduction in blood flow and metabolism in both hemispheres has been shown to occur following unilateral cerebral lesions, both vascular and neoplastic in origin. A summary of evidence on diaschisis was given by Smith (1975) while Goulet and Sieroff (1995) have discussed the notion of diaschisis in relation to the interpretation of neuropsychological studies.

Attention and the right hemisphere

The concept of attention is a complex one embracing increased physiological responsiveness, preparation for action and response selectivity. Heilman (1982) has argued that the right hemisphere plays a greater role for these processes and thus can be considered dominant for attention. This would explain why neglect phenomena are seen more frequently and are more severe with right hemisphere lesions. Evidence from studies on patients with hemispheric lesions and on normal subjects is consistent with this hypothesis. The reaction time of brain damaged subjects is generally reduced with lesions of either hemisphere but right-sided lesions have shown a greater effect than those in the left hemisphere in some studies (De Renzi & Faglioni 1965, Howes & Boller 1975). On the other hand, decision making aspects of responding, such as the accuracy of responses, may be differentially affected by left hemisphere lesions (Tartaglione et al 1991).

Patients with right parieto-temporal lesions and neglect have shown less arousal when compared with patients with left hemisphere lesions with aphasia (Heilman et al 1978). Finally, Heilman and Van Den Abell (1980) tested a measure of attention in normal subjects. This consisted of presenting lateralized visual stimuli to 12 normal subjects and checking alpha desynchronization in the EEG. This phenomenon, formerly called *alpha blocking*, has been known to be an indicator of attention or orientation to a stimulus ever since the pioneering work of Berger. These normal subjects showed alpha desynchronization in the left parietal region, mainly to right-sided stimuli, but the right parietal region showed desynchronization to both right- or left-sided stimuli. Heilman (1982) offered other converging but less direct evidence in support of this proposal. More recently, similar evidence in favour of right hemisphere attentional dominance has come from PET studies (Corbetta et al 1993, Gitelman et al 1996).

Finally, there are rare cases of a pure right hemisphere syndrome occurring in non-right-handed individuals with a left-sided lesion (Padovani et al 1992).

Familiarity

One unusual claim concerning asymmetry of function is that of Van Lancker (1991), whose review proposes that the right hemisphere may play a more important role than the left in things which are of personal relevance to the subject, covering a wide range of functions including emotion, preference, familiarity and recognition of formerly relevant material.

HEMISPHERECTOMY

The operation of hemispherectomy might more correctly be termed hemidecortication, since not all the hemisphere is removed in most instances. Usually parts of the deep nuclear masses such as the thalamus and striate complex remain untouched. The nature of the operation varies according to the indication for operation, the two major conditions to date being (i) infantile hemiplegia, and (ii) extensive invasion of the hemisphere by neoplastic disease; because of the very great difference between these two types of cases they are treated separately here.

Infantile hemiplegia

The earliest report of removal of a very considerable proportion of one hemisphere for the treatment of uncontrollable epilepsy associated with hemiparesis of early onset appears to be that of McKenzie (1938). This was followed by a series reported by Krynauw from Johannesburg (1950). The complex problems posed by using such material to provide evidence about brain function is indicated by the following description of indications for operation given by Carmichael (1966) and cited in Dimond (1972). 'The patient must first of all have a hemiplegia. This should affect the arm more profoundly than the leg, and the patient usually suffers from fits which do not prove amenable to medical treatment. The patient frequently has behaviour disturbances in the nature of being difficult to handle, personality problems, temper tantrums and rages.'

The most striking feature of early reports, apart from clinical improvement, was the absence of mental deterioration that might be expected on a priori grounds from such massive removal of cortical tissue. Krynauw's first report (1950) described 12 cases with 'improvement of mentality' as adjudged by clinical evidence, though no psychometric evidence was presented in support. Cairns and Davidson (1951) reported three cases with no evidence of intellectual loss but rather an improvement in scores on tests such as the Wechsler-

Bellevue and Stanford-Binet scales. Such improvement strongly supported the frequent claim by Hebb and others mentioned earlier (see Ch. 4) that the deficits seen after operations on the brain might often result from the effect of residual pathological tissue rather than simply loss of brain substance. Presumably, where the pathological tissue was radically removed, as in the cases of hemispherectomy, there was no longer any interference effect so that residual healthy brain tissue was permitted to function at an optimal level, thus providing an explanation for the seemingly 'paradoxical' effect that the brain could perform better after hemidecortication than before. In the decade which followed, this point of view received further support in the finding that these cases of infantile hemiplegia seemed to benefit much more from complete hemispherectomy than from partial removal (McFie 1961).

One of the most influential reports was that of Basser (1962) who described the outcome in 35 cases of hemispherectomy – 17 with the left hemisphere removed and 18 with the right. 25 patients had sustained their lesions before the advent of speech and 10 after. This report showed that sensorimotor functions, praxis and language were largely preserved whichever hemisphere was removed. Thus it seemed that either hemisphere was capable of mediating most functions, though mental activity usually remained at a fairly low level with lack of drive and initiative.

Gardner et al (1955) attempted a comparison of residual function following hemispherectomy for tumour in adults and for infantile epilepsy in children, claiming more devastating deficits in the adult cases. However, data were supplied on only one infantile case. The study of McFie (1961), using small groups of patients with lesions dating from different ages, concluded that patients who sustained their lesions before 1 year of age recovered better than those injured later.

Thus there emerged a piece of neuropsychological dogma which has been endlessly restated without regard to a critical appraisal of the evidence. This dogma states that differentially better recovery can be expected the earlier the onset of injury. While many have left this as a vague generalization, others have been more specific. The age beyond which the *plasticity* might not be expected can be termed the critical period, and estimates have varied from 1 year through to 15 years (McFie 1961, Obrador 1964, Lenneberg 1967, Netley 1972, Krashen 1973). Contrary evidence, e.g. the data in Griffith and Davidson's report (1966), which appear to show better recovery for those injured after 1 year than those injured before, are seldom cited. Two long term follow-up studies are worth reporting in some detail.

The first is a case of left hemispherectomy performed for epilepsy at the age of 5½ years and reported 21 years later by Smith and Sugar (1975). This case provides impressive evidence of the brain's ability to utilize residual tissue in the remaining hemisphere as the basis for high level ability in both the verbal and non-verbal spheres. Before operation at 5½ the patient's mental age was 4.0 years, with marked speech defect but normal verbal comprehension. Four months after operation his mental age was close to his chronological age and his speech 'which earlier had been practically unintelligible, had rapidly become normal'. When tested at 8 years 8 months, his mental age was 7 years 10 months. After that time he made further progress and his scores on a wide variety of tests, both verbal and non-verbal, were in, and in some cases

Table 8.3 Test performances after left hemispherectomy (condensed from Smith & Sugar 1975)

Age	21	26½
Postoperative interval (years)	15½	21
WAIS Weighted Scores		
Information	13	16
Comprehension	19	19
Arithmetic	9	15
Similarities	12	15
Digit Span	7	9
Digit Symbol	8	10
Block Design	11	9
Picture Arrangement	10	9
Object Assembly	8	12
Verbal IQ	113	126
Performance IQ	98	102
Full scale IQ	107	116
Peabody Picture Vocabulary	125	137+
Benton Visual Retention	7	8

well above, the normal range. Some extracts from Smith and Sugar's table of his test performances 15 and 21 years after hemispherectomy are shown in Table 8.3.

In addition to these and other good performances on psychometric measures, the patient's performance in all language modalities at these two examinations was normal (speech, comprehension, reading and writing).

The second case is one studied over many years by Damasio and colleagues (1975). This patient was not a case of infantile hemiplegia, but had a normal development until the age of 5 years, at which time she sustained a severe head injury resulting in left hemiplegia. She developed left focal seizures 7 years after injury and these increased in frequency; some 13 years after injury she was showing aggressive and disturbed behaviour. Two years later right hemispherectomy was performed for frequent uncontrollable seizures. The result of surgical intervention was 'dramatic relief of intractable epilepsy, the recovery of personal independence, and...remarkable improvement of motor and sensory capabilities'. Such a case demonstrates that alternative systems may be brought into play even when the lesion has occurred as late as 5 years. Damasio et al comment: 'Removal of the right diseased hemisphere rid our patient of a squalid nuisance, stopping its deleterious effect on the rest of the brain and disclosing a normal, partially duplicated left hemisphere'. The partial duplication of function is evidenced by the patient's normal performance on a number of tasks of a visuoperceptive, visuospatial and visuoconstructive nature normally thought to be dependent upon the integrity of the right hemisphere.

It should be pointed out that the essential difference between this case and those of infantile hemiplegia is the presence of perfectly healthy tissue in both hemispheres for some years prior to a major lesion of one side. The case presents a number of other features in the adaptation after operation which need further study, but it is obvious that age of occurrence should not in itself be a contraindication to operation.

Later, St James-Roberts (1981) re-examined the available hemispherectomy data from a wide range of studies on operated cases who had sustained injury in infancy, childhood or adulthood, and found that the data failed to support the plasticity model, being explained more parsimoniously in terms of other factors.

Hemispherectomy for infantile hemiplegia has decreased with time though most reports have shown improvement after operation (French et al 1966, Breschi et al 1970, Wilson 1970, Verity et al 1982). A surgical modification (Adams 1983) that promises to minimize the late complications which led to abandonment of the operation may result in reintroduction of the procedure.

Adult hemispherectomy

The first reports of removal of most of one hemisphere for tumour were made by Dandy (1928, 1933). A case reported by Zollinger (1935) showed that not all language was lost with dominant hemispherectomy. Zollinger's patient retained an elementary vocabulary which was partially increased by speech training. No other formal neuropsychological examination was carried out partly because of the patient's adynamia or unwillingness. Death of the patient 17 days postoperatively prevented follow-up. A second case of dominant hemispherectomy reported by Crockett and Estridge (1951) survived 4 months and, although severely impaired, also showed improving capacity for speech as well as verbal comprehension.

These findings were supported by the more detailed examination of a case followed for more than 7 months by Smith (Smith 1966, Smith & Burklund 1966). Immediately after the operation the patient showed the anticipated signs of right hemiplegia, right hemianopia and severe aphasia. On later examinations the patient showed continuing recovery of language functions, not the total abolition which might have been expected on the belief that the left hemisphere played the 'dominant' role in such functions. 'Since these functions are not abolished, and since speaking, reading, writing and understanding language show continuing improvement in E.C. after left hemispherectomy, the right hemisphere apparently contributes to all these functions, although in varying proportions (i.e. receptive language functions were initially less impaired and have shown greater recovery than expressive language)' (Smith 1966, p. 470). The patient preserved the ability to sing old songs, suggesting that the right hemisphere plays an important role in this area. This finding would be in keeping with evidence from studies of restricted lesions and from brain stimulation mentioned earlier.

Smith's patient also showed preserved learning ability, as shown by an increased score of 2½ years on two testings with the Porteus Maze Test at a 10-day interval some 6 months after operation. The patient was also able to solve abstract as well as concrete mathematical problems and was close to normal on non-language tests of higher mental functions. Smith and Burklund (1966) took these good performances to indicate 'either that these functions are not exclusively or predominantly "localized" in the adult dominant hemisphere, or that, following removal of this hemisphere, the right hemisphere has the capacity to amplify previously smaller contributions to these functions…'.

A second patient followed by Smith (Burklund & Smith 1977) showed even more rapid and extensive recovery of language and singing until his rapid decline following recurrence of the tumour and death 18 months postoperatively.

A case of hemispherectomy for epilepsy of late onset described by French, Johnson and Adkins (1966) similarly supports the cases operated for tumour in demonstrating capacity for both language comprehension and some expression after removal of the so-called dominant hemisphere.

Hemispherectomy on the right (non-dominant) side has been carried out much more frequently. Early reports such as those of Dandy (1928, 1933) and Rowe (1937) commented on the sparing of intellectual ability, at least with clinical tests and the standard intelligence tests of the day. Rowe's case showed a postoperative intelligence quotient on the Stanford-Binet scale in the 'superior adult' range, not greatly different from that which she showed before operation. As with other reports there was also return of considerable motor function and some sensory function on the opposite side of the body. The mental changes noted in this case included impairment of recent memory, emotional instability and loss of inhibition. Mensh et al (1952) were impressed with the extreme variation in performance of their patient with non-dominant hemispherectomy as well as the numerous disturbances reflected in psychological tests. Though verbal facility and vocabulary remained good, their patient showed 'concreteness and perseveration of ideas, confused and psychotic-like thinking, clang associations, mingling of old and new information,...self-reference...and extremely compulsive behaviour'. Smith (1967) also noted extreme variability in one case of right and one of left hemispherectomy and pointed to this as a common finding in the clinical reports of some 40 non-dominant hemispherectomies to that time. Improvement in contralateral motor function was also frequently reported. In 1969, Smith reported on three non-dominant cases examined from 1 year to 30 years after operation. All three cases showed specific non-language defects, in keeping with similar reports by Austin and Grant (1955) and Bruell and Albee (1962). Smith notes that while impairment of language functions after dominant hemispherectomy is more severe than the deficits of non-language functions after non-dominant resection, the impairment is still 'sub-total'. 'In all reported cases, no single specialized hemispheric function was totally abolished'. The finding of relatively greater impairment (of speech) with left hemispherectomy than the impairment (non-verbal) after right hemispherectomy confirms a greater degree of specialization for speech functions.

There is a major difference between the effects of partial hemisphere lesions and hemispherectomy, which has implications for theories of brain dysfunction. This difference is seen with regard to both motor function and speech. If one assumes that a gain in function is never produced by removal of cerebral tissue, the most plausible explanation seems to be that the improvement is produced by removal of interference or inhibition. One of Smith's three cases (1969) had been totally unable to lift his leg from the bed and was barely able to move the left arm on command for 1 month before operation. Immediately after recovering from anaesthesia he promptly lifted his left leg on command. His voluntary arm movements were also improved though still impaired. Smith commented 'This suggests that the more severe or total defects in other specialized hemispheric functions or the presence of unique defects reported in certain cases with lateralized lesions may reflect interference with or inhibition of the role of the opposite hemisphere or of caudally inferior ipsilateral structures in such functions'. The presence of speech after left hemispherectomy demonstrates (though the evidence is scanty) that the non-dominant hemisphere may have limited command over the executive apparatus of speech if the inhibiting influence of the dominant hemisphere is removed. A few hints from the commissurotomy evidence in support of this notion have already been mentioned in the literature.

Finally, the report of Gott (1973) of three hemispherectomy cases, all with memory quotients below normal, suggests that two communicating hemispheres are probably necessary for normal memory functioning. The similar claim of Sperry with regard to the poor memory of some commissurotomy patients is mentioned below.

A 20-year review of the cognitive effects of hemidecortication in cases of both early onset and late onset epilepsy is given by Vargha-Khadem and Polkey (1992).

CEREBRAL COMMISSUROTOMY

Around the turn of the 20th century, neurologists had described clinical syndromes which they felt were caused by lesions of the corpus callosum. The best known of these were the syndromes of alexia without agraphia (Déjérine 1892) and that of left-hand apraxia (Liepmann 1906). The first disorder has been described in Chapter 7, and the disconnection theory argues that the syndrome is explained by an isolation of the speech areas of the left hemisphere from the right visual cortex. The second disorder was described in Chapter 3, and finds a similar explanation in terms of isolation of the dominant hemisphere language centres from the right motor cortex. Only a few reports of this kind were available until the introduction of surgical division of the corpus callosum for the prevention of the lateral spread of an epileptic discharge (van Wagenen & Herren 1940). The first commissurotomy operation involved section of the corpus callosum together with bilateral section of the fornix. The operation proved beneficial in some cases, and a considerable number of psychological studies of the effect of partial (15 cases) or complete division (9 cases) of the corpus callosum were soon reported by Akelaitis (1940, 1941a–c, 1942a, b, 1943, 1944, Akelaitis et al 1941, 1942, 1943). These were completely negative, i.e. they provided no support for the concept of a hemisphere disconnection syndrome. This state of affairs remained until Myers began the now classic studies on callosal section in animals (Myers 1955, 1956, 1959, 1961, 1965). Beginning with cats, callosal experiments continued with monkeys and chimpanzees and, finally, specially designed tests were applied by Sperry's group to human patients who had undergone division of the main commissures of the brain for the relief of epilepsy. The principal findings of the Sperry group are set out below.

In keeping with the findings of Akelaitis, split-brain animals behaved quite normally in most of their activities. However, the story was quite different if steps were taken to restrict information to one hemisphere at a time. With tactile information this can be achieved readily because the information is conveyed almost exclusively to the contralateral hemisphere. With vision the fact that each eye presents information to both cerebral hemispheres (Fig. 8.3A) presents a problem if the principal aim is to restrict information to one hemi-

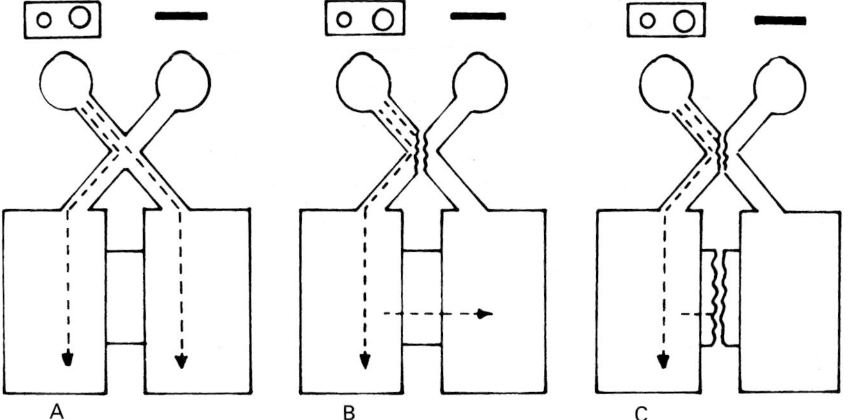

Fig. 8.3 Split-brain experiments in animals. A, normal animal; B, optic chiasma divided; C, optic chiasma and commissure divided.

sphere only, for the purpose of studying the single hemisphere's capabilities. In animals, this was simply achieved by dividing the optic chiasma in the midline so that direct transmission of information from each eye to the contralateral hemisphere was no longer possible (Fig. 8.3B).

The first experiments of this kind were carried out by Myers (1955, 1956) and may be described as follows: (i) the chiasma sectioned animal had one eye occluded while it learned a visual discrimination via the other (Fig. 8.3B); (ii) after discrimination training the occluded eye was uncovered and the 'training' eye was occluded; and (iii) the animal showed very rapid discrimination learning via the 'untrained' eye.

In a second stage the same procedure was repeated, this time with commissurotomy (callosal division) added to splitting of the optic chiasma (Fig. 8.3C). In this second stage the animal reacted as if it had not seen the problem before, i.e. transfer of memory and learning from one hemisphere to the other was prevented by division of the corpus callosum. It took the animal just as long to learn the discrimination with the second eye as it had with the first.

Of course, splitting the optic chiasma does not form part of the commissurotomy operation in man. The operation is generally restricted to division of the two major forebrain commissures, the corpus callosum and the anterior commissure, together with the interthalamic connection (or massa intermedia) where this exists. This latter structure is not a commissure but consists of grey matter. It is a variable structure seen only in a proportion of human brains and its exact role is uncertain.

In man, study of response to visual information by each hemisphere is achieved by taking advantage of the orderly projection of fibres from the two halves of each retina (Fig. 8.4).

It can be seen that, with eyes fixated on a central point, information to the left of this point is projected by each eye only to the right hemisphere (A), while stimuli to the right of the midline project only to the left hemisphere (B). This is, of course, true only for the moment of fixation. In normal viewing the presence of both voluntary and involuntary eye movements would mean that

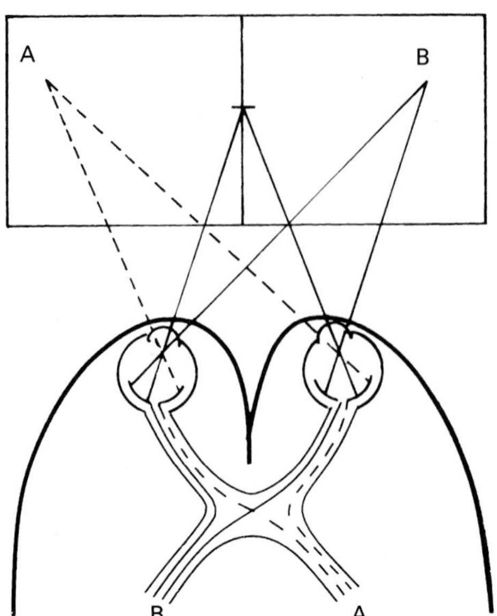

Fig. 8.4 Projection of information from left and right visual fields to the hemispheres.

stimuli to either side of the midline would be transmitted to *both* hemispheres. In order to prevent this, the technique of half-field (or hemiretinal) projection has been used. With the subject fixating a central point the stimuli to be studied are projected to either half-field at an exposure so brief (tachistoscopic) that eye movement is not possible. This achieves a functional split of the optic projection in much the same way as achieved by surgical division of the chiasma in animals. It should be stressed that the projection in the studies which follow is to the half-field, left or right (hence to the corresponding contralateral hemisphere), and not to the left eye or right eye.

The use of such specialized techniques in the study of commissurotomized man was first reported by Sperry (1961, 1964), and Gazzaniga, Bogen and Sperry (1962). The discrepancy between the early studies of Akelaitis and those of Sperry's group may be accounted for by a number of factors, among which the more important would appear to be difference in completeness of section of the corpus callosum and sophistication of the experimental techniques used in postoperative testing. Goldstein and Joynt (1969) carried out a follow-up of one of Akelaitis' patients who had been operated upon some 27 years earlier, and found lasting defects in interhemispheric transfer of information with no evidence of any reorganization of function.

Despite the small number of patients who have been studied with 'split brain' techniques, the extensive testing, often ingenious, which has been carried out has led to a fairly consistent picture of the hemisphere disconnection syndrome. The peculiar anatomical condition of the brain has allowed a variety of hypotheses concerning brain function to be tested in a way that would not otherwise be possible. While the review that follows attempts to present the general tenor of findings it is important to know the precise details of commissure sections carried out in individual cases since different results may depend on the exact extent and positions of the disconnections made at operation (Gazzaniga et al 1989).

There have been recent challenges to the disconnection syndrome position outlined in the following sections. However, specific testing of the notion in three commissurotomy subjects by Seymour et al (1994) lends support to the traditional view.

Visual perception

Using the tachistoscopic half-field technique a marked difference is noted between the two sides. Material which is presented to the right half-field (left hemisphere) can be read or described at about the preoperative level. Material in the left half-field can not be described in speech or in writing. This has held true over hundreds of replications for tachistoscopic presentations of 100 milliseconds or less. 'This is not true if objects are merely held in the left field or shown with longer exposure times, presumably because very rapid eye movements bring stimuli on the left into the right half field. Failure to find the foregoing left field defect in the Akelaitis studies seems best ascribed to the fact that tachistoscopic projection was not used in visual testing' (Sperry et al 1969).

Though commissurotomy patients could not speak about what was in the left half-field they could use non-verbal responses such as pointing to a matching stimulus or selecting the name of the object from a list. There is no hemianopia. The right hemisphere is unable to utilize the apparatus of speech for responding.

Earlier experiments revealed the independence of the two visual fields in memory as well as perception. The dissociation between things falling in the two half-fields has been utilized to great effect in the elegant 'chimera' experiments described below.

In the early experiments where two objects were presented simultaneously on the screen, one in each field, the response was shown to be dependent on the request made. If subjects were asked to reach behind the screen and retrieve the object from a number of others with the left hand they would select the object presented to the left half-field (right hemisphere / left hand). If asked to name the object they would invariably name that in the right half-field. This occurred even when the subject was still in the process of retrieving the object with the left hand. 'When asked to confirm verbally what item was selected by left hand subject names incorrectly the *right* field stimulus' (Sperry et al 1969). Such gross discrepancy attests powerfully to the independence of the two hemisphere-eye combinations.

Chimeric figures

One of the most subtle techniques for testing the perceptual abilities and control of motor response by each hemisphere is the method of chimeric stimuli described by Levy et al (1972). The technique is based on the observation by Trevarthen and Kinsbourne that commissurotomy patients tend to complete material across the midline in a similar way to some hemianopic patients (Ch. 7). For example, when only half a stimulus was presented in such a way that the edge of the half-stimulus coincided with the vertical meridian, the commissurotomy patient often responded as though perceiving a whole

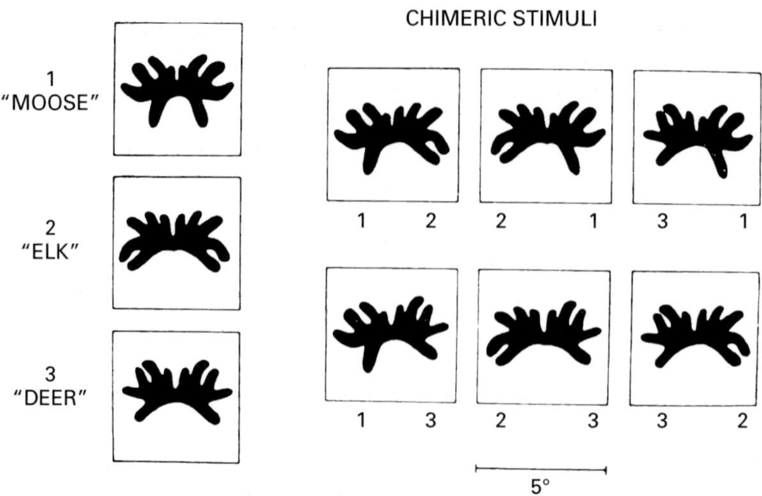

Fig. 8.5 Chimeric figures (from Levy et al 1972).

stimulus. This completion process was particularly strong in completion to the left when verbal report was used and in completion to the right where the subject was asked to draw the stimulus (Trevarthen 1974a, b). Chimeric stimuli consist of a composite joined at the vertical midline comprising the right half of one stimulus and the left half of another, e.g. the left half of one face and the right half of another. Other stimuli constructed by Levy et al were 'antler' patterns, line drawings of common objects and chain patterns (Fig. 8.5).

The composite stimuli were exposed briefly in a tachistoscope and the subject was asked to indicate what he had seen. Three modes of response were used: (i) pointing with the left hand; (ii) pointing with the right hand; and (iii) naming the stimulus.

When using pointing responses, the subject had available an array of the original stimuli from which the chimeras had been constructed. In the case of naming, the choice stimuli were removed, the subject having been taught assigned names for each of the faces and the different types of 'antlers'.

Levy and her colleagues pointed out that 'recognition of faces appears to be strongly Gestalt-like in nature and a face is relatively resistant to analytical verbal description'. They also noted the clinical finding that most patients with difficulty in facial recognition seem to have lesions in the right hemisphere. This suggested that the disconnected right hemisphere might be superior at this type of task. This hypothesis of asymmetry of function favouring the right hemisphere was strongly supported for all four sets of stimuli (faces, antlers, drawings and patterns) *irrespective of which hand was used for pointing*. When the response was changed to verbal naming, however, there was a reversal in favour of the visual information going to the left hemisphere. When pointing was employed, the 'completed' stimulus from the left half of the visual field was favoured, while naming was significantly biased in favour of the right visual field. The asymmetry of function when naming faces, while significant, was not as striking as with pointing, and there was a higher proportion of errors. The authors commented 'It was evident in the hesitancy and incidental comments of the subjects as well, that the left hemisphere found this kind of task extremely difficult and *was inclined to describe the distinctive features of the right field face instead of naming it as a unit*' (Levy et al 1972, p. 66; italics added by present authors).

The implication of this set of experiments is of such significance that the authors' summary is worth presenting in full:

> Visual testing with composite right-left chimeric stimuli shows that the two disconnected hemispheres of commissurotomy patients can process conflicting information simultaneously and independently. Which hemisphere dominates control of the read-out response was found to be determined primarily by the central processing requirement rather than by the nature of the stimuli or whether the response is ipsilaterally or contralaterally mediated. Where the task needs no more than visual recognition, a visual encoding ensues, mediated by the right hemisphere and based on the form properties of the stimulus as such rather than on separate feature analysis. On the other hand, where some form of verbal encoding is specifically required, the left hemisphere takes over and attempts a visual recognition based on nameable analytical features of the stimulus. Stimuli having no verbal labels stored in long term memory and which are resistant to feature analysis were found to be extremely difficult for the left hemisphere to identify. We conclude that each of the disconnected hemispheres has its own specialized strategy of information processing, and that whether a hemisphere is dominant for a given task under the test conditions depends upon which strategy is the more proficient. (Levy et al 1972, pp. 75–76)

Visuospatial functions

One of the striking pieces of information supporting the notion of lateral differences in visuospatial functions came from early reports of studies on two commissurotomy patients (Gazzaniga et al 1962, Bogen & Gazzaniga 1965, Bogen 1969a). Both these patients were able to write with either hand before surgery, the left being the non-preferred hand. After commissurotomy both patients lost the ability to write with the left hand, but preserved the ability to write with the right hand. There was, however, a dissociation between their writing and drawing abilities. Though both patients could copy drawings better with the right hand before operation, after surgery they were each better at this task when using the left hand. This visuospatial superiority of the so-called minor hemisphere was also seen in better performance of Block Design problems with the left hand. Where verbal instructions were used superiority reverted to the right hand.

To make clear the distinction between drawing to instructions (dysgraphia) Bogen (1969a) coined the parallel term *dyscopia* to mean a difficulty in following a 'visual instruction (that is copying from a model) rather than drawing from verbal instructions'.

Further insight into the nature of the right hemisphere's superiority was provided by three experiments by Nebes which demonstrated that the effect extends to the tactile modality as well as the visual and also to the synthesis of information between these modalities. Nebes (1974a) put forward the hypothesis that the right hemisphere 'attends to the overall configuration of the stimulus situation, synthesizing the fragmentary chunks of perceptual data received from sampling of the sensory surround into a meaningful percept of the environment. The right hemisphere is thus viewed as giving spatial context to the detailed analysis carried out by the major hemisphere' (p. 156).

In the first experimental test of this hypothesis (Nebes 1971) the subject was required to judge from visual or tactile appreciation the size of circle from which arcs of various size (80°, 120°, 180°, 280°) had come. Tactile-visual, visual-tactile and tactile-tactile conditions were employed. Four of the five commissurotomized patients tested performed significantly better with their left hand on all three versions, i.e. both on intramodal and cross-modal tasks. In a second experiment (Nebes 1972) the subject was required to select from a number of tactually presented shapes the one which would be formed from a visually presented fragmented figure. These visual figures each depicted a geometric shape that had been cut up and the pieces drawn apart, maintaining, however, their original orientations and relative positions. Once again commissurotomized subjects proved far more accurate with their left hand than with their right. Control experiments showed that neither difficulty with tactile discrimination nor the intermodal nature of the tasks were significant factors determining the poor performance but rather the 'Gestalt' requirement of the task. The third experiment (Nebes 1973) utilized the well known Gestalt principle of proximity. Here an alteration in the spacing of the uniform stimulus units gives rise to two differing percepts, e.g. in Figure 8.6 the figure on the left is perceived as columns of dots whereas the figure on the right is seen as rows.

Commissurotomy subjects (three in number) were presented tachistoscopically with one of these figures to either the left or right half-field of vision and were required to signal either vertical or horizontal organization by finger movements. All three subjects were more accurate with displays in the left half of the visual field 'suggesting that in man the right hemisphere is more competent than the left in perceiving the overall stimulus configuration inherent in the spatial organization of its parts' (p. 285).

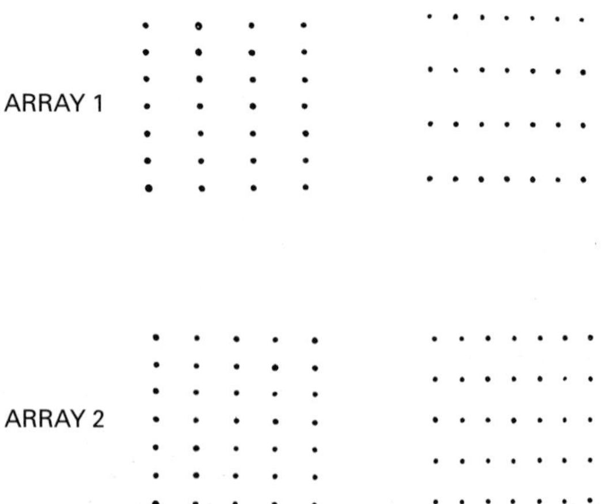

Fig. 8.6 Gestalt figure (Fig.1, p. 286 Nebes 1973, courtesy of Pergamon Press).

Such experiments provide strong support for the position that the right hemisphere functions much more efficiently in situations where synthesis of configurations is required from fragmentary information. Nebes (1974b) considered that this ability of the right hemisphere 'can be viewed as a spatial function in which, from limited data, we infer the structure and organization of our environment without having to submit the whole sensory array to a detailed analysis' (p. 12). Nebes pointed out that the results of his experiments taken together with the data from the chimera experiments suggest that it is the type of information processing required in a given situation which determines whether one hemisphere or the other will be 'dominant' or function in a superior manner. 'If only visual recognition is called for, even if the material is verbal, it is the right hemisphere which acts. If, however, a verbal transformation is demanded, even if the material is non-verbal it is handled by the left hemisphere.' If this suggestion is true (and there is much experimental support for it), then it will enable us to understand why certain contradictions in the lesion literature have arisen on the basis of patients' performance on 'verbal' versus 'non-verbal' tasks. It will also enable tests to be designed which should have greater value in the prediction of laterality of localized lesions in either hemisphere.

Finally, although many callosal experiments have used the 'restriction to hemisphere' techniques described above, the use of free field methods may still reveal differential responses from the two hands according to the nature of the material being processed (Loring et al 1989).

Corballis (1995) has reviewed the integration of visual information with the split brain.

Tactile perception

Here the task of object recognition (stereognosis) gave similar results to those in vision. Objects felt with the right hand (but not seen) could be named and described. Using the left hand the patient could recognize the presence of an object but was never able to name or describe it. Experimenters found that it was important to control for auditory cues such as those arising from moving the object on the table surface thus producing information which could alert the left hemisphere to the nature of the object which could then be named, the so-called *cross cueing*.

As with vision, a variety of tests demonstrated that the object felt with the left hand had been perceived and remembered by the right hemisphere. The subject could retrieve an object previously felt by the left hand from a mixed group of objects even after several minutes. The problem then is not one of stereognosis or tactile object agnosia but a unilateral anomia. 'This deficit has been present and persistent in every right-handed patient with complete commissurotomy' (Bogen 1985a, p. 104).

The commissurotomy patient is also unable to copy with one hand a configuration of the fingers of the other hand which has been arranged by the examiner.

The independence of the two hemispheres for tactile information is shown clearly where integration is required for solution of a problem such as the simple jigsaw puzzles of Gazzaniga (1970) (Fig. 8.7).

INTERMANUAL TACTILE COMPARISON

	JIGSAW PATTERN	ONE PATTERN IN EACH HAND		BOTH IN LH	BOTH IN RH
		LH	RH		
1	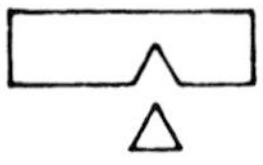	Not Completed		Correct	Correct
2	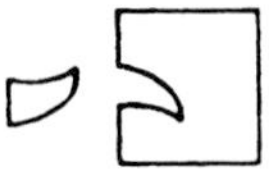	"		"	"
3	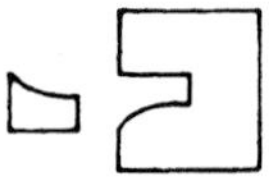	"		"	"

Fig. 8.7 Intermanual tactile comparison (Fig. 28, p. 87 Gazzaniga 1970, courtesy of Plenum Publications).

The subjects could fit together simple two piece jigsaw puzzles with either hand separately but not when intermanual collaboration was required by placing one piece in each hand. It is noteworthy that when stylus maze learning problems were used there was complete intermanual transfer.

When information has to be integrated between two modalities such as vision and touch the commissurotomy patient only succeeds where the information is processed in the same hemisphere. The subject cannot retrieve an object with the right hand if it is flashed to the left visual field. This tactile-visual match is not possible since the information from the two sense modalities is divided between the two hemispheres. For the same reason other forms of intermodal association are impossible.

Intermanual conflict and the 'alien hand' syndrome

In this syndrome one of the patient's hands appears to have a life of its own. The limb performs actions 'that are experienced as involuntary and frequently contrary to the patient's stated intention' (Feinberg et al 1992). The condition has been described in naturally occurring lesions and is seen regularly in the early weeks after commissurotomy, tending to lessen greatly with the passage of time (Bogen 1985b). In an early report of studies of the corpus callosum, Akelaitis (1944) called the phenomenon '*diagonistic apraxia*' (the term highlighting its two fold nature coupled with conflict between the two sides, i.e. agonistic aspects). Numerous reports have been made after callosotomy since that time (e.g. Wilson et al 1977).

With naturally occurring lesions, quite early case descriptions have appeared, though no descriptive term was derived nor was an attempt made to account for the observation in neuropathological terms. In rereading Liepmann's paper on motor asymboly or dyspraxia, the present author noted statements such as, 'His wife stated that he repeatedly used his right hand to bring down his left hand, which he would raise to scratch the back of his neck' (Liepmann 1900). Other facts in the case would place this in the same category.

In a recent quite detailed review, Feinberg et al (1992) reported descriptions by Goldstein (1908, 1909) of a patient who complained that her left hand was out of control and which even attempted to choke her. Their own patient described his right hand as 'having a mind of its own' and it was 'always trying to get into the act'. Both patients had vascular lesions.

The term alien hand syndrome (*la main étrangère*) was coined relatively recently by Brion and Jedynak (1972) who saw it as a sign of callosal disconnection in three patients with callosal tumours. 'The patient who holds his hands one in the other behind his back does not recognize that his left belongs to him.' They stress that this is not a matter of failed tactile recognition but a failure on the patient's part to recognize that the hand he is holding actually belongs to himself. Two patients when asked to write with their left hand were able to do so but expressed amazement and were unwilling to believe that they themselves had done the writing.

The anatomical basis of the disorder is still uncertain in its detail: the lesions often affect one mesial frontal region and / or the anterior portion of the corpus callosum (Banks et al 1989, Goldberg & Bloom 1990, Kuhn et al 1990, Hanakita & Nishi 1991, Gasquoine 1993, Trojano et al 1993, Giroud & Dumas 1995, Papagno & Marsile 1995), though the sign may appear in posterior lesions without an apparent callosal component (Marcos Delado et al 1995, Ventura et al 1995), and may even appear in repeated bursts over time (Leiguarda et al 1993) with both anterior and posterior lesions. One case has been noted with Alzheimer's disease (Ball et al 1993). With the clinical variability and the number of anatomical sites implicated, Dolado et al (1995) suggest the term 'alien hand sign' rather than syndrome should be used.

Infarction of the anterior cerebral artery which supplies the medial aspect of the frontal lobe, medial portions of the parietal lobe and the rostral two thirds of the corpus callosum produces a variety of disordered movements including the alien hand sign (McNabb et al 1988, Kuhn et al 1990). Both these sets of authors implicate the supplementary motor area. Feinberg and colleagues (1992) argue that there may be two forms of the disorder. In both pathological and postoperative cases the disorder tends to wane with the passage of time. These authors postulate two types of syndrome: (i) a frontal or fronto-callosal version in which the patient shows 'reflexive grasping, groping, and compulsive manipulation of tools'; and (ii) an anterior callosal type characterized by intermanual conflict.

Apart from after callosotomy, studied cases with circumscribed lesions of the corpus callosum with the alien hand syndrome are rare. Examination of one such recent case supports the notion of interhemispheric motor disconnection as the essential feature of the disorder (Geschwind et al 1995).

Auditory perception

Differences have been noted in the testing of commissurotomy subjects under dichotic conditions. Firstly, there is a marked lowering in the number of digits correctly reported from the left ear (Milner et al 1968, Sparks & Geschwind 1968). This difference is also seen after right temporal lobectomy though to a less marked degree. On monaural stimulation, subjects showed equal efficiency for the two ears. Milner and her co-workers extended this finding by presenting pairs of competing instructions simultaneously to each ear. The subject was told, for example, to pick up an object from a group of objects hidden from view, but on each occasion separate objects were named to the left and right ears. Under these conditions the subjects showed a strong preference to pick up objects named through the left ear with a relative neglect of items named in the right ear. This suppression or neglect of information coming to the right ear varied from subject to subject and with the conditions of testing. Subjects also had some difficulty with naming the objects picked up with the left hand. They tended to misname them and often gave the name which had been simultaneously presented to the right ear. The authors conclude that the 'dissociation between verbal and left-hand stereognostic response indicates a right-left dichotomy for auditory experience in the disconnected hemispheres'.

The suppression of ipsilateral signals under dichotic presentation, which is so marked for speech sounds, does not occur for dichotically presented pure tones (Efron et al 1977). It is likely that pitch information is combined at some central subcortical site.

Language

Language comprehension

Much interest has centred on the non-dominant hemisphere's capacity for language comprehension. The use of auditory material is complicated by the fact that both ears present information almost equally to both hemispheres and it is not possible to devise an auditory procedure analogous to the half-field visual technique. It is possible that, since the dominant hemisphere hears the same material as the non-dominant hemisphere, it may facilitate the latter by some means other than the major commissures.

With this reservation in mind, it does seem that the non-dominant hemisphere possesses a fair degree of language comprehension. Patients are able to retrieve with their left hand objects named or even described by function. They may also be able to indicate which name read aloud corresponds to an object flashed in the left half-field.

Comprehension of written material has also been tested by the split-field technique. The right hemisphere appears to comprehend limited word classes, particularly concrete nouns.

Gazzaniga (1970) noted that, while object nouns appeared to be comprehended best of any words flashed in the left visual field, nouns derived from verbs were not comprehended at all. Words containing more than one morpheme also presented difficulty for the right hemisphere. Caplan, Holmes and Marshall (1974) failed to confirm this hypothesis, namely that, while simple nouns are represented in the right hemisphere, agentive (verb-derived) nouns or bi-morphemic nouns are not.

One of Sperry's patients was studied by Sugishita (1978) some 12 years after operation. The subject was given a series of objects to feel with the left hand and then asked to select from a visual array of words a corresponding word using the left hand. She was able to do this if the words were related by category or by function or even by an occupation associated with the object, but she could not select words representing abstract concepts related to the object. Patients did not comprehend verbs in the left half-field nor were they able to act upon simple one-word verbal commands such as 'nod'.

Bogen (1985a) reported a considerable increase in the number of single words recognized by the right hemisphere with the passage of years, but this is rarely accompanied by speech, and the syntactic capabilities remain rudimentary at best (Zaidel 1978). There are a few exceptions. One 15-year-old normally right-handed male patient with total callosotomy (but sparing of the anterior commissure) could carry out verbal and pictorial commands presented visually and could write clumsily with his left hand the name of objects presented to the right hemisphere (Gazzaniga et al 1977).

The major hemisphere always shows normal comprehension of all orally and visually presented material in the commissurotomy subjects.

At first sight the commissurotomy evidence appears to be at variance with large numbers of lesion studies, e.g. left hemisphere lesion cases with aphasia often seem to have less verbal comprehension that one might expect from the commissurotomy studies.

Relatively small lesions confined to the left hemisphere have been described as producing word-blindness or word-deafness (Geschwind 1965, 1970, Luria 1970, Gazzaniga 1972). It might have been expected that if the right hemisphere was intact the patient should show at least the amount of comprehension shown by the right hemisphere in commissurotomy subjects. Two explanations have been offered. The first and more plausible explanation suggests interference with right hemisphere function from the left-sided lesion by way of the commissural pathways. The second explanation suggests that, because of their long-standing epilepsy, commissurotomy subjects may have developed a stronger bilateral representation of language.

Language expression

Extensive examinations of commissurotomy patients seemed to give very strong support to the contention that the right hemisphere is mute. 'Information perceived exclusively or generated exclusively in the minor (right) hemisphere could be communicated neither in speech nor in writing; it has to be expressed entirely through nonverbal responses' (Gazzaniga 1970, p. 125). This led Levy and her colleagues to ask the question, 'Does the minor hemisphere suffer from expressive aphasia because it cannot wrest control of the linguistic expressive mechanisms from the left hemisphere, or is the right hemisphere simply incapable of thinking of words?' (Levy 1974b, p. 165).

In an earlier experimental study, Levy, Nebes and Sperry (1971) tested the ability of the surgically separated right hemisphere to spell out words. Two commissurotomy patients were asked to use their hidden left hand to rearrange plastic letters to form a meaningful word. Both patients were able to arrange the letters into words but were unable to name the word they had 'spelled out'. They performed very poorly when asked to write the name of an object felt with the left hand, whereas they were able to draw the object readily. These patients were also inferior in left-handed writing of verbs as compared with nouns. Levy and her colleagues considered that there were two major factors accounting for poor performance in expression (here written expression) by the right hemisphere: (i) dominance by the major hemisphere over the motor mechanisms for expression; and (ii) an intrinsic limitation in the processing of language. They comment, 'Our results suggest that though there are two aspects of language expression – central conceptual dominance and peripheral motor dominance – there is a fairly direct relationship between the two. When a hemisphere is intrinsically better equipped to handle some task, it is also easier for that hemisphere to dominate motor pathways' (Levy et al 1971, p. 58). When the effect of the dominant hemisphere is removed, as in dominant hemispherectomy, the positive but limited power of the minor hemisphere over expression becomes apparent.

In the early studies, evidence for vocalization originated by the minor hemisphere in commissurotomy patients was almost non-existent. Butler and Norrsell (1968) reported one patient tested 3 years after total section of both major commissures who was able at times to name simple words presented in the left visual field. Other workers (Trevarthen 1969, Milner & Taylor 1970, Teng & Sperry 1973) have mentioned situations in which the right hemisphere has appeared to initiate fragmentary utterances in split-brain testing. Gazzaniga and Hillyard (1971) could find no confirmation for expressive capacity in the right hemisphere. There was, moreover, virtually no syntactic ability shown by their tests, even the limited amount of comprehension by the right hemisphere on pictorial-verbal matching tasks being limited to the affirmative-negative dimension.

Two cases of complete callosotomy with the anterior commissure intact have shown limited speech, apparently controlled from the right hemisphere (Gazzaniga et al 1979, Sidtis et al 1981, Gazzaniga 1982, Gazzaniga et al 1982, McKeever et al 1982). Both patients showed right hemisphere comprehension but no speech for approximately 1 year. Then utterances of one word were noted. At this stage if both hemispheres were shown stimuli simultaneously and asked to name them the left hemisphere dominated, but the right hemisphere could write (but not speak) the name of the stimulus presented to it. By about 3 years instances occurred of the reverse phenomenon, i.e. the left hemisphere could write but not name while the right hemisphere responded with speech. These two patients developed the ability to integrate verbal material presented separately to *either* hemisphere. Gazzaniga gives the following example: 'If two pictures or two words are sequentially flashed to the left or right visual field and the choice available requires an inference to be made from the two words, both hemispheres of P.S. and V.P. can perform the task… In one study, for example, if the words 'pin' and 'finger' are to be assessed, the correct response would be the word 'bleed'' (1982, p. 17). This inference capability has been seen only in the *left* hemisphere of other commissurotomy patients, including the small number who have developed a fair degree of semantic competence though no speech.

Two conclusions flow from these observations: (i) there is the possibility of paracallosal transfer of language information; and (ii) 'when a right hemisphere does acquire the capacity to speak, it appears to be remarkably like the left brain in general cognitive capacity' (Gazzaniga op cit, p. 16).

In 1987 Gazzaniga et al described a callosotomy patient who, under special test conditions, could both name and write about information coming to the right hemisphere, but this appeared to be an instance of the right hemisphere programming the left hemisphere to respond rather than a direct expression from the right hemisphere.

Unilateral agraphia

The ability to write with the left hand is lost after commissurotomy, though the patient may be able to carry out other skilled fine movements such as drawing or copying with the same hand (Bogen & Gazzaniga 1965, Zaidel & Sperry 1977). It is noteworthy that a patient of Sugishita et al (1980) had unilateral agraphia after section of only the posterior half of the corpus callosum during removal of an arteriovenous malformation. This patient showed no unilateral apraxia or tactile anomia.

Hemialexia

This refers to the loss of the ability to read in one visual half-field where there is no concurrent homonymous hemianopia. It follows section of the splenium of the corpus callosum for whatever reason and is a rare occurrence (Trescher & Ford 1937, Maspes 1948, Gazzaniga et al 1965, Gazzaniga & Sperry 1967, Sugishita et al 1978). Sugishita and co-workers (1978) found that their three patients with division of the splenium for pineal tumours had hemialexia postoperatively for both versions of the Japanese language, i.e. Kana (syllabograms) and Kanji (ideograms). Two or three years later the hemialexia was relatively restricted to Kana with improvement in the ability to read the ideograms.

Unilateral apraxia

All of Bogen's patients showed unilateral (left-sided) apraxia after operation (Bogen 1985a). There was some improvement with time but even many years later some degree of apraxia could still be elicited (Zaidel & Sperry 1977). This disorder is included here since, strictly speaking, it is a language related disorder being in essence a unilateral ideomotor apraxia.

Memory

Numerous studies by Sperry and his associates have demonstrated that each hemisphere has the capacity to store information for subsequent retrieval, and this capacity is directly related to the specialization of each hemisphere. This does not mean, however, that the memory abilities of split-brain subjects remain normal. Milner and Taylor (1972) tested the tactile recognition memory of commissurotomy patients by asking them to feel an object then select it tactually from a group of four after delays of up to 2 minutes. Two classes of objects were used: (i) everyday objects to which verbal labels could be readily attached – rubber band, key, coin, scissors; and (ii) 'non-verbal' tactile nonsense shapes. In six out of the seven subjects there was a marked superiority for the left hand. This was taken to mean that complex perceptual information can be remembered without the necessity for verbal encoding, and it is the right hemisphere which specializes in this regard.

The combination of these two findings seems to imply that 'both cerebral hemispheres normally participate in such tasks, but with the right playing the preponderant role'. Milner (1974) pointed out that concentration on the evidence of hemispheric specialization derived from commissurotomy studies and the parallel studies of asymmetry in normal subjects using similar experimental techniques may lead to an overemphasis of the functional differences between the two hemispheres. She reminds us that unilateral lesion studies have demonstrated that there is a parallel organization of function on the two sides of the brain which is in danger of being overlooked. Zaidel and Sperry (1974) examined a total of 10 commissurotomy patients on six standardized tests of memory. An examination of the data suggested that the processes which mediate the initial encoding as well as the retrieval of contralateral engrams involve co-operation between the hemispheres and so depend upon the commissural connections. More recently, Phelps and associates (1991) compared the effects of anterior versus complete commissure division. A deficit of both visual and verbal recall was found in those with complete sections, but not in the partial (anterior) cases. The authors stress the known importance of the hippocampus and its connections in memory processes. Complete sections tend to include these structures while the partial ones do not.

The present selection of commissurotomy evidence has focused on those areas which have been most closely examined. Other areas which have been less systematically explored include emotion, volition and consciousness. Incidental reports related to these have occurred throughout many of the studies mentioned. Much of the earlier material was reviewed by Lishman (1971).

Finally, Simernitskaia and Rurua (1989) have described what appears to be a distinct and unusual form of memory difficulty following surgical damage to the genu of the corpus callosum in operations for regional aneurysms. Such changes have not been reported in partial anterior callosotomy for epilepsy (Provinciali et al 1990), nor in three cases of spontaneous partial anterior callosal disconnection from haemorrhage reported by Leiguarda et al (1989). This leads to the possibility that any memory difficulties may be related more to interference with the blood supply to memory circuits than with the corpus callosum *per se*.

AGENESIS OF THE CORPUS CALLOSUM

On rare occasions the major neocortical commissure, the corpus callosum, fails to develop, a condition termed agenesis. A summary of the early literature with representative cover of much of the literature in neuropsychological studies has been provided by Dimond (1972). Apart from the rarity of the condition, the usefulness of this material in the study of hemispheric asymmetry is restricted by a number of factors, such as the completeness or otherwise of the agenesis and the presence of associated abnormalities of the cerebrum. The fact that no dramatic manifestations may be present during life is demonstrated by the cases where the agenesis is revealed for the first time at post mortem. Furthermore, most of the cases described in the literature until recently have failed to use sophisticated examination procedures (such as those developed in the study of commissurotomy) which would allow disconnection effects to be demonstrated if present. Some authors (e.g. Russell & Reitan 1955) have felt that this was probably the case for most of the earlier studies which claimed an absence of symptoms unless the callosal agenesis was associated with other brain anomalies. The question of clinico-pathological correlation in these cases was re-examined by Loeser and Alvord (1968a, b), and the advent of MRI has recently provided a powerful tool in establishing which parts of the interhemispheric systems are present or deficient (Jinkins 1991), thus allowing a stronger position from which to argue about neuro-behavioural correlations.

Since the 1960s detailed examination of a small number of cases of agenesis has been carried out. Jeeves (1965a) examined three acallosal cases with particular reference to tasks requiring bimanual manipulation and co-ordination. All three subjects were inferior to suitably matched controls on a variety of such tasks, and the ante-mortem evidence, including radiological studies, seemed to suggest that absence of the callosum was the major anomaly present. Other cases of partial or complete agenesis studied by Jeeves (1965b) varied in their ability on motor co-ordination tasks. Even where the everyday level of motor ability of some of these subjects was close to the norm for their age, sensitive tests involving integration of the two hands showed a poorer performance for acallosal subjects.

A single case studied by Solursh et al (1965) confirmed the difficulty of integrating tactile or proprioceptive information across the midline. Like commissurotomy subjects, this boy could identify by touch with the corresponding (contralateral) hand, objects presented to either hemisphere (i.e. to either half visual field) but was unable to do so with the ipsilateral hand. Despite this, fairly clear indication of transfer of information presented solely to one hemisphere was obtained in other situations. Incomplete compensation for the lack of the major organ of transfer of learning seems to have taken place. Extracallosal pathways appear to be limited in the ability to which they can enter into the transmission of information from one side to the other. This position is reinforced by the study of Karnath et al (1991).

In another patient with complete absence of the corpus callosum, Saul and Sperry (1968) could find no evidence of callosal symptoms despite the use of tests developed in the study of split-brain subjects. However, they also found indications that absence of the callosum hampered the patient 'in those activities in which the specialized nonverbal and spatial facilities of the minor hemisphere would normally reinforce, complement and enhance the verbal and volitional performances of the major hemisphere' (Sperry et al 1969, p. 288).

Ettlinger and his colleagues (1972, 1974), in a comparison of patients having partial or total developmental absence of the corpus callosum with control subjects, found a conspicuous lack of impairment in the acallosal subjects. Their tests included the following: intermanual tactile matching; depth perception; tachistoscopic visual identification and matching; spatial localization and dichotic listening. Further negative studies support these findings (Ferriss & Dorsen 1975, Gott & Saul 1978, Jeeves 1979). The absence of a pronounced laterality effect which had been found in commissurotomy subjects had also been reported by Bryden and Zurif (1970). The fact that their subject performed in a manner very similar to a group of normal subjects suggested that alternative pathways for adequate listening could be developed in cases of agenesis.

The heterogeneous nature of the clinical material means that it would be unwise to speculate about the mechanisms and alternate pathways used for compensation. However, the observed enlargement of the anterior commissure in a small number of callosal subjects led some authors (Saul & Sperry 1968, Ettlinger et al 1974) to speculate that at least some of the tasks, such as cross-matching, might utilize this tract. The principal argument against this is that most of the total split-brain picture is seen after callosotomy in which the anterior commissure is spared (Gazzaniga & Le Doux 1978, McKeever et al 1981). This statement should, however, be qualified by noting the age at operation. Using intra- and inter-manual tasks, Lassonde et al (1991) found that two subjects whose callosal sections were performed in childhood performed as well as normals when tested later, while three subjects operated in adolescence or adulthood showed typical disconnection effects. They hypothesize that there is probably a critical period favouring the development of alternative neural connections.

Finally, in spite of what appears to be conflicting evidence cited above, Lassonde et al (1995) studied eight subjects with complete agenesis together with subjects having partial or complete commissurotomy and found the acallosal subjects to be impaired on all tasks requiring integration of sensory or tactile information across the midline.

The intelligence of callosal subjects covers a wide range. The majority are below the norm on intellectual measures, with a few cases at or above normal. Once again, it is difficult to disentangle the contribution of any associated cerebral abnormalities and there does not appear to be any common pattern in the small amount of psychometric data available. The common depression of intellectual measures would lead many to agree with Dimond's suggestion '...in the early stages of development the absence of the corpus callosum places the individual at a disadvantage for which it is difficult subsequently to compensate. This condition does depress intellectual function and the employment of subsidiary pathways cannot totally compensate for this disadvantage' (Dimond 1972).

Critical reviews covering numerous aspects of callosal agenesis have been given by Ferriss and Dorsen (1975), Jeeves (1979), Milner and Jeeves (1979) and Chiarello (1980). A good starting point for the student of agenesis and partial callosotomy is provided by Jeeves (1991).

FUNCTIONAL ASYMMETRY IN NORMAL SUBJECTS

The hemispheric asymmetry of function demonstrated in lesion studies and after commissurotomy has been supported by studies, particularly of auditory and visual perception, in normal subjects. In the years since the first edition of this book, this area has stimulated such a proliferation of studies that one eminent neuropsychologist has referred to it as 'a PhD industry'. Students might refer to the following books and review articles on cerebral asymmetry which deal comprehensively with studies and theories of brain function based on normal subjects (Beaumont 1982, Bryden 1982, Bradshaw & Nettleton 1983, Corballis 1983, Hellige 1983, Segalowitz 1983, Young 1983, Springer & Deutsch 1985).

DOMINANCE REVISITED

As evidence has accumulated regarding the specialized functions of the two

Table 8.4 Some dichotomies distinguishing between the two hemispheres (from Bogen 1969b)

	Dominant (left) hemisphere	Minor (right) hemisphere
Jackson (1864)	Expression	Perception
Jackson (1874)	Audito-articular	Retino-ocular
Jackson (1876)	Propositioning	Visual imagery
Milner (1958)	Verbal	Perceptual or non-verbal
Zangwill (1961)	Symbolic	Visuospatial
Bogen and Gazzaniga (1965)	Verbal	Visuospatial
Levy-Agresti and Sperry (1968)	Logical or analytic	Synthetic perceptual
Bogen (1969b)	Propositional	Appositional

hemispheres, attempts have been made to characterize the different contributions of each hemisphere. Bogen (1969b) traced the emergence of the various dichotomies from the time of Hughlings Jackson (Table 8.4).

Bogen pointed out the difficulty which we have in the present state of our knowledge in characterizing the ability of the right hemisphere. An earlier dichotomy of Bogen's (a combination of those of Milner and Zangwill) was abandoned because of the evidence of some verbal capacity in the right hemisphere. Bogen proposed the use of the provisional term 'appositional' for right hemisphere function. 'This term implies a capacity for opposing or comparing of perceptions, schemas, engrams, etc. but has, in addition, the virtue that it implies very little else. If it is correct that the right hemisphere excels in capacities as yet unknown to us, the full meaning of 'appositional' will emerge as these capacities are further studied and understood' (Bogen 1969b, p. 149). Though much more information has accumulated since then, it is still difficult to select a pair of terms to epitomize the lateral differences in function. Perhaps this is just as well since, as Milner (1974) points out, it would be wrong in studying hemispheric differences in function to overlook the large amount of evidence from both neurological and neuropsychological studies which demonstrate that 'similarities as well as differences exist between corresponding areas, in the two hemispheres', i.e. there is what she aptly terms a complementary specialization of the two hemispheres with regard to psychological functions. The question then is one of relative rather than absolute dominance. Benton expressed this in the following way: 'Dominance denotes *asymmetry* in hemispheric function, i.e. the two hemispheres subserve particular functions to an unequal degree. Theoretically the degree of inequality with respect to a particular function might be either *absolute* (one hemisphere exclusively mediating the function) or *relative* (one hemisphere being the more important in the mediation of the function). All available evidence suggests that absolute inequality is rare, the more common relationship being one of relative inequality' (Benton 1975, p. 9). Some authors would prefer to specify the particular function being considered rather than speak of one hemisphere as 'the dominant one' (e.g. Poeck 1975).

Finally, the evidence from some commissurotomy studies, coupled with studies of normal subjects, has supported the notion that one of the major differences between the functioning of the two hemispheres lies not so much in the specialization for different types of information or for different psychological functions but rather in the different strategies and modes of central processing which each hemisphere employs.

In summarizing the evidence on asymmetry of function in the brain to that time Levy concluded:

> the human cerebral hemispheres exist in a symbiotic relationship in which both the capacities and motivations to act are complementary. Each side of the brain is able to perform and chooses to perform a certain set of cognitive tasks which the other side finds difficult or distasteful or both. In considering the nature of the two sets of functions, it appears they may be logically incompatible. The right hemisphere synthesises over space. The left hemisphere analyzes over time. The right hemisphere notes visual similarities to the exclusion of conceptual similarities. The left hemisphere does the opposite. The right hemisphere perceives form, the left hemisphere, detail. The right hemisphere codes sensory input in terms of images, the left hemisphere in terms of linguistic descriptions. The right hemisphere lacks a phonological analyser; the left hemisphere lacks a Gestalt synthesizer… (Levy 1974a, p. 167)

This description of hemispheric behaviour suggests that the Gestalt Laws of Perceptual Organisation pertain only to the mute hemisphere. If so, the adaptive functions served by these organizational principles are likewise restricted to the mute hemisphere, just as the adaptive functions served by language are restricted to the verbal hemisphere.

With the passage of time the *analytic versus holistic* processing model received widespread support, and writers such as Bradshaw and Nettleton (1983) drew attention to the body of evidence in psychology in support of two distinctly different forms of mental organization which have arisen quite independently of any consideration of cerebral asymmetry. These have been given very similar names to those employed in the asymmetry literature.

The concept of cerebral dominance or laterality has come a long way since the days of Paul Broca. Nothing illustrates better the way in which the concept has permeated every aspect of brain-dependent functions than the comprehensive, and at times speculative, reviews of Geschwind and Galaburda (1985a–c). Much of their theorizing relates to planum temporale asymmetry, but more recent imaging studies of handedness demonstrate other asymmetries such as that of the parietal operculum, and the two major asymmetries produce different subtypes, though the co-occurrence of both temporal and parietal asymmetries is very strongly associated with right-handedness (Habib et al 1995). Le Doux (1983) reminds us that many have been so carried away by work on the differential capacities of the separate and separated hemispheres that they 'treat the normal brain as though it were split', an almost tacit disregard of interhemispheric integration. His caution is a fitting conclusion to this chapter. 'No one cognitive function is completely dependent on one hemisphere or the other. Complex psychological processes reflect the functioning of both sides of the brain at all levels of the neuraxis, and a theory of how these processes relate to brain mechanisms must account for the integrated functioning of the nervous system. Any model which focuses on cerebral compartmentalisation at the expense of integration would seem to be misdirected' (Le Doux 1983, p. 212).

References

Adams C B T 1983 Hemispherectomy – a modification. Journal of Neurology, Neurosurgery and Psychiatry 46: 617–619

Akelaitis A J 1940 A study of gnosis, praxis and language following partial and complete section of the corpus callosum. Transactions of the American Neurological Association 66: 12–15

Akelaitis A J 1941a Psychobiological studies following section of the corpus callosum. American Journal of Psychiatry 97: 1147–1157

Akelaitis A J 1941b Studies on the corpus callosum. VIII. American Journal of Psychiatry 98: 409–414

Akelaitis A J 1941c Studies on the corpus callosum. II. Archives of Neurology and Psychiatry 45: 788–796

Akelaitis A J 1942a Studies on the corpus callosum. V. Archives of Neurology and Psychiatry 47: 971–1008

Akelaitis A J 1942b Studies on the corpus callosum. VI. Archives of Neurology and Psychiatry 48: 914–937

Akelaitis A J 1943 Studies on the corpus callosum. VII. Journal of Neuropathology and Experimental Neurology 2: 226–262

Akelaitis A J 1944 Studies on the corpus callosum. I. Diagonistic dyspraxia in epileptics following partial and complete section of the corpus callosum. American Journal of Psychiatry 101: 594–599

Akelaitis A J, Risteen W A, Van Wagenen W P 1941 A contribution to the study of dyspraxia following partial and complete section of the corpus callosum. Transactions of the American Neurological Association 67: 75–78

Akelaitis A J, Risteen W A, Van Wagenen W P 1942 Studies on the corpus callosum. III. Archives of Neurology and Psychiatry 47: 971–1007

Akelaitis A J, Risteen W A, Van Wagenen W P 1943 Studies on the corpus callosum IX. Archives of Neurology and Psychiatry 49: 20–25

Ardila A 1984 Right hemisphere participation in language. In: Ardila A, Ostrosky-Solis F (eds) The right hemisphere: neurology and neuropsychology. Gordon and Breach, New York

Arroyo S, Lesser R P, Gordon B et al 1993 Mirth, laughter and gelastic seizures. Brain 116: 757–780

Austin G M, Grant F C 1955 Observations following total hemispherectomy in man. Surgery 38: 239–258

Babinski J 1914 Contribution a l'étude des troubles mentaux dans l'hémiplegie organique cérébrale. Revue Neurologique 1: 845–848

Bakar M, Kirshner H S, Wertz R T 1996 Crossed aphasia. Functional brain imaging with PET or SPECT. Archives of Neurology 53: 1026–1032

Ball J A, Lantos P L, Jackson M, Marsden C D, Scadding J W, Rossor M N 1993 Alien hand sign in association with Alzheimer's histopathology. Journal of Neurology, Neurosurgery and Psychiatry 56: 1020–1023

Banks G, Short P, Martinez J, Latcjaw R, Ratcliff G, Boller F 1989 The alien hand syndrome. Clinical and postmortem findings. Archives of Neurology 46: 456–459

Basser L S 1962 Hemiplegia of early onset and the faculty of speech with special reference to the effects of hemispherectomy. Brain 85: 427–460

Battersby W S, Krieger H P, Pollack M, Bender M B 1953 Figure ground discrimination and the abstract attitude in patients with cerebral tumors. Archives of Neurology and Psychiatry 70: 703–712

Bear D M 1982 Hemispheric specialization and human emotional functions. In: Katsuki S, Tsubaki T, Toyokura Y (eds) Neurology. Proceedings of the 12th World Congress of Neurology, Kyoto, Japan. Excerpta Medica, Amsterdam, pp 63–82

Beaumont J G (ed) 1982 Divided visual field studies of cerebral organization. Academic Press, London

Belmont I, Karp E, Birch H G 1971 Hemispheric inco-ordination in hemiplegia. Brain 94: 337–348

Benowitz L I, Bear D M, Rosenthal R, Mesulam M M, Zaidel E, Sperry R W 1983 Hemispheric specialization in nonverbal communication. Cortex 19: 5–11

Benton A L 1965 The problem of cerebral dominance. Canadian Psychologist 6: 332–348
Benton A L 1972 The 'minor' hemisphere. Journal of the History of Medicine and Allied Sciences 27: 5–14
Benton A L 1975 On cerebral localization and dominance. Bulletin of the International Neuropsychological Society, July
Benton A L 1982 Spatial thinking in neurological patients: historical aspects. In: Potegal M (ed) Spatial abilities: Development and physiological foundations. Academic Press, New York, ch 11
Benton A L, Hannay J, Varney N R 1975 Visual perception of line direction in patients with unilateral brain disease. Neurology 25: 907–910
Benton A L, Varney N R, Hamsher K de S 1978 Visuospatial judgment. A clinical test. Archives of Neurology 35: 364–367
Benton A L, Hamsher K de S, Varney N R, Spreen O 1983 Contributions to neuropsychological assessment. Oxford University Press, New York
Blakemore C B, Falconer M A 1967 Long-term effects of anterior temporal lobectomy on certain cognitive functions. Journal of Neurology, Neurosurgery and Psychiatry 30: 364–367
Bogen J E 1969a The other side of the brain. I: Dysgraphia and dyscopia following cerebral commissurotomy. Bulletin of the Los Angeles Neurological Societies 34: 73–105
Bogen J E 1969b The other side of the brain. II. An appositional mind. Bulletin of the Los Angeles Neurological Societies 34: 135–162
Bogen J E 1985a Split-brain syndromes. In: Vinken P J, Bruyn G W, Klawans H L (eds) Handbook of clinical neurology, New Series l. Elsevier, Amsterdam, vol 45, pp 99–106
Bogen J E 1985b The stabilized syndrome of hemisphere disconnection. In: Benson D F, Zaidel E (eds) The dual brain. Hemisphere specialization in humans. Guildford Press, New York
Bogen J E, Gazzaniga MS 1965 Cerebral commissurotomy in man: minor hemisphere dominance for certain visuospatial functions. Journal of Neurosurgery 23: 394–399
Bogousslavsky J 1994 Frontal stroke syndromes. European Neurology 34: 306–315
Boller F, De Renzi E 1967 Relationship between visual memory defects and hemispheric locus of lesion. Neurology 17: 1052–1058
Bradshaw J L, Nettleton N 1983 Human cerebral asymmetry. Prentice-Hall, Englewood Cliffs, N J
Brain R 1941 Visual disorientation with special reference to lesions of the right hemisphere. Brain 64: 244–272
Branch C, Milner B, Rasmussen T 1964 Intracarotid sodium amytal for the lateralization of cerebral speech dominance. Journal of Neurosurgery 21: 399–405
Breschi F, D'Angelo A, Pluchino F 1970 Résultat a distance de l'hémisphèrectomie dans 13 cas d'hémiatrophie cérébrale infantile épileptogene. Neurochirurgie 16: 397–411
Brewer W F 1969 Visual memory, verbal encoding and hemispheric localization. Cortex 5: 145–151
Brion S, Jedynak CP 1972 Troubles du transfert interhémisphèrique. Le signe de la main étrangère. Revue Neurologique 126: 257–266
Bruell J H, Albee G W 1962 Higher intellectual functions in a patient with hemispherectomy for tumors. Journal of Consulting Psychology 26: 90–98
Bryden M P 1982 Laterality: Functional asymmetry in the intact brain. Academic Press, New York
Bryden M P, Zurif E B 1970 Dichotic listening performance in a case of agenesis of the corpus callosum. Neuropsychologia 8: 371–377
Burklund C W, Smith A 1977 Language and the cerebral hemispheres. Neurology 27: 627–633
Butler S R, Norrsell W 1968 Vocalization possibly initiated by the minor hemisphere. Nature 220: 793–794
Butters N, Soeldner C, Fedio P 1972 Comparison of parietal and frontal lobe spatial deficits in man: extra-personal vs personal (egocentric) space. Perceptual and Motor Skills 34: 27–34
Cairns H, Davidson M A 1951 Hemispherectomy in the treatment of infantile hemiplegia. Lancet 2: 411–415
Caltagirone C, Ekman P, Friesen W et al 1989 Posed emotional expression in unilateral brain damaged subjects. Cortex 25: 653–663

Cancelliere A E B, Kertesz A 1990 Lesion localization in acquired deficits of emotional expression and comprehension. Brain and Cognition 13: 133–147
Caplan D, Holmes J M, Marshall V C 1974 Word classes and hemispheric specialization. Neuropsychologia 12: 331–337
Carmichael A E 1966 The current status of hemispherectomy for infantile hemiplegia. Clinical Proceedings of the Children's Hospital D.C. 22: 285–293
Carmon A 1971 Sequenced motor performance in patients with unilateral cerebral lesions. Neuropsychologia 9: 445–449
Carmon A, Nachson I 1971 Effect of unilateral brain damage on perception of temporal order. Cortex 7: 410–418
Charles P D, Abou Khalil R, Abou Khalil B et al 1994 MRI asymmetries and language dominance. Neurology 44: 2050–2054
Chesher E D 1936 Some observations concerning the relatedness of handedness to the language mechanism. Bulletin of the Neurological Institute of New York 4: 556–562
Chiarello C 1980 A house divided? Cognitive functioning with callosal agenesis. Brain and Language 11: 125–158
Cogan D G 1960 Hemianopia and associated symptoms due to parieto-temporal lobe lesions. American Journal of Ophthalmology 50: 1058–1066
Conrad K 1949 Uber aphasische sprachtochungen bei hirnverletzen Linksaendeia. Nervenarzt 20: 148–154
Corballis M C 1983 Human laterality. Academic Press, New York
Corballis M C 1995 Visual integration in the split brain. Symposium on neuropsychological and developmental studies of the corpus callosum, Edinburgh. Neuropsychologia 33: 937–959
Corbetta M, Miezin F M, Shulman G L, Petersen S E 1993 A PET study of visuospatial attention. Journal of Neuroscience 13: 1202–1226
Corkin S H 1964 Somesthetic function after cerebral damage in man. Unpublished doctoral dissertation, McGill University
Corkin S 1965 Tactually-guided image learning in man. Effect of unilateral cortical excisions and bilateral hippocampal lesions. Neuropsychologia 3: 339–351
Corkin S, Milner B, Rasmussen T 1964 Effects of different cortical excisions on sensory thresholds in man. Transactions of the American Neurological Association 89: 112–116
Critchley M 1962 Speech and speech-loss in relation to the duality of the brain. In: Mountcastle V B (ed) Interhemispheric relations and cerebral dominance. Johns Hopkins University Press, Baltimore
Crockett H G, Estridge N M 1951 Cerebral hemispherectomy. Bulletin of the Los Angeles Neurological Society 16: 71–78
Damasio A R, Lima P A, Damasio H 1975 Nervous function after right hemispherectomy. Neurology 24: 89–93
Dandy W E 1928 Removal of right cerebral hemisphere for certain tumours with hemiplegia. JAMA 90: 23–25
Dandy W E 1933 Physiological studies following extirpation of the right cerebral hemisphere in man. Johns Hopkins Hospital Bulletin 53: 31–51
Darby D G 1993 Sensory aprosodia: a clinical clue to lesions of the inferior division of the right middle cerebral artery? Neurology 43: 567–572
Déjérine J 1892 Contribution a l'étude anatomo-pathologique et clinique des différents variétés de cécité verbale. Comptes Rendus, Société de Biologie 4: 61–90
Denes G, Caldognetto E M, Semenza C, Vagges K, Zettin M 1984 Discrimination and identification of emotions in human voice by brain-damaged subjects. Acta Neurologica Scandinavica 69: 154–162
Denny-Brown D, Meyer J S, Horenstein S 1952 The significance of perceptual rivalry resulting from parietal lesions. Brain 75: 433–471
De Renzi E 1982 Disorders of space exploration and cognition. Wiley, New York
De Renzi E, Faglioni P 1962 Il disorientamento spatiale da lesione cerebrale. Sistema Nervoso 14: 409–436
De Renzi E, Faglioni P 1965 The comparative efficiency of intelligence and vigilance tests in detecting hemispheric cerebral damage. Cortex 1: 410–433
De Renzi E, Spinnler H 1966 The influence of verbal and non-verbal defects on visual memory tasks. Cortex 2: 322–335

De Renzi E, Faglioni P, Scotti G 1971 Judgment of spatial orientation in patients with focal brain damage. Journal of Neurology, Neurosurgery and Psychiatry 34: 489–495
Dimond S J 1972 The double brain. Churchill Livingstone, London
Dimond S J, Beaumont J G 1974 Hemispheric function in the human brain. Elek Science, London
Dolado A M, Castrillo C, Urra D G, Varela de Seijas E 1995 Alien hand sign or alien hand syndrome? Journal of Neurology, Neurosurgery and Psychiatry 59: 100–101
Efron R 1963a The effect of handedness on the perception of simultaneity and temporal order. Brain 86: 261–284
Efron R 1963b Temporal perception, aphasia, and déjà vu. Brain 86: 403–424
Efron R, Bogen J E, Yund E W 1977 Perception of dichotic chords by normal and commissurotomized human subjects. Cortex 13: 137–149
Eisenson J 1962 Language and intellectual modifications associated with right cerebral damage. Language and Speech 5: 49–53
Ettlinger G, Warrington E, Zangwill O L 1957 A further study of visual-spatial agnosia. Brain 80: 335–361
Ettlinger G, Blakemore C B, Milner A D, Wilson J 1972 Agenesis of the corpus callosum: A behavioural investigation. Brain 95: 327–346
Ettlinger G, Blakemore C B, Milner A D, Wilson J 1974 Agenesis of the corpus callosum: A further behavioural investigation. Brain 97: 225–234
Falzi G, Perrone P, Vignolo L A 1982 Right-left asymmetries in anterior speech region. Archives of Neurology 39: 239–240
Feinberg T E, Schindler R J, Flanagan N G, Haber L D 1992 Two alien hand syndromes. Neurology 42: 19–24
Ferriss G S, Dorsen M M 1975 Agenesis of the corpus callosum: 1. Neuropsychological studies. Cortex 11: 95–122
Fischer R S, Alexander M P, Gabriel C, Gould E, Milione J 1991 Reversed lateralization of cognitive functions in right handers. Exceptions to classical aphasiology. Brain 114: 245–261
Fisher M 1956 Left hemiplegia and motor impersistence. Journal of Nervous and Mental Disease 123: 201–218
French L A, Johnson D R, Adkins G A 1966 Cerebral hemispherectomy for intractable seizures. A long-term follow-up. Lancet 1: 58–65
Gainotti G 1972 Emotional behaviour and hemispheric side of lesion. Cortex 8: 41–55
Gainotti G 1984 Some methodological problems in the study of the relationships between emotions and cerebral dominance. Journal of Clinical Neuropsychology 6: 111–121
Galaburda A M, Le May M, Kemper T L, Geschwind N 1978a Right-left asymmetries in the brain. Science 199: 852–856
Galaburda A M, Sanides F, Geschwind N 1978b Cytoarchitectonic left-right asymmetries in the temporal speech region. Archives of Neurology 35: 812–817
Gardner W J, Karnosh L J, McClure C C, Gardner A K 1955 Residual function following hemispherectomy for infantile hemiplegia. Brain 87: 487–502
Gasparrini W G, Satz P, Heilman K, Coolidge F L 1978 Hemispheric asymmetries of affective processing as determined by the Minnesota Multiphasic Personality Inventory. Journal of Neurology, Neurosurgery and Psychiatry 41: 470–473
Gasquoine P G 1993 Alien hand sign. Journal of Clinical and Experimental Neuropsychology 15: 653–667
Gazzaniga M S 1970 The bisected brain. Appleton-Century-Crofts, New York
Gazzaniga M S 1972 One brain – two minds? American Scientist 60: 311–317
Gazzaniga M S 1982 Cognitive functions of the left hemisphere. In: Katsuki S, Tsubaki T, Toyokura Y (eds) Neurology. Proceedings of the 12th World Congress of Neurology, Kyoto, Japan. Excerpta Medica, Amsterdam, pp 11–19
Gazzaniga M S, Hillyard S A 1971 Language and speech capacity of the right hemisphere. Neuropsychologia 9: 273–280
Gazzaniga M S, Le Doux J E 1978 The integrated mind. Plenum, New York
Gazzaniga M S, Sperry R W 1967 Language after section of the cerebral commissures. Brain 90: 131–148
Gazzaniga M S, Bogen J E, Sperry R W 1962 Some functional effects of severing the cerebral commissures in man. Proceedings of the National Academy of Science 48: 1765–1769
Gazzaniga M S, Bogen J E, Sperry R W 1965 Observations on visual perception after disconnexion of the cerebral hemispheres in man. Brain 88: 221–236

Gazzaniga M S, Le Doux J E, Wilson D H 1977 Language, praxis, and the right hemisphere: clues to some mechanisms of consciousness. Neurology 27: 1144–1147
Gazzaniga M S, Volpe B J, Smylie C S, Wilson D H, Le Doux J E 1979 Plasticity in speech organization following commissurotomy. Brain 102: 805–815
Gazzaniga M S, Sidtis J J, Volpe B T, Smylie C, Holtzman J Wilson D H 1982 Evidence for paracallosal verbal transfer after callosal section. A possible consequence of bilateral language organization. Brain 105: 53–63
Gazzaniga M S, Holtzman J D, Smylie C S 1987 Speech without conscious awareness. Neurology 37: 682–685
Gazzaniga M S, Kutas M, Van Petten C, Fendrich R 1989 Human callosal function: MRI-verified neuropsychological functions. Neurology 39: 942–946
Geffen G, Quinn K 1984 Hemispheric specialization and ear advantages in processing speech. Psychological Bulletin 96: 273–291
Geschwind D H, Iacoboni M, Mega M S et al 1995 Alien hand syndrome: interhemispheric motor disconnection due to a lesion in the midbody of the corpus callosum. Neurology 45: 802–808
Geschwind N 1965 Alexia and colour-naming disturbance. In: Ettlinger G (ed) Functions of the corpus callosum. Churchill, London, pp 95–101
Geschwind N 1970 The organization of language and the brain. Science 170: 940–944
Geschwind N, Galaburda A M 1985a Cerebral lateralization. Biological mechanisms, associations and pathology: I. A hypothesis and a program for research. Archives of Neurology 42: 428–459
Geschwind N, Galaburda A M 1985b Cerebral lateralization II. Archives of Neurology 42: 521–552
Geschwind N, Galaburda A M 1985c Cerebral lateralization III. Archives of Neurology 42: 634–654
Geschwind N, Levitsky W 1968 Human brain: left-right asymmetries in temporal speech region. Science 161: 186–187
Giroud M, Dumas R 1995 Clinical and topographical range of callosal infarction: a clinical and radiological correlation study. Journal of Neurology, Neurosurgery and Psychiatry 59: 238–242
Gitelman D R, Alpert N M, Kosslyn S, Daffner K, Scinto L, Thompson W, Mesulam M M 1996 Functional imaging of human right hemispheric activation for exploratory movements. Annals of Neurology 39: 174–179
Goldberg G, Bloom K K 1990 The alien hand sign. Localization, lateralization and recovery. American Journal of Physical Medicine and Rehabilitation 69: 228–238
Goldstein K 1908 Zur Lehre der motorischen Apraxie. Journal für Psychologie und Neurologie 11: 169–187
Goldstein K 1909 Der makroskopische Hirnbefund in meinem Falle von linksseitiger motorischer Apraxie. Neurologisches Zentralblatt 28: 898–906
Goldstein K 1927 Die lokalisation in der grosshirnrinde. In: Bethe A, Fischer E (eds) Handbuch der Normalen und Pathologischen Physiologie. Springer, Berlin
Goldstein K 1939 The organism. American Book, New York
Goldstein M N, Joynt R J 1969 Long-term follow-up of a callosal-sectioned patient. Archives of Neurology 20: 96–102
Gorelick P B, Ross E D 1987 The aprosodias: further functional-anatomical evidence for the organisation of affective language in the right hemisphere. Journal of Neurology, Neurosurgery and Psychiatry 50: 553–560
Gott P S 1973 Cognitive abilities following right and left hemispherectomy. Cortex 9: 266–274
Gott P S, Saul R E 1978 Agenesis of the corpus callosum: limits of functional compensation. Neurology : 28: 1272–1279
Goulet P, Sieroff E 1995 The impact of research methods in human neuropsychology as illustrated with the study of diaschisis. Revue de Neuropsychologie 5: 129–160
Griffith H, Davidson M 1966 Long-term changes in intellect and behavior after hemispherectomy. Journal of Neurology, Neurosurgery and Psychiatry 29: 571–576
Habib M, Robichon F, Levrier O et al 1995 Diverging asymmetries of temporo-parietal cortical areas: a reappraisal of Geschwind / Galaburda theory. Brain and Language 48: 238–258
Hanakita J, Nishi S 1991 Left alien hand sign and mirror writing after left anterior cerebral artery infarction. Surgical Neurology 35: 290–293

Hécaen H 1969 Aphasic, apraxic and agnosic syndromes in right and left hemisphere lesions. In: Vinken P J, Bruyn G W (eds) Handbook of clinical neurology. North-Holland, Amsterdam, vol 4, ch 15
Hécaen H, Sauguet J 1972 Cerebral dominance in left handed subjects. Cortex 8: 19–48
Hécaen H, Ajuriaguerra J de, Massonet J 1951 Les troubles visuo-constructifs par lésion pariéto-occipitale droite. Encephale 40: 122–179
Heilman K M 1982 Right hemisphere dominance for attention. In: Katsuki S, Tsubaki T, Toyokura Y (eds) Neurology. Proceedings of the 12th World Congress of Neurology, Kyoto, Japan. Excerpta Medica, Amsterdam, pp 20–26
Heilman K M, Van Den Abell T 1980 Right hemisphere dominance for attention: The mechanism underlying hemispheric asymmetries of inattention (neglect). Neurology 30: 327–330
Heilman K M, Scholes R, Watson R T 1975 Auditory affective agnosia. Journal of Neurology, Neurosurgery and Psychiatry 38: 69–72
Heilman K M, Schwartz H D, Watson R T 1978 Hypoarousal in patients with the neglect syndrome and emotional indifference. Neurology 28: 229–232
Heilman K M, Bowers D, Speedie L, Coslett H B 1984 Comprehension of affective and nonaffective prosody. Neurology 34: 917–921
Hellige J B 1983 Cerebral hemisphere asymmetry: method, theory, and application. Praeger, New York
Hellige J B, Bloch M I, Eng T L, Eviatar Z, Sergent V 1994 Individual variation in hemispheric asymmetry: multitask study of effects to handedness and sex. Journal of Experimental Psychology General 123: 235–256
Helmstaedter C, Kurthen M, Linke D B, Elger C E 1994 Right hemisphere restitution of language and memory functions in right-hemisphere dominant patients with left temporal lobe epilepsy. Brain 117: 729–737
Hier D B, Mondlock J, Caplan L R 1983 Behavioral abnormalities after right hemisphere stroke. Neurology 33: 337–344
Hines D, Satz P 1971 Superiority of right visual half-fields in right handers for recall of digits presented at varying rates. Neuropsychologia 9: 21–25
Howes D, Boller F 1975 Simple reaction time: evidence for focal impairment from lesion of the right hemisphere. Brain 98: 317–322
Jackson J H 1864, 1874, 1876 See Taylor J (ed) 1958 Selected writings of John Hughlings Jackson. Basic Books, New York
Jeeves M A 1965a Psychological studies of three cases of congenital agenesis of the corpus callosum. In Ettlinger E G (ed) Functions of the corpus callosum. Churchill, London, pp 73–94
Jeeves M A 1965b Agenesis of the corpus callosum: physiopathological and clinical aspects. Proceedings of the Australian Association of Neurology 3: 41–48
Jeeves M A 1979 Some limits to interhemispheric integration in cases of callosal agenesis and partial commissurotomy. In: Russell I S, Van Hof M W, Berlucchi G (eds) Structure and function of cerebral commissures. University Park Press, Baltimore, ch 37
Jeeves M A 1991 Stereo perception in callosal agenesis and partial callosotomy. Neuropsychologia 29: 19–34
Jinkins J R 1991 The MR equivalents of cerebral hemispheric disconnection: a telencephalic commissuropathy. Computerized Medical Imaging and Graphics 15: 323–331
Joynt R J, Goldstein M N 1975 Minor cerebral hemisphere. In: Friedlander W J (ed) Advances in Neurology. Raven Press, New York, vol 7
Joynt R L, Benton A L, Fogel M L 1964 Behavioral and pathological correlates of motor impersistence. Neurology 12: 876–881
Karnath H O, Schumacher M, Wallesch E W 1991 Limitations of interhemispheric extracallosal transfer of visual information in callosal agenesis. Cortex 27: 345–350
Kimura D 1963 Right temporal lobe damage: perception of unfamiliar stimuli after damage. Archives of Neurology 8: 264–271
Kinsbourne M, Smith W L 1974 Hemisphere disconnection and cerebral function. Thomas, Springfield, Illinois
Kleist K 1934 Gehirnpathologie. Barth, Leipzig
Krashen S 1973 Lateralisation, language learning and the critical period: some new evidence. Language and Learning 23: 63–74

Krynauw R A 1950 Infantile hemiplegia treated by removing one cerebral hemisphere. Journal of Neurology, Neurosurgery and Psychiatry 13: 243–267
Kuhn M J, Shekar P C, Schuster J, Buckler R A, Couch S M 1990 CT and MR findings in a patient with alien hand sign. American Journal of Neuroradiology 11: 1162–1163
Lansdell H 1962 Laterality of verbal intelligence in the brain. Science 135: 922–923
Lassonde M, Sauerwein H, Chicoine A J, Geoffroy G 1991 Absence of disconnexion syndrome in callosal agenesis and early callosotomy: brain reorganization or lack of structural specificity during ontogeny? Neuropsychologia 29: 481–495
Lassonde M, Sauerwein H C, Lepore F 1995 Extent and limits of callosal plasticity: Presence of disconnection symptoms in callosal agenesis. Neuropsychologia 33: 989–1007
Le Doux J E 1983 Cerebral asymmetry and the integrated function of the brain. In: Young A W (ed) Functions of the right cerebral hemisphere. Academic Press, New York
Leiguarda R, Starkstein S, Berthier M 1989 Anterior callosal haemorrhage. A partial interhemispheric disconnection syndrome. Brain 112: 1019–1037
Leiguarda R, Starkstein S, Nogues M et al 1993 Paroxysmal alien hand syndrome. Journal of Neurology, Neurosurgery and Psychiatry 56: 788–792
Le May M 1976 Morphological cerebral asymmetries in modern man, fossil man, and non human primates. In: Harnad S R, Steklis H, Lancaster J (eds) Origins and evolution of language and speech. Annals of the New York Academy of Sciences 280: 349–366
Le May M, Culebras A 1972 Human brain morphologic differences in the hemispheres demonstrable by carotid arteriography. New England Journal of Medicine 287: 168–170
Le May M, Kido D K 1978 Asymmetries of the cerebral hemispheres on computed tomograms. Journal of Computer Assisted Tomography 2: 471–476
Lenneberg E H 1967 Biological foundations of language. Wiley, New York
Levin H S 1973 Motor impersistence and proprioceptive feedback in patients with unilateral cerebral disease. Neurology 23: 833–841
Levy J 1974a Psychobiological implications of bilateral asymmetry. In: Dimond S J, Beaumont J G (eds) Hemisphere function in the human brain. Elek Science, London, ch 6
Levy J 1974b Cerebral asymmetries as manifested in split-brain man. In: Kinsbourne M, Smith W L (eds) Hemisphere disconnection and cerebral function. Thomas, Springfield, Illinois, ch 9
Levy J, Nebes R D, Sperry R W 1971 Expressive language in the surgically separated minor hemisphere. Cortex 7: 49–58
Levy J, Trevarthen C B, Sperry R W 1972 Perception of bilateral chimeric figures following hemispheric deconnection. Brain 95: 61–78
Levy-Agresti J, Sperry R W 1968 Differential perceptual capacities in major and minor hemispheres. Proceedings of the National Academy of Science 61: 1151
Liepmann H 1900 The syndrome of apraxia (motor asymboly) based on a case of unilateral apraxia. Monattschrift für Psychiatrie und Neurologie 8: 15–44. Translated in: Rottenberg D A, Hochberg F H (eds) 1977 Neurological classics in modern translation. Hafner Pres, New York
Liepmann H 1906 Der Weitere. Krankheitsverlauf bei dem einsitig Apraktischen und der Gehirnbefund auf Grund von Serienschnitten. Monatsschrift für Psychologie und Neurologie 19: 217–243
Lishman W A 1971 Emotion, consciousness and will after brain bisection in man. Cortex 7: 181–192
Loeser J D, Alvord E C 1968a Agenesis of the corpus callosum. Brain 91: 553–570
Loeser J D, Alvord E C 1968b Clinico-pathological correlations in agenesis of the corpus callosum. Neurology 1: 745–756
Loring D W, Meador K J, Lee G P 1989 Differential-handed response to verbal and visual spatial stimuli: evidence of specialized hemispheric processing following callosotomy. Neuropsychologia 27: 811–827
Luria A R 1970 The functional organization of the brain. Scientific American 222: 66–78
Mammucari A, Caltagirone C, Ekman P et al 1988 Spontaneous facial expression of emotions in brain-damaged patients. Cortex 24: 521–533
Marcos Delado A, Castrillo C, Urra D G, Varela de Seijas E 1995 Alien hand sign or alien hand syndrome? Journal of Neurology, Neurosurgery and Psychiatry 59: 100–101
Marie P, Behague P 1919 Syndrome de désorientation dans l'espace consécutif aux plaies profondes du lobe frontal. Revue Neurologique 26: 1–14

Marie P, Bouttier H, van Bogaert L 1924 Sur un cas de tumeur préfrontale droite. Troubles de l'orientation dans l'espace. Revue Neurologique 31: 209–221

Maspes P E 1948 Le syndrome expérimental chez l'homme de la section du splenium du corps calleux. Revue Neurologique 80: 100–113

McFarland R A, Kennison R 1989 Handedness affects emotional valence asymmetry. Perceptual and Motor Skills 68: 435–441

McFie J 1961 The effects of hemispherectomy on intellectual functioning in cases of infantile hemiplegia. Journal of Neurology, Neurosurgery and Psychiatry 24: 240–249

McFie J, Piercy M F, Zangwill O L 1950 Visual spatial agnosia associated with lesions of the right cerebral hemisphere. Brain 73: 167–190

McKeever W F, Sullivan K F, Ferguson S M, Rayport M 1981 Typical cerebral hemisphere disconnection deficits following corpus callosum section despite sparing of the anterior commissure. Neuropsychologia 19: 745–755

McKeever W F, Sullivan K F, Ferguson S M, Rayport M 1982 Right hemisphere speech development in the anterior commissure-spared commissurotomy patient. A second case. Clinical Neuropsychology 4: 17–22

McKenzie K G 1938 Cited in Williams D J, Scott J W 1939 The functional response of the sympathetic nervous system of man following hemidecortication. Journal of Neurology and Psychiatry 2: 313–322

McNabb A W, Carroll W M, Mastaglia F L 1988 Alien hand and loss of bimanual coordination after dominant anterior cerebral artery territory infarction. 51: 218–222

Mehta Z, Newcombe F 1991 A role for the left hemisphere in spatial processing. Cortex 27: 153–167

Mehta Z, Newcombe F, Damasio H 1987 A left hemisphere contribution to visuospatial processing. Cortex 23: 447–461

Mensh I N, Schwartz H G, Matarazzo R R, Matarazzo J D 1952 Psychological functioning following cerebral hemispherectomy in man. Archives of Neurology and Psychiatry 67: 787–796

Meyer V, Yates A J 1955 Intellectual changes following temporal lobectomy for psychomotor epilepsy. Journal of Neurology, Neurosurgery and Psychiatry 18: 44–52

Miller E 1972 Clinical neuropsychology. Penguin Books, Harmondsworth, Middlesex

Milner A D, Jeeves M A 1979 A review of behavioural studies of agenesis of the corpus callosum. In: Russell I S, Hof M W, Berlucchi G (eds) Structure and function of the cerebral hemispheres. Macmillan, London

Milner B 1958 Psychological defects produced by temporal lobe excision. Research Publications, Association for Research in Nervous and Mental Disease 36: 244–257

Milner B 1965 Visually-guided maze learning in man: effects of bilateral hippocampal, bilateral frontal and unilateral cerebral lesions. Neuropsychologia 3: 317–338

Milner B 1967 Brain mechanisms suggested by studies of temporal lobes. In: Darley F L (ed) Brain mechanisms underlying speech and language. Grune and Stratton, New York

Milner B 1968 Visual recognition and recall after right temporal lobe excision in man. Neuropsychologia 6: 191–209

Milner B 1971 Interhemispheric difference in the localization of psychological processes in man. British Medical Bulletin 27: 272–277

Milner B 1974 Hemispheric specialization scope and limits. In: Schmitt F O, Worden F G (eds) The neurosciences third study. MIT Press, Cambridge, Massachusetts, ch 8

Milner B, Taylor L B 1970 Somesthetic thresholds after commissural section in man. Paper presented at the American Academy of Neurology meeting, Miami

Milner B, Taylor L 1972 Right-hemisphere superiority in tactile pattern-recognition after cerebral commissurotomy: evidence for nonverbal memory. Neuropsychologia 10: 1–15

Milner B, Teuber H L 1968 Alteration of perception and memory in man: reflections on methods. In: Weiskrantz L (ed) Analysis of behavioral change. Harper and Row, New York, ch 11

Milner B, Branch C, Rasmussen T 1966 Evidence for bilateral speech representation in some non-right handers. Transactions of the American Neurological Association 91: 306–308

Milner B, Taylor L, Sperry R W 1968 Lateralized suppression of dichotically-presented digits after commissural section in man. Science 161: 184–186

Mountcastle V B (ed) 1962 Interhemispheric relations and cerebral dominance. Johns Hopkins Press, Baltimore

Musolino A, Dellatolas G 1991 Asymmetries of human cerebral cortex assessed in vivo by stereotaxic-stereoscopic angiography. Anatomo-functional correlations. Revue Neurologique 147: 35–45
Myers R E 1955 Interocular transfer of pattern discrimination in cats following section of crossed optic fibres. Journal of Comparative and Physiological Psychology 48: 470–473
Myers R E 1956 Functions of corpus callosum in interocular transfer. Brain 79: 358–363
Myers R E 1959 Interhemispheric communication through the corpus callosum: Limitations under conditions of conflict. Journal of Comparative and Physiological Psychology 52: 6–9
Myers R E 1961 Corpus callosum and visual gnosis. In: Fessard A et al (eds) Brain mechanisms and learning. Blackwell, Oxford
Myers R E 1965 The neocortical commissures and interhemispheric transmission of information. In: Ettlinger E G (ed) Functions of the corpus callosum. Churchill, London
Nebes R D 1971 Superiority of the minor hemisphere in commissurotomized man for the perception of part-whole relations. Cortex 7: 333–349
Nebes R D 1972 Dominance of the minor hemisphere in commissurotomized man on a test of figure unification. Brain 95: 633–638
Nebes R D 1973 Perception of spatial relationships by the right and left hemispheres in commissurotomized man. Neuropsychologia 11: 285–289
Nebes R D 1974a Dominance of the minor hemisphere for the perception of part-whole relationships. In: Kinsbourne M, Smith W L (eds) Hemispheric disconnection and cerebral function. Thomas, Springfield, Illinois, ch 7
Nebes R D 1974b Hemispheric specialization and commissurotomized man. Psychological Bulletin 81: 1–14
Netley C 1972 Dichotic listening performance of hemispherectomized patients. Neuropsychologia 10: 233–240
Newcombe F 1969 Missile wounds of the brain. Oxford University Press, Oxford
Newcombe F, Ratcliff G, Damasio H 1987 Dissociable visual and spatial impairments following right posterior cerebral lesions: clinical, neuropsychological and anatomical evidence. Neuropsychologia 25: 149–161
Newcombe F, de Haan E H, Ross J, Young A W 1989 Face processing, laterality and contrast sensitivity. Neuropsychologia 27: 523–538
Obrador S 1964 Nervous integration after hemispherectomy in man. In: Schaltenbrand G, Woolsey C N (eds) Cerebral localization and integration. University of Wisconsin Press, Madison, pp 133–146
Orgass B, Poeck K, Kerschensteiner M, Hartje W 1972 Visuo-cognitive performances in patients with unilateral hemispheric lesions. Zeitschrift für Neurologie 202: 177–195
Padovani A, Pantano P, Frontoni M et al 1992 Reversed laterality of cerebral function in a non-right-hander: neuropsychological and SPECT findings in a case of 'atypical' dominance. Neuropsychologia 30: 81–89
Papagno C, Marsile C 1995 Transient left-sided alien hand with callosal and unilateral fronto-mesial damage: a case study. Neuropsychologia 33: 1703–1709
Paterson A, Zangwill O L 1944 Disorders of visual space perception associated with lesions of the right cerebral hemisphere. Brain 67: 331–358
Paterson A, Zangwill O L 1945 A case of topographical disorientation associated with a unilateral cerebral lesion. Brain 68: 188–212
Phelps E A, Hirst W, Gazzaniga M S 1991 Deficits in recall following partial and complete commissurotomy. Cerebral Cortex 1: 492–498
Piercy M, Hécaen H, Ajuriaguerra J de 1960 Constructional apraxia associated with unilateral cerebral lesions – left and right sided cases compared. Brain 83: 225–242
Poeck K 1975 In editorial – On cerebral localization and dominance. Bulletin of the International Neuropsychological Society, July
Poeck K 1985 Temporal lobe syndromes. In: Vinken P J, Bruyn G W, Klawans H L (eds) Handbook of clinical neurology, New Series l. Elsevier, Amsterdam, vol 45, pp 43–48
Poeck K, Orgass B 1966 Gerstmann's syndrome and aphasia. Cortex 2: 421–437
Poeck K, Kerschensteiner M, Hartje W, Orgass B 1973 Impairment in visual recognition of geometric figures in patients with circumscribed retrorolandic brain lesions. Neuropsychologia 11: 311–317
Poppelreuter W 1917 Die psychischen schadigungen durch kopfschuss im Kriege 1914–1916. Voss, Leipzig

Primavera A, Bandini F 1993 Crossed aphasia: analysis of a case with special reference to the nature of the lesion. European Neurology 33: 30–33
Provinciali L, Del Pesce M, Censori B et al 1990 Evolution of neuropsychological changes after partial callosotomy in intractable epilepsy. Epilepsy Research 6: 155–165
Ratcliff G 1987 Spatial cognition in man: evidence from cerebral lesions. In: Ellen P, Tinus-Blanc C (eds) Cognitive processes and spatial orientation in animal and man. Martinus Nijhoff, Dordrecht, vol 2
Ratcliff G, Newcombe F 1973 Spatial orientation in man: effects of left, right, and bilateral posterior lesions. Journal of Neurology, Neurosurgery and Psychiatry 36: 448–454
Rey G J, Levin B E, Rodas R, Bowen B C, Nedd K 1994 A longitudinal examination of crossed aphasia. Archives of Neurology 51: 95–100
Ross E D 1981 The aprosodias: functional-anatomic organization of the affective components of language in the right hemisphere. Archives of Neurology 38: 561–569
Rowe S N 1937 Mental changes following the removal of the right cerebral hemisphere for brain tumor. American Journal of Psychiatry 94: 605–614
Rubens A B, Mahowald M W, Hutton J T 1976 Asymmetry of the lateral (sylvian) fissures in man. Neurology 26: 620–624
Rubino C A 1970 Hemispheric lateralization of visual perception. Cortex 6: 102–130
Russell J R, Reitan R M 1955 Psychological abnormalities in agenesis of the corpus callosum. Journal of Nervous and Mental Disease 121: 205–214
Russo M, Vignolo L A 1967 Visual figure-ground discrimination in patients with unilateral cerebral disease. Cortex 3: 113–127
Sackeim H A, Greenberg M S, Weiman A L, Gur R C, Humgerbuhler J P, Geschwind N 1982 Hemispheric asymmetry in the expression of positive and negative emotions. Archives of Neurology 39: 210–218
Saul R, Sperry R W 1968 Absence of commissurotomy symptoms with agenesis of the corpus callosum. Neurology 18: 307
Schlaug G, Jäncke L, Huang Y, Steinmetz H 1995 In vivo evidence of structural brain asymmetry in musicians. Science 267: 699–701
Schmitt F O, Worden F G (eds) 1974 The neurosciences third study program. The MIT Press, Cambridge, Massachusetts
Searleman A 1977 A review of right hemisphere linguistic abilities. Psychological Bulletin 84: 503–528
Searleman A 1983 Language capabilities of the right hemisphere. In: Young A W (ed) Functions of the right cerebral hemisphere. Academic Press, New York
Segalowitz S J 1983 Two sides of the brain: brain lateralization explored. Prentice-Hall, Englewood Cliffs, New Jersey
Semmes J 1965 A non-tactual factor in astereognosis. Neuropsychologia 3: 295–315
Semmes J, Weinstein S, Ghent L, Teuber H L 1960 Somatosensory changes after penetrating brain wounds in man. Harvard University Press, Cambridge, Massachusetts
Seymour S E, Reuter-Lorenz P A, Gazzaniga M S 1994 The disconnection syndrome. Basic findings reaffirmed. Brain 117: 105–115
Sidtis J J, Volpe B T, Wilson D H, Rayport M, Gazzaniga M S 1981 Variability in right hemisphere language function after callosal section. Evidence for a continuum of generative capacity. Journal of Neuroscience l: 323–331
Simernitskaia E G, Rurua V G 1989 Memory disorders in lesions of the corpus callosum in man. Zhurnal Vysshei Nervnoi Deiatelnosti Imeni I. P. Pavlova 39: 995–1002
Smith A 1966 Speech and other functions after left (dominant) hemispherectomy. Journal of Neurology, Neurosurgery and Psychiatry 29: 467–471
Smith A 1967 Nondominant hemispherectomy: Neuropsychological implications for human brain functions. Proceedings of the 75th Annual Convention, American Psychological Association
Smith A 1969 Nondominant hemispherectomy. Neurology 19: 442–445
Smith A 1974 Diaschisis and neuropsychology. Bulletin of the International Neuropsychological Society, pp 2–3
Smith A 1975 Neuropsychological testing in neurological disorders. In: Friedlander W J (ed) Advances in neurology. Raven Press, New York, vol 7, pp 49–110
Smith A, Burklund C W 1966 Dominant hemispherectomy: preliminary report on neuropsychological sequelae. Science 153: 120–122

Smith A, Sugar O 1975 Development of above normal language and intelligence 21 years after left hemispherectomy. Neurology 25: 813–818
Smith B D, Meyers M, Kline R, Bozman A 1987 Hemispheric asymmetry and emotion: Lateralized parietal processing of affect and cognition. Biological Psychology 25: 247–260
Smith B D, Kline R, Meyers M 1990 The differential hemispheric processing of emotion: a comparative analysis in strongly lateralized sinistrals and dextrals. International Journal of Neuroscience 50: 59–71
Solursh L P, Margulies A I, Ashem B, Stasiak E A 1965 The relationship of agenesis of the corpus callosum to perception and learning. Journal of Nervous and Mental Disease 141: 180–189
Soper H V, Cicchetti D V, Satz P, Light R, Orsini D L 1988 Null hypothesis disrespect in neuropsychology: dangers of alpha and beta errors. Journal of Clinical and Experimental Neuropsychology 10: 255–270
Sparks R, Geschwind N 1968 Dichotic listening in man after section of the neocortical commissures. Cortex 4: 3–16
Sperry R W 1961 Cerebral organization and behavior. Science 133: 1749–1757
Sperry R W 1964 The great cerebral commissure. Scientific American 210: 42–52
Sperry R W, Gazzaniga M S, Bogen J E 1969 Interhemispheric relationships: the neocortical commissures; syndromes of hemispheric disconnection. In: Vinken P J, Bruyn G W (eds) Handbook of clinical neurology. North-Holland, Amsterdam, vol 4, ch 14
Springer S P, Deutsch G 1985 Left brain, right brain. Revised edn. Freeman, New York
St. James-Roberts I 1981 A reinterpretation of hemispherectomy data without functional plasticity of the brain. Brain and Language 13: 31–53
Subirana A 1958 The prognosis in aphasia in relation to cerebral dominance and handedness. Brain 81: 415–425
Subirana A 1969 Handedness and cerebral dominance. In: Vinken P J, Bruyn G W (eds) Handbook of clinical neurology. North Holland, Amsterdam, vol 4, ch 13
Sugishita M 1978 Mental association in the minor hemisphere of a commissurotomy patient. Neuropsychologia 16: 229–232
Sugishita M, Iwata M, Toyokura Y, Yoshioka M, Yamada R 1978 Reading of ideograms and phonograms in Japanese patients after partial commissurotomy. Neuropsychologia 16: 417–426
Sugishita M, Toyokura Y, Yoshioka M, Yamada R 1980 Unilateral agraphia after section of the posterior half of the truncus of the corpus callosum. Brain and Language 9: 215–225
Tartaglione A, Inglese M L, Bandini F, Spadavecchia L, Hamsher K, Favale E 1991 Hemispheric asymmetry in decision making abilities. An experimental study in unilateral brain damage. Brain 114: 1411–1456
Taylor A M, Warrington E K 1973 Visual discrimination in patients with localized cerebral lesions. Cortex 9: 82–93
Teng E L, Sperry R W 1973 Interhemispheric interaction during simultaneous bilateral presentation of letters or digits in commissurotomized patients. Neuropsychologia 11: 131–140
Teuber H L, Rudel R G 1962 Behavior after cerebral lesions in children and adults. Developmental Medicine and Child Neurology 4: 3–20
Teuber H L, Weinstein S 1956 Ability to discover hidden figures after cerebral lesions. Archives of Neurology and Psychiatry 76: 369–379
Teuber H L, Battersby W S, Bender M B 1951 Performance of complex visual tasks after cerebral lesions. Journal of Nervous and Mental Disease 114: 413–429
Trescher J H, Ford F R 1937 Colloid cyst of the third ventricle. Archives of Neurology and Psychiatry 37: 959–973
Trevarthen C B 1969 Cerebral midline relations reflected in split-brain studies of the higher integrative functions. Paper presented at the 19th International Congress of Psychology, London
Trevarthen C 1974a Analysis of cerebral activities that generate and regulate consciousness in commissurotomy patients. In: Dimond S J, Beaumont J G (eds) Hemispheric function in the human brain. Paul Elek, London, ch 9
Trevarthen C 1974b Functional relations of disconnected hemispheres with the brain stem and with each other: monkey and man. In: Kinsbourne M, Smith W L (eds) Hemisphere disconnection and cerebral function. Thomas, Springfield, Illinois, ch 10

Trojano L, Crisci C, Lanzillo B et al 1993 How many alien hand syndromes? Follow-up of a case. Neurology 43: 2710–2712
Van Lancker D 1991 Personal relevance and the human right hemisphere. Brain and Cognition 17: 64–92
Van Wagenen W P, Herren R Y 1940 Surgical division of the commissural pathways in the corpus callosum; relation to spread of an epileptic attack. Archives of Neurology and Psychiatry 44: 740–759
Vargha-Khadem F, Polkey C E 1992 A review outcome after hemidecortication in humans. Advances in Experimental Medicine and Biology 325: 137–151
Ventura M G, Boldman S, Hildebrand J 1995 Alien hand syndrome without a corpus callosum lesion. Journal of Neurology, Neurosurgery and Psychiatry 58: 735–737
Verity C M, Strauss E H, Moyes P D, Wada J A, Dunn H G, Lapointe J S 1982 Long-term follow-up after cerebral hemispherectomy: Neurophysiologic, radiologic, and psychological findings. Neurology 32: 629–639
Von Monakow C 1911 Lokalisation der Hirnfunktionen. Journal für Psychologie und Neurologie 17: 185–200
Wada J 1949 A new method for the determination of the side of cerebral speech dominance. A preliminary report on the intracarotid injection of sodium amytal in man. Igaku to Siebutsugaku 14: 221–222
Wada J A, Clarke R, Hamm A 1975 Cerebral hemispheric asymmetry in humans. Archives of Neurology 32: 239–246
Wapner W, Hamby S, Gardner H 1981 The role of the right hemisphere in the apprehension of complex linguistic materials. Brain and Language 14: 15–33
Warrington E K, James M 1967 Tachistoscopic number estimation in patients with unilateral cerebral lesions. Journal of Neurology, Neurosurgery and Psychiatry 30: 468–474
Warrington E K, Pratt R T C 1973 Language laterality in left-handers assessed by unilateral ECT. Neuropsychologia 11: 423–428
Warrington E K, Rabin P 1970 Perceptual matching in patients with cerebral lesions. Neuropsychologia : 475–487
Warrington E K, Rabin P 1971 A preliminary investigation between visual perception and visual memory. Cortex 6: 87–96
Weekes B 1995 Right hemisphere writing and spelling. Aphasiology 9: 305–319
Weinstein S 1965 Deficits concomitant with aphasia or lesions of either hemisphere. Cortex 1: 154–169
Weinstein S, Sersen E A 1961 Tactual sensitivity as a function of handedness and laterality. Journal of Comparative and Physiological Psychology 54: 665–669
Whitty C W M, Newcombe F 1965 Disabilities associated with lesions in the posterior parietal region of the nondominant hemisphere. Neuropsychologia 3: 175–186
Wilson D H, Reeves A, Gazzaniga M, Culver C 1977 Cerebral commissurotomy for intractable seizures. Neurology 27: 708–715
Wilson P J 1970 Cerebral hemispherectomy for infantile hemiplegia, a report of 50 cases. Brain 93: 147–180
Witelson S F, Pallie W 1973 Left hemisphere specialization for language in the newborn. Neuro-anatomical evidence of asymmetry. Brain 96: 641–646
Young A W 1983 Functions of the right cerebral hemisphere. Academic Press, New York.
Zaidel D, Sperry R W 1974 Memory impairment after commissurotomy in man. Brain 97: 263–272
Zaidel D, Sperry R W 1977 Some long-term motor effects of commissurotomy in man. Neuropsychologia 15: 193–204
Zaidel E 1978 Lexical organization in the right hemisphere. In: Buser P, Rougeul-Buser A (eds) Cerebral correlates of conscious experience. Elsevier, Amsterdam
Zangwill O 1960 Cerebral dominance and its relation to psychological function. Thomas, Springfield, Illinois
Zangwill O L 1961 Asymmetry of cerebral hemisphere function. In: Garland H (ed) Scientific aspects of neurology. Livingstone, London
Zollinger R 1935 Removal of left cerebral hemisphere: report of a case. Archives of Neurology and Psychiatry 34: 1055–1064
Zurif E B, Bryden M P 1969 Familial handedness and left-right difference in auditory and visual perception. Neuropsychologia 7: 179–187

9

The interbrain

Three major subdivisions of the brain emerge during embryological development. These are the forebrain or *prosencephalon,* the midbrain or *mesencephalon,* and the hindbrain or *rhombencephalon*. The latter is continuous with the spinal cord. The forebrain itself becomes subdivided, the cranial portion being termed the *telencephalon,* and the caudal portion the *diencephalon*. The side walls of the *telencephalon* produce the two cerebral hemispheres, each with a lateral ventricle. In broad terms the *diencephalon* corresponds to the third ventricle and the structures which bound it. Thus the diencephalon stands at the junction of the prosencephalon and the mesencephalon and so merits the title the 'interbrain'. The term *thalamencephalon* has also been used for this region.

The preceding chapters have been concerned exclusively with the major derivatives of the *telencephalon,* namely the cerebral hemispheres, especially the neocortical areas and their connections. In relatively recent times it has become obvious that the functional anatomical systems subserving at least certain important higher functions extend deep into the diencephalon. This helps to reinforce the central concept of this text which might be stated as follows: *every complex psychological process has as its neural substrate aggregations of nerve cells both cortical and subcortical joined together by a three-dimensional set of nerve fibres*. Studies of psycho-anatomical relationships in cases where the points of disruption are clearly known help to establish the details of such networks.

It has become clear that major functional disruptions can be produced by diencephalic lesions, and the crucial sites needed to produce such changes are emerging. Before outlining these disorders, particularly the common and much studied *diencephalic amnesia,* it will be helpful to review the general structure of the region.

THE DIENCEPHALON

The diencephalon is a midline structure with symmetrical right and left halves. Crossing the lateral wall of the third ventricle is a groove, the *hypothalamic sulcus,* which varies in its prominence and extends from the *interventricular*

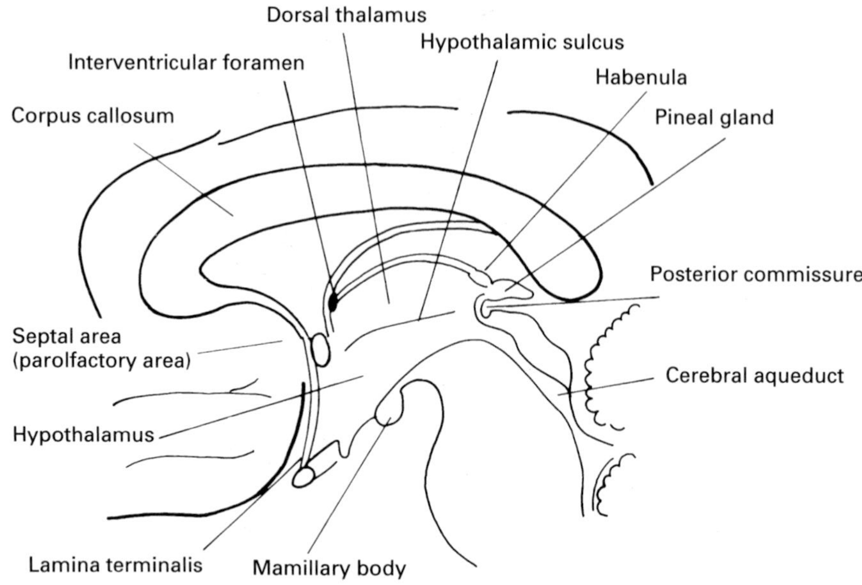

Fig. 9.1 Lateral view of the diencephalon seen in mid-sagittal section.

foramen to the *cerebral aqueduct*. This divides the diencephalon into a dorsal or upper part and a ventral or lower part (Fig. 9.1).

The dorsal part of the diencephalon consists of three parts: (i) the *dorsal thalamus* which is commonly called simply the thalamus by many anatomists and most clinicians; (ii) the *metathalamus* made up of the medial and lateral geniculate bodies; and (iii) a collection of structures, including the pineal gland, in the caudal part of the roof, which are termed the *epithalamus*.

The ventral part of the thalamus includes (i) the *hypothalamus* and (ii) the *ventral thalamus*. The hypothalamus extends from the *lamina terminalis* to a vertical plane just caudal to the *mamillary bodies* and downwards from the hypothalamic sulcus to include the structures in the side wall and floor of the third ventricle. These include the mamillary bodies themselves. One of the major tracts from the mamillary bodies terminates in the anterior nucleus of the thalamus and is called the *mamillo-thalamic tract*.

The nuclei of the thalamus were described in Chapter 2 and readers may wish to consult the illustrations of the thalamic nuclei and their cortical projections (Figs 2.22–2.24) when reading clinical papers on thalamic lesions. The relationships of the main components of the diencephalon are shown in Figures 9.1 and 9.2.

It must be stressed that the above is an anatomical description and all of the structures in the diencephalon have connections which cross these descriptive boundaries into other areas. Thus, while some structures in the diencephalon form important nodal points and connections in the neural substrate of memory and learning, the latter includes most subdivisions of the forebrain. It is also important to realize that even fairly discrete lesions, such as small infarcts, are likely to affect more than one thalamic nucleus and the blood supply to this region is such that adjacent non-thalamic areas are often involved. Masdeu (1985) has provided a brief but excellent review of

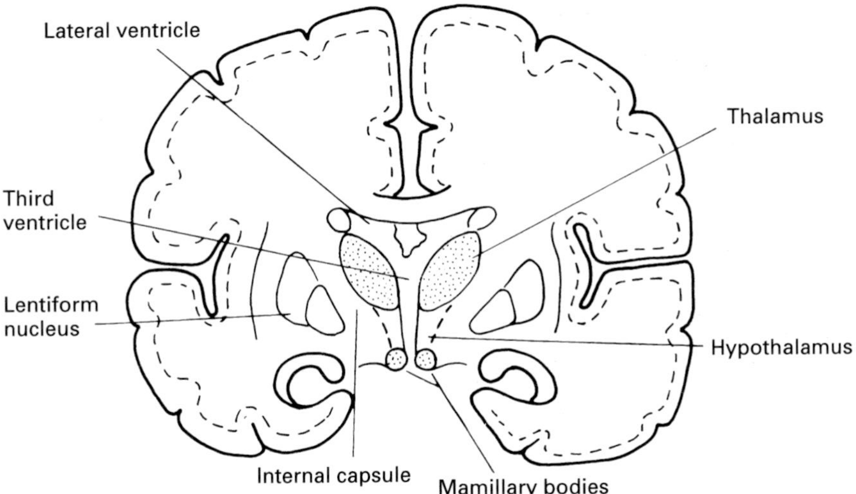

Fig. 9.2 Coronal section of the brain at the level of the mamillary bodies showing the principal features of the diencephalon.

the anatomy of the thalamus and its connections, including the all-important blood supply. An extremely detailed treatment of the anatomy of the thalamus is also given by Jones (1985).

FUNCTIONAL DISORDERS

Diencephalic amnesia

There are two distinct forms of lasting amnesia, bitemporal (see Ch. 5) and diencephalic. The latter appears in association with vascular, traumatic and neoplastic lesions. In one of the first observations, von Gudden (1896) commented on the association of memory disorders with lesions in the mesial regions of the thalamus. Since that time there have been numerous reports of amnesia implicating structures in the medial thalamus, particularly the dorsomedial nucleus. Occasionally anatomical evidence is available (e.g. McEntee et al 1976). In recent times, studies of patients with paramedian thalamic infarction show promise of adding to our understanding of the basis of the amnesias. More anatomical detail for these cases is being provided by recent imaging studies, such as MRI and CT scans (see Stuss et al 1988, Graff-Radford et al 1990).

Nevertheless, the association between structure and function remains somewhat unclear. One of the principal reasons is that the diencephalon contains a number of separate nuclei and their connections, all within a small space, so that it is difficult to determine just which structures are critical for the production of amnesia. Not only the particular nuclei involved, but also the degree of their involvement may be of importance in producing amnesia (Kritchevsky et al 1987). The anatomical evidence is reviewed by Markowitsch (1988).

Furthermore, by far the largest group of studies in recent decades has concerned patients with amnesia of alcoholic aetiology (Korsakoff psychosis), whose pathology includes usually the dorsal thalamus and mamillary bodies, though other widespread associated pathology is the rule.

An overview of the main questions associated with diencephalic amnesia is given by Butters and Stuss (1989).

Korsakoff's amnesia

In 1881 Wernicke first described three cases of the syndrome which bears his name. The salient features were ataxia, ocular symptoms and mental confusion. Two of the cases were alcoholic. It was later established that the condition was related to poor nutrition, the specific deficiency being that of thiamine or vitamin B_1. This accounts for its frequent appearance in undernourished alcoholics, though it also appears in other circumstances which produce thiamine avitaminosis.

In a series of reports from 1887 to 1891, Korsakoff reported the association of various mental disorders with polyneuritis. Sometimes the patient retained clear consciousness but was agitated, while in others the agitation was part of a confusional state. In most of the patients an amnesic disorder was a prominent feature. Soon after these initial observations Korsakoff, along with others, noted that the amnesic syndrome could be seen without the polyneuritis. As with Wernicke's encephalopathy, the most common association was with alcoholism and malnutrition.

Although a close association between Wernicke's disease and Korsakoff's psychosis was recognized by a number of writers around 1900, the intimate clinical relationship was established by Bonhoeffer (1904), though pathological confirmation was not established firmly for about three more decades (see Victor et al 1971). Following resolution of the acute episode of Wernicke's encephalopathy, patients were found to be suffering from the Korsakoff amnesic syndrome. Moreover, the pathological lesions appear to be identical in the two conditions. Because of the nature of the populations studied it is not always possible to ascertain whether Korsakoff patients have suffered from one or more episodes of Wernicke's disorder, though this is usually the case. Most workers would agree with Victor (1976) that Korsakoff's psychosis is the psychic manifestation of Wernicke's disease.

Neuropathology. The main features of the pathology of the Korsakoff syndrome were provided by the earlier reviews of Brierley (1977) and Horel (1978) together with the classical description of the Wernicke-Korsakoff lesions by Victor et al (1971) and Victor (1976). In the Wernicke-Korsakoff group the mamillary bodies are affected in virtually every case (Harper 1982). This is in keeping with numerous early studies which implicated these structures (Gamper 1928, Grunthal 1939, Remy 1942, Gruner 1956, Hécaen & de Ajuriaguerra 1956, Malamud & Skillicorn 1956). In some cases with mamillary body lesions cited by Victor et al (1971), there had been no amnesia apparent in life. Victor favoured the dorsomedial nucleus as the vital site. However, the two cases of Mair, Warrington and Weiskrantz (1979) showed mamillary body lesions but no major thalamic pathology. Also the claim that amnesia followed operative lesions of the dorsal thalamus is not borne out by the evidence (Orchinik 1960). All argument is confounded by the widespread pathology (Harper 1982, Harper et al 1985).

Neuroimaging (e.g. Squire et al 1990) shows a dissociation in the neuropathology associated with diencephalic versus temporal lobe amnesic syndromes. The former show very small mamillary nuclei with normal temporal lobe structures, while in the latter there is marked hippocampal reduction with little change in mamillary nuclei.

Clinical features

1. There is a profound difficulty or total inability in acquiring new material. This deficit encompasses both verbal and non-verbal material and is also independent of the sense modality through which the material is presented. For this reason the term general amnesic syndrome is used to distinguish it from the material-specific amnesias seen with unilateral lesions of the temporal lobes. Clinical tests demonstrate that material which appears to have been apprehended cannot be recalled after the passage of an unusually brief period which, in severe cases, may be down to minutes. As nothing new is learned there develops an increasing period of anterograde amnesia.

2. There is less complete agreement about the presence of retrograde amnesia, but all agree that the Korsakoff patient has a profound difficulty of spontaneous recall of prior events. In endeavouring to extract a personal chronology from the patient several things are noticeable: (i) much more information can be elicited by direct questioning than the patient can recall spontaneously; (ii) the amount of information decreases as questions move closer in time to the present; and (iii) some of the information has no 'time tags', i.e. its temporal relations to other happenings appear to have been lost. This 'achronogenesis' has been stressed by several writers (see Barbizet 1970) and its presence should suggest very strongly an alcoholic aetiology. Apart from these difficulties, the patient will, in the advanced stages, tend to wander off the subject. Janet (1928) referred to the core of this difficulty as the 'problem of narration'.

Many clinical writers have described a temporal gradient in the sparing of memories, with those of childhood and early adult life being less affected than those of later periods. A test of the temporal gradient hypothesis by Sanders and Warrington (1971) found that the duration of the retrograde defect was very long indeed. However, later studies with larger samples and improved methodology tended to give strong support to a temporal gradient theory (Seltzer & Benson 1974, Marslen-Wilson & Teuber 1975, Albert et al 1979). It may be that the severity of the condition plays a major role. Korsakoff himself noted that while remote sparing was often seen, in other cases 'even the memory of remote events may be disturbed' (Victor & Yakovlev 1955). Victor (1976) agreed that 'memories of the distant past are impaired in practically all cases of Korsakoff's psychosis and seriously impaired in most of them'. The recent review of the Korsakoff syndrome by Kopelman (1995) supports the notion that disruption of circuits involving the mamillary bodies, mamillo-thalamic tract and the anterior thalamus is critical for anterograde amnesia in this group, while retrograde amnesia may be related to the frontal lobes. It may be that the severity of associated frontal damage may determine the degree of retrograde amnesia.

3. An essential feature is the preservation of immediate memory, the audioverbal and visual spans being around seven.

4. Many aspects of learned behaviour are preserved. Clinical examination

reveals no difficulties with speech, language, gesture and well-practised skills. There are no problems with the basic activities of daily living. However, outside a familiar environment, Korsakoff patients will get into difficulties, especially if they need to incorporate new information for their behaviour to become adapted to a novel situation.

5. Confabulation had earlier been considered as necessary for the diagnosis of Korsakoff's psychosis, but it is by no means a constant feature. It appears to be seen mainly in the acute state together with some confusion. Confabulation has been defined by Berlyne (1972) as 'a falsification of memory occurring in clear consciousness in association with an organically derived dementia'. It appears to be as common in dementia as it is in Korsakoff's disease and is also seen in other neurological disorders. There is some evidence that at least one form of confabulation may be related to associated pathology in the frontal lobes (Stuss et al 1978, Kapur & Coughlan 1980). A study by Mercer et al (1977) using objective tests found that confabulation 'proved to be strongly related to the inability to withhold responses, to monitor one's own responses, and to provide verbal self-corrections'. Such a description would fit well with what is known of frontal lobe dysfunction. This is closely akin to the observation of experienced clinicians that confabulation is directly related to the absence of insight (Zangwill 1978, personal communication). Certainly, confabulation is not a marked feature of the chronic state.

6. The patient often exhibits a lack of initiative and spontaneity, together with a blunting of affect.

With regard to terminology, preoccupation with clinical and experimental studies of general amnesic syndromes has led many to write as if the terms *Korsakoff amnesic syndrome* and *Korsakoff psychosis* were *synonymous*. This is far from the case. While Korsakoff patients preserve many aspects of learned behaviour, they demonstrate other cognitive deficits, particularly those of adaptive behaviour (Bolter & Hannon 1980, Walsh 1991). On the other hand, patients with amnesia from diencephalic lesions not related to alcohol may be free of these other cognitive deficits.

Finally, because it is relatively common, this form of amnesia has contributed much to the evaluation of specific aspects of memory in the area of cognitive neuropsychology and the basic material in this chapter should be reinforced from this source.

Bilateral thalamic lesions

Amnesia has often been reported with tumours around the third ventricle (Smythe & Stern 1938, Delay et al 1964, Kahn & Crosby 1972, McEntee et al 1976, Ziegler et al 1977, Lawrence 1984, Lobosky et al 1984). More widespread cognitive deficits are often seen with communicating hydrocephalus as well as pressure on the diencephalon. Because of their complex physiological effects, these cases are unhelpful in differentiating brain-behaviour relationships.

More helpful are a number of single case reports of bilateral paramedian thalamic infarcts in which severe non-specific anterograde amnesia has dominated the clinical picture (Mills & Swanson 1978, Cramon & Zihl 1979, Schott et al 1980, Barbizet et al 1981, Walsh 1982, 1991, Winocur et al 1984). CT scans have confirmed the presence of symmetrical infarcts and in the author's case autopsy evidence was available. It is probable that the bilateral infarcts arise because of the origin in some cases of the two paramedian thalamo-subthalamic arteries from a common trunk (Percheron 1976, Castaigne et al 1981). Except in two or three cases neuropsychological evidence is scanty. The free recall of one case (Winocur et al 1984) was nil at 5 minutes over many testings, but recognition on a multiple-choice test was always 'rapid and perfect' even after delays exceeding 24 hours. A second case, followed over several years (Walsh 1982, 1991), demonstrated marked dissociation between free recall and cued recall suggestive of relatively spared recognition memory. However, the patient performed differently on sundry measures of recognition memory compared with normal subjects, though not nearly as poorly as the typical Korsakoff patient. In another study, persistent anterograde amnesia appeared to be related to damage to specific structures exclusively (Graff-Radford et al 1988).

Aneurysmal amnesia

Amnesia following subarachnoid haemorrhage has been reported in a small percentage of cases since 1921 (Flateau 1921, Tarachow 1939, Walton 1953), but its specific association with anterior communicating artery aneurysms came much later (Norlén & Olivecrona 1953, Lindqvist & Norlén 1966, Logue et al 1968, Sengupta et al 1975, Luria 1976). After a period of confusion and subsequent anterograde amnesia many patients go on to complete recovery. A few are left with lasting severe amnesia. Detailed specification of the form of amnesia has been attempted in only a few instances (Talland et al 1967, Brion et al 1968, Luria 1976), the clearest being that of Volpe & Hirst (1983). Apart from the 'core' symptoms of preserved immediate memory and a non-specific anterograde amnesia, the cases are marked by great susceptibility to proactive interference and differentially better recognition memory than free recall with some benefit from cued recall. However, a study of seven such patients (Kinsella & Clausen 1982), employing the material and methods of a previous study of Korsakoff amnesics (Cermak et al 1974), showed a clear qualitative difference between the two groups. Unlike the Korsakoff patients, the aneurysmal cases employed semantic encoding in much the same way as normal subjects.

This form of amnesia is considered here for convenience, although the lesions may lie in part or in whole outside the diencephalon. The review of Gade (1982) implicates the penetrating vessels which supply deep midline structures as the probable mechanism. It may be that both septal and diencephalic structures are involved.

Transient global amnesia

This disorder, described in Chapter 5, is known to occur with discrete lesions in the thalamus (Gorelick et al 1988, Goldenberg et al 1991, Raffaele et al 1995). Transient autobiographic amnesia has been reported with loss of personal information transiently, bilateral temporal and parietal hypoperfusion on SPECT and no psychiatric disorder (Venneri & Caffarra 1998).

Amnesic syndrome – one or many?

It is now clear that lesions in several sites in the brain can cause difficulty with memory and learning. While these cases of differing aetiologies and different lesion sites share the core features of a general amnesia, there is growing evidence that the Gestalt of deficits varies significantly with the locus of the lesion (Whitty & Zangwill 1977, Moscovitch 1982, Butters et al 1984). 'The unitary character of the organic amnesic syndrome was always a rather dubious assumption and it is now seriously in question' (Piercy 1977, p. 145). The fact that different aspects of memory and learning processes may be dissociated by lesions in different locations is the clearest evidence for such a position. It will not be practicable to review all the evidence, but some of the highlights will be presented. This will do a disservice to the complexity of the evidence, especially as it refers to different theoretical positions regarding the amnesic syndrome or syndromes. For the latter, such reviews as that of Meudell and Mayes (1982) are recommended. The following brief sketch will outline only some of the major features of clinico-pathological relationships.

The problem of classification of amnesias has much in common with the classification of other disorders, e.g. aphasia, where many cases share common features but characteristic patterns of the basic disorder vary with different anatomical lesion sites. Whether the different configurations should be designated as independent syndromes or as subtypes of a general amnesic disorder is perhaps a matter of terminology. Knowledge of these emerging differences will not only inform us about the regional contributions to different processes in the complex acts of memorization and recall but might also suggest appropriate strategies for management and remediation of amnesic patients. This biological factor analysis depends on detailed examination of cases with 'anatomically clean' lesions, an unfortunately rare event.

The first important difference between amnesic groups was reported by Lhermitte and Signoret (1972). Following Zangwill's early suggestion (1943) that different forms of the amnesic syndrome might exist according to the locus of the lesion, they compared post-encephalitic patients (hippocampal damage) with Korsakoff patients (thalamic or mamillo-thalamic damage) on a series of tasks. Two of these required the learning of the position of 9 stimuli in a 3 by 3 array. In the first form of the tasks (Spatial Arrangement) the stimuli were pictures of common objects, while the second (Logical Arrangement) consisted of geometrical shapes ordered according to a logical matrix of colour, shape and number. The two groups showed clear differences which we have replicated on numerous occasions. On the first task both groups showed poor acquisition and virtually no free recall even with a short delay. However, the alcoholic subjects benefited markedly with the type of cued recall used, while the encephalitic subjects showed no such benefit. On the other hand the encephalitic subjects learned the logical matrix with the ease of normal subjects whereas the alcoholic subjects were totally unable to do so, and there were further differences on the other tasks used.

While it was suggested that the differences were related to the two major anatomical sites, it is just as plausible to link the observed differences to the presence of associated pathology in the Korsakoff group which gives rise to the difficulty with conceptual operations which form an essential part of the requirements for the Logical Arrangement task and other tasks employed (Talland 1965, Bolter & Hannon 1980, Walsh 1991). The encephalitic group, being free of such pathology, had no difficulty with the conceptual tasks. This proposal is strengthened by our own observation that the Logical Arrangement task presents great difficulty for alcoholic subjects in the absence of clinical or experimental evidence of memory disorder.

Other studies have confirmed the presence of simultaneous deficits in two or more independent psychological processes in the alcohol-related amnesic disorder (Mattis et al 1978, Kovner et al 1981, Squire 1981).

Perhaps the most consistent group difference has been with measures of forgetting, where Korsakoff patients have appeared to differ from other types (see below).

Finally, different groups of amnesic subjects differ in the degree to which remote memory is affected. HM showed only a limited deficit (Scoville & Milner 1957, Milner 1966, 1970), as did patients following ECT (Cohen & Squire 1981, Squire 1981, Squire & Cohen 1982) and cases NA, RB, and LN (Walsh 1991) with localized diencephalic lesions. Post-encephalitic patients vary greatly, some showing little and others marked retrograde amnesia. Thus lesions restricted to the diencephalon or hippocampus may produce relatively short retrograde amnesia, and the longer retrograde amnesia of the Korsakoff patient and some post-encephalitics may reflect more widespread pathology in these conditions. As yet there is little anatomical information on the few unusual cases claiming prolonged retrograde amnesia in the absence of any considerable anterograde deficit, so-called 'focal retrograde amnesia' (Goldberg et al 1981, Evans et al 1996, Venneri & Caffarra 1998). From available evidence, it would seem likely that responsible lesions must involve at least one temporal lobe, perhaps superiorly, with disruption of an interconnected network of multiple non-axial cortical regions (Evans et al 1996).

Recent work in concussed elite football players, where premorbid testing has been performed and video-taped records prior to collision allow accurate verification of reported memories, is perhaps the most promising method of understanding components of retrograde amnesia. Yarnell and Lynch (1970, 1973) originally reported that retrograde amnesia was less extensive when examination was made immediately after concussion, but increased within minutes to a maximum and subsequently shrank with recovery. Recently, McCrory (1998, personal communication) has described a consistent pattern of retrograde loss at three time periods after concussion in 19 Australian football players. Immediately after recovery from loss of consciousness or impact, there is an irreversible loss of a mean of 0.7 minutes of recent memories. By 10 minutes after impact, the duration has increased to a mean retrograde loss of 21 minutes. By 24 hours, mean retrograde loss reduces to 3.5 minutes. Thus some memories are lost irretrievably immediately after impact, but duration of retrograde loss is not maximal. Thereafter, memories are progressively unavailable for recall, implying a secondary progressive process (perhaps oedema) which impairs retrieval mechanisms for progressively more distant memories. Some of these return over the next 24 hours, the 'shrinking retrograde amnesia', presumably with resolution of the secondary process, but a proportion of the most recently experienced memories remain unavailable for recall despite apparent recovery. Consolidation of memories is therefore a complex process with several mechanisms whose fractionation will be the subject of future research.

The multiple dissociations within the amnesias have been reviewed by Moscovitch (1982). The general tenor of the evidence would support a distinction between two patterns of amnesic disorder, one hippocampal which may affect storage of information, and the other diencephalic which may affect encoding or acquisition (Winocur et al 1984). This point of view is well supported in the comprehensive review of Parkin (1984).

It appears that memory may be affected differently by lesions in different locations and that we are still far from clear as to which structures, or sets of structures, form the essential substrate for particular aspects of the total process. Though it has been argued that certain structures such as the hippocampus, mamillary bodies and dorsal thalamic nuclei are vital, there are enough negative instances, i.e. where damage to these structures did not produce amnesia, to hold a simplistic view; for review see Markowitsch (1984). All we may say with certainty is that lasting amnesia commonly follows bilateral damage to certain of the structures shown in the crude diagram (Fig. 9.3). What is perhaps most surprising is the absence of amnesic disorder with bilateral severing of such major fibre pathways as the fornix.

Preservation and dissociation

The terminology in the amnesias varies according to the model being espoused and it is important for those entering the field to have an early grasp of these terms even before studying the details of the cognitive neuropsychology of amnesia. Much of the stimulus for model building and the derivation of new terms has come from the study of dissociations in amnesic patients, i.e. what is lost and what is preserved. 'It is now widely held that the key to the amnesic syndrome lies in a model or theory that gives priority to the preserved/impaired character of the syndrome' (McCarthy & Warrington 1990). The understanding of preserved capabilities is also fundamental to the planning of rehabilitation.

Early studies focused on rates of forgetting. The subjects were predominant-

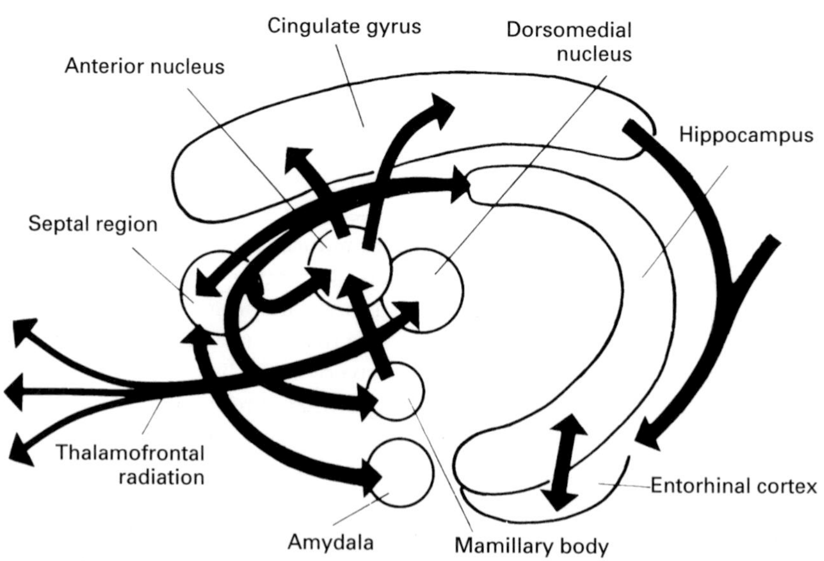

Fig. 9.3 Some of the structures which are involved in the neural substrate of memory.

ly those with an alcoholic Korsakoff syndrome, studies sometimes comparing these with small numbers from other categories of amnesia.

Huppert and Piercy (1979, 1982) compared the speed of forgetting of Milner's patient HM, whose lesions were wholly or largely hippocampal, with Korsakoff patients where all subjects were equated on their level of initial learning. The Korsakoff group showed that once the material was learnt subsequent forgetting was at a normal rate, whereas HM showed a higher rate of forgetting. However a later study of HM using Huppert and Piercy's methodology and pictorial material found no difference from normal forgetting (Freed et al 1987). Others have confirmed the normal forgetting of Korsakoff groups (Squire 1981, Martone et al 1986).

Squire (1981) also found a normal forgetting rate for his patient with a stab wound of the diencephalon (case NA, mentioned below). His study of patients following ECT, however, showed rapid forgetting, for which he postulated hippocampal dysfunction. Similarly, while confirming the normal forgetting rate for Korsakoff patients, Kopelman (1985) demonstrated rapid forgetting in Alzheimer patients. Whether this latter finding is related to presumed limbic (hippocampal) pathology in the Alzheimer group is open to confirmation. Finally, RB, a patient of Butters et al (1984), who suffered from 'aneurysmal amnesia' showed a 'precipitous decline' in recall though he had actually been superior to the controls at a very short interval.

A remarkable preservation in nearly all amnesics is the ability to acquire and retain visuomotor and visuoperceptual skills (Cermak et al 1973, Brooks & Baddeley 1976, Cohen & Squire 1980, Martone et al 1984). Cohen and Squire saw this as a dissociation between *procedural* or skill-based knowledge versus *declarative* or information-based knowledge. This terminology provided a useful shorthand for some time but further experimentation showed that it failed to do justice to the emerging elaboration of just what was preserved and what was compromised.

Butters and Stuss (1989) see this preservation of procedural knowledge as a reflection of the dissociation in amnesics between their largely preserved *implicit* memory and very poor *explicit* memory. Implicit here refers to the fact that previous experiences may facilitate performance without the individual being consciously aware, while explicit refers to conscious attempts to acquire knowledge.

The demonstration of the preservation of implicit memory or the effect of prior learning on subsequent retention stems back to the studies of Warrington and Weiskrantz (1968, 1970, 1974) and Gardner et al (1973). Subsequently, the topic was researched by such workers as Schacter, utilizing a variety of paradigms to explore the basis in greater detail (Schacter 1987a, b, Schacter et al 1988). A recent case of diencephalic amnesia following bilateral thalamic infarction also showed a clear dissociation between poor performance on both verbal and non-verbal tests of declarative memory with adequate performance on non-declarative memory tasks (Daum & Ackermann 1995).

In turn the efficacy of implicit memory has been shown to depend on, or to be closely related to, semantic knowledge (Winocur & Weiskrantz 1976, Shimamura & Squire 1984, Cermak et al 1985).

This brings out the third set of terms reflecting a dissociation in amnesics, namely that between *episodic memory* (memory for events) and *semantic memory* (memory for words and their meanings).

This distinction was introduced by Tulving (1973) and discussed in detail by Schacter and Tulving (1982) and Wood et al (1982). While the distinction accounts for further facts such as the details of retrograde amnesia, like the procedural/declarative distinction it cannot account for many experimental findings. These three major notions or models of memory, and others, are clearly summarized in McCarthy and Warrington (1990).

Recently a rather different approach to memory has come to the fore. It utilizes the concept of *working memory* (Baddeley 1986, 1992), stressing the close interaction of 'memory' with other systems, such as those devoted to attention and perception and the simultaneous processing that is proceeding in all modules. The conceptualization may prove productive, though we are still far from a definitive model to cope with the heterogeneous data subsumed under the word memory.

Thalamic dementias

These conditions form a group of disorders which are unlikely to be seen by neuropsychologists. They are caused by extensive bilateral damage to the thalamus. There are several familial forms, one of which represents the thalamic form of Creutzfeldt-Jakob disease (Petersen et al 1992, Iwasaki et al 1994, Kornfeld & Seelinger 1994), or the dementia may result from bilateral thalamic infarction (Sener et al 1993). In all cases there is a devastating combination of marked disorders of attention, memory, language, movement and affect.

Thalamic amnesia

Memory disturbance often accompanies thalamic aphasia, the usual cause of which is intracerebral haemorrhage (see below). Discrete lesions, most frequently infarctions, may also produce amnesia and this follows the material specificity shown with unilateral medial temporal lobe lesions outlined in Chapter 5. Speedie and Heilman (1982) reported a case of unilateral infarction in the left thalamus in a 33-year-old man. Following the sudden onset of confusion and disorientation the patient was unable to remember anything. The confusion cleared leaving him with a severe verbal anterograde amnesia with normal visual recognition memory. Some 'frontal' signs were present. Though isolated thalamic infarcts are uncommon, such pure verbal amnesia with unilateral left thalamic lesions is well documented (Parkin et al 1994, Rousseaux et al 1995, Sodeyama et al 1995). Sodeyama et al (1995) also review the anatomical sites involved in reported cases of persisting verbal amnesia. As in their own case, the structures most involved appeared to be the mamillothalamic tract, ventrolateral nucleus, lower portion of the medial nucleus and the internal medullary lamina.

Descriptions of non-verbal amnesia with right-sided infarcts are less common. One early case with right unilateral thalamic infarction affecting most of the dorsomedial nucleus (Speedie & Heilman 1983) showed an anterograde amnesia for visuospatial material with preserved verbal acquisition. This case also showed frontal signs. One recent case of right thalamic infarction showed a non-specific amnesia in the acute stage, but this reduced to a lasting, solely non-verbal amnesia in the chronic phase (Takamatsu et al 1990).

Five cases of thalamic infarction, three left-sided and two right-sided, reported by Graff-Radford et al (1984) support the differential role of the two thalami in specific memory functions, though the cases were all accompanied by other abnormalities of intellect and personality and best fit into the category of thalamic dementia.

Further reports supporting lateral specialization have come from Ghidoni et al (1989), Ino et al (1989) and Okada et al (1991). However, one case with a left medial thalamic haematoma showed difficulty with several figural memory tasks as well as the expected marked verbal memory deficit (Brown et al 1989).

A unique case of a stab wound involving the left dorsal thalamus was reported over many years (Teuber et al 1968, Squire & Slater 1978, Squire & Moore 1979). The evidence of lesion location is derived from CT scan so that precise anatomical definition is not possible. Nevertheless, the case shows sparing of perception, cognition and vigilance in the presence of a largely verbal-specific amnesia. This patient also showed paralysis of upward gaze, as reported in many bilateral thalamic infarcts with memory loss, arguing for a similar location of lesion. This case and that of Speedie and Heilman (1982) showed difficulty with complex non-verbal material (the Rey Figure) but not with simple material. Such a difficulty has also been described with amnesia arising from left posterior cerebral artery lesions (Signoret & Lhermitte 1976). It may be caused largely by a deficit in verbal encoding used when the material becomes complex. The study of patients undergoing thalamotomy for movement disorders provides added support for dissociation of function between the two sides of the thalamus (Krayenbuhl et al 1965, Ojemann et al 1968, Shapiro et al 1973). Likewise, stimulation at the time of operation lends further support (Ojemann & Fedio 1968, Ojemann 1971, 1977, 1979, 1981, Ojemann et al 1971, Fedio & Van Buren 1975). A comprehensive review is provided by Mateer and Ojemann (1983). As in all laterality relationships, however, there are exceptions and amnesia has been described occasionally following right-sided lesions (Akiguchi et al 1987, Tsoi et al 1987).

Finally, we are constantly reminded of the intimate relationship between the thalamus and the frontal lobes, as in a case of Daum and Ackermann (1994). Here a man with a right thalamic lesion showed not only specific (visuospatial) memory loss but also characteristics of frontal memory problems and frontal behavioural characteristics, such as irritability and disinhibition. Further instances continue to be reported (Eslinger et al 1991, Sandson et al 1991, Hashimoto et al 1995). Such cases probably occur more frequently than their appearance in the literature might suggest.

Thalamic aphasia

There had been a number of early reports of language disturbance with thalamic haemorrhage but the systematic examination of thalamic aphasia possibly dates from the paper of Fisher (1959). Though relatively rare, various studies of *left* thalamic haemorrhage and infarct in the past 40 years have confirmed the presence of aphasia (which is not normally seen with *right* thalamic haemorrhage), and clarified the characteristics of the disorder (Bugiani et al 1969, Ciemins 1970, Fazio et al 1973, Samarel et al 1976, Walshe et al 1977, Elghozi et al 1978, Cappa & Vignolo 1979, Demeurisse et al 1979, Mazaux et al 1979,

Reynolds et al 1979, Damasio et al 1982, Mazaux & Orgogozo 1982). One case of aphasia with right thalamic haemorrhage has been described in a left-handed person (Kirschner & Kistler 1982).

It has been argued that the more widespread effects with haemorrhagic lesions compared with those following infarction may be responsible for the more global aphasia rather than purely thalamic disruption, and this is supported by the observation that aphasia in some cases improved with time though the prognosis for full recovery after haemorrhage is poor. A review of global aphasia with thalamic haemorrhage is given by Kumar et al (1996). More instructive on the role of the thalamus are the cases of ischaemia or infarction in the left thalamus, though these instances are rare (Elghozi et al 1978, Speedie & Heilman 1982, 1983, Graff-Radford et al 1984). Blood flow studies are beginning to support the hypothesis that aphasia (as well as other disorders) may be produced by disturbance of thalamo-cortical connections (e.g. de la Sayette et al 1992, Megens et al 1992). In general, pathological studies (e.g. Lazzarino et al 1991) suggest that the paramedian nuclei, particularly the dorsomedial nucleus, play a major role.

In thalamic aphasia the emphasis is on expressive speech. While comprehension may be affected it is seldom a major feature. At the outset there may be complete arrest of speech but this soon disappears to leave a condition where the patient has difficulty with volume control. The patient speaks softly and there is verbal adynamia whereby the patient volunteers little or nothing, replying only to direct questions. There are semantic paraphasias both in spontaneous speech and on attempting to name objects. Disruption of the ordering of ideas coupled with perseveration of words and phrases may render speech incoherent. Some authors (e.g. Naeser et al 1982, Graff-Radford et al 1984) suggested that there may be a relation between type of aphasic symptomatology and anatomical location. Though little supporting evidence emerged (Robin & Schienberg 1990), the notion continues to be put forward: for example, Kennedy and Murdoch (1993) suggested that a range of aphasic disorders may be due to extra-thalamic lesions such as striato-capsular involvement, and claimed to be able to distinguish two separate syndromes, one thalamic and the other striato-capsular (Kennedy & Murdoch 1994).

There are isolated cases of agraphia, or alexia and agraphia, with preservation of oral language (Araki et al 1990, Aiba et al 1991).

Some improvement of language is the rule after subcortical lesions, but verbal adynamia and sometimes the associated verbal memory deficit may persist.

Thalamic neglect

Although unilateral neglect has been studied over a long period (see Ch. 6), contralateral neglect was first reported in three cases with right thalamic haemorrhage by Watson and Heilman (1979). The patients also showed limb akinesia, visuospatial disorders, anosognosia and emotional flattening. Soon after, Cambier and colleagues (1980) reported three more cases, two with haemorrhage and one with infarction of the right thalamus, all of whom had 'massive left visual neglect' without aphasia. The cases did, however, show 'excessive spontaneous verbalization and luxuriant answers to the most trivial question' (Cambier & Graveleau 1985, p. 88). We have observed this phenomenon in some right hemisphere cases with lesions affecting the right posterior cerebral artery territory. Cambier et al (1982) attribute the multimodal neglect seen with infarction from right posterior cerebral artery occlusion to the thalamus.

In summarizing this brief review one might say that there is emerging evidence that the asymmetry of function so characteristic of the cerebral hemispheres extends to embrace the interbrain and thus lends further support to the notion of extended functional systems. Much more remains to be learned about the role of cortico-subcortical connections in the functions discussed in this chapter.

References

Aiba E, Souma Y, Kulita I, Kishida K 1991 Two cases of pure agraphia developed after thalamic haemorrhage. No To Shinkei 43: 275–281

Akiguchi I, Ino T, Nabatama H et al 1987 Acute-onset amnestic syndrome with localized infarct on the dominant side – comparison between anteromedial thalamic lesion and posterior cerebral artery territory lesion. Japanese Journal of Medicine 26: 15–20

Albert M L, Butters N, Levin J 1979 Temporal gradients in the retrograde amnesia of patients with alcoholic Korsakoff's disease. Archives of Neurology 36: 211–216

Araki S, Kawamura M, Isono O, Honda H, Shiota J, Hirayama K1990 Reading and writing deficit in cases of localized infarction of the left anterior thalamus. No To Shinkei 42: 65–72

Baddeley A 1986 Working memory. Oxford University Press, Oxford

Baddeley A 1992 Working memory. Science 255: 556–559

Barbizet J 1970 Human memory and its pathology. Freeman, San Francisco

Barbizet J, Degos J D, Louarn S, Nguyen J P, Mas J L 1981 Amnésie par lésion ischémique bi-thalamique. Revue Neurologique 137: 415–424

Berlyne N 1972 Confabulation. British Journal of Psychiatry 120: 31–39

Bolter J F, Hannon R 1980 Cerebral damage associated with alcoholism: A re-examination. The Psychological Record 30: 165–179

Bonhoeffer K 1904 Der Korsakowsche Symptomenkomplex in seinen Beziehungen zu den verschieden Krankheitsformen. Allgemeine Zeitschrift für Psychiatrie 61: 744–752

Brierley J 1977 The neuropathology of amnesic states. In: Whitty C W M, Zangwill O L (eds) Amnesia, 2nd edn. Butterworths, London, pp 199–223

Brion S, Derome P, Guiot G, Teitgen Mme 1968 Syndrome de Korsakoff par anevrysme de l'artère communicante antèrieure: le problème des syndromes de Korsakoff par hémorragie meningée. Revue Neurologique 118: 293–299

Brooks D N, Baddeley A D 1976 What can amnesic patients learn? Neuropsychologia 14: 111–122

Brown G G, Kieran S, Patel S 1989 Memory functioning following a left medial thalamic hematoma. Journal of Clinical and Experimental Neuropsychology 11: 206–218

Bugiani O, Conforto C, Sacco G 1969 Aphasia in thalamic hemorrhage. Lancet 1: 1052

Butters N, Stuss D T 1989 Diencephalic amnesia. In: Bolter C, Grafman J (eds) Handbook of neuropsychology. Elsevier, Amsterdam, vol 3, ch 5, pp 107–148

Butters N, Milliotis P, Albert M S, Sax D S 1984 Memory assessment: evidence of the heterogeneity of amnesic symptoms. In: Goldstein G (ed) Advances in clinical neuropsychology. Plenum, New York, vol 1, pp 127–159

Cambier J, Graveleau T 1985 Thalamic syndromes. In: Vinken P J, Bruyn G W, Klawans H L (eds) Handbook of clinical neurology, New series l. Elsevier, Amsterdam, vol 45, pp 87–98

Cambier J, Elghozi D, Strube E 1980 Lésions du thalamus droit avec syndrome de l'hémisphère mineur. Discussion du concept de négligence thalamique. Revue Neurologique 136: 106–166

Cambier J, Masson M, Graveleau T, Elghozi D 1982 Sémiologie de négligence lors de lésions ischémiques dans le territoire de l'artère cérébrale postérieure droite. Revue Neurologique 138: 631–648

Cappa S F, Vignolo L A 1979 'Transcortical' features of aphasia following left thalamic hemorrhage. Cortex 15: 121–130

Castaigne P, Lhermitte F, Buge A, Escourolle R, Hauw J J, Lyon-Caen O 1981 Paramedian thalamic and midbrain infarcts: clinical and neuropsychological study. Annals of Neurology 10: 127–148

Cermak L S, Butters N, Gerrein J 1973 The extent of the verbal encoding ability of Korsakoff patients. Neuropsychologia 11: 85–94

Cermak L S, Butters N, Moreines J 1974 Some analyses of the verbal encoding deficit of alcoholic Korsakoff patients. Brain and Language 1: 141–150

Cermak L S, Talbot N, Chandler K, Wolbarst L R 1985 The perceptual priming phenomenon in amnesia. Neuropsychologia 23: 615–622

Ciemins V A 1970 Localized thalamic haemorrhage: a cause of aphasia. Neurology 20: 776–782

Cohen N J, Squire L R 1980 Preserved learning and retention of patterning skill in amnesia: dissociation of knowing how and knowing what. Science 210: 207–209

Cohen N J, Squire L R 1981 Retrograde amnesia and remote memory impairment. Neuropsychologia 19: 337–356

Cramon D von, Zihl J 1979 Roving eye movements with bilateral symmetrical lesions of the thalamus. Journal of Neurology 221: 105–112

Damasio A R, Damasio H, Rizzo M, Varney N, Gersh F 1982 Aphasia with nonhemorrhagic lesions in the basal ganglia and internal capsule. Archives of Neurology 39: 15–24

Daum I, Ackermann H 1994 Frontal type memory impairment associated with thalamic damage. International Journal of the Neurosciences 77: 187–198

Daum I, Ackermann H 1995 Dissociation of declarative and nondeclarative memory after bilateral thalamic lesions: A case report. International Journal Of Neuroscience 75: 153–165

de la Sayette V, Le Doze F, Bouvard G et al 1992 Right motor neglect associated with dynamic aphasia, loss of drive and amnesia: case report and cerebral blood flow study. Neuropsychologia 30: 109–121

Delay J, Brion S, Derouesné C 1964 Syndrome de Korsakoff et étiologie tumorale: étude anatomo-clinique de trois observations. Revue Neurologique 111: 97–133

Demeurisse G, Derouck M, Coekaerts M J et al 1979 Study of two cases of aphasia by infarction of the left thalamus, without cortical lesion. Acta Neurologica Belgica 79: 450–459

Elghozi D, Strube E, Signoret J L, Cambier J, Lhermitte F 1978 Quasi-aphasie lors de lésions du thalamus. Revue Neurologique 134: 557–574

Eslinger P J, Warner G C, Grattan L M, Easton J D 1991 "Frontal lobe" utilization behavior associated with paramedian thalamic infarction. Neurology 41: 450–452

Evans J J, Breen E K, Antoun N, Hodges J R 1996 Focal retrograde amnesia for autobiographical events following cerebral vasculitis: a connectionist account. Neurocase 2: 1–11

Fazio L, Sacco G, Bugiani O 1973 The thalamic haemorrhage. An anatomo-clinical study. European Neurology 9: 30–43

Fedio P, Van Buren J M 1975 Memory and perceptual deficits during electrical stimulation in the left and right thalamus and parietal subcortex. Brain and Language 2: 78–100

Fisher C M 1959 The pathological and clinical aspects of thalamic hemorrhage. Transactions of the American Neurological Association 84: 56–59

Flateau E 1921 Sur les hémorragies meningées idiopathiques. Gazette des Hôpitaux 94: 1077–1081

Freed D, Corkin S, Cohen N 1987 Forgetting in H.M.: a second look. Neuropsychologia 25: 461–471

Gade A 1982 Amnesia after operations on aneurysms of the anterior communicating artery. Surgical Neurology 18: 46–49

Gamper E 1928 Zur Frage der Polioencephalitis der chronischen Alkoholiker. Deutsche Zeitschrift für Nervenheilkunde 102: 122–129

Gardner H, Boller F, Moreines J, Butters N 1973 Retrieving information from Korsakoff patients; effects of categorical cues and reference to the task. Cortex 9: 165–175

Ghidoni E, Pattacini F, Galimberti D, Aguzzoli L 1989 Lacunar thalamic infarcts and amnesia. European Neurology 29 (suppl 2): 13–15

Goldberg E, Antin S P, Bilder R M, Gerstman L J, Hughes J E O 1981 Retrograde amnesia: possible role of mesencephalic reticular activation in long-term memory. Science 213: 1392–1394
Goldenberg G, Podreka I, Pfaffelmeyer N, Wessely P, Deecke L 1991 Thalamic ischemia in transient global amnesia: a SPECT study. Neurology 41: 1748–1752
Gorelick P B, Amico L L, Ganellan R, Benevento L A 1988 Transient global amnesia and thalamic infarction. Neurology 38: 496–499
Graff-Radford N R, Eslinger P J, Damasio A R, Yamada T 1984 Nonhemorrhagic infarction of the thalamus. Behavioral, anatomic, and physiological correlates. Neurology 34: 14–23
Graff-Radford N R, Tranel D, Brandt J 1988 Anatomical and neuropsychological characteristics of amnesia from bilateral thalamic infarcts. Neurology 38 (suppl 1): 171
Graff-Radford N R, Tranel D, Van Hoesen G W, Brandt J P 1990 Diencephalic amnesia. Brain 113: 1–25
Gruner J E 1956 Sur la pathologie des encéphalopathies alcooliques. Revue Neurologique 94: 682–689
Grunthal E 1939 Uber das Corpus mamillare und den Korsakowschen symptomencomplex. Confinia Neurologica 2: 64–95
Harper C 1982 Neuropathology of brain damage caused by alcohol. Medical Journal of Australia 2: 277–282
Harper C G, Kril J J, Holloway R L 1985 Shrinkage in chronic alcoholics: a pathological study. British Medical Journal 20: 501–504
Hashimoto R, Yoshida M, Tanaka Y 1995 Utilization behavior after right thalamic infarction. European Neurology 35: 58–62
Hécaen H, Ajuriaguerra J de 1956 Les encéphalopathies alcooliques subaiguées et chroniques. Revue Neurologique 94: 528–555
Horel J A 1978 The neuroanatomy of amnesia. A critique of the hippocampal memory hypothesis. Brain 107: 403–445
Huppert F A, Piercy M 1979 Normal and abnormal forgetting in organic amnesia: effect of locus of lesion. Cortex 15: 385–390
Huppert F A, Piercy M 1982 In search of the functional locus of amnesic syndromes. In: Cermak L S (ed) Human memory and amnesia. Erlbaum, Hillsdale, N J
Ino T, Akiguchi I, Nabatame H, Kameyama M 1989 Left antero-medial thalamic infarction and symptoms of amnesia, aphasia, and dementia. Rinsho Shinkeigaku 29: 693–700
Iwasaki Y, Ikeda K, Tagaya N, Kinoshita M 1994 Magnetic resonance imaging and neuropathological findings in two patients with Creutzfeldt-Jakob disease. Journal of the Neurological Sciences 126: 228–231
Janet P 1928 L'évolution de la mémoire et la notion du temps. Chahine, Paris
Jones E G 1985 The thalamus. Plenum Press, New York
Kahn E A, Crosby E C 1972 Korsakoff's syndrome associated with surgical lesions involving the mamillary bodies. Neurology 22: 117–125
Kapur N, Coughlan A K 1980 Confabulation and frontal lobe dysfunction. Journal of Neurology, Neurosurgery and Psychiatry 43: 461–463
Kennedy M, Murdoch B E 1993 Chronic aphasia subject to striato-capsular and thalamic lesions in the left hemisphere. Brain and Language 44: 284–295
Kennedy M, Murdoch B E 1994 Thalamic aphasia and striato-capsular aphasia as independent aphasic syndromes: A review. Aphasiology 8: 303–313
Kinsella G, Clausen H 1982 Amnesia following rupture of an anterior communicating artery aneurysm. In: Stanley G V, Walsh K W (eds) Brain Impairment. Proceedings of the Seventh Brain Impairment Conference, University of Melbourne, pp 121–130
Kirschner H S, Kistler K H 1982 Aphasia after right thalamic haemorrhage. Archives of Neurology 39: 667–669
Kopelman M 1985 Rates of forgetting in Alzheimer-type dementia and Korsakoff's syndrome. Neuropsychologia 23: 623–638
Kopelman M D 1995 The Korsakoff syndrome. British Journal of Psychiatry 166: 154–173
Kornfeld M, Seelinger D F 1994 Pure thalamic dementia with a single focus of spongiform change in cerebral cortex. Clinical Neuropathology 13: 77–81
Kovner R, Mattis S, Gartner J, Goldmeier E 1981 A verbal semantic deficit in the alcoholic Korsakoff syndrome. Cortex 17: 419–426

Krayenbuhl H, Siegfried J, Kohenhof M, Yasargil M G 1965 Is there a dominant thalamus? Confinia Neurologica 26: 246–249

Kritchevsky M, Graff-Radford N R, Damasio A R 1987 Normal memory after damage to medial thalamus. Archives of Neurology 44: 959–962

Kumar R, Masih A K, Pardo J 1996 Global aphasia due to thalamic haemorrhage: a case report and review of the literature. Archives of Physical Medicine and Rehabilitation 77: 1312–1315

Lawrence C 1984 Testing for memory disorder. Editorial comment. Australian and New Zealand Journal of Psychiatry 18: 207–210

Lazzarino L G, Nicolai A, Valassi F, Biasizzo E 1991 Language disturbances from mesencephalo-thalamic infarcts. Identification of thalamic nuclei by CT reconstructions. Neuroradiology 33: 300–304

Lhermitte F, Signoret J L 1972 Analyse neuro-psychologique ed différenciation des syndromes amnésiques. Revue Neurologique 126: 161–178

Lindqvist G, Norlén G 1966 Korsakoff's syndrome after operation on ruptured aneurysm of anterior communicating artery. Acta Psychiatrica Scandinavica 42: 24–34

Lobosky J M, Vangilder J C, Damasio A R 1984 Behavioural manifestations of third ventricular colloid cysts. Journal of Neurology, Neurosurgery, and Psychiatry 47: 1075–1080

Logue V, Durward M, Pratt T R C et al 1968 The quality of survival after rupture of an anterior cerebral aneurysm. British Journal of Psychiatry 114: 137–160

Luria A R 1976 The neuropsychology of memory. Winston and Sons, Washington

Mair W G, Warrington E K, Weiskrantz L 1979 Memory disorder in Korsakoff's psychosis: a neuropathological and neuropsychological investigation of two cases. Brain 102: 749–783

Malamud N, Skillicorn S A 1956 Relationship between the Wernicke and Korsakoff syndrome. Archives of Neurology and Psychiatry 76: 585–596

Markowitsch H J 1984 Can amnesia be caused by damage to a single structure? Cortex 20: 27–45

Markowitsch H J 1988 Diencephalic amnesia: a reorientation towards tracts? Brain Research 472: 351–370

Marslen-Wilson W D, Teuber H L 1975 Memory for remote events in anterograde amnesia: recognition of public figures from news photographs. Neuropsychologia 13: 347–352

Martone M, Butters N, Payne M, Becker J T 1984 Dissociations between skill learning and verbal recognition in amnesia and dementia. Archives of Neurology 41: 965–970

Martone M, Butters N, Trauner D 1986 Some analyses of forgetting of pictorial material in amnesic and demented patients. Journal of Clinical and Experimental Neuropsychology 8: 161–178

Masdeu J C 1985 The anatomic localization of lesions in the thalamus. In: Brazis P W, Masdeu J C, Biller J (eds) Localization in clinical neurology. Little Brown, Boston, ch 17

Mateer C A, Ojemann G A 1983 Thalamic mechanisms in language and memory. In: Segalowitz S J (ed) Language functions and brain organization. Academic Press, New York, pp 171–191

Mattis S, Kovner R, Goldmeier E 1978 Different patterns of mnemonic deficits in two organic amnesic syndromes. Brain and Language 6: 171–191

Mazaux J M, Orgogozo J M 1982 Etude analytique et quantitative des troubles du langage par lésion du thalamus gauche: l'aphasie thalamique. Cortex 18: 403–406

Mazaux J M, Orgogozo J M, Henry P, Loiseau P 1979 Troubles du langage au cours des lésions thalamiques. Revue Neurologique 135: 59–64

McCarthy R A, Warrington E K 1990 Cognitive neuropsychology. A clinical introduction. Academic Press, San Diego

McEntee W J, Biber M P, Perl D P, Benson D F 1976 Diencephalic amnesia: a reappraisal. Journal of Neurology, Neurosurgery and Psychiatry 39: 436–441

Megens J, van Loon J, Goffin J, Gybels J 1992 Subcortical aphasia from a thalamic abscess. Journal of Neurology, Neurosurgery and Psychiatry 55: 319–321

Mercer B, Wapner W, Gardner H, Benson D F 1977 A study of confabulation. Archives of Neurology 34: 429–433

Meudell P, Mayes A 1982 Normal and abnormal forgetting: some comments on the human amnesic syndrome. In: Ellis A W (ed) Normality and pathology in cognitive function. Academic Press, London, pp 203–237

Mills R P, Swanson P D 1978 Vertical oculomotor apraxia and memory loss. Annals of Neurology 4: 149–153
Milner B 1966 Amnesia following operations on the temporal lobes. In: Whitty C W M, Zangwill O L (eds) Amnesia. Butterworth, London
Milner B 1970 Memory and the medial temporal regions of the brain. In: Pribram K H, Broadbent D E (eds) Biology of memory. Academic Press, New York, pp 29–50
Moscovitch M 1982 Multiple dissociations of function in amnesia. In: Cermak L S (ed) Memory and amnesia. Erlbaum, Hillsdale, N J
Naeser M A, Alexander M P, Helm-Esterbrooks N, Levine H L, Laughlin S A, Geschwind N 1982 Aphasia with predominantly subcortical lesion sites: description of three capsular / putaminal aphasia syndromes. Archives of Neurology 39: 2–14
Norlén G, Olivecrona H 1953 The treatment of aneurysms of the circle of Willis. Journal of Neurosurgery 10: 414–415
Ojemann G 1971 Alteration in nonverbal short-term memory with stimulation in the region of the mamillothalamic tract in man. Neuropsychologia 9: 15–201
Ojemann G 1977 Asymmetric function of the thalamus in man. Annals of the New York Academy of Science 299: 380–396
Ojemann G 1979 Altering human memory with human ventrolateral thalamic stimulation. In: Hitchcock E, Ballantine H, Myerson B (eds) Modern concepts in psychiatric surgery. Elsevier, Amsterdam, pp 103–109
Ojemann G 1981 Interrelationship in the localization of language, memory and motor mechanisms in human cortex and thalamus. In: Thomson R (ed) New perspectives in cerebral localization. Raven Press, New York, pp 157–175
Ojemann G, Fedio P 1968 Effect of stimulation of the human thalamus and temporal white matter on short term memory. Journal of Neurosurgery 29: 51–59
Ojemann G, Hoyenga K, Ward A 1968 Prediction of short-term memory disturbances after ventrolateral thalamotomy. Journal of Neurosurgery 35: 203–210
Ojemann G, Blick K, Ward A 1971 Improvement and disturbance of short-term verbal memory with ventrolateral thalamic stimulation. Brain 94: 225–240
Okada V, Sadoshima S, Fujii K, Ichiya Y, Fujishima M 1991 Cerebral blood flow and metabolism in an amnestic patient with left thalamic infarction – a positron emission study. Japan Journal of Medicine 30: 367–372
Orchinik C W 1960 Some psychological aspects of circumscribed lesions of the diencephalon. Confinia Neurologica 20: 292–310
Parkin A J 1984 Amnesic syndrome: a lesion-specific disorder? Cortex 20: 479–508
Parkin A J, Rees J E, Hunkin N M, Rose P E 1994 Impairment of memory following discrete thalamic infarction. Neuropsychologia 32: 39–51
Percheron G 1976 Les artères du thalamus humain. II. Artères et territoires thalamiques paramédians de l'artère basilaire communicante. Revue Neurologique 132: 309–324
Petersen R B, Tabaton M, Berg L et al 1992 Analysis of the prion protein gene in thalamic dementia. Neurology 42: 1859–1863
Piercy M F 1977 Experimental studies of the amnesic syndrome. In: Whitty C W M, Zangwill O L (eds) Amnesia, 2nd edn. Butterworth, Woburn, Massachusetts, pp 1–52
Raffaele R, Tornali C, Genezzani A A, Vecchio I 1995 Transient global amnesia and cerebral infarct: A case report. Brain Injury 9: 815–818
Remy M 1942 Contribution a l'étude de la maladie de Korsakow. Monatsschrift für Psychiatrie und Neurologie 106: 128–144
Reynolds A F, Turner P T, Harris A B, Ojemann G A, Davis L E 1979 Left thalamic haemorrhage with dysphasia: A report of 5 cases. Brain and Language 7: 62–73
Robin D A, Schienberg S 1990 Subcortical lesions and aphasia. Journal of Speech and Hearing Disorders 55: 90–100
Rousseaux M, Cabaret M, Benaim C, Steinling M 1995 Deficit of verbal recall caused by left dorso-lateral thalamic infarction. Revue Neurologique 151: 34–46
Samarel A, Wright T L, Sergay S, Tyler R H 1976 Thalamic hemorrhage with speech disorder. Transactions of the American Neurological Association 101: 283–285
Sanders H I, Warrington E K 1971 Memory for remote events in amnesic patients. Brain 94: 661–668
Sandson T A, Daffner K R, Carvalho P A, Mesulam M M 1991 Frontal lobe dysfunction following infarction of the left-sided medial thalamus. Archives of Neurology 48: 1300–1303

Schacter D L 1987a Implicit memory: history and current status. Journal of Experimental Psychology. Memory, Learning and Cognition 13: 501–518
Schacter D L 1987b Implicit expressions of memory in organic amnesia: learning new facts and associations. Human Neurobiology 6: 107–118
Schacter D L, Tulving E 1982 Memory, amnesia and the episodic semantic distinction. In: Isaacson R L, Spear N E (eds) Expression of knowledge. Plenum, New York
Schacter D L, McAndrews M P, Moscovitch M 1988 Access to consciousness: dissociations between implicit and explicit knowledge in neuropsychological syndromes. In: Weiskrantz L (ed) Thought without language. Oxford University Press, New York, pp 242–277
Schott B, Mauguiere F, Laurent B, Serclerat O, Fischer C 1980 L'amnésie thalamique. Revue Neurologique 136: 117–130
Scoville W B, Milner B 1957 Loss of recent memory after bilateral hippocampal lesions. Journal of Neurology, Neurosurgery and Psychiatry 20: 11–21
Seltzer B, Benson D F 1974 The temporal pattern of retrograde amnesia in Korsakoff's disease. Neurology 24: 527–530
Sener R N, Alper H, Yunten N, Dundar C 1993 Bilateral acute thalamic infarcts causing thalamic dementia. American Journal of Roentgenology 161: 678–679
Sengupta R P, Chiu J S P, Brierly H 1975 Quality of survival following direct surgery for anterior communicating artery aneurysms. Journal of Neurosurgery 43: 58–64
Shapiro D Y, Sadowsky D, Henderson W, Van Buren J 1973 An assessment of cognitive function in post-thalamotomy Parkinson patients. Confinia Neurologica 35: 144–166
Shimamura A, Squire L R 1984 Paired-associate learning and priming effects in amnesia: a neuropsychological study. Journal of Experimental Psychology 113: 556–570
Signoret J L, Lhermitte F 1976 The amnesic syndrome and encoding process. In: Rosenzweig M R, Bennett E L (eds) Neural mechanisms of learning and memory. MIT Press, Cambridge, Massachusetts, pp 67–75
Smythe G E, Stern K 1938 Tumours of the thalamus - a clinico-pathological study. Brain 61: 339–374
Sodeyama N, Tamaki M, Sugishita M 1995 Persistent pure verbal amnesia and transient aphasia after left thalamic infarction. Journal of Neurology 242: 289–294
Speedie L J, Heilman K M 1982 Amnestic disturbance following infarction of the left dorsomedial nucleus of the thalamus. Neuropsychologia 20: 597–604
Speedie L J, Heilman K M 1983 Anterograde memory deficits for visuospatial material after infarction of the right thalamus. Archives of Neurology 40: 183–186
Squire L R 1981 Two forms of human amnesia: an analysis of forgetting. Journal of Neuroscience l: 635–640
Squire L R, Cohen N 1982 Remote memory, retrograde amnesia and the neuropsychology of memory. In: Cermak L (ed) Human memory and amnesia. Lawrence Erlbaum, Hillsdale, New Jersey, pp 275–303
Squire L R, Moore R Y 1979 Dorsal thalamic lesion in a noted case of human memory dysfunction. Annals of Neurology 6: 503–506
Squire L R, Slater P C 1978 Bilateral and unilateral ECT: effects on verbal and nonverbal memory. American Journal of Psychiatry 135: 1316–1320
Squire L R, Amaral D G, Press G A 1990 Magnetic resonance imaging of the hippocampal formation and mammillary nuclei distinguish temporal lobe and diencephalic amnesia. Journal of Neuroscience 10: 3106–3107
Stuss D T, Alexander M P, Lieberman A, Levine H 1978 An extraordinary form of confabulation. Neurology 28: 1166–1172
Stuss D T, Guberman A, Nelson R, Larochelle S 1988 The neuropsychology of paramedian thalamic infarction. Brain and Cognition 8: 348–378
Takamatsu K, Yamamoto M, Ohno F 1990 A case of amnestic syndrome due to right thalamic infarction. Japanese Journal of Medicine 29: 301–304
Talland G 1965 Deranged memory. Academic Press, New York
Talland G A, Sweet W H, Ballantine H T 1967 Amnesic syndrome with anterior communicating artery aneurysm. Journal of Nervous and Mental Disease 145: 179–192
Tarachow S 1939 The Korsakoff psychosis in spontaneous subarachnoid haemorrhage. Report of three cases. American Journal of Psychiatry 5: 887–899
Teuber H L, Milner B, Vaughan H G 1968 Persistent anterograde amnesia after stab wound of the basal brain. Neuropsychologia 6: 267–282

Tsoi M M, Huang C Y, Lee A O, Yu Y L 1987 Amnesia following right thalamic haemorrhage. Clinical and Experimental Neurology 23: 201–207
Tulving E 1973 Episodic and semantic memory. In: Tulving E, Donaldson W (eds) Organization of memory. Academic Press, New York
Venneri A, Caffarra P 1998 Transient autobiographic amnesia: EEG and single-photon emission CT evidence of an organic etiology. Neurology 50: 186–191
Victor M 1976 The Wernicke-Korsakoff syndrome. In: Vinken P J, Bruyn G W (eds) Handbook of clinical neurology. North-Holland, Amsterdam, vol 28, ch 9
Victor M, Yakovlev P I 1955 S.S. Korsakoff's psychic disorder in conjunction with peripheral neuritis. A translation of Korsakoff's original article with brief comments on the author and his contribution to clinical medicine. Neurology 5: 394–406
Victor M, Adams R D, Collins G F 1971 The Wernicke- Korsakoff syndrome. Davis, Philadelphia
Volpe B T, Hirst W 1983 Amnesia following the rupture and repair of an anterior communicating artery aneurysm. Journal of Neurology, Neurosurgery, and Psychiatry 46: 704–709
von Gudden B 1896 Klinische und anatomische Beiträge zur Kenntnis der multiphen Alkoholneuritis nebst Bemerkungen über die Regenerationsvorgange im peripheren Nervensystem. Archiv für Psychiatrie und Nervenkrankenheiten 28: 643–741
Walsh K W 1982 Thalamic amnesia: A key to the problem of memory disorders? In: Stanley G V, Walsh K W (eds) Brain impairment. Proceedings of the Seventh Brain Impairment Workshop, University of Melbourne, pp 96–120
Walsh K W 1991 Understanding brain damage. A primer of neuro psychological evaluation. 2nd edn Churchill Livingstone, Edinburgh
Walshe J M, Davis K R, Fischer C H 1977 Thalamic haemorrhage: a computed tomographic clinical correlation. Neurology 27: 217–222
Walton J N 1953 The Korsakov syndrome in spontaneous subarachnoid haemorrhage. Brain 99: 521–530
Warrington E K, Weiskrantz L 1968 New method of testing long-term retention with special reference to amnesic patients. Nature 217: 972–974
Warrington E K, Weiskrantz L 1970 Amnesic syndrome: consolidation or retrieval? Nature 228: 628–630
Warrington E K, Weiskrantz L 1974 The effect of prior learning on subsequent retention in amnesic patients. Neuropsychologia 12: 419–428
Watson R T, Heilman K M 1979 Thalamic neglect. Neurology 2: 60–64
Whitty C W M, Zangwill O L 1977 Amnesia, 2nd edn. Butterworth, London
Winocur G, Weiskrantz L 1976 An investigation of paired-associate learning in amnesic patients. Neuropsychologia 14: 97–110
Winocur G, Oxbury S, Roberts R, Agnetti V, Davis C 1984 Amnesia in a patient with bilateral lesions to the thalamus. Neuropsychologia 22: 123–143
Wood F, Ebert V, Kinsbourne M 1982 The episodic-semantic distinction in memory and amnesia. In: Cermak L (ed) Human memory and amnesia. Erlbaum, Hillsdale, N J, pp 167–193
Yarnell P R, Lynch S 1970 Retrograde memory immediately after concussion. Lancet 1: 863–864
Yarnell P R, Lynch S 1973 The "ding": amnestic states in football trauma. Neurology 23: 196–197
Zangwill O L 1943 Clinical tests of memory impairment. Proceedings of the Royal Society of Medicine 36: 576–580
Ziegler D K, Kaufman A, Marshall H E 1977 Abrupt memory loss associated with thalamic tumor. Archives of Neurology 34: 545–548

10

Neuropsychological assessment

GENERAL CONSIDERATIONS

Some conceptual problems

Brain damage

The search for tests of 'organicity' or 'brain damage' is now only of historical interest to most neuropsychologists. Earlier reviews dealt adequately with the shortcomings of this approach (Yates 1954, Meyer 1957, Smith 1962, Yates 1966, Kinsbourne 1971, Reitan & Davison 1974) though the controversy is by no means ended. Examples of opposing views can be seen in Mapou (1988) versus Kane et al (1989).

The argument against single or group tests of 'brain damage' does not mean that cerebral lesions do not have generalized or non-specific effects. Long ago, Yates (1966) pointed out that brain damage may produce different types of effect in any individual: (i) a general deterioration in all aspects of functioning; (ii) differential (group) effects, depending on the location, extent and other characteristics of the damage; and (iii) highly specific effects in certain locations. Each of these needs to be taken into account when inferring the reason for poor test performance.

Clinical validation

A test validated on clearly defined groups (e.g. brain damaged versus normal) may have low predictive validity. If it can identify 'only those subjects whose brain damage is obvious, then the test serves no useful purpose, since it confirms what needs no confirmation' (Yates 1966). 'A crucial study would be one in which the neurological group is made up entirely of subjects for whom neurologists disagree as to diagnosis or are unable to make a diagnostic statement at all at the time the psychological measure is obtained and for whom retrospective diagnosis is possible' (Heilbrun 1962, p. 513). One such study is that of Matthews, Shaw and Kløve (1966) who showed that some measures held up in this predictive validity situation, while others did not. Further treatment of this topic with illustrative cases is given in Walsh (1991).

Determinants of performance

Another shortcoming of studies relates to the principle of multiple determination. 'Behavioural deficits are defined in terms of impaired test performance. But impaired test performance may be a final common pathway for expression of quite diverse types of impairment' (Kinsbourne 1972). Smith (1975) commented about a commonly used test, the Digit-Symbol Substitution Test, in similar vein, 'the responses are the end product of the integration of visual perceptual, oculomotor, fine manual motor and mental functions'. It is therefore important to be aware that low scores on such complex tasks may be caused by a disturbance in any of the functions involved or any combination of them.

If complex tests must be used, two methods of clarification are possible: (i) to observe the sharing of variance between a patient's performance on sundry tests; and (ii) to test hypotheses about the various possible reasons for failure (see below). In the latter instance the practitioner will be helped by a sound understanding of the corpus of knowledge in neuropsychology.

A notion closely allied to multiple determination is that of multiple pathways to the goal. Many psychological tests are concerned solely with whether or not the subject can reach the goal. 'The flexibility of cerebral mechanisms is such that the solution of most test items can be reached by many devious routes. The method the subject uses in tackling a problem will in general provide more information as to the character of a skill or of a psychological deficit than will the knowledge as to the subject's success or failure' (Elithorn 1965). Qualitative observations are of paramount value and no amount of quantification will, at times, override the importance of the psychologist as an observer of behaviour.

Face validity and the seductive inference

There is a danger in assuming that if a patient fails on a test then that patient has a deficiency in the psychological function stated by the manual to be what the test measures; however, 'most tests have only an indirect relationship with the variables they are supposed to measure' (Shapiro 1973).

A simple example of making the wrong inference might be as follows: the patient produces a poor score on a memory for designs test, e.g. the Benton Visual Retention Test, and this is then reported as a 'visual memory deficit' and this may be extended to the further inference that 'the patient shows poor visual memory suggesting impairment of the right hemisphere' or even more specifically 'the patient shows differentially poor visual memory with normal verbal memory suggesting impairment of the right temporal region'. However, in the form given, the memory for designs test may have relied on the patient drawing the remembered stimulus. Thus one of the possible reasons for failure could be an executive or graphic difficulty, i.e. the reason for failure is the same as the reason the patient fails on other tasks with a constructional element. Awareness of such a possibility would prompt the use of a task where the constructional element has been removed, e.g. the multiple choice version of the BVRT. Here the subject is shown a design and then must select it some time later from a multiple choice array which contains the item plus three distractors. The same logic applies, *mutatis mutandis*, to the examination of other possible causes for poor performance, e.g. perceptual difficulties.

In summary, many tests are multifactorial in their composition and hypotheses about the possible reasons for poor performance need to be examined. This process may involve the use of other tasks, but may also be solved by noting the performance of the subject on tests already performed. The multifactorial determination of test scores is one of the stumbling blocks of deriving inferences from group data since 'Different individuals may obtain the same test score on a particular test for very different reasons' (Ryan & Butters 1980).

Miller (1983) nicely refers to the process as 'paralogical thinking'. He cites one study which argued that since normal elderly subjects did less well on tests which have been shown to be sensitive to right hemisphere pathology, the right hemisphere ages more rapidly than the left. He emphasizes that while a lesion located at a particular point may produce a test deficit, this does not mean that the converse follows. 'In fact the logical status of this argument is the same as arguing that because a horse meets the test of being a large animal with four legs that any newly encountered large animal with four legs must be a horse. The newly encountered specimen could of course be a cow or hippopotamus and still meet the same test' (Miller 1983, p 131).

Further examples of incorrect inferences are given in Walsh (1995).

Sharing of variance

On the other hand, multiple failures on seemingly disparate tests may reflect a common disorder. The magnitude of the failure on separate tests will be a reflection of the degree to which the disturbed function is represented in their composition. In most situations only a small number of functional disturbances will account for the many observed deficits in performance. In attempting to explain them it is wise to remember that the law of parsimony has never been repealed.

Summarizing measures

A further difficulty with tests is that the frequently used aggregate indices may bury the very data which are of significance in understanding the patient's difficulties (see Lezak 1988, Walsh 1991). A subject may obtain a Memory Quotient on the Wechsler Memory Scale above 120, an apparently superior memory performance. However, in some cases the subject may show by consistent failure of all 'hard' items of the Associate Learning subtest that he has a severe new learning or amnesic disorder which is confirmed by the clinical history substantiated by extended testing.

The same logic extends to the summing of items *within* a test. In both cases certain critical item or subtest failures of key significance can be obscured. A classical example in pseudoneurological cases is the failing of easy items accompanied by passes on the more difficult, although the summed score is 'within normal limits' or 'fails to meet the cutting point'. In such cases failure on simple problems is most unlikely to be due to neural incapacity and raises the possibility of role enactment. For detailed examples see Pankratz et al (1975), Pankratz (1979, 1983), Binder & Pankratz (1987), Pankratz et al (1987), Pankratz & Paar (1988), Walsh (1991).

If one invokes the simple notion that the difficult subsumes the easy, then combined scores means that this key to understanding of the individual case may be lost. Internal consistency with regard to item difficulty is an important element of the interpretation of test performance.

Finally, a summary score may lead some to assume that it has the same significance in the neurologically impaired as it has in the intact subject. For example, two equally gifted individuals sustain head injuries. After the acute phase one individual tests higher on an intelligence scale, leading some to believe that the prospects for rehabilitation in that case are better. However, the individual with the higher score has features of the dysexecutive or frontal syndrome, rendering occupational rehabilitation difficult or impossible, while the individual with the lower score does not have such features and can be rehabilitated, albeit at a lower level of work than before.

Symptoms and syndromes

The significance of a patient's symptoms and signs can be understood in the context of the notion of a functional system (Ch. 1). A functional system in the brain consists of a number of parts of the brain, particularly but not exclusively cortical, together with their fibre connections. The system operates in a concerted manner to form the substratum of a complex psychological function. This systemic concept allows a new approach to the use of psychological tests in the diagnosis or assessment of neurological conditions, an approach which parallels the study of other bodily systems.

It will be apparent that if a psychological process is served by an anatomical system which is spread out in the brain then the psychological process will be vulnerable at a number of different points, some of which may be widely separated. Such a finding was, in fact, one of the seemingly powerful arguments used against the early localizationists. If, for example, speaking or writing or perceiving could be altered by lesions in sundry locations, then these functions could not be localized. The argument turns, of course, on what is meant by 'localized'.

The modern notion of a functional system also incorporates the notion of regional specialization within the system and it is this which increases its value both in theoretical explanation as well as application to the individual case. While damage anywhere in the system will lead to some change in the function which the system subserves, the *nature* of the change will be dependent upon the particular part of the system which is damaged or the set of connections which has been disrupted, since each part contributes something characteristic to the whole. It is thus necessary to look carefully at the *nature* of the changes in a psychological function to determine how they are related to the location and character of the lesion.

This multiple significance of what appears at first to be the same symptom or symptom complex begins to render meaningful the apparently conflicting findings of many early studies and, at the same time, allows symptoms or signs to have localizing value. To take a common example, psychologists have long observed that the Kohs block design test is often performed poorly by many, but certainly not all, brain damaged subjects. Poor performance on this test could result from a disruption of what might rather loosely be termed constructional praxis. It could also be performed poorly because of visual and other difficulties but if these are excluded and poor performance of the block design task is taken as an operational definition of constructional apraxia, the regional significance still remains to be determined. Here *qualitative* observations are of help. For example, constructional deviations where the patient fails to conform to the square framework are observed most strikingly in patients with posterior lesions, particularly right-sided. Constructional deviations are particularly prominent in right hemisphere lesions and markedly so where there is a posterior locus. Ben-Yishay and his colleagues (1971) described these errors in terms of deviation from the square format of the design to be copied – 'broken squares; rectangles; linearly placed horizontally, vertically, diagonally; irregular shapes – patterns wherein the individual blocks are improperly aligned with respect to one another and with the horizontal and vertical planes'.

An equally poor score on the block design test may be obtained by a second patient with a frontal lesion. However, such a patient will usually show few constructional deviations and the difficulty may be shown to be dependent upon incomplete preliminary investigation of the problem as in the case examined by Luria and Tsvetkova (1964) cited in Chapter 4. In this case the frontal patient is helped by the provision of a design card upon which the outlines of the four (or more) constituent blocks have been drawn. On the other hand, right parietal patients tend to benefit little from this procedure. The 'partially solved' block design problem apparently has no more meaning in their shattered visuospatial world than the original. As mentioned elsewhere, the nature of the observations which will be of value and the tests which will be applied must rest on a knowledge of the findings emerging from research studies.

The neuropsychological syndrome

Deriving as it does largely from the broad base of clinical neurology, the concept of a syndrome plays a central role in the thinking of clinical neuropsychology. Central to the concept of the syndrome is the sense of a unique constellation of signs and symptoms which occur together frequently enough to suggest a particular underlying process. However, not all the signs and symptoms are of equal importance and the weighting of the different elements is often an idiosyncratic process 'being unformulated outcome of the interaction of medical instruction and clinical experience' (Kinsbourne 1971).

It is now several decades since English workers suggested that the syndrome concept should be used in the area of cerebral impairment:

> The assessment of intellectual deterioration calls, not for single valid standardization test, but rather for a flexible test procedure and awareness of the relevant syndromes. This view is justified by a consideration of the multiform effects on intellectual performance of focal and diffuse cerebral lesions and also by a consideration of the focal disturbance of intellectual function already recognized by neurologists and utilized in diagnosis. (Piercy 1959)

> As far as cases of suspected cerebral lesion are concerned, the psychologist can tell the neurologist whether or not the patient's performances resembles that of a typical case of a lesion in one of the major cerebral lobes; and the neurologist can combine the information with evidence from other procedures in arriving at his assessment. (McFie 1960)

> Neuropsychologists should be concerned with pattern of impairment, and

as their knowledge of syndromes increases they will, when confronted with certain symptoms and signs, look for the association of the other features to confirm or disconfirm the presence of a particular syndrome. This is the medical model of *differential diagnosis*.

For the method to work effectively in clinical practice knowledge is required in three areas: (i) the corpus of fact in human neuropsychology; (ii) an acquaintance with relevant principles and details of allied clinical neurosciences, especially clinical neurology, neuroanatomy and neuropathology; and (iii) psychological test theory and practice.

Syndromes also vary a good deal in their degree of specificity or vagueness. The frontal lobe syndrome is a much more general working term than, say, the general amnesic syndrome. One of the reasons for this generality may be the grouping together of a number of functionally different areas, particularly if these are affected simultaneously by one pathological process. However, if the term syndrome is used in an extremely broad sense then it fails to have meaning. One such usage was the earlier term 'chronic brain syndrome'. Geschwind (1978) commented: 'My objection to the term is that it carries an implication, however many qualifications are put on it, that there is such a thing as a single organic brain syndrome, something for which there is no evidence. The brain is the most complicated organ in the body, and thus one can expect many syndromes with different manifestations'.

Finally, it is essential to stress that it is the total configuration or Gestalt which imparts significance. A syndrome is, indeed, more than (or other than) the sum of its individual constituents. It is a useful working fiction which allows us to create some order out of the complexity of the patient's subjective complaints and the findings of our examinations. Knowledge of a variety of syndromes allows us to generate hypotheses about the nature of the disruptions of function in the individual case.

The method of extreme cases

Training in differential diagnosis is best done by what Kraepelin called 'the method of extreme cases' (Zangwill 1978, personal communication). The trainee neuropsychologist is introduced to syndromes in their clear-cut form, i.e. classical or 'extreme' cases. Later, more subtle and complex cases are introduced to teach the range of variation that might be encountered in clinical practice. We have found that this method facilitates the recognition of syndromes in their less dramatic or latent forms and makes it possible to detect characteristic patterns of neuropsychological deficit in their early stages of development.

HYPOTHESIS TESTING IN THE SINGLE CASE

Qualitative information

One serious drawback to almost every purely quantitative approach to neuropsychological evaluation is the loss of information. Shapiro (1951) quoted Schafer 'A test response is not a score; scores, where applicable, are abstractions designed to facilitate intra-individual and inter-individual comparisons, and as such they are extremely useful in clinical testing. However, to reason –

or do research – only in terms of scores or score patterns is to do violence to the nature of the raw material. The *scores do not communicate the responses in full'* (emphasis added). Reitan's (1964) study mentioned in Chapter 4 shows clearly that, utilizing the same test data, clinical prediction can be superior to formal or psychometric methods. This may have been because of loss of qualitative features in individual responses or complex *intra-individual* patterns of response lost when only levels of performance were used. More recently Goldberg and Costa 1986 restated this truism: 'The behavior that generates scorable responses is, however, far richer and more varied than any scoring system will allow'. While it is desirable to use quantification where possible, some clinically relevant information does not lend itself readily to such quantification.

One way of coping with the limitations of scores alone is by recording the quality and patterning of responses noted during evaluation, 'information about the neuropsychological processes which underlie a subject's performance can only be provided by a detailed qualitative analysis' (Ryan & Butters 1980). This position is supported in the approaches of Kaplan and her colleagues (Kaplan 1988, Kaplan et al 1991) where task- or process-specific sample qualitative responses are provided in the test material.

Hypothesis testing

Shapiro has pointed out also some of the major difficulties and limitations inherent in the application of standardized validated tests in the clinical diagnostic setting. These comments remained pertinent and, after two more decades, Shapiro was still able to point to the absence of any serious attempts in the intervening period to overcome these difficulties by application of the recommended solution, namely, the experimental investigation of the single case (Shapiro 1973). After reminding us of the scientific concept of error in psychological measurement, Shapiro argued that while this should prevent us from making unwarranted generalizations from the data it should not prevent us from using observations in a systematic way to advance our understanding of the individual case.

> The awareness of error makes us look upon any psychological observation not as something conclusive but as the basis of one or more hypotheses about the patient. One's degree of confidence in any hypothesis suggested by an observation would depend upon the established degree of validity of that observation and upon other information about the patient concerned. If one or more hypotheses are suggested by an observation, then steps must be taken to test them. In this way further observations are accumulated in a systematic manner. It should then become possible to arrive at a psychological description in which we can have greater confidence. The additional observations may in turn suggest new hypotheses which have in turn to be tested. We are thus led to the method of the systematic investigation as a means of improving the validity of our conclusions about an individual patient. (Shapiro 1973, p. 651)

Working hypotheses may arise from generalizations which have emerged from the research literature. Clinical neuropsychology is becoming very rich in this regard as evidenced by the sample provided in Chapters 4 to 9 which, while representative, is far from exhaustive. As this work grows, converging lines of evidence make the generalizations more secure and thus facilitate the implementation of crucial tests of the various hypotheses, e.g. the evidence on asymmetry of hemispheric function has made the testing of laterality of lesions more open to systematic investigation.

Despite his forceful advocacy, even Shapiro considered that this method might not have strong appeal since it could tend to be time consuming. In practice, however, it tends to be more economical than the application of a fixed battery of tests, since many of these prove irrelevant to the questions being asked. Since in clinical practice certain questions tend to recur frequently, trainees quite soon recognize the most likely hypotheses and the most productive tests to be used in particular situations. Subsequent case evaluation in the light of neurological or neurosurgical knowledge continually improves the process.

In busy clinical practice, time is an expensive commodity and on some occasions the clinician has to tender an opinion after a less than ideal examination of the patient. In this situation the report should make it clear to the referring source that the opinion consists 'of the hypotheses which the applied scientist thinks best account for the data at his disposal, and which he would choose to test next time if he had sufficient time and suitable means' (Shapiro 1973, p. 652). The term 'suitable means' often takes the form of appropriate tests. In some cases these do not exist but this situation is becoming rare as neuropsychology develops, and clinicians working in a particular field are likely to acquire the tests which prove useful in answering the most common hypotheses. Very popular standardized tests such as the Wechsler Memory Scale may well provide the central hypothesis which can then be tested by other procedures. Sometimes the whole or part of the answer lies in testing that has already been carried out with standardized tests. Psychologists trained in one of the psychometric traditions often ask what are the newest or latest tests for brain damage. It can be pointed out that they already have significant information in the tests they commonly employ but, being largely unaware of the developments in neuropsychology, they are unable to recognize its significance.

As Ley (1970) comments, the criticism that the method is time-consuming is valid 'only in so far as one thinks that: (i) the method will produce findings of sufficient value; and (ii) that there are more valuable things for clinical psychologists to do'. Economy of time must be seen in relation to the importance of the question being asked.

As referring agencies become more sophisticated in their awareness of neuropsychology, they are more likely to present quite specific hypotheses for investigation. The following example from the companion volume (Walsh 1991) illustrates such a referral. The neurologist wrote: 'Does this patient have an amnesia to which she is not entitled?'. Though it is not expressly stated, the neuropsychologist is being asked to study the patient's hospital file. Perusal of this record revealed the following: A 56-year-old housewife had a history of episodes of sudden detachment from reality, staring eyes and lack of awareness of her surroundings, each episode lasting about 2 minutes. The episodes had commenced shortly after a head injury 15 years before when she was struck on the right temple. EEG recordings had consistently shown the presence of a left temporal focus with no electrical abnormality on the right side. All attempts to control the attacks with drug therapy had failed and the patient was proposed as a candidate for left unilateral temporal lobectomy. Depth electrodes strongly confirmed the presence of a left medial temporal focus. It was at this stage that the referral question was posed.

The question thus placed in its context assumes that the neuropsychologist is familiar with the literature related to the question. The neurologist will not be surprised if the patient shows a differentially weaker verbal than non-verbal memory performance in line with the proven double dissociation shown with lateralized temporal lobe lesions between verbal and non-verbal material. This would be a deficit to which the patient would be 'entitled' by virtue of a left medial temporal lesion. However, a 'non-entitled' deficit of *non-verbal* memory would signal a possible dysfunction in the right temporal region. This dysfunction might be silent to neurological examination since, in the case of an atrophic lesion, the area may be electrically silent, i.e. a normal EEG on the right side would not exclude pathology.

The import of finding a *non-entitled* neuropsychological deficit would have the utmost significance since surgical ablation of the electrically active focus in the left temporal lobe would be added to the previously unsuspected atrophic damage in the right side. Functionally, this would be equivalent to bilateral medial temporal damage, a condition which produces a general, profound and lasting amnesic syndrome. Hence, the finding of an amnesia to which the patient was 'not entitled' would be a clear contraindication to surgery.

In this case the neuropsychological examination did show minor difficulty with one aspect of new verbal learning though verbal short-term memory, memory for prose material and other verbal intelligence measures were at an appropriate level. However, the patient clearly had much more difficulty with non-verbal memory together with evidence of constructional dyspraxia because of more widespread right hemisphere disruption of function. It seemed that the proposed surgery ran the risk of producing a general amnesic syndrome. At this stage the patient died suddenly and at autopsy the site of the left-sided irritative focus was of normal appearance while the electrically silent right side was atrophic in the hippocampal region. To operate would have been to produce a devastating amnesic disorder.

History

The most important information in deriving hypotheses usually comes from a carefully elicited history. 'Extra time spent on the history is likely to be more profitable than extra time spent on the examination' (Hampton et al 1975, p. 489). A good history can only be obtained if the neuropsychologist has a significant grasp of allied disciplines such as neurology, otherwise crucial factors will be overlooked.

In most cases temporal aspects of the disorder must be included. In many instances, it is absolutely essential that a careful history be taken from a spouse, other relative or caregiver, such that differences in historical accounts can be appreciated. In many neurological disorders affecting cognition, the patient may be unaware of the reasons for referral, true nature of the disability or its consequences, frequency of failures, quality of performance or relevant examples. On the other hand, in many psychiatric or psychological conditions the patient is painfully aware of perceived deficits, which do not accord with objective performance. Textbooks of neurology are essential sources of reference for further details (e.g. Adams & Victor 1993).

Selecting the tools

Knowledge of syndromes and brain-behaviour relationships is the principal factor in determining the selection of tools. Certain of these will be employed on an almost daily basis in answering commonly occurring questions. However, there will be questions or hypotheses which will require 'special' tools to produce pathognomonic data. Test selection should be germane to the questions asked, so that the experienced neuropsychologist will gradually develop quite a large armamentarium from which to choose. While developing this arsenal, beginning practitioners will find an encyclopaedic source of test data and wisdom in Lezak (1995). To this and other textual sources they should add a personal store of further qualitative observations. Such test familiarity is necessary for the rapid and economic evaluation associated with the branching decision-making process which is the basis of clinical evaluation using a flexible or individualized method. In the case extracts which follow only a few well-known tests are cited but this merely exemplifies the way in which assessment can proceed.

The selection of tests may entail a one step process, i.e. a group of tests is chosen in the belief that these will provide the information needed to answer the questions. Sometimes the issues remain unresolved but observations derived from the primary set of tests may suggest that further specific tests may provide the answer, i.e. a stepwise approach will be used by many. Much of the efficacy of this method turns on the selection of the primary group of tests, since the use of tests which do not touch the problem at all will give apparently negative results. In reporting such negative results it is important to inform the referral agency that 'nothing abnormal was detected with the tests used'. It is of help to colleagues familiar with psychological tests to specify exactly which were used. These should certainly be documented in hospital practice and in medico-legal cases. Unfortunately, negative reports are often written which contain the implication that no impairment is present. We should bear in mind Teuber's dictum 'absence of evidence is not evidence of absence' (of impairment). Russell (1982) points out that the entire controversy between fixed versus flexible test methodology hinges on a single rather obvious principle that is axiomatic to neuropsychology: *'one cannot determine whether a certain function of the brain is impaired unless that function is tested'*.

Reporting

Reports not only record the neuropsychologist's findings but should be conveyed in a way that increases the understanding by other professionals of the settings in which neuropsychology can be useful. Clearly written reports should contain both the data and conclusions and, where relevant, the arguments used in support of such conclusions. They should comment not only on the qualitative and quantitative findings but also on such matters as the congruence between similar measures of the same function and between test performance and reported behaviour. This process may appear time-consuming but proves helpful in forcing the examiner to exteriorize thinking processes thus leading to further development of clinical competence.

The sequential nature of the problem solving process with neurobehavioural disorders often means that brief verbal interchanges with professionals in related fields will modify the next step in the investigation procedures of both parties, leading to economy of time and effort. For further detail see Walsh (1991, 1992, 1995) and the forensic neuropsychology section in Chapter 11.

CASE EXAMPLES

In applying the hypothesis method to 'clinical' cases neuropsychologists will encounter different types of situation. They are commonly asked to confirm the likelihood that the features presented by the patient or client represent a particular disorder or syndrome. This is often the case in referral from medical or psychologist colleagues.

On other occasions the matter is presented as a puzzle or problem for which an appropriate hypothesis is sought. In such situations the neuropsychologist needs to generate a number of possible explanations or hypotheses and test between them.

Finally, the neuropsychologist may become involved in deciding between opposing hypotheses being put forward (often very strongly) by different parties, as is often the case in medico-legal disputation (see Ch.11). This latter situation offers an excellent opportunity for expounding the advantages of the proposed philosophy of evaluation. Such a case is exemplified in the first of the cases which follow.

Choosing between hypotheses

Case: NG

This 45-year-old marketing executive was severely injured in a motor vehicle accident in which the driver of the other vehicle and two passengers were killed. On arrival at a small town hospital some 30 minutes after the crash NG was unconscious and did not regain consciousness for another 4 hours but was confused and required sedation for 3 days. Radiological examination revealed a fracture of the maxilla and a fractured humerus but no skull fracture. Imaging was not available. Neurological examination showed no localizing signs. A week after the event NG was transferred to a metropolitan rehabilitation centre where he was found to be correctly oriented but mildly disinhibited. CT scan at 10 days after injury was unremarkable and patient was considered fit for discharge home by the end of 3 weeks.

Personal history. The patient's past history was elicited from him and from members of his family. He had a Master's degree in business studies and was a member of the board of his company. His family commented that he now seemed less reserved than before and on several occasions had made crude comments which were atypical for him. He was described by himself and his family as a social drinker, consuming on average about four or five standard drinks a day, and only exceeded this on rare occasions such as family celebrations.

At later interviews some 3 and 4 months after injury NG's wife and son both commented spontaneously on his 'personality change' which they described as a brashness and marked lack of sensitivity which was in contrast to his pre-accident state and they mentioned that he had alienated many of his former friends and colleagues. His wife was concerned by the resulting isolation but it appeared not to concern NG.

He returned to work at 4 months and coped with his work adequately though he now made errors which he had not done before and was intolerant of criticism. His firm moved him to a less demanding position and one where he had fewer dealings with clients. A promotion which was about to be given at the time of his accident was deferred.

About 2 years after the accident NG was referred for neuropsychological evaluation in support of a claim being made that he had suffered changes caused by brain impairment as a result of the event. It was learned that opposing legal argument centred on the position that any changes observed in NG were caused by alcohol-related brain damage, a position supported by opinions given by a psychologist and a psychiatrist who had examined him several times in the period dating from 18 months to 2 years after the event.

At interview, NG admitted to the neuropsychologist that he was aware that he had changed but showed incomplete insight into the effect these changes had on others. He admitted that he no longer seemed as good at his job but could not explain the difficulty and tended to play this down.

Neuropsychological examination. Several examinations were conducted in the period from $1^1/2$ to 3 years after the accident. His performances were stable over these examinations. The WAIS results shown are taken from an examination 2 years after the accident by the psychologist who had offered alcohol as the cause of any deficits which the subject might have.

Information	13	Picture Completion	14
Comprehension	13	Object Assembly	10
Arithmetic	12	Block Design	12
Digit Span	12	Digit-Symbol	13
Similarities	14	Picture Arrangement	12
Vocabulary	13		
VIQ	119	PIQ	126
Full scale IQ	124		

The principal hypothesis suggested by the history was that the clinical changes seemed characteristic of closed head injury affecting the anterior portions of the brain. Since the personality changes alone appeared almost pathognomonic, the examination was designed to confirm the hypothesis by evaluating aspects of adaptive behaviour with appropriate and sensitive measures described in the literature (see Ch. 5, Walsh 1991).This was imperative, since an alternate cause, namely alcohol-related brain damage, had been suggested by a psychiatrist and supported by a clinical psychologist.

Milner pathway on the Austin Maze Test (Walsh 1991). Several examinations over time showed essentially the same pattern. The following represents the examination at 2 years.

Over the first ten trials NG reduced his errors consistently.

Trial	1	2	3	4	5	6	7	8	9	10
Errors	15	6	9	5	5	4	3	3	2	1

Nevertheless, he continued to make errors on further trials, even after he had achieved two (non-consecutive) errorless trials. He appeared only mildly frustrated and applied himself, saying that he was keen to succeed.

Trial	11	12	13	14	15	16	17	18	19	20
Errors	2	1	6	4	0	2	1	1	1	0

Trial	21	22	23	24	25	26	27	28	29	30
Errors	1	2	2	1	2	1	1	1	1	1

This is a classical pattern whereby patients with anterior damage from whatever reason find it difficult if not impossible to eradicate all errors from their programmes of behaviour to produce a *stable error-free performance* (Walsh 1991). Moreover, he made different errors on different occasions, cursing mildly and chiding himself when he did so.

Tested again at 3 years, he made only one error on the third trial but over 30 trials was never able to gain more than two successive error free trials.

Rey Figure. The copy was complete but the recall at 3 minutes was sparse (Fig. 10.1).

After 3 minutes delay there was considerable impoverishment of his reproduction from memory. He also recalled two features but stated that he did not know where they should be placed in the whole and was asked to draw these in the margins of the paper. The performance seemed characteristic of those patients with frontal pathology.

Verbal Fluency. He managed to average only 11 words for the three letters (F–12; A–7; S–14), which would place him just below the 25th percentile, considerably below expectation based on his educational and social history and his fluent use of language in normal conversation and his score on the

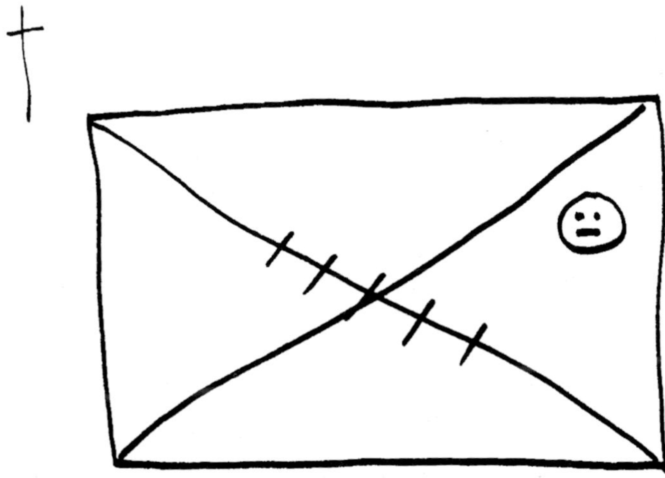

Fig. 10.1 Case NG. Recall of Rey Figure at 3 minutes.

Vocabulary subtest of the WAIS. He also broke the rules several times though he was able to repeat these rules when asked. This did not prevent him from breaking them again subsequently.

Tower of London (Shallice 1982, 1988). The first four problems were solved quickly. He solved problem five slowly and seven only when he *insisted* on 'having another try' and failed on item six and the final four items. In discussion after the task he made quite intelligent comments about solution demonstrating the frontal 'dissociation between knowing and doing' (see Ch. 4 above).

Trail Making Test. Part A was performed accurately and rapidly (25 seconds) but he was considerably slower on Part B (119 seconds), though he made no errors.

Colour-Form Sorting Test. He spontaneously announced the two principles of 'shape' and 'colour' but then sorted immediately according to form and did so again. When asked what he was supposed to be doing he spontaneously made the shift to colour. Once again he seemed to show a mild dissociation between conceptualization and action or 'inability to shift' as described in the earliest literature on frontal lobe damage.

WMS Form I

Information	6	Digits Total	12 (7,5)
Orientation	5	Visual Reproduction	14
Mental Control	9	Associate Learning	11
Memory Passages	11	(6,2; 6,3; 6,4)	
MQ	122		

On this test his performance seemed close to expectation. After 30 minutes' delay he recalled 9 of the 10 pairs in the Associate Learning subtest. He was then given the Rey Auditory Verbal Learning Test. This consists of 5 learning trials of a 15 word list followed by one recall and one recognition trial after a single trial of an interpolated list of the same length.

RAVLT

	List A					*List B*	*List A*	*List A*
Trials	1	2	3	4	5	Recall	Recall	Recognition
Correct	8	12	13	12	13	7	10	15

This performance seemed below expectation for an obviously intelligent man and, again, he seemed unable to perfect his learning. From the second to the fifth trial both the order of responses and the missing words differed from trial to trial.

Discussion. In general, the severity of closed head injury has been related to the length of the period of unconsciousness or, preferably, to the period of post-traumatic amnesia (PTA) (see Walsh 1991, Ch. 5). The longer the period of PTA, the more likely it is that the person will have lasting deficits. However, while this generalization is clinically useful there are exceptions, e.g. some cases with relatively short periods of PTA have demonstrated radiological changes of considerable damage, particularly in the frontal regions, and invariably reveal deficits of personality and cognition (Levin et al 1989).

From the scanty records this man appears to have been unconscious for a few hours and confused for approximately 4 days. His wife said that his memory was poor for at least 10 days, but this estimate came over 1 year later.

General argument

Head injury. It is not unusual to see preservation of high scores on standard psychometric measures following head injury in formerly intelligent subjects. This does not signify preservation of 'effective intelligence' since the disorders of adaptive ability which are so debilitating in these patients are not revealed except in severe cases. Intelligent individuals develop programmes of behaviour which allow them to deal with a variety of everyday situations. On the other hand, they have difficulty both in generating new programmes for behaviour and adapting prior programmes to meet changing contingencies.

NG did show the consistent and characteristic learning and executive difficulties described in those with anterior brain damage (Austin Maze, Rey Figure, Tower of London, RAVLT). These features accompanied personality changes, particularly disinhibition of the type reported almost invariably with trauma to the frontal parts of the brain. The present patient was indifferent to his own errors and the effect of his behaviour on others. Both sets of changes appeared for the first time immediately after the injury and there was no evidence of attempts to exaggerate or enact other deficits.

The alcohol impairment hypothesis. Features which militate against this are:

None of the observed changes of personality or cognition was reported by any observers to be present before the injury, even in retrospect. Changes with alcohol-related brain damage are slow and insidious, never of sudden onset.

The type of change in personality is uncharacteristic of alcohol-related brain impairment but highly characteristic of traumatic damage.

While changes in adaptive behaviour and problem solving largely dependent on cognitive loss are a feature of alcohol damage, they occur against a background of more widespread cognitive deterioration. In all cases in our experience these changes lead to a lowering of some subtests of the Performance Scale, in particular Object Assembly, Block Design and Picture Arrangement (for examples see Walsh 1991, Ch. 2).

While it is often difficult to gain a true estimate of the degree of an individual's drinking, there was no evidence of the usual sort put forward even by those supporting this hypothesis, i.e. prolonged heavy drinking (often combined with inadequate nutrition).

Mild atrophy which had been seen in the CT scan might be consistent with alcohol damage as well as traumatic damage, but there was also a localized area in the front of the brain more consistent with trauma (though, of course, head injuries are very common in alcoholics).

The court ruled in favour of head injury as the cause of the man's changes. Certainly the *post hoc ergo propter hoc* argument is strong in such cases, especially if evidence can be produced of absence of deficits in the period immediately prior to the event.

A second situation is that of conflicting or uncertain diagnosis.

Functional versus organic

Case: WN

A 53-year-old woman was the caretaker of a house which caught fire. Although no serious damage occurred the incident was upsetting for the 'house minder'. One week later Mrs N was having dinner when she experienced a 5 minute period of chest pain with nausea together with 5 minutes of difficulty in enunciating her words. She also complained of weakness of her left upper limb which persisted; some hours later her friend took her to hospital where the examining neurologist felt that this might represent a right-sided cortical event. The neurologist also felt that there were few signs consistent with organic impairment and several suggesting that the weakness of her left hand could be functional. The neurobehavioural examination included a request to draw a bicycle. Her attempt is shown in Figure 10.2. The drawing was rudimentary and included the dotted figure as an afterthought. She described the figure as 'a man who puts one leg on each wheel'.

With an 'hysterical' disorder as a possible diagnosis, the neurologist also administered the 15 item memory test of Rey. (The stimuli for this test are shown in Fig.10.13.) The patient's first response was to continue the alphabet in columns of three underneath the correct first line A B C and, when shown the stimuli again and asked to reproduce them from memory a few seconds later, she began with the number one and continued the numerical series until stopped by the examiner.

A psychiatric opinion was sought 5 days after the event because of the possibility of a non-neurological basis for her difficulties. It is noteworthy that a CT scan taken soon after admission was reported as being within normal limits.

There was no previous psychiatric history. She was described as being alert, co-operative, attentive and correctly oriented. She did, however, evince errors in speech and perseveration. She was able to give internally consistent details of her background and history and at this time told the examiner of how the recent fire had brought to mind a tragic event of her childhood when at the age of 5 or 6 years her younger brother of some 2 years was burned to death, an event which she had witnessed.

The psychiatrist commented that her disorganized mental state appeared to have a considerable functional element, but he also felt that an organic cause for her left arm weakness needed vigorous investigation.

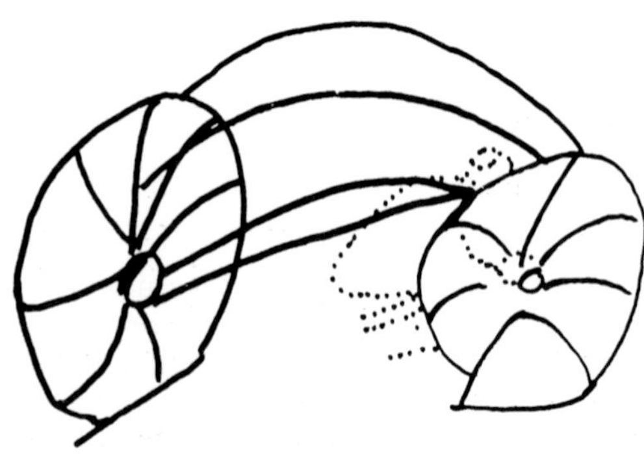

Fig. 10.2 Case WN. Drawing of a bicycle.

After a further few days she was noted to have no difficulty speaking but the weakness in her left hand persisted. The neurologist on that occasion admitted that he could not decide whether her problems were 'functional or organic'.

About a week after admission the speech pathologist described her as having non-specific speech and language problems most consistent with frontal lobe pathology sparing the major language areas. However, she said that she could not rule out a functional element. The major signs included perseveration, poor self-monitoring, difficulty learning new material, reduced verbal fluency with inappropriate responses and verbal paraphasias.

The neurologist was puzzled by this case and sought advice from the Department of Neuropsychology. On seeing her drawings, which included the Complex Figure of Rey done 2 days after admission (Fig. 10.3), and hearing the story, the neuropsychologist suggested a number of tests, the first one of which was the Colour-Form Sorting Test, an extremely simple but rewarding task.

The examination was videotaped and shown to the consulting neuropsychologist who pointed to the presence of all the qualitative features which have been shown on this test by patients with frontal lobe pathology. The patient also showed a poverty of response on the Verbal Fluency Test and the characteristic features shown by patients with left or bilateral frontal lesions on such tasks. This confirmed the findings of the speech pathologist's earlier examination. Other tasks sensitive to frontal pathology, such as the Porteus Maze Test, were performed poorly. The Rey Figure was again disorganized (Fig. 10.4). The opinion was that the patient had significant frontal pathology with clear evidence of left hemisphere involvement and that this could account for all the test findings and the patient's clinical presentation. The numerous qualitative observations did not support a separate or additional diagnosis of a functional disorder.

Concurrently with the neuropsychological examination, a repeat CT scan revealed a left-sided frontal infarct (Fig. 10.5). The reason for apparent weakness on the 'wrong' side, i.e. ipsilateral to the lesion, never became clear. The weakness had resolved by the end of one week.

With the emphasis on quantitative measures in much of neuropsychological evaluation there is a great need for articles such as that of Goldberg and Costa (1986) which add a rich description of the qualitative features characteristic of certain types and locations of pathology. The most effective way by far to convey this material to trainees is videotape but such material is unfortunately sparse.

A medley of case extracts

The following medley may serve to exemplify a few of the range of questions asked of neuropsychologists. The extracts are of necessity brief. In each case the presented data are restricted mostly to a few widely known tests. Often many other tests were employed. It is difficult to do justice to even the most straightforward case in a brief span, but each case has a point to make. As such experience accumulates the clinician develops an ever widening and consolidating frame of reference against which to make future judgments.

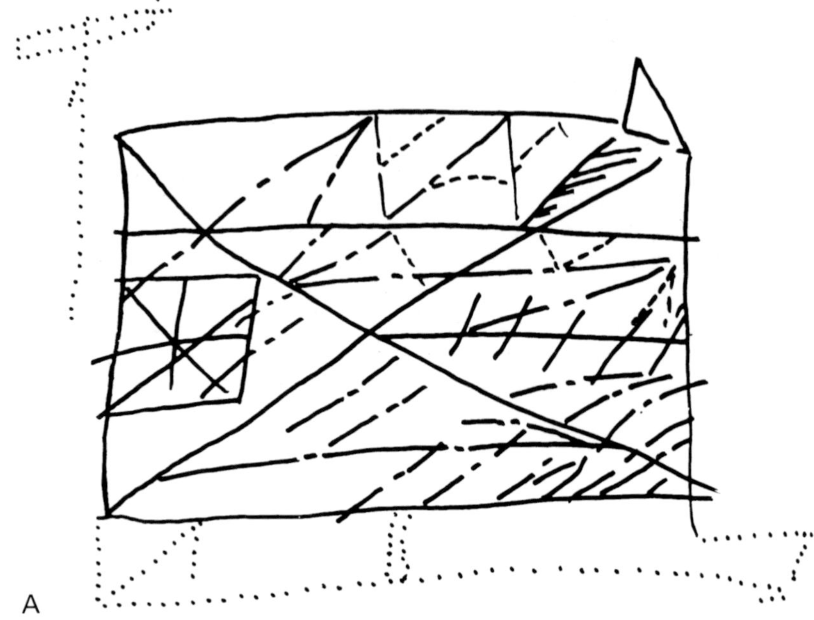

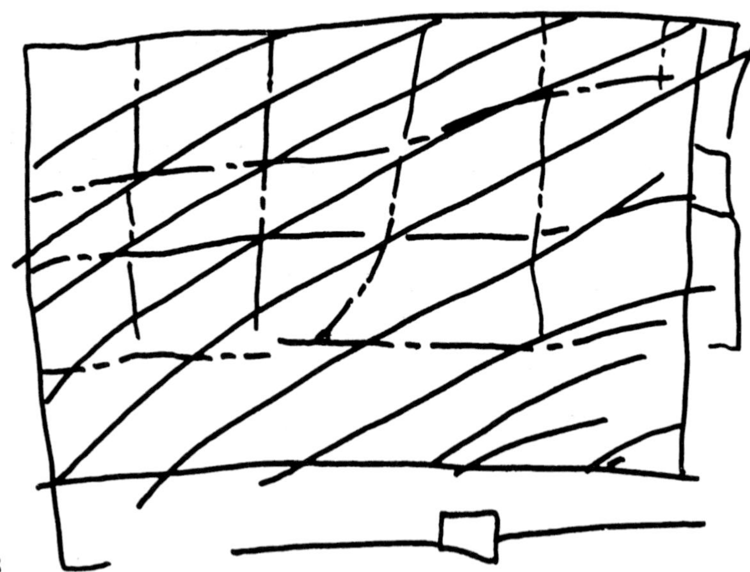

Fig. 10.3 Case WN. A, Copy and B, Recall of the Rey Figure two days after admission. (Order of drawing is indicated by solid lines followed by progressively more broken lines).

Korsakoff psychosis

Case: YW

A year before his assessment, YW, a 49-year-old teacher, had suffered a 'ner-

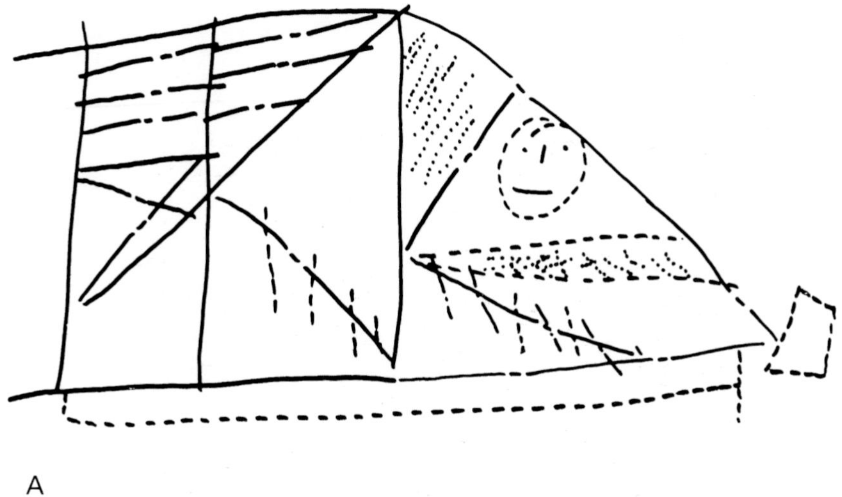

A

B

Fig. 10.4 Case WN. A, Copy and B, Recall of the Rey Figure 7 days after admission.

vous breakdown' when he was unable to remember certain commitments as head of a rural school. Soon after hospitalization a CT scan revealed cerebral atrophy, a diagnosis of Korsakoff psychosis was made, he was hospitalized for treatment of his alcoholism and had been abstinent since that time. Neuropsychological assessment was requested as part of the decision as to whether he might be able to return to work or whether he should be retired.

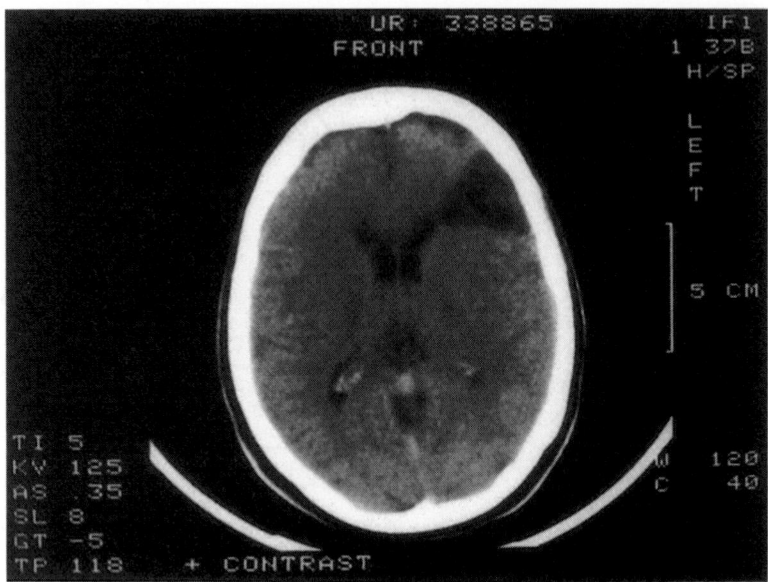

Fig. 10.5 Case WN. CT scan showing wedge shaped infarct.

YW began drinking in his early twenties and gradually increased his consumption of beer on a daily basis in the rural towns where he spent his professional life. He had never appreciated that he was drinking to excess and managed to obtain higher teaching certificates over the years. He was never absent from work until the final episode which brought him under attention. At this time he was consuming more than 2 litres of wine per day.

He presented as an alert co-operative man, well aware of his condition over which he showed realistic concern. He said he was strongly motivated to return to work but knew that his memory was poor though somewhat improved since he became abstinent. He wrote down everything he had to remember, but there was no evidence of how effective this strategy had been. He had been abstinent for several months at this examination.

The Wechsler Memory Scale (WMS) and the Wechsler Adult Intelligence Scale (WAIS) immediately revealed the extent of his difficulties.

WMS Form I

Information	3	Digits Total	13 (7,6)
Orientation	5	Visual Reproduction	8
Mental Control	9	Associate Learning	9
Memory Passages	4.5 (5,4)	(5,0; 6,0; 5,1)*	
MQ	94		

* The designation (5,0; 6,0; 5,1) refers to performance on the learning of the 10 pairs of the verbal paired associate learning task where 6 pairs have logical associations requiring the relearning of old associations (e.g. baby – cries) and 4 pairs require the learning of novel associations (e.g. crush – dark). Thus a perfect score would be '6,4'. In the present case, which is quite typical of verbal-specific or general amnesic syndromes, the patient shows a marked dissociation between the 'old' and 'new' learning.

This revealed the features of a general amnesic syndrome. YW was well oriented, though confused on questions about current political leaders. In keeping with preservation of insight into his deficits he showed no confabulation. Automatic mental operations were performed speedily without error and immediate memory span was normal. However, there was a clear anterograde amnesia (Memory Passages, Visual Reproduction, Associate Learning).

The amnesic difficulty was strongly confirmed by the Rey Auditory Verbal Learning Test.

RAVLT

	List A					*List B*	*List A*	*List A*
Trials	1	2	3	4	5	Recall	Recall	Recognition
Correct	5	7	8	8	11	5	3	14

YW performed a little better on the fifth trial than many with alcohol-related memory deficits, but considerably below that expected from his background. The results also show a characteristic retroactive inhibition or interference effect, shown by a score of only 3 after the interpolated list. He also showed interference by intruding words from the previously administered associate learning subtest. As with most Korsakoff patients, the recognition trial was significantly better than any of the recall trials.

The complex Figure of Rey showed a very good copy, followed by an attempt at recall which rated a score of zero when the patient attempted to draw the figure from memory *only 3 minutes later* (Fig. 10.6).

WAIS Scaled Scores

Information	12	Digit Symbol	12
Comprehension	18	Block Design	8
Similarities	14	Object Assembly	7

An indication of YW's premorbid intellectual ability can be gained from the three verbal subtests. These would suggest a prior level in the vicinity of

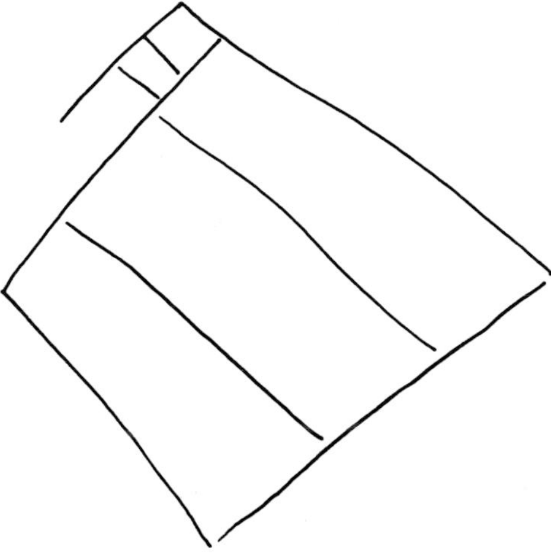

Fig. 10.6 Case YW. Recall of Rey Figure at 3 minutes.

130 IQ. In contrast, the two tests requiring planning and problem solving were significantly inferior. On Block Design he showed inappropriate strategies, attempting to solve the problems using faces of the blocks having only one colour, rotating them at odd angles to achieve a diagonal effect. There was also a disinclination to alter placements which he clearly recognized as being incorrect. He was, however, upset with not being able to succeed on tasks which he knew would clearly have been well within his ability.

Three months later another examination was requested before the final decision was taken on his re-employment or retirement. No measurable improvement had taken place and the testing was terminated when he became distressed after failing totally to make the slightest improvement after 10 trials on the Milner pathway of the Austin Maze Test.

Trial	1	2	3	4	5	6	7	8	9	10
Errors	19	10	15	17	11	19	15	15	23	15

This case not only illustrates most of the commonly found features of an alcohol-related disorder, but also shows how advanced cognitive deficit may become in certain situations before action is prompted.

YW shows a general amnesic syndrome together with other non-amnesic cognitive deficits. These latter have been termed 'the adaptive behaviour syndrome' (Walsh 1991) and may predate the emergence of an amnesic disorder by years or may be seen without amnesia in the well-nourished alcoholic.

Amnesia complicating arteriography

Case: DD

Following an adverse reaction to angiography at another centre, this 54-year-old accountant was admitted to the emergency ward in a semi-comatose condition. Over the preceding 8 weeks he had suffered a number of sudden attacks of dizziness and inco-ordination with weakness of the left arm and leg, each attack lasting 2 to 3 minutes. On occasion he also reported numbness of the left side of the face. Apparently the examining physician felt that carotid arteriography was indicated but, for reasons which never became clear, a *vertebral* injection was made instead and a large dose of contrast material was used. Shortly after the injection the patient lost consciousness for a few minutes then roused sufficiently to realize that he was blind. He was confused and showed retrograde amnesia for events over the past few days. Neurological examination revealed no other localizing signs but it was apparent that DD also had a severe anterograde amnesia. At this stage he was transferred to a large metropolitan hospital's department of neurology. As with idiopathic cases of transient global amnesia (without blindness) he continually posed the same questions about what had happened to him. Over the next 12 hours he slowly improved but was confused, irritable and disoriented and constantly complained of poor vision but was unaware of his recent episode of blindness.

The first neuropsychological examination was carried out 18 hours after angiography. By this time he was able to distinguish objects and could describe a person at 4 feet (1.22 m). His memory had improved sufficiently for him to recall an interview with the psychologist which took place 1 hour before. The Wechsler Memory Scale was administered at this time and comparisons are given when he was re-examined at 72 hours and 4 weeks after the event.

WMS	*18 hours*	*72 hours*	*4 weeks*
Information	6	6	6
Orientation	3	5	5
Mental Control	9	8	9
Memory Passages	6	12	10
Digits Total	13	15	15
Visual Reproduction	1	10	11
Associate Learning	7.5	10	14
	5,0; 5,0; 5,0	4,0; 6,1; 6,1	6,0; 6,3; 6,2
MQ	89	122	132

At 18 hours. The WMS suggested a general amnesic syndrome, though it was difficult to interpret the poor performance on Visual Reproduction because of the patient's visual problem. Associative verbal fluency was given but he was able to give only 2 words on the letter F in 60 seconds, and none on the letters A and S. He was able to read words and name objects and colours and showed no other difficulties.

At 72 hours. This examination showed marked improvement in DD's memory. The improvement in visual reproduction was confirmed by the Benton Visual Reproduction Test where he scored 7 correct out of 10 with only 4 errors. Despite this, DD's recall of the Rey Figure fell to only 8, 3 minutes after he had scored 32 out of a possible 36 for his copy. His vision had returned to normal but he was very anxious about a possible return of his blindness. Once again he found it very difficult to find words according to their beginning letter. He managed only 4 for F, 5 for A, and 7 for S despite a Verbal Intelligence Quotient (WAIS) of 131 and he had had much difficulty with the paired associate learning subtest of the WMS. His memory weakness hampered his acquisition of the Milner pathway on the Austin Maze Test where there was no significant reduction of errors from the 3rd to the 11th trial. In sharp contrast, DD's performance on the Spatial and Logical Arrangement Tasks of Lhermitte (see Appendix, Walsh 1991) were performed perfectly on the first trial. There were no conceptual difficulties on several other tests.

At 5 days. CT scan revealed no evidence of cerebral infarction.

At 4 weeks. Further improvements were shown though, once again, his difficulty with paired associate learning was apparent and he managed to reach only the 40th percentile on the word fluency task, a considerable deficit for a very intelligent man as shown by an extended examination. The parallel form of the Rey Figure (Taylor Figure) was recalled almost perfectly after 3 minutes. Finally, as it was considered that there was still some verbal memory difficulty, the Rey Auditory Verbal Learning Test was given.

RAVLT

	List A					*List B*	*List A*	*List A*
Trials	1	2	3	4	5	Recall	Recall	Recognition
Correct	8	11	13	9	11	6	9	4

This was thought to be well below par and the poor recognition memory was somewhat surprising.

DD had returned to work and was not concerned about his memory but remained very apprehensive about having another attack of blindness and was still concerned over this when he visited the hospital a year later with another unrelated complaint.

Amnesic stroke

Case: XD

This successful businessman was 65 and had been in good health until 6 months prior to his admission. He had suddenly became blind while driving his car but stopped the vehicle without mishap. The blindness was total but resolved after 10 minutes. During this time XD noted difficulty with his memory.

Following this episode XD suffered many attacks of blurring of vision, associated vertigo and memory loss lasting 15–30 minutes. Although he improved greatly after each attack he felt that there had been a general deterioration in his memory and he had become very tired in recent months.

Neurological examination revealed no observable deficits and no carotid bruits were noted. The clinical history prompted angiographic examination. The main abnormality was a very hypoplastic right vertebral artery and a smooth walled left vertebral with a gross stenosis at its origin. There was also a plaque on the right internal carotid artery.

Neuropsychological examination was requested prior to vertebral endarterectomy since poor vertebrobasilar perfusion appeared to be the likely cause of his troubles.

On examination he was alert, oriented and co-operative, with a clear insight into the presence of his stable memory disorder.

WMS Form I

Information	4	Digits Total	9 (6,3)
Orientation	5	Visual Reproduction	5
Mental Control	9	Associate Learning	6.5
Memory Passages	2	(3,0; 5,0; 5,0)	
MQ	87		

There was no confabulation despite the extreme poverty of his verbal recall, and on the second card of the Visual Reproduction subtest he failed to gain even one point. The RAVLT showed the same features as in the preceding case of the general amnesic syndrome, though much more severe, namely poor acquisition, retroactive inhibition and good recognition score.

RAVLT

	List A					List B	List A	List A
Trials	1	2	3	4	5	Recall	Recall	Recognition
Correct	4	4	4	4	7	4	0	15

A perfect copy of the Rey Figure was followed by a much impoverished recall at 3 minutes with only the basic outline retained (Fig. 10.7).

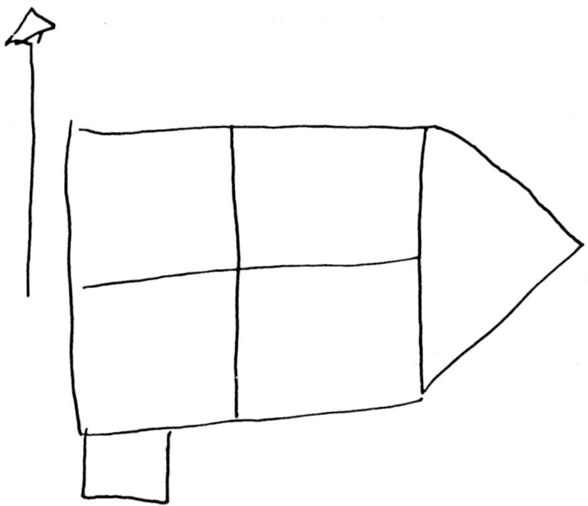

Fig. 10.7 Case XD. Recall of Rey Figure at 3 minutes.

Sundry subtests of the WAIS showed the patient to be in the normal to bright normal range with no qualitative features suggestive of deficit other than the amnesia.

Re-examination. 5 weeks after endarterectomy XD was re-examined with parallel forms of the tests given before operation. There was no change in either direction, and added memory tests only served to confirm the presence and severity of the amnesic disorder.

A final examination after the lapse of another 6 months showed the condition to be stable. XD was anxious and frustrated because of the pervasive nature of his memory loss coupled with retention of full insight into his condition. He had suffered no further attacks of visual difficulty and his visual fields were normal.

An open verdict

Case: IJ

IJ, who was a 64-year-old motor mechanic, was admitted after experiencing several episodes of recurrent 'surges' of sensation which commenced in the legs, progressed rapidly up the trunk and reached a climax in the head. The sensory experience was accompanied by unusual smells. The episodes typically lasted from 30 to 60 seconds and were followed by a brief period of confusion but there was no loss of consciousness. His memory was defective for some time after the events but returned to normal a few hours later. There were no abnormal movements, auditory or visual hallucinations or feelings of derealization or depersonalization. He had never been incontinent. There was no clear precipitating event and he had sometimes had attacks while driving. The attacks had begun 1 year before but had become more frequent in recent times. His medications had included aspirin and trifluoperazine.

During the 2 days prior to admission he had had 7 attacks. He volunteered the information that his memory had deteriorated over the past 2 years – he had to rely constantly on his notebook – and it is possible that memory difficulty pre-dated the onset of the sensory episodes. Over the past year he had admitted to an examining psychiatrist that he was disturbed by certain recurring thoughts but there was no detail as he requested them not to be recorded.

At the time of neuropsychological examination the reason for the attacks remained unclear. Differential diagnosis had included transient ischaemic attacks, temporal lobe epilepsy, psychosis and early dementia. Clinical examinations rendered the diagnosis of transient ischaemia or psychosis most unlikely and neuropsychological assessment was sought as an aid to diagnosis.

It was evident from his account of his past history that his remote memory was intact and a screening of his immediate and recent memory was performed.

WMS Form I

Information	4	Digits Total	11 (7,4)
Orientation	4	Visual Reproduction	6
Mental Control	7	Associate Learning	6
Memory Passages	4	(1,0; 5,0; 6,0)	
MQ	89		

Despite having a good immediate memory, IJ did poorly on the three tests of new learning (Logical Memory, Visual Reproduction, Associate Learning). He recalled little of either memory passage and was unable to recall any more when asked specific questions. The pattern of performance was strongly suggestive of a general amnesic disorder.

As one of the possibilities raised was an early dementing process, it was necessary to find out if his memory disorder was accompanied by other signs of intellectual decline. The WAIS was administered over two sessions and the high level and quality of his performances overall threw the poor memory performance into sharp contrast. Dementia was now excluded.

WAIS Scaled Scores

Information	13	Digit Symbol	10
Comprehension	16	Picture Completion	12
Arithmetic	15	Block Design	12
Similarities	12	Picture Arrangement	11
		Object Assembly	10
VIQ prorated	128	PIQ	123

Further evidence of IJ's memory problem was revealed by the Complex Figure of Rey. His copy was well planned and executed with a maximum score of 36, while the recall at 3 minutes was rudimentary (Fig. 10.8).

A CT scan following this assessment revealed no abnormalities. EEG scalp recordings showed normal alpha activity present bilaterally. There was bilateral excess of theta components which was considered to be more marked on the left but there was no clear lateralization. At this stage a diagnosis of temporal lobe epilepsy was made and the patient was commenced on carbamazepine.

The relationship of what appears to be a clear-cut and quite severe general amnesic syndrome and temporal lobe epilepsy remains unclear. Certainly in a

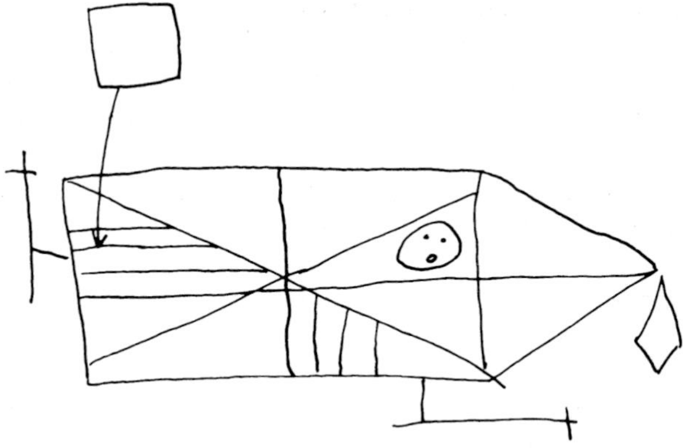

Fig. 10.8 Case IJ. Recall of Rey Figure at 3 minutes.

large number of younger cases we have not seen instances of an axial amnesia, though material specific deficits are not uncommon. IJ's epilepsy may have had a more sinister cause but he has not presented again at our hospital in the ensuing years. As is not infrequently the case, an open verdict must be entered.

The silence of the right frontal lobe

The following case illustrates that there is at least one area of the brain where extensive damage may take place without significant change on the wide range of cognitive tests currently employed in neuropsychological assessment. The following resumé covers only part of the detailed investigation of this case.

Case: WS

WS was a 14-year-old student who was admitted to hospital with multiple injuries when a home-made bomb he was constructing exploded with a devastating result. He remained conscious despite a penetrating wound above the right eye into the cranial vault, a penetrating chest wound, a penetrating abdominal wound with protruding bowel, lacerations to the hands and minor injuries to the legs and genitalia.

In numerous emergency surgical procedures fragments of bone and metal were removed from the right frontal lobe though other fragments remained deep in the lobe (Fig. 10.9). The extent of the damage can be gauged from the CT scan.

WS remained conscious, alert and orientated most of the time. Apart from the primary surgery, a mediastinal abscess was later drained together with a pericardial effusion. Despite these harrowing experiences, WS was able to be moved to a general ward only 2 weeks after admission. At this time he was grossly uninhibited in a fluctuating manner, at times being polite and accommodating, and at others grossly unco-operative, abusive, manipulative and carrying out numerous unsavoury acts such as throwing faeces at the staff. This behaviour moderated sufficiently over the next 2 weeks to enable efforts at rehabilitation to commence, though he lacked motivation and varied in his concentration span. His first neuropsychological assessment was carried out 3 weeks after his admission. Because of his many injuries, which caused pain and discomfort, and a tendency either to fatigue or become bored, the exami-

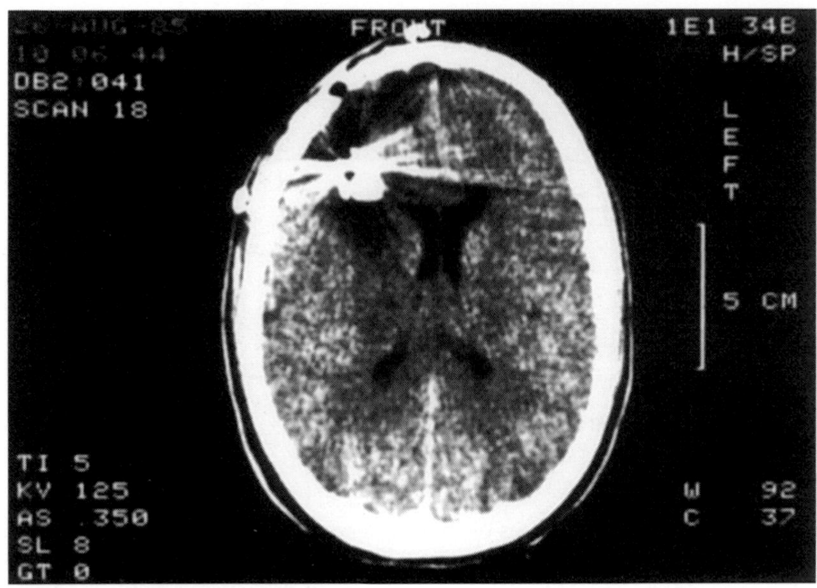

Fig. 10.9 Case WS. CT scan showing shrapnel in the right frontal lobe.

nation was carried out in several short sessions. Each time he was pleasantly co-operative, though flat in affect, and at times mildly adynamic. At other times he was highly distractible.

By this time it was known that WS had had a long history of an antisocial conduct disorder; little detail was to be had from the parents who, however, felt that there had been little personality change since the explosion.

WISC-R Age Scaled Scores

Information	10	Picture Completion	10
Similarities	12	Picture Arrangement	7
Arithmetic	12	Block Design	7
Vocabulary	9	Object Assembly	8
Comprehension	10	Mazes	13
Digit Span	9		
VIQ	114	PIQ	92

Much of the poor performance on the three items from the Performance Scale was caused by slowness resulting from lack of dexterity secondary to his hand lacerations. A minor analytical difficulty was apparent on the Block Design subtest.

WMS Form I

Information	4	Digits Total	10 (6,4)
Orientation	4	Visual Reproduction	13
Mental Control	9	Associate Learning	19
Memory Passages	11 (13,9)	(6,2; 6,4; 6,4)	

No suggestion of memory deficit was seen in this excellent set of performances, which was commensurate with his VIQ.

Corsi Block Tapping Test. Immediate memory span: 8.

Complex Figure of Rey. A complete but somewhat careless copy was made which was well planned. At this stage WS appeared bored and his poor recall was difficult to interpret.

Austin Maze (Milner pathway). WS enjoyed this game-like test, mastering it in only 5 trials, a very superior performance (for further information see Walsh 1991). He then insisted on being allowed to try it backwards, making only one error at his first attempt and none on his second. Next day he asked to do it again with exactly the same result. Complex learning of this type was clearly unaffected.

Tower of London Test (Shallice 1982). This was included in a series of tests usually shown to be sensitive to left frontal lobe damage since it was possible that damage might have been sustained in areas other than the primary site of impact. Here again WS turned in a first rate performance:

Average preparation time	5.7 seconds
Average execution time	11.5 seconds
Correct	10 of 12 correct with 3 errors, two of which were recognized and corrected

Several other tests suggested intact cognitive processes at a level in keeping with his above average intelligence.

Finally, this case provided an opportunity to check the finding that design fluency might prove a sensitive measure of right frontal lobe function comparable to that of verbal fluency for the left frontal lobe (Jones-Gotman & Milner 1977). Data from this study are shown in comparison to WS, who appeared to have no difficulty in generating drawings under both conditions.

WS	*Normal*	*Right*	*Frontal*
Free condition	17	16.2	8.0
Fixed condition	15	19.7	7.0

When WS was seen at 5 months after injury extensive examinations revealed some improvement in speed of information processing, but an otherwise stable set of cognitive performances. On the Taylor version of the Rey Figure his recall score reached the 100th percentile. The analytical problem on the Block Design items was still in evidence but only on the most difficult items.

Unfortunately WS was still causing concern because of his antisocial conduct. He still retained his old group of friends and mixed well with his peer group. It was impossible to tell whether his psychosocial difficulties had been exacerbated by his injuries. His mother at this stage described him as 'a deviant little brat' who had not been worsened by the event.

Carbon monoxide poisoning

Case: QT

This 45-year-old bank manager was admitted to hospital following a suicide attempt involving motor vehicle exhaust fumes. He was confused and disoriented for 4 days and his first clear memories were of a family visit 5 days after admission, though he subsequently recalled isolated events from the third and fourth days. He was amnesic for the incident but recalled setting out in his car. EEG and CT scan on the third day were both normal. The reason for his attempt remained unclear but may have been related to difficulties with his second marriage.

On examination on the sixth day he was pleasantly co-operative and seemingly unconcerned with the fact that he had tried to commit suicide. He complained of a severe memory difficulty.

As amnesic deficit looms large in many cases of carbon monoxide poisoning, testing commenced with the Wechsler Memory Scale Form I.

WMS Form I

Information	5	Digits Total	14 (7,7)
Orientation	5	Visual Reproduction	12
Mental Control	7	Associate Learning	8
Memory Passages	7	(2,0; 4,2; 6,0)	

QT had particular difficulty with new verbal learning. We have found the 'difficult' items on Paired Associate learning to be particularly sensitive in these cases. However, we have usually found a general amnesia in previous instances of carbon monoxide poisoning so the good performance on Visual Reproduction was unexpected, though we have seen such a sparing in cases of alcohol-related amnesia which have all the features of Korsakoff psychosis (see Ch. 2, Walsh 1991).

RAVLT

	List A					*List B*	*List A*	*List A*
Trials	1	2	3	4	5	Recall	Recall	Recognition
Correct	6	5	7	8	8	6	3	7

The RAVLT performance was marked by virtually no extension beyond his immediate memory span (7), a marked interference effect, and poor recognition memory.

Copy of the Complex Figure of Rey was complete and well organized, but only the main outline was recalled at 3 minutes (score 10/36).

Finally, four subtests of the WAIS-R showed a relatively poor performance on only Object Assembly.

Similarities	11	Block Design	12
Digit Span	12	Object Assembly	8

Testing was terminated because of lack of time, with the impression of an amnesic disorder largely uncomplicated by more widespread intellectual loss. Prognosis was reserved as we have seen varying degrees of recovery in amnesic disorders following carbon monoxide poisoning and hypoxic events.

A second neuropsychological assessment was performed at 1 month. With one exception, the repeated testing – WMS (Form II), RAVLT and Rey Figure – produced almost identical results. There was still a discrepancy between a good performance on Visual Reproduction and measures of verbal learning. This dissociation was confirmed by the Benton Visual Retention Test given with a 15 second delay. QT had no difficulty: 8 of 10 correct with only 2 errors. The clear difference noted was on the RAVLT. While the poor acquisition and interference effect were identical to the early examination, the Recognition score had risen from 7 to 13 of a possible 15.

Other subtests of the WAIS-R produced a level of performance as before.

Arithmetic	14	Picture Completion	10
Digit Symbol	12	Picture Arrangement	12

A third examination was made at 3 months. The patient said his memory was still poor but had improved somewhat as he was now able to recall some telephone numbers and addresses. Testing was restricted to memory as there had been no indication of other cognitive deficits. In keeping with his subjective report there were slight gains over the 2 month period though a sizeable memory deficit still remained.

WMS Form I

Memory Passages	6
Visual Reproduction	14
Associate Learning (6,0; 6,1; 6,2)	12

RAVLT

	List A					*List B*	*List A*	*List A*
Trials	1	2	3	4	5	Recall	Recall	Recognition
Correct	4	7	8	9	9	6	5	13

The great difficulty with spontaneous recall and the marked interference effect remained as serious as before, and the prognosis began to look gloomy. In an endeavour to see whether logical structure of the material to be learned influenced learning and retention, two of the tests of Lhermitte and Signoret (1972) were given (see Walsh 1991). The test of Spatial Arrangement was mastered in 4 trials, a normal performance, and an even better performance of only 2 trials to criterion on the test of Logical Arrangement suggested that memory retraining might be advantageous in this case since there was reason to believe that visual memory was relatively spared and the ability to benefit from logical structure to aid learning was clearly present. Follow-up was suggested but the patient failed to keep the next appointment.

Alcohol and error utilization

Case: ZS

This man had always worked as an unskilled labourer and had a long history of alcohol abuse dating back at least 20 years. His own (possibly conservative) estimate was at least 12 standard drinks per day. His alcoholism had caused the breakdown of his marriage 7 years before and he was reduced to relying on charitable institutions for lodging and support. At this stage he realized that he needed professional help and entered a recovery project for those with alcohol problems. He had been sober for 5 months when he was sent for an evaluation of his cognitive abilities, such assessment forming part of the planning of his rehabilitation. ZS also stated his concern to his doctor that he was unintelligent but his doctor did not consider this to be the case. He was highly motivated to attend for assessment and to do well. He saw it as a means of finding out whether he had any worthwhile abilities. He was also quite worried about the possibility of brain damage after such a long period of alcohol abuse.

Tests of memory and new learning were carried out first.

WMS Form I

Information	5	Digits Total	10 (6,4)
Orientation	5	Visual Reproduction	11
Mental Control	6	Associate Learning	16
Memory Passages	9	(6,1; 6,2; 6,4)	
MQ	114		

The relative ease with which he handled the tasks sensitive to disorders of new learning (Logical Memory, Visual Reproduction and Associate Learning) was immediately reinforcing to ZS.

RAVLT

	List A					*List B*	*List A*	*List A*
Trials	1	2	3	4	5	Recall	Recall	Recognition
Correct	5	7	7	9	9	6	8	13

This performance was surprisingly unexpected in view of his good performances on the WMS, but it is not uncommon in such patients where the pathological process or processes resulting from alcohol abuse often result in difficulty with complex learning, especially where subjects must generate strategies of learning and recall for themselves.

A short version of the WAIS-R was used to estimate current levels of functioning in a variety of areas and an estimate of probable premorbid ability based on subtests such as Information and Comprehension, which appear relatively stable in the face of years of heavy drinking. It was thought that after a long period of abstinence ZS's intellectual functioning would be stable.

WAIS-R Scaled Scores

Information	11	Block Design	9
Comprehension	11	Object Assembly	10
Similarities	9	Digit Symbol	5

Apart from a non-specific slowing affecting the Digit Symbol Substitution subtest, there were no quantitative or qualitative features to suggest unsuspected cognitive deficits.

Despite the apparent preservation of memory and intellectual abilities at a level consonant with premorbid expectations, we have found that patients with a history such as that of ZS often have a serious problem with any degree of new learning that involves benefiting from experience (see Ch. 4 and Walsh 1991).

Austin Maze (Milner pathway)

Trial	1	2	3	4	5	6	7	8	9	10
Errors	22	30	15	14	11	10	12	6	7	5
Trial	11	12	13	14	15	16	17	18	19	20
Errors	5	5	5	4	5	6	4	5	5	4

Trial	21	22	23	24	25	26	27	28	29	30
Errors	2	1	3	3	4	2	1	1	1	1

Trial	31	32	33	34	35	36	37	38	39	40
Errors	2	1	1	2	1	1	1	1	1	1

Discontinued after 40 trials.

ZS applied himself diligently to the task, insisting that he would get it right eventually. A stable, error-free performance might be expected in 15 trials or less in someone of his estimated premorbid ability. His performance exemplifies very clearly the problem of 'error utilization' or inability to perfect the learning of a novel, relatively complex procedure requiring integration over time. In this case the single error on each of the last six trials was made at a different choice point.

This learning difficulty may easily escape notice unless appropriate tests are used. Such tests need to have the following characteristics: (i) novelty; (ii) complexity; (iii) self-direction; and (iv) integration over time.

We have found this imperfect learning disorder to correlate highly with success or failure in job retraining and getting back into stable employment in individuals such as ZS, and the prognosis in these cases should be guarded. Further examination usually reveals the presence of other indices of reduction in adaptive behaviour.

The case of the elderly parachutist

Case: YQ
Age: 60
Education: Postgraduate diploma
Occupation: Property management consultant

Following the death of his wife a few years before, this successful 60-year-old businessman had taken up parachuting. Several of his jumps were not well executed and on one of them he was badly shaken though apparently not unconscious.

After this incident (28 December 1983), YQ developed severe left-sided headaches, drowsiness, vomiting, poor concentration and photophobia. During the next 2 weeks, however, he continued his parachute jumping despite persistent headaches and concentration difficulties. He was involved in three minor car accidents on 2 January 1984. On 3 January 1984 he eventually sought medical attention, and was admitted to hospital where CT scan revealed a subdural haematoma. At operation a mixture of old and fresh blood was evacuated from the left fronto-temporal region.

Postoperatively there was motor aphasia and mild right arm weakness but these were almost normal on discharge 2 weeks later.

At neuropsychological assessment at 2 months, YQ was co-operative although somewhat flippant and facetious. He said that his memory, which was poor for some weeks, had returned to normal but he still had mild word finding difficulties when tired.

WMS Form I

Information	6	Digits Total	13 (8,5)

Orientation	5	Visual Reproduction	12
Mental Control	7	Associate Learning	8.5
Memory Passages	13	(4,0; 5,1; 6,0)	
MQ	122		

The principal finding of marked difficulty with the 'hard' pairs of Asssociate Learning was further investigated with the Rey Auditory Verbal Learning Test.

RAVLT

	List A					*List B*	*List A*	*List A*
Trials	1	2	3	4	5	Recall	Recall	Recognition
Correct	5	5	7	7	7	5	3	12

This test highlighted a verbal learning difficulty of some severity. Apart from the very low level of acquisition, the unsystematic order of recall over successive trials suggested a 'frontal amnesia' (see Ch. 4).

Because of this deficit and the known location of the lesion, the ensuing assessment included several tests often found to be sensitive to frontal lobe dysfunction together with several subtests of the WAIS-R.

WAIS-R Scaled Scores

Information	14	Object Assembly	10
Similarities	10	Digit Symbol	8
Block Design	10		

Apart from a generalized slowing on all tests which robbed him of time credits, YQ showed a concept level on the Similarities subtest lower than expected for his educational and occupational background.

Verbal Fluency Test 1: (F, 11; A, 10; S, 12). This was well below expectation and thought to be consistent with residual dysfunction in the left frontal region.

Complex Figure of Rey

Copy: Score 34/36 but poorly organized.

Recall: Score 19/36. A considerable reduction in keeping with the provisional diagnosis of frontal amnesia.

Austin Maze (Milner pathway)

Trial	1	2	3	4	5	6	7	8	9	10	11	12
Errors	26	21	7	12	6	6	4	5	7	5	5	2
Trial	13	14	15	16	17	18	19	20	21	22	23	24
Errors	3	3	1	1	2	4	1	2	3	2	1	1
Trial	25	26	27	28	29	30	31	32	33	34		
Errors	1	1	1	2	2	1	1	1	0	0		

YQ's performance strongly supported the hypothesis of residual frontal lobe dysfunction. After making only 4 errors on trial 7, a person of his premorbid competence should have reached a stable error-free performance in the next few trials, yet it took him more than 25 further trials to reduce his errors to zero and there is no guarantee in such a case that he would be able to maintain this error-free condition. The difficulty demonstrates very clearly what was termed in Chapter 4 *the problem of error utilization*.

Advice was given on the possible disruptive effects of his brain injury on his work performance.

A second assessment was made at 8 months. YQ had returned to his former position as national manager of a major corporation. He described a number of personality changes which he dated to the time of his injury. He described himself as more 'laid back' at work and less committed, preferring to delegate work. He reported being more forthright and outspoken than before. Apart from some minor difficulty recalling names he reported no significant memory problems. His minor word finding difficulty persisted.

To check any recovery of cognitive functioning parallel forms of tests previously used were employed where possible.

WMS Form II. Despite a rise in MQ from 122 to 132 from small improvements on several subtests, YQ still showed no facility in learning the new or difficult pairs of the Associate Learning subtest: score 11 (6,0; 6,1; 6,1). There was modest gain on the RAVLT, but this was still considerably below par for a man of his premorbid ability.

RAVLT

List A						*List B*	*List A*	*List A*
Trials	1	2	3	4	5	Recall	Recall	Recognition
Correct	5	7	7	10	11	5	9	15

Complex Figure of Rey. The copy score was again 34, but the organization poor. The recall score was even less than before and showed several features described with frontal lobe lesions (see Messerli et al 1979). YQ could not resist the impulse to draw a house (possibly aroused by the figure) which he then scribbled out (Fig. 10.10).

Verbal fluency had increased only marginally, from a mean of 11 to a mean of 12.3.

Austin Maze (Milner pathway)

Trial	1	2	3	4	5	6	7	8	9	10	11
Errors	37	18	15	14	9	13	10	4	4	4	7
Trial	12	13	14	15	16	17	18	19	20	21	22
Errors	7	3	3	1	2	5	3	1	1	0	0

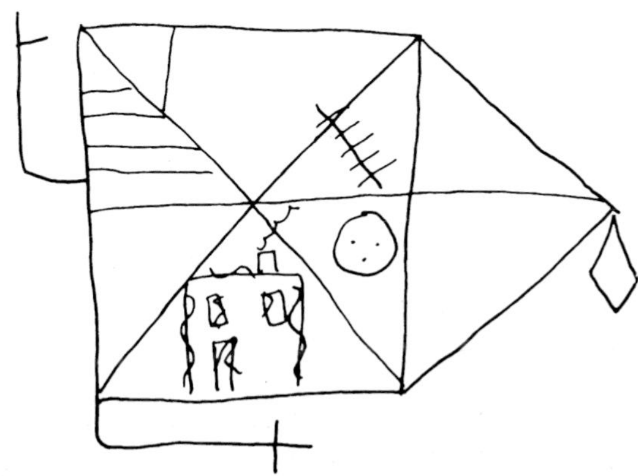

Fig. 10.10 Case YQ. Frontal dysfunction in recall of Rey Figure.

Once again, while there might be some improvement, there was still a significant problem of error utilization some considerable time after injury. It also became clear at this second examination that YQ had little or no insight into the nature and extent of his deficits.

Postscript. At neurosurgical review 2 months later, YQ expressed a strong desire to retire from work as he felt that he was not able to perform intellectually as well as he had prior to his accident. His superior, obviously aware of the subtle but pervasive changes wrought by the frontal injury, supported the suggestion of immediate retirement. The patient was still keen, however, to continue his parachute jumping. One can only surmise why he took this on in the first place.

Dementia variants

Case: QS

This 56-year-old male, right-handed, formerly high-functioning general practitioner was referred with a presumptive diagnosis of Alzheimer's disease after experiencing more than a year of slowly progressing vocational difficulties.

The initial symptoms were regarded as memory difficulties. He reported being surprised that commonly used drug names no longer meant anything to him. When required to re-prescribe medications, he found that he no longer recognized many specific drugs. Occasionally he would ask patients the indications for these medications and, when told, found that such prompts did not cue any additional familiarity. He created notes on medical topics and specific drugs to aid him. Patients began to complain that he seemed 'confused' and hesitant at times.

His wife had noticed difficulties at least 2 years previously. While overseas, he seemed less able to cope with the busy schedule, becoming withdrawn, easily frustrated and reserved. He was found spending more time reading professional material than formerly. He had been an eloquent orator, but a recent wedding speech was regarded as uncustomarily simple, and he had found it difficult to spell or construct words during games of Scrabble. His wife also commented that his powers of logic seemed affected, though his personality was similar and temporal orientation and knowledge of current affairs were preserved. Personal hygiene, grooming, driving and social independence remained normal. No unusual medical symptoms were present.

There was no other past, family or social history of note. He had never smoked and at most drank a single glass of whisky or wine each day.

He was initially referred to a neurologist, who reported no elementary neurological or general abnormalities and then referred him to a psychiatrist. He noted no formal psychiatric or mood disorder, but found prominent language difficulties, particularly with word selection, recall and usage, together with slow speed of information processing, organizational and abstraction impairments, and difficulty encoding and recalling verbal information with impoverished recall of complex visual information. The psychiatrist considered that such widespread deficits made Alzheimer's disease the most likely diagnosis and that neuroimaging was not necessary. QS was referred to our unit for neuropsychological screening prior to experimental drug trials.

Neuropsychological examination. QS was alert, co-operative, well-groomed, polite, appropriate in affect and, although correcting himself repeatedly, was oriented to time and location and knew political figures and current events. His initial verbal responses were frequently incorrect though within the correct semantic category. He would then show frustration and attempt to correct his answer, usually only ceasing when correct. Hesitations and word finding problems dominated his performances. Premorbid verbal intelligence was predicted to be in the superior range (New Adult Reading Test 7 errors, predicted Verbal IQ 122, Nelson & O'Connell 1978).

He could repeat 5 digits forwards and 4 backwards. Routine mental operations were performed more poorly than expected, e.g. counting from 20 to 1 in 31 seconds, reciting months of the year forwards in 4 seconds but backwards in 73 seconds, and during serial addition of 3 he hesitated, forgot current numbers and made repetitions. He appeared to have difficulty keeping task instructions as well as current items in mind simultaneously.

Language tasks were particularly impaired. Spontaneous language was fluent, grammatical and adequate for conversational expression, though with occasional semantic paraphasias. Repetition was preserved. Confrontation naming was severely impaired. He was only able to name correctly the highest frequency items of the Boston Naming Test, and was not assisted by semantic or phonemic cues. He could not correctly complete the sentence: 'a tool to tighten a nut on a bolt is a...'. Definitions of telescope, barometer and periscope were slow and laborious. Comprehension was intact for passive and relational constructions, names of fingers and sides of the body; writing, although slow, was correct. Mental arithmetic was very poor, e.g. 6 + 5 is '...11', 13 − 7 is '...don't know', 20 − 7 is '...13', 17 × 3 is '...don't know'.

Verbal fluency was markedly impaired, particularly for semantic categories, e.g. animals 2 ('parrot, dog...'), vegetables 3, supermarket items 4. His performance for word generation using initial letters was poor (F, 7; A, 5; S, 8). For animals, he stated 'parrot, dog...' and then could not think of any others for the entire minute. He could recall the route home correctly in terms of direction of consecutive turns, but not all the names of important streets along the way.

RAVLT

	List A					*List B*	*List A*	*List A*
Trials	1	2	3	4	5	Recall	Recall	Recognition
Correct	3	5	5	6	3	3	7	12 (+ 6)

He was not able to improve his recall of the 15 words of the RAVLT significantly beyond his verbal span, showing little attempt at organizing his recall or success in the middle words of the list. When attempting to listen to the words, he commented 'they disappear...go straight through'. Retroactive interference was prominent, and recognition relatively better, though with multiple intrusions.

His copy of the Rey-Osterreith Complex Figure was poorly organized (score 30/36, 20th percentile) and recall markedly impoverished (score 9/36, < 10th percentile).

Simpler measures of encoding and recall, e.g. the Three Words Three Shapes Test (see Lezak 1995) and memory for three objects in three locations, were more easily encoded but he showed greater difficulty recalling verbal than visual material after interpolated tasks. Multiple choice presentation did not noticeably improve his recall for verbal items. On the other hand, visual material was recalled accurately even 2 hours later, suggesting that language difficulties may underlie these many failures, rather than a general amnesic syndrome.

Simple visuoconstructive tasks were performed well, and he was able to point out multiple hidden figures in an embedded figures test, but more complex tasks tended to be poorly organized and executed. Other executive deficits were also present, suggesting that visuospatial impairments were secondary to executive, not visuoperceptive difficulties. On part B of the Trail Making Test he reverted to connecting consecutive letters. He could not correctly perform conflicting motor tasks with both hands, or reproduce simple hand positions without verbal assistance. He could not complete the Milner pathway of the Austin Maze.

Austin Maze (Milner pathway)

Trial	1	2	3	4	5	6	7	8	9	10
Errors	14	7	9	7	6	6	4	3	4	7

Trial	11	12	13
Errors	2	1	3...gave up

Although he indicated understanding of the task and approached it in a logical manner, he quickly forgot the location of central choice points, making both the same and new errors repeatedly, and became too frustrated to continue. In addition, although he evinced frustration with some of his performances, he appeared less concerned than expected.

Discussion. On the basis of these performances, it was clear that he was performing well below the level expected. The history of insidious onset, gradual progression and early and disproportionate difficulties with language-based tasks suggested an intrinsic brain disease asymmetrically affecting his dominant hemisphere. His language deficits resembled a transcortical sensory aphasia, with very severe semantic difficulties suggesting a lesion in the left posterior or inferior temporal region. His initial difficulties recalling medical terms resembled 'alienation du mot' (estrangement of word meaning, see Poeck & Luzzatti 1988). Executive deficits were mild but suggested added anterior involvement. Those functions which were relatively spared included phonology, syntax, syntactic comprehension, autobiographical and episodic memory, visuospatial abilities and non-verbal memory.

A similar clinical pattern has been reported within the spectrum of *primary progressive aphasia* (Basso et al 1988, Weintraub et al 1990, Weintraub & Mesulam 1993, Kertesz 1997, Mesulam et al 1997). Others have separately classified the grammatically fluent form as 'semantic dementia' (Snowden et al 1989, Hodges et al 1992, Talbot et al 1995), emphasizing the dissolution of semantic information stores including the lexicon, but relative preservation of other cognitive abilities. Specific asymmetrical left inferior temporal neocortical atrophy is a reported feature of semantic dementia (Chawluk et al 1986, Hodges et al 1992, Mesulam et al 1997), so neuroimaging studies were recommended.

MRI showed predominant inferolateral left temporal lobe atrophy. Positron emission tomography confirmed asymmetrical hypometabolism of both temporal lobes extending into the left frontal cortex. The hypometabolism appeared to spare the superior and middle temporal gyri, making it atypical for Alzheimer's disease. These findings, as well as the patient's clinical features, accorded well with those reported in semantic dementia.

It is important to differentiate this condition from Alzheimer's disease. The pathology underlying semantic dementia is variable and may include non-specific superficial neuronal loss, gliosis and spongiform degeneration or Alzheimer's disease (Weintraub & Mesulam 1993, see Neary 1997). Inclusion of such patients in trials of Alzheimer's disease related medications may confound results. Patients with semantic dementia tend to present at around the age of 55 years, resembling more the epidemiological spectrum seen with frontotemporal dementia (see Ch. 3), and there may be similar genetic implications. The prognosis may also be different - some patients show several years of relative stability and preserved non-language functions, making their quality of life dramatically better than modal Alzheimer's disease patients. The progression of deficits is also different, on average taking a longer course for the non-Alzheimer's disease patient. Counselling should take this into account, particularly the prospect of progressive language dissolution out of proportion to other intellectual deficits, or the development of additional executive impairment.

Course. Over the next 2 years, QS continued to show cognitive deterioration. His lexical knowledge deteriorated dramatically with simplification of his conversational speech, frequent hesitations and word finding pauses, and confusion of simple medical terms, e.g. using 'sphygmomanometer' for stethoscope and denying any knowledge of the word 'cystitis' or specific antibiotics. Past acquaintances were forgotten completely, as were the associations of old photographs, to which he started adding subtitles. His spelling deteriorated markedly, so that he tended to write with letters poorly differentiated. He became confused in conversations involving several people. His insight deteriorated further, as did his awareness of social mores; his wife could no longer take him to live concerts since he was apt to be noisier or talk abruptly without the usual regard. He became more rigid in his manner, more impulsive and short-tempered. He once became angry with their pet labrador, and threw him bodily out of the back door. At times he was child-like, following his wife around. He remains physically active but is continuing to deteriorate.

Hysterical pseudodementia

Case: XW

This 60-year-old woman had worked as a technical assistant in a laboratory until a few years before her referral for possible dementia.

The difficulties began in 1981 when she suddenly became unable to write; when seen in 1983 she was unable to write even her own name. The onset of this difficulty was not accompanied by any other signs of neurological deficit. Neither she nor her husband reported any major medical or psychological problems prior to this sudden onset. She did have a history of hypertension but this was well controlled on medication. There had been no history of other neurological symptoms apart from left-sided headaches, particularly during times of stress.

Since the onset of her writing difficulties, XW reported that she had experienced increasing difficulties with her memory and in carrying out daily tasks. She reported rapid forgetting, being unable to remember where she put things and hanging up the telephone and immediately forgetting the message or reason for the call. She stated that she was unable to remember day-to-day events or even what day it was. She was unable to cook a simple meal, do the shopping, handle money, knit or sew her own clothes, tasks she had previously performed with ease. Her husband reported that if his wife attempted any routine tasks she would just 'dither' and become upset. Consequently, he had taken over the majority of the domestic responsibilities.

XW described herself as a perfectionist. She stated that she found it extremely distressing, frustrating and even frightening when she found herself unable to perform everyday tasks. Her degree of insight seemed surprising in view of the described severity of her complaint. During the assessment she was pleasantly co-operative but this was punctuated by periodic bouts of uncontrolled weeping. After each of these she rapidly regained her composure and was quite willing to carry on. Throughout the session she displayed apparent comprehension and word finding difficulties.

WMS Form I			
Information	4	Digits Total	4 (4,0)
Orientation	0	Visual Reproduction	0
Mental Control	2	Associate Learning	4
Memory Passages	0.5	(3,0; 3,0; 2,0)	
MQ	57		

The validity of what appears to be a very severe amnesic difficulty was called into question since the level of performance was out of keeping with her presentation during examination. Despite scoring zero on Orientation she showed clear evidence of recording ongoing events. While unable to give her date of birth and other well learned information she was able to recall the names of current and former political figures with ease. On the two prose passages she produced only one piece of information, and questioning produced no additions. Fragments of the three cards of Visual Reproduction produced another score of zero (Fig. 10.11). Finally, unlike most patients with moderate dementia she was unable to produce even a modest number of responses to the 'easy' associations of the Paired Associate subtest.

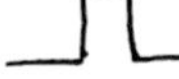

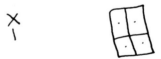

Fig. 10.11 Case XW. Recall of the 3 cards of the Wechsler Memory Scale, Form I.

It seemed to the examiner that this might reflect an attempt to enact the role of 'sicker than the sickest' and a possible differential diagnosis of hysterical pseudodementia was entertained. This very simple examination took over an hour because of extreme slowness, complaints of not being able to understand the simplest instructions, and time out for bouts of weeping.

Next an attempt was made at supraspan learning using only five digits. Despite 10 trials XW showed no evidence of even approximating the series. Testing was then abandoned.

During the second examination, despite the passage of 4 weeks without significant change, XW spontaneously recalled the examiner's name. When asked to write her name and a simple sentence to dictation she produced a small amount of illegible scrawl (Fig. 10.12).

To check the presence of a pseudoneurological memory disorder, XW was given the 15 item 'memory' task of Rey cited in Lezak (1976, p. 476 f, 1983). 'The principle underlying it is that the patient who consciously or unconsciously wishes to appear impaired will fail at a task that all but the most severely brain damaged or retarded patients will perform easily.' Her performance seemed consistent with a pseudodementia (Fig. 10.13).

Finally, XW's reading was characterized not only by dysfluency but also by the insertion of material that was not in the original text.

During this second visit further evidence came to hand of inconsistencies in

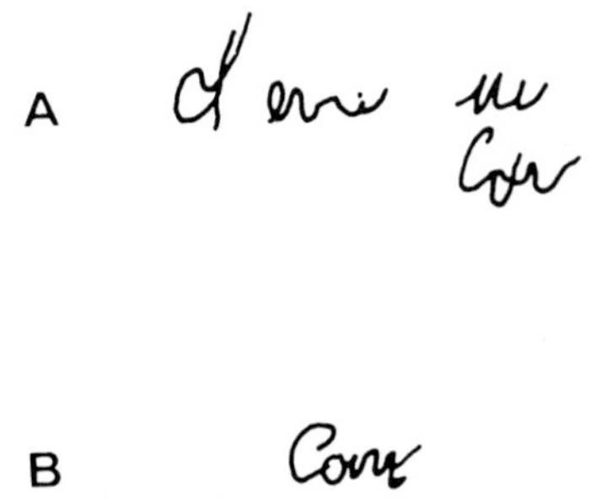

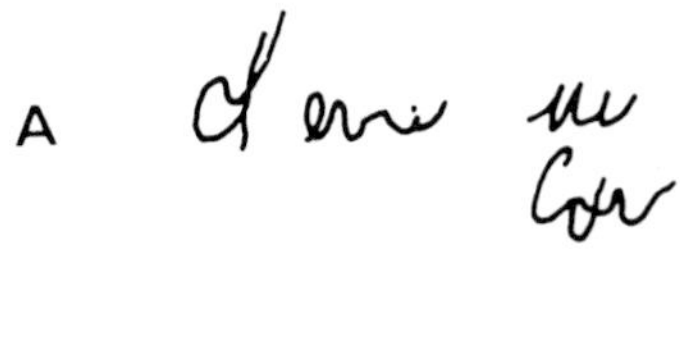

B

Fig. 10.12 Case XW. Writing to dictation: A, Attempts to write her name; B, the sentence 'The cat ate the fish'.

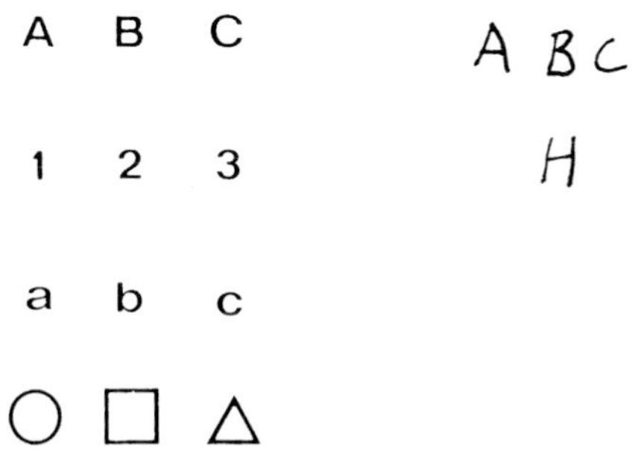

A B C   A B C

1 2 3   H

a b c

○ □ △

Fig. 10.13 Case XW. Response to Rey's 15 item memory test.

her behaviour; for example, while she was unable to knit or cook a simple meal she was quite able to drive herself into the country to visit friends.

Psychiatric opinion concurred with the diagnosis of hysterical pseudo-dementia and treatment was commenced. Neurological examination and CT scan carried out between the two testing sessions had been normal.

References

Adams R D, Victor M 1993 Principles of neurology, 5th edn. McGraw-Hill, New York

Basso A, Capitani E, Laiacona M 1988 Progressive language impairment without dementia: a case with isolated category specific semantic defect. Journal of Neurology, Neurosurgery and Psychiatry 51: 1201–1207

Ben-Yishay Y, Diller L, Mandelberg I, Gordon W, Gerstman L J 1971 Similarities and differences in Block Design performance between older normal and brain-injured persons. A task analysis. Journal of Abnormal Psychology 78: 17–25

Binder L, Pankratz L 1987 Neuropsychological evidence of a fictitious memory complaint. Journal of Clinical and Experimental Neuropsychology 9: 167–171

Chawluk J B, Mesulam M-M, Hurtig H et al 1986 Slowly progressive aphasia without generalized dementia: studies with positron emission tomography. Annals of Neurology 19: 68–74

Elithorn A 1965 Psychological tests. An objective approach to the problem of task difficulty. Acta Neurologica Scandinavica, Supplementum 13 Part 2: 661–667

Geschwind N 1978 Organic problems in the aged: Brain syndromes and alcoholism. Journal of Geriatric Psychiatry 11: 161–166

Goldberg E, Costa L D 1986 Qualitative indices in neuropsychological assessment. In: Grant I, Adams K M (eds) Neuropsychological assessment of neuropsychiatric disorders. Oxford University Press, New York, pp 48–64

Hampton J R, Harrison M J G, Mitchell J R A, Pritchard J S, Seymour C 1975 Relative contributions of history taking, physical examination, and laboratory investigation to diagnosis and management of medical out-patients. British Medical Journal ii: 486–489

Heilbrun A B 1962 Issues in the assessment of organic brain damage. Psychological Reports 10: 511–515

Hodges J R, Patterson K, Oxbury S, Funnell E 1992 Semantic dementia: progressive fluent aphasia with temporal lobe atrophy. Brain 115: 1783–1806

Jones-Gotman M, Milner B 1977 Design fluency: the invention of nonsense drawings after focal cortical lesions. Neuropsychologia 15: 673–674

Kane R L, Goldstein G, Parsons O A 1989 A response to Mapou. Journal of Clinical and Experimental Psychology 11: 589–595

Kaplan E 1988 A process approach to neuropsychological assessment. In: Boll T, Bryant B K (eds) Clinical neuropsychology and brain function: research, measurement and practice. American Psychological Association, Washington, pp 129–167

Kaplan E, Fein D, Morris R, Delis D 1991 WAIS-R NI Manual. Psychological Corporation, San Antonio

Kertesz A 1997 Frontotemporal dementia, Pick disease, and corticobasal degeneration: one entity or 3? 1. Archives of Neurology 54: 1427–1429

Kinsbourne M 1971 Cognitive deficit: experimental analysis. In: McGaugh J L (ed) Psychiobiology. Academic Press, New York, ch 7

Kinsbourne M 1972 Contrasting patterns of memory span decrement in ageing and aphasia. Journal of Neurology, Neurosurgery and Psychiatry 35: 192–195

Levin H S, Eisenberg H M, Benton A L (eds) 1989 Mild head injury. Oxford University Press, New York

Ley P 1970 Acute psychiatric patients. In: Mittler P (ed) The psychological assessment of mental and physical disorders. Tavistock Publications, London, ch 7

Lezak M D 1976 Neuropsychological assessment. Oxford University Press, New York

Lezak M D 1983 Neuropsychological assessment, 2nd edn. Oxford University Press, New York

Lezak M D 1988 IQ: RIP. Journal of Clinical and Experimental Neuropsychology 10 : 351–361

Lezak M D 1995 Neuropsychological assessment, 3nd edn. Oxford University Press, New York
Lhermitte F, Signoret J L 1972 Analyse neuropsychologique et différenciation des syndromes amnésiques. Revue Neurologique 126: 161–178
Luria A R, Tsvetkova L D 1964 The programming of constructive activity in local brain injuries. Neuropsychologia 2: 95–108
Mapou R L 1988 Testing to detect brain damage: An alternative to what may no longer be useful. Journal of Clinical and Experimental Neuropsychology 10: 271–278
Matthews C G, Shaw D J, Kløve H 1966 Psychological test performances in neurologic and 'pseudo-neurologic' subjects. Cortex 2: 244–253
McFie J 1960 Psychological testing in clinical neurology. Journal of Nervous and Mental Diseases 131: 383–393
Messerli P, Seron X, Tissot P 1979 Quelques aspects de la programmation dans le syndrome frontal. Archives Suisses de Neurologie, Neurochirurgie et de Psychiatrie 125: 25–35
Meyer V 1957 Critique of psychological approaches to brain damage. Journal of Mental Science 103: 80–109
Mesulam M-M, Johnson N, Grujic Z, Weintraub S 1997 Apolipoprotein E genotypes in primary progressive aphasia. Neurology 49: 51–55
Miller E 1983 A note on the interpretation of data derived from neuropsychological tests. Cortex 19: 131–132
Neary D 1997 Frontotemporal dementia, Pick disease, and corticobasal degeneration: one entity or 3? 3. Archives of Neurology 54: 1425–1427
Nelson H E, O'Connell A 1978 Dementia: the estimation of premorbid intelligence levels using the new adult reading test. Cortex 14: 234–244
Pankratz L 1979 Symptom validity testing and symptom retraining: Procedures for the assessment and treatment of functional sensory deficits. Journal of Consulting and Clinical Psychology 47: 409–410
Pankratz L 1983 A new technique for the assessment and modification of feigned memory deficit. Perceptual and Motor Skills 57: 367–372
Pankratz L, Paar G H 1988 A test of symptom validity in assessing functional symptoms. Zeitschrift fur Klinische Psychologie, Psychopathologie und Psychotherapie 36: 130–137
Pankratz L, Fausti S A, Peed S 1975 A forced choice technique to evaluate deafness in the hysterical or malingering patient. Journal of Consulting and Clinical Psychology 43: 421–422
Pankratz L, Binder L M, Wilcox L M 1987 Evaluation of an exaggerated somatosensory deficit with symptom validity testing. Archives of Neurology 44: 798
Piercy M F 1959 Testing for intellectual impairment – some comments on tests and testers. Journal of Mental Science 105: 489–495
Poeck K, Luzzatti C 1988 Slowly progressive aphasia in three patients: the problem of accompanying neuropsychological deficit. Brain 111: 151–168
Reitan R M 1964 Psychological deficits resulting from cerebral lesions in man. In: Warren J M, Akert K (eds) The frontal granular cortex and behavior. McGraw Hill, New York, ch 14
Reitan R M, Davison L A (eds) 1974 Clinical neuropsychology: current status and applications. Wiley, New York
Russell E W 1982 Theory and developments of pattern analysis methods related to the Halstead-Reitan Battery. In: Logue P E, Shear J M (eds) Clinical neuropsychology: a multidisciplinary approach. Thomas, Springfield, Illinois, pp 50–98
Ryan C, Butters N 1980 Learning and memory impairment in young and old alcoholics: Evidence for the premature aging hypothesis. Alcoholism: Clinical and Experimental Research 4: 288–293
Shallice T 1982 Specific impairments of planning. Philosophical Transactions of the Royal Society of London 298: 199–209
Shallice 1988 From neuropsychology to mental structure. Cambridge University Press, Cambridge
Shapiro M B 1951 Experimental studies of a perceptual anomaly. 1: Initial experiments. Journal of Mental Science 97: 90–100
Shapiro M B 1973 Intensive assessment of the single case: an inductive deductive approach. In: Mittler P (ed) The psychological assessment of mental and physical handicaps. Tavistock Publications, London, ch 21

Smith A 1962 Ambiguities in concepts and studies of 'brain damage' and 'organicity'. Journal of Nervous and Mental Disease 135: 311–326

Smith A 1975 Neuropsychological testing in neurological disorders. In: Friedlander W J (ed) Advances in neurology. Raven Press, New York, vol 7, pp 49–110

Snowden J S, Goulding P J, Neary D 1989 Semantic dementia: a form of circumscribed cerebral atrophy. Behavioral Neurology 2: 167–182

Talbot P R, Snowden J S, Lloyd J J, Neary D, Testa H J 1995 The contribution of single photon emission tomography to the clinical differentiation of degenerative cortical brain disorders. Journal of Neurology 242: 579–586

Walsh K W 1991 Understanding brain damage. A primer of neuropsychological evaluation, 2nd edn. Churchill Livingstone, Edinburgh

Walsh K W 1992 Some gnomes worth knowing. The Clinical Neuropsychologist 6: 119–133

Walsh K W 1995 A hypothesis-testing approach to assessment. In: Mapou R L, Spector J (eds) Neuropsychological assessment of cognitive function. Plenum, New York

Weintraub S, Mesulam M M 1993 Four neuropsychological profiles in dementia. In: Boller F, Spinnler H (eds) Handbook of neuropsychology, vol 8. Elsevier, Amsterdam

Weintraub S, Rubin N, Mesulam M-M 1990 Primary progressive aphasia: longitudinal course, neuropsychological profile and language features. Archives of Neurology 47: 1329–1335

Yates A 1954 The validity of some psychological tests of brain damage. Psychological Bulletin 51: 359–380

Yates A J 1966 Psychological deficit. Annual Review of Psychology 17: 111–144

11

Brain and behaviour: the broader context

A MAJOR ORIENTATION

The subtitle of the present work highlights the fact that it is restricted to a particular approach, namely improving the brain-behaviour model. Elsewhere the author has referred to this central orientation as 'the psycho-anatomical method' (Walsh 1992). This term stresses the need to amplify our knowledge of the way in which the details of anatomy relate to psychological processes such as perception, attention, memory and learning, speech, affect and the intellectual regulation of behaviour. This is seen as a major building block, not the whole of neuropsychology, but that aspect which could be most helpful to practitioners seeking an understanding of clinical cases.

The basic notion of this approach to brain-behaviour relationships, namely the functional system, was developed in the many works of Luria and was briefly outlined in Chapter 1. A preferred term might be the 'distributed anatomical system'. Such a term would emphasize that every complex psychological process has as its underpinning collections of nerve cells, both in the cerebral cortex and subcortex, linked together through fibre pathways which are usually of great complexity. Each of these anatomical systems has extensive connections with numerous other systems. Mesulam (1981) has expressed the major features clearly as follows:

> (1) components of a single complex function are represented within distinct but interconnected sites which collectively constitute an integrated network for that function;
> (2) individual cortical areas contain the neural substrate for components of several complex functions and may therefore belong to several partially overlapping networks;
> (3) lesions confined to a single cortical region are likely to result in multiple deficits;
> (4) severe and lasting impairments of an individual complex function usually involve the simultaneous involvement of several components in the relevant network; and
> (5) the same complex function may be impaired as a consequence of a

lesion in one of several cortical areas, each of which is a component of an integrated network for that function.

It should also be made explicit that the integrated working of distributed anatomical systems will be disrupted by lesions which interfere with the fibrous connections between neuronal collections (either cortical or subcortical) that form the 'functional' elements of the systems. Neurological lesions can interfere with systems in one of two ways. Firstly, changes may be wrought by breaking connections in the system, thus interfering with its integrated action. This was discussed in Chapter 1 and dramatic examples are provided in the 'split-brain' material in Chapter 8. There has been much less systematic study of the second form of interference whereby pathological tissue may exert an inimical influence on intact tissue to which it is still connected. Such influence can operate between one part of a system and another or between systems. In this latter case this so-called 'diaschisis' effect may operate at a distance, even from one hemisphere to another (see Ch. 8). The delineation of psycho-anatomical systems has been based on what an earlier writer referred to as 'biological factor analysis'. Naturally occurring lesions in different locations have diverse effects on various psychological functions enabling an increasing sophistication in the understanding of the range of neural structures that comprise the systems. Crucial in this exercise has been the study of so-called 'unique cases', especially where there was sound evidence that the lesion was delimited to a circumscribed area. Much of the early work depended on autopsy evidence with its limitations. The advent of imaging techniques has vastly improved this situation, allowing an appreciation of neural dysfunction concurrent with neuropsychological evaluation

Acceptance of this general notion is easy to convey to the beginning student who is already conversant with the concept of integrated circuits from electronics. It is a major step from the idea of cortical localization with its tacit assumption that psychological functions resided in different bits of cortex.

In the two decades since the publication of the first edition of this text there has been considerable evolution of the field of neuropsychology. While the classical association between disorders of psychological function and the anatomical divisions of the brain continues to be refined, there has also been a very active and rapid parallel development of the use of clinical material to further our understanding of cognitive processes in general. This development is termed cognitive neuropsychology. A further development has been the attempt to utilize the knowledge from clinical and cognitive neuropsychology to plan therapeutic and adjustment manoeuvres on a basis of these two main branches of neuropsychology.

At the same time the development of interaction with other professions concerned with behavioural change has not been as great. The relationship with neurology has increased steadily since the advent of neuropsychology and it is hoped that this will continue, especially with the emergence of the separate speciality of behavioural neurology. On the other hand, the relations with neuropsychiatry are in their infancy but should be fostered by the dialogue made possible by conjoint journals such as *Neuropsychiatry, Neuropsychology and Behavioral Neurology*, and *Neurocase.* A brief comment on each of these two disciplines is given later.

RELATED DISCIPLINES

Cognitive neuropsychology

Most students of clinical neuropsychology have their basic training in psychology, thus many of them will already be familiar with the orientation and some of the detail of experimental studies of cognition in brain impaired subjects. The following brief résumé will merely serve to outline some of the major features of cognitive neuropsychology for others.

The central notion of cognitive neuropsychology is nicely summarized in the title of one major textbook, *From Neuropsychology to Mental Structure* (Shallice 1988). The principal aim is an understanding of mental processes: 'In modern cognitive neuropsychology, data from pathology are used mainly for model-building purposes...' (Sartori 1988, p. 59). 'Cognitive neuropsychologists...tend to infer the functional characteristics of normal cognition from the exploration of the deficient and spared cognitive capabilities of brain-damaged patients, and they look for clinical evidence permitting to adjudicate between alternative models of normal cognitive mechanisms' (Denes et al 1988). 'The goal is to propose a set of statements about the processing components that define normal cognition and the neuroanatomical (and neurophysiological) substrates of these processes in the normal brain' (Caramazza 1984).

Much of the literature shows a preoccupation with the first part of this last statement with only secondary consideration being given to the latter part.

While some psychologists concerned with the study of cognition have reservations about using brain impairment data, most would agree with McShane et al (1992) that the 'natural fractionations' produced by lesions 'has allowed for detailed studies of complex systems in relative isolation. In such cases one obtains a privileged insight into the structure of the information processing system. Evidence from the study of neurological damage can shed light on what is being computed and how it is being computed' (p. 252).

An early example of studies in the field is that of McCarthy and Warrington (1987). As these authors point out, it is not necessary to have anatomical reference in using the fractionation method to understand a function, though such reference would contribute to the understanding of brain-behaviour relationships. The growth of cognitive neuropsychology can be gauged not only by the emergence of major texts (e.g. Ellis & Young 1988, McCarthy & Warrington 1990, Shallice 1988, Margolin 1992) and journals in recent years, but by texts on special topics within the field (e.g. Colthart et al 1987, Riddoch & Humphreys 1994).

One of the arguments for using pathological case material in theorizing about normal function centres around the emergence of qualitatively different data in the latter material. 'In fact, the investigation of neuropsychological disturbances forces one to ask questions that are often very different from those arising with respect to normal subjects or artificial systems. Neurological diseases are accidents of nature that are blind with respect to our epistemic perspectives. Investigating such impairments of cognition can, therefore, direct our attention to the relevance of phenomena that we might otherwise overlook' (Semenza et al 1988, p. 15).

Processing theory

The development of this division of neuropsychology has been promoted by experimental scientists, many of whom have had a background in experimental studies of cognition in normal subjects. The processing models which arose in psychology from the 1960s onwards have been particularly influential and form a recognizable common core for the speciality. However, despite their having a broad orientation in common, there is still much controversy over basic issues among the foremost workers in the field. One of the strongest arguments in favour of cognitive neuropsychology is that it produces 'data which could not easily be obtained from other sources' (McShane et al 1992).

Case study methodology

This refers to the use of single or 'unique' cases for inferring normal function. Even before the emergence of cognitive neuropsychology, the basic concepts and difficulties in making inferences from clinical material had been argued by earlier theorists such as Shapiro and his colleagues (Shapiro 1966, 1973, Shapiro et al 1973). The issue was discussed in the first volume of the *Journal of Clinical Neuropsychology* (Shallice 1979). While there was much resistance to the single case approach over the next decade, acceptance had become widespread: 'The critical point is that the results of single case studies have become as legitimate a type of evidence with which to support or criticise a theory as the results of group studies. Moreover, it is held in cognitive neuropsychology that the individual case study is much more likely to produce strong evidence for discriminating among theories of normal function' (Shallice 1988).

The understanding produced by cognitive neuropsychology should be applicable both to normal and disordered function. It should lead to the evolution of procedures to assist patients by designing methods by which individuals may compensate for deficits through utilizing obviously intact portions of functional systems or, where this is not possible, by designing methods which utilize other systems which may carry out a function, albeit in a less than efficient manner. In any case, the therapeutic attempt would be based on a model which could be tested objectively.

Group studies

The use of data from group studies of patient populations to draw inferences about normal function has been strongly criticized. The fact that the data may be difficult if not impossible to interpret or may be misleading has been put most strongly by Caramazza (1984, 1986). However, others such as Shallice (1988) and Zurif and colleagues (1989) would allot a secondary role to group studies for a number of reasons, not the least of which is that it may be difficult to generate sufficient data in single case form to explore particular functional systems.

While they always entail much time, effort and personnel, group studies have some positive features, e.g. they obviate the practice effects which necessarily arise from the repeated study of individual cases.

Dissociation and fractionation

These two terms are closely linked in cognitive neuropsychology. The basic concept of double dissociation has already been referred to in Chapter 1. While it is widely accepted in the field, its implicit or explicit definition varies and even its validity in allowing inferences to be drawn has been questioned by some (see Caramazza 1986). Shallice (1988) has greatly clarified the situation by delineating three subtypes of dissociation. He warns of the practice of taking complementary dissociations in two patients as the model, i.e. where one patient performs better on one task than on a second while the second patient performs better on the second task than on the first. He proposes a more stringent formulation: 'The valid formulation of the double dissociation...is that on task I, patient A performs significantly better than patient B, but on task II, the situation is reversed... This form of the classic double dissociation logic is therefore a satisfying means of falsifying a model where the two tasks are critically dependent on the same subsystem, even where the tasks differ in their degree of difficulty' (p. 235).

Normal psychology

Study of disordered function must interact with studies of function in normal subjects to produce a theory which will account for all observations. However, while cognitive neuropsychology may produce increased understanding of psychological functions in normal subjects, the reverse may not hold true. Kertesz (1983b) warned: 'The functional analysis of normal cognitive systems may not provide enough background to test the damaged or reorganized functions in patients. The behavior observed after the lesion may not be analysable in terms of normal function'.

Behavioural neurology

The editor of the new journal *Behavioural Neurology* commented in the first issue: 'Broadly, Behavioural Neurology includes the study of disorders of mood, personality, intelligence, perception and arousal and is concerned with the structural basis of normal and abnormal behaviour. In addition to the conventional foundation stones of the neurosciences: neuroanatomy, neurophysiology and neurochemistry, it is dependent on the practical skills of neuropsychology and social anthropology' (Lees 1988). In the same year the editor of another new journal, *Neuropsychiatry, Neuropsychology and Behavioral Neurology*, commented that neuropsychology was 'the basic science of behavioral neurology' being 'concerned with understanding the relationships between cognitive functions (e.g. memory, perception, thinking), behavior, and brain structure. It forms the bridge between neuropsychiatry and behavioral neurology' (Taylor 1988).

The common ground between neuropsychology and behavioural neurology is so great on a wide variety of topics that it is difficult in some areas to define the difference. Texts on behavioural neurology (e.g. Mesulam 1985, Kirshner 1986, Hier et al 1987) reinforce this view. Some major works in 'neuropsychology' have been edited and written by neurologists (see e.g. Kertesz 1983a). The major difference would appear to be preparatory training, specifically medical and neurological versus psychological. Each deploys methods of assessment, theoretical models and analysis deriving primarily from their background, supplemented by postgraduate and collaborative clinical experience.

Behavioural neurologists, like neuropsychologists, are also contributors in all disciplines where behaviour is perturbed, including neurological interfaces with psychiatry, speech pathology and rehabilitation, with additional therapeutic responsibilities. They are usually found in multidisciplinary clinics alongside neuropsychologists where there is great potential for mutually enhancing the richness of the diagnostic and management environment for both patients and staff.

Neuropsychiatry

The relationship between psychiatry and neurology has a long history. Some of the difficulties were spelled out in an article entitled 'The bridge between neurology and psychiatry' by Hill in 1964 and, in a volume bearing the same title, dedicated to him 25 years later (Reynolds & Trimble 1989), many of the issues remain unsolved. Collaborative research and clinical problem solving have only recently begun to gain momentum.

One of the major gulfs stems from the very different levels of discourse of psychiatrists and neuroscientists. Lishman (1992), a long-time proponent of organic (or biological) psychiatry, says that the psychiatrist 'deals with abnormalities of mood, qualities of thought disorder, false beliefs, and abnormal subjective experiences…' and '…tries to relate his clinical information to a knowledge of "mental diseases" but these are far from clearly defined'. This situation is far more difficult than that of neuropsychology where complex processes can be readily broken down into subcomponents, e.g. memory can be divided into short or long term and further qualified as material specific or modality specific and studied with regard to spontaneous recall or recognition. Many such notions can be given operational definitions which will assist in systematic experimental study. This fractionation can then be related to subdivisions of neurological systems. Such a model is difficult to apply in the more complex situation which holds in neuropsychiatry, though some progress has been made in recent years, particularly in the increasing interaction between psychiatry and neuropathology (Lishman 1995). To the excellent texts such as those of Lishman, now in its 20th year (Lishman 1987), and Cummings (1985) have been added the recent works of Yudovsky and Hales (1992, 1994), Cummings and Trimble (1995), Fogel et al (1994) and Joseph (1996). Growth in interest in the speciality is also reflected in texts on specific topics, e.g. on the neuropsychiatry of traumatic brain injury (Silver et al 1994).

Much of the advance can be traced to increased communication – both in shared journals and multidisciplinary conferences. Speaking of the effectiveness of such collaboration Hebb (1958) commented on: 'the stimulation to new ideas, the criticism and guidance when workers with different background and skills effectively understand each other's language and modes of thought' (p. 451). In the case of neuropsychiatry the practitioner needs to be conversant with several other languages and modes of thought since the speciality embraces information from numerous branches of neuroscience, e.g. electrophysiology, neuropharmacology, neuropathology, neuroradiology and neurochemistry. This communication is being fostered by the new *Journal of Neuropsychiatry and Clinical Neurosciences*. At the same time neuropsychology is providing a *lingua franca* for neurology and psychiatry, at least in those areas which Miller (1986) called psychiatric neuropsychology.

Misidentification disorders – a confluence of disciplines

This set of disorders from neuropsychiatry has been chosen both because it is a fine example of how a number of streams of brain-and-behaviour science converge over a particular problem, and also because the subject has received increasing interest in recent times.

Phenomenology

The term 'misidentification' is as old as psychiatry itself; the various named syndromes date back to the 1920s, but their amalgamation as a loosely related set of disorders has received consistent exploration only very recently. The modern term *delusional misidentification syndromes* attempts to link a set of disorders, all of which relate to distortions or changes in familiarity, usually of persons but sometimes of objects of significance to the patient. Brief descriptions of the more commonly described symptoms or behaviour changes will illustrate common features which allow them to be discussed under the collective term.

Reduplicative paramnesia

This term was coined by Pick (1903) to designate a particular form of disturbance, though it had been described in the literature as far back as 1788. The term paramnesia had been used to indicate a disturbance of memory in which reality and fantasy were confused. In the reduplicative form, the patient inappropriately relocates the present environment to another location, generally close to home. In simple terms, it is the replacement of something unfamiliar by something familiar. It is the misidentification most frequently associated with neuropathology (Forstl et al 1991a), often an acute infarction that involves the right frontal and parietal regions.

Capgras' syndrome

This was first noted by Capgras and Reboul-Lachaux in 1923, the condition they termed 'l'illusion des sosies'. The subject believes that a closely associated person has been replaced by an identical-appearing impostor or double. In the original case, that of a 53-year-old woman, the 'doubles' concerned members of her family, the police and her neighbours. Using simple terms again, this is the replacement of something familiar by something unfamiliar.

On occasions only one person may be misidentified, on others there may be what Todd (1957) called 'a delirium of doubles'. Repeated episodes of Capgras' phenomenon occur in some individuals, some with sudden onset and termination (e.g. Lipkin 1988). Recurrent cases encountered by the authors have shown persistent delusional denial even when confronted by videotape evidence of themselves confirming the identity of the subject of their current delusion.

At the outset, much of the early literature was in the French language, and it should be pointed out that there is no French word 'délusion' – the word employed for the English word delusion is 'illusion'. This is mentioned since English translations have appeared, even recently, rendering the French term as its English homonym and thus altering in a significant way the sense of the translated passage.

At first the phenomenon was thought to be confined to females, a point of significance for the preponderantly psychoanalytical theorizing of the period (e.g. Coleman 1933). Murray first described a male victim in 1936, and many more cases have been noted since, especially in the elderly. Murray's 26-year-old patient claimed that the man who visited him in hospital was not his father, but 'had no difficulty in recognizing other people, such as the doctors and nurses. *Indeed he has shown acute memory for faces*' (emphasis added). For a long time the condition was said to be 'typically seen in psychotic females who are saturated with suspicion, but have clear sensoria' (Todd 1957). This author described seven cases covering a rich variety of symptomatology both individually and collectively, and this spectrum has since been confirmed in many cases. The more recent case description by Crichton and Lewis (1990) provides an excellent example of how the term Capgras' syndrome has often been used to label a wide spectrum of delusion.

The age of the patients varies widely from young adults to the very elderly, including a 90-year-old woman who had no evidence of dementia though she did have the characteristic neuropsychological deficits outlined below (Burns 1985). The disorder is a particular burden for caregivers (Forstl et al 1994b).

One of the major difficulties in determining the aetiology of Capgras' syndrome and its congeners is that they appear in psychiatric disorders, particularly schizophrenia and depression, as well as in a wide variety of medical conditions. The cases with depression are said to be more superficial than those with schizophrenia (Christodoulou 1991) and clear with treatment. Some cases have localized cerebral disorders such as cortical infarction, temporal lobe epilepsy and neoplasms, while others have disorders with more widespread brain effects such as Alzheimer's disease, severe head injury and encephalitis of different forms. Oddities such as a case with pituitary tumour and another with AIDS have been published. Misidentification disorders have also been seen with medical conditions such as diabetes, hepatic encephalopathy, hypothyroidism and vitamin B12 deficiency. Treatment of both medical and psychiatric conditions often leads to remission of the Capgras symptoms (Enoch & Trethowan 1991). This treatment includes ECT in those cases associated with depression, though ECT actually precipitated Capgras' symptomatology on two occasions in a case of depression (Hay et al 1974, Hay 1986). Disappearance of the disorder may be reflected in resolution of some abnormalities such as is seen on serial CT scanning (e.g. Crichton & Lewis 1990).

To help clarify some of the complexity, Malloy et al (1992) have advised the use of the common distinction in psychiatry between 'primary' and 'secondary' types, the distinction resting on the presence or absence of an 'identifiable neurologic disorder'. The phenomenology does not appear to differ significantly between primary and secondary types. Having noted the unusual association of an organic and a behavioural disorder in what they felt was the first organic case (one of severe head injury), Weston and Whitlock (1971) considered that such cases might be of use in understanding the aetiology of delusional states. Owing to their singularity, the secondary cases might also be over-represented (Forstl et al 1991a).

Many primary cases are of paranoid schizophrenia with gradual onset before the age of 40 with good neuroleptic response. Malloy et al (1992) provide details of one case of each type. Their conclusion that there is a relative absence of violence in the secondary cases is not borne out by the evidence presented below. The psychiatric cases occur in clear consciousness, but those of organic origin may have mild confusion and show other features, particularly of the neurological condition. In a schizophrenic group (Silva & Leong 1992) the delusion was focused most often on the parents but covered a wide range of other individuals. In rare cases the focus is solely on inanimate objects (Abed & Fewtrell 1990); this individual, who evinced no neurological or neuropsychological deficits, was also thought not to be schizophrenic. Other cases have a range of misidentifications which include inanimate things (Anderson 1988). One depressive patient swore that someone had replaced her spectacles with an identical pair which she refused to wear (Rastogi 1990). A schizophrenic patient of Thomson et al (1980) believed that each time he came home from hospital he did so to one of a number of 'impostor cities', each having duplicates of his family members. Another patient suffering from drug intoxication felt his home town had been duplicated in Asia (Ball & Exworthy 1990), while a third believed that the entire city of Los Angeles had a double (Kiriakos & Ananth 1980).

The question of the relation of Capgras' phenomena to schizophrenia is a difficult one. A survey 20 years ago pointed out that the average age of schizophrenic patients with Capgras' symptoms was higher than those without (Merrin & Silberfarb 1976), but these authors commented about their own case that 'in the absence of the Capgras delusion one would be hard pressed to diagnose schizophrenia'. This led them to enquire whether Capgras' syndrome was 'one end of the schizophrenic spectrum, or a special diagnostic category with multiple etiological variables?'. Certainly follow-up studies are needed to trace the future behaviour of these older 'schizophrenic' subjects.

A review of 133 cases of Capgras' syndrome with an extensive bibliography is given by Berson (1983). Part of the theoretical discussion appears below.

Variants of Capgras' syndrome. A 'reverse' Capgras' syndrome was described by Signer (1987) in which the patient believed that his or her identity had been substituted or radically changed. The *Frégoli* delusion is the delusional belief that one or more familiar persons, usually persecutors following the patient, repeatedly change their appearance. They are all psychologically identical though physical appearances differ. The delusion was named by Courbon and Fail in 1927 in honour of a great Italian mimic of the French music halls, Frégoli, who had remarkable skill in changing his facial appearance. A review of 34 cases is given by Mojtabai (1994). *Intermetamorphosis* is a somewhat rarer variant of Capgras' syndrome described by Courbon and Tusques (1932). The patient believes that others have interchanged their appearance and psychological identity. These others are often described as tormentors. In a typical case reported by Bick (1984) a woman believed that her husband and son had changed themselves into other people, e.g. her husband changed himself into one of her neighbours. A strong co-occurrence of this and other misidentifications with the Capgras' disorder has long been noted (Atwal & Khan 1986, Signer 1987, Silva et al 1991).

Another variant, *subjective doubles delusion,* was first described by Christodoulou in 1978. This belief is that there exists a double who carries out independent actions. There may be confusion with what in the past has been termed the Doppelganger which is a complex hallucinatory experience of one's own body projected into external visual space and is seen in epilepsy, migraine and on direct brain stimulation. The projection may be in whole or in part, black and white or coloured, but the face is always included. It is generally recognized by the subject to be a pathological event. This clearly separates it from the delusions, where belief in the reality of the experience is very strongly held.

Delusional misidentification symptoms (DMS)

Although the term misidentification has been used in psychiatry for decades, it was only recently realized that not only are the above and various similar delusions frequently seen together in one subject, but they appear to share certain features and so are now most often grouped together in discussion to distinguish them as a class from other delusions. Quite early in the history of Capgras' disorder, Coleman (1933) had separated delusional from other forms of misidentification: 'Here perception of the object is unimpaired and memory is intact, but misidentification results because a judgment, based on a subjective evaluation rather than on objective findings, is made a priori'. A decade later, though Vié (1944) allied the Capgras', Frégoli and intermetamorphosis disorders with failure to perceive illness (anosognosia), there was no discussion in the English literature. Vié had earlier outlined a variation on Capgras' syndrome; he classed Capgras' syndrome as a delusion of negative doubles (since he felt that the perception of non-existent differences gave rise to a negation of identity) whereas, in the variant which he termed the delusion of positive doubles, an identity was proposed on the basis of 'imaginary resemblances' (Vié 1930). Frégoli's syndrome was thought of as an example of the latter.

Eleven different syndromes of misidentification were brought together by Joseph (1986a) and are listed in Cutting (1991). Unfortunately, the increasing use of this collective term has meant that specific details of particular cases are not always spelled out, with resulting shortcomings for researchers.

These delusional states are seldom seen in a pure form and all of the symptoms gathered under the rubric of DMS may each be accompanied by one (or more) of the others, and also by other disparate psychiatric and neuropsychological disorders, particularly disturbance of memory functions. However, certain observations warn of the danger of considering DMS as anything but a loose collective noun: e.g. (i) a particular DMS may persist while the other psychiatric symptoms improve; (ii) the DMS may disappear though the other psychiatric symptoms remain; and (iii) two or more DMS conditions may occur together but one may clear while the other does not. An entire issue of the journal *Psychopathology* (1994) has been given over to the topic of DMS while the *British Journal of Psychiatry* (Sims 1991) devoted a *Supplement* to 'Delusions and awareness of reality'.

Dangerousness and violent behaviour.

The extent to which conduct is affected by the presence of delusions is, however, very variable. In some cases patients under the influence of persecutory ideas will commit serious assaults upon their imagined enemies, and become a source of great danger to the community. In a very large number of cases, on the other hand, the delusion seems to have no direct effect upon the patient's behaviour. Often, indeed, belief and conduct are completely divorced from one another, or even grotesquely inconsistent. (Hart 1912)

The present decade has seen an awareness of the fact that patients with DMS often evince violent behaviour and so constitute a danger to the object of their delusions and occasionally to others around them. It is seldom mentioned that Courbon and Fail's original Frégoli patient was hospitalized for assaulting her employer whom she accused of being a famous actress of the period. The seriousness of the problem is shown in recent surveys. Forstl et al (1991a) noted reports of violent behaviour in 41 of 260 cases of DMS, while 50 out of 80 cases reviewed by Silva et al (1994b) had physically attacked others. The violence occurs in those cases with an obvious organic basis (Silva et al 1994b) as well as in 'psychiatric' cases. An hypothesis aimed at explaining this violence in misidentification states has been attempted by Silva et al (1993a, 1994a). However, de Pauw and Szulecka (1988) point out that a multitude of factors needs to be taken into account when considering whether a delusional patient may be violent.

While violence may occur in all delusional states, patients with misidentification delusions seem less likely to attack with weapons than others (Silva et al 1995).

Neuropathological associations

Although Capgras' syndrome may occur without obvious neuropathology and may have spontaneous remissions and recurrences over a long period, there is a sufficiently high proportion of organic cases to suggest a rigorous neurological examination if the symptoms are seen. Very early on, Vié (1930) had suggested that the Capgras syndrome could be an organic delusional state.

Furthermore, a diagnosis of schizophrenia does not preclude an organic basis for DMS which may even be similar to that seen in cases where there is an obvious connection between localized neuropathology and delusional symptomatology, though it may not be demonstrable by current techniques.

Lateralization and localization. The association of reduplication phenomena with the right hemisphere was remarked by very early articles, such as that of Weinstein et al (1952). Later studies have confirmed this; for example, Forstl et al (1991a) looked at 260 misidentification subjects – about half had schizophrenia but 46 had demonstrable organic causes. Those with reduplicative paramnesia were mainly suffering from the effects of head injury or cerebral infarction, and both CT and neuropsychological testing implicated the right hemisphere. The survey of Feinberg and Shapiro (1989) agrees with the strong right hemisphere association but also reports a small percentage of left hemisphere cases. The misidentification of place, as against face, seemed more often associated with an organic cause, especially in the right hemisphere. They further reviewed the cases with neurological involvement (69 cases of reduplication and 26 of Capgras' phenomenon). The strong right hemisphere preponderance was again reported and the pattern of results comparing left, right or bilateral involvement was about the same for the two conditions, with the trend to the right hemisphere. There was a high percentage of bilateral involvement for both types (62% for Capgras versus 41% for reduplication). The review of Ellis (1994) also strongly favours an association between Capgras' symptomatology and the right hemisphere.

The recent review of the greater majority of cases in the French and English literature (Signer 1994) permits an outline to be drawn of the findings to date on location of lesions:

1. Of 750 cases, 200 appeared to have an organic contributor; in 79 of the latter cases a major role could be assigned to one hemisphere.
2. Of these 79 cases, 13 had bilateral lesions, all but one of which were in the frontal and temporal regions.
3. 16 cases were classified as of 'unknown' lobar location but were assigned to one or other hemisphere – 11 to the left and 5 to the right.
4. Of the 63 cases with 'known location', almost 90% were frontal or temporal as compared to 11% of parietal or occipital lesions.
5. Finally, of the 50 cases with a single lobe siting, the most frequent locations were right frontal and left temporal.

These data, gathered from a variety of sources with differing degrees of care in case description, allow only broad conclusions but one of these seems to be the emphasis on anterior rather than posterior regions. This conclusion has significance for generating hypotheses about the aetiology of misidentification delusions. The data also confirm that this class of disorder must have a wide neuro-anatomical basis if it can be produced by lesions in separate discrete locations, for example the case of Kapur et al (1988) involved haemorrhage restricted to the right frontal lobe, while a Capgras' syndrome case of Ardila and Rosseli (1988) had a cysticercum in the left temporal lobe. Reduplicative paramnesia is more often considered neurological than neuropsychiatric.

Even in cases of DMS with widespread brain damage, a strongly focal feature may also be in evidence: DMS is sometimes seen in recovery from severe head injury, again implicating right hemisphere function and often with frontal lobe features (e.g. Benson et al 1976, Staton et al 1982, Forstl et al 1993). The frontal accentuation of the disturbance is seen with other conditions, even a case of migraine (Fuller et al 1993), while the case of Kapur et al (1988) involved haemorrhage restricted to the right frontal lobe.

In the investigation of two patients with extensive right hemisphere damage and a marked tendency for misidentification and false recognition, Rapcsak et al (1994) reported widespread difficulties with facial recognition tasks. Like other authors they point out that reliable facial identification depends on the processing of configural information which is the prime mode of the right hemisphere, while the left hemisphere processing of individual features is prone to errors. The case of Silva et al (1993b), with right frontal gunshot wound and subsequent violent misidentification, also showed severe impairment of facial recognition on the Benton Test. Faces are a fine example of Gestalten which confer uniqueness or identity. These workers also postulate a vital role for the frontal lobes in decision making as well as processing mode, resolving ambiguities which may arise during processing when the right frontal lobe may play a more important role. These two factors, viz. the right hemisphere and frontal lobe involvement, have been postulated by other writers.

Dementia and DMS. Misidentifications are common in established Alzheimer's disease. One prospective study of 128 Alzheimer patients revealed 40 with Capgras' symptoms; the common CT finding was enlargement of the right anterior horn of the lateral ventricle and larger left than right frontal lobes (Forstl et al 1991b). A later study by this group (Forstl et al 1994a) confirmed a rate of around 30%. Other studies confirm the high incidence of misidentification in Alzheimer's disease (Mendez et al 1992). In a series of 50 Alzheimer patients, Forstl et al (1993) found that those with paranoid delusions and hallucinations deteriorated faster than those with delusional misidentification.

Capgras' and related symptoms are also recognized as a precursor of dementia. Lipkin (1988) reported the case of a 71-year-old woman who developed a misidentification delusion about her second husband, the misidentification coming in episodes lasting several days with subsequent remission. Early CT scan was normal but slow waves were seen bilaterally in the EEG. Nine months later she was admitted to hospital with clear signs of dementia and CT then showed mild general atrophy with slight ventricular dilatation. An elderly man with no signs of dementia on extensive neuropsychological testing at the onset of Capgras' syndrome later progressed to dementia (Diesfeldt & Troost 1995).

In Alzheimer's disease, EEG has shown an increase in delta waves over the right hemisphere and CT scans demonstrate greater atrophy in the right frontal than in other areas (Forstl et al 1994a).

Neuropsychological evaluation

Numerous factors, including clinical rarity and the difficulties involved in the examination of deluded patients, mean that published neuropsychological test findings are much rarer than case reports; even when they do appear, they may be restricted merely to brief statements of a few abnormal findings.

Face processing impairments. Attention has been focused on visual perceptual tasks with an accent on configural processing. The data come from incidental observations on neuropsychological examination, from specific testing of DMS subjects and from experimental comparisons between groups. An example of the first category is the patient of Crichton and Lewis (1990) who showed 'a specific visuospatial deficit for recall of patterns not available for verbal encoding…'. More specifically, Young and colleagues and others have tested DMS subjects on various face processing tasks: the results ranged from borderline performance to clear-cut deficits (Young et al 1990, 1993, Wright et al 1993). A typical example is that of Young et al (1993) where two DMS cases both had difficulty on: (i) the ability to identify familiar faces; (ii) the ability to determine facial expression; and (iii) matching unfamiliar faces. Neither had difficulty with word recognition tasks. Though they scored poorly on facial recognition, they both rejected 20 out of 20 of the unfamiliar faces in the sets. Other studies report similar failures by delusional patients on tasks such as the Benton Facial Recogniton Test and the facial component of the Warrington Recognition Memory Test (Warrington 1984). Another case of Silva et al (1992) with multiple delusions concerning his self but with a negative CT scan gave a borderline performance on the Benton Facial Recognition Test but only reached the 6th percentile on the Faces subtest of the Warrington Recognition Memory Test

(Warrington 1984). Another patient with the Frégoli delusion, though also performing well on the Benton Visual Retention Test and the Mini Mental State, reached only the 7th percentile on the Warrington task (de Pauw et al 1987).

Taking a broad series of 18 neurologically based cases from the recent literature, Malloy et al (1992) commented: 'Patients tended to display executive/self-regulatory, visuospatial, and memory deficits (usually nonverbal worse than verbal), or generalized abnormalities (in cases with diffuse diseases such as degenerative dementia). The focal findings were consistent with CT and EEG results in indicating right frontotemporal localization'. Ten psychiatric cases of Tzavaras et al (1986) also appeared to use a so-called left hemisphere (analytical) mode of visual processing as well as showing signs suggestive of frontal lobe impairment.

Negative neuropsychological test findings have also been reported with Capgras' phenomena (e.g. Merrin & Silberfarb 1976, Dally & Gomez 1979, Abed & Fewtrell 1990). Few if any have produced data relative to the 'right hemisphere hypothesis' of recent times (see below), though the absence of such changes can be inferred from the use of certain named tests.

Models and theories

The symptomatology of these misidentification disorders is so distinctive and clinically indistinguishable between so-called primary and secondary types that for many it suggests a common neuropathological basis. While this may not be at the macroscopic level, in all cases the disturbance of a shared underlying physiological mechanism must be considered. Furthermore, the sudden onset and clearing of symptoms, and even complete remission in some cases also suggest that all cases cannot be caused by lasting structural damage.

To date there have been two types of hypotheses – the psychodynamic and the organic – and, at the outset, one can say that neither alone seems capable of explaining the wealth of behaviour manifestations. Even where misidentification appears in the setting of a proven organic condition such as Alzheimer's disease, the fact that the symptoms may be modified by the patient's mood state underlines the interplay between psychological and organic factors (Molchan et al 1990). This interactive view is shared by others (e.g. Mendez et al 1992).

Psychodynamic theories. These are beyond the scope of the present work but readers should peruse at least a sample of views (Berson 1983, Enoch & Trethowan 1991). Many would agree with Berson's view that 'the organic factors in themselves, however, seem neither necessary nor sufficient to explain the particular and peculiar content of the delusion', and a distinction should be made between misrecognition and delusional denial which are not synonymous terms.

Organic approaches. A number of neuropsychological features have been emphasized. Mendez (1992) in looking at 7 cases of dementia with misidentification noted that all had as a prominent feature a loss of the sense of familiarity. Silva and Leong (1992) remind us that brain stimulation in the temporal lobe areas has given rise to illusions of familiarity or of unfamiliarity suggesting that damage to these areas may provide a basis in some cases for delusional misidentification phenomena.

Person misidentification may rest in large part on a mismatch of new perceptions with past memories, a concept which lends itself to neuropsychological testing. These authors point to three possibilities but acknowledge that there are probably other factors in sustaining the state: (i) disturbed present perception may not match recorded knowledge; (ii) damage in the temporal areas, a frequent occurrence, may not permit normal perceptions to be linked with past memories; (iii) 'defective new memory formation may result in a failure of perceptions of a person to correspond to established memories of how the person should appear' (Ardila & Rosseli 1988).

A similar position has been taken by others: 'Thus, by reason of a functional disconnection between the central visual system and the temporolimbic lobe, a correct perception fails to evoke the normal affective memories tied to it' (Lewis 1987).

One might also speculate on the relation between disturbance of emotional behaviour dependent on the integrity of the limbic system and some aspects of delusional behaviour. This type of explanation is supported by Young and colleagues (1993) who feel that the basis of the Capgras' delusion may lie 'in damage to neuro-anatomical pathways responsible for appropriate emotional reactions to familiar visual stimuli'. This disruption could of course lie in different parts of the limbic system in different cases. The central notion of familiarity, i.e. recognizing personally relevant phenomena, emotional associations and other related issues which impinge on the relationships within the brain, in particular the right hemisphere, are ably discussed by Van Lancker (1991). To understand misidentification phenomena one needs to tackle the work cited in such articles.

The emphasis to date in neuropsychology has been solely on cognition, and then only on standardized tests. There is a good deal more to psychology than this.

Prosopagnosia. This term is frequently encountered in discussions of misidentification since the term also has to do with facial recognition. The term itself is a misnomer since there is no lack of knowing. A patient can recognize that a face is a face but not to whom the face belongs though the person may be well known. The phenomenon is seen with other categories such as animals and classes of inanimate objects (see Ch. 7). It is always associated with large posterior lesions, most frequently vascular. Although some writers have tried to link DMS in theoretical models with prosopagnosia, many patients have been specifically tested and found to be free of it.

Cognitive neuropsychology. In this branch of neuropsychology the data about the spared and deficient cognitive performances of subjects with neuropathology are utilized to formulate models or theories about how cognitive processes are carried out in normal subjects. Essentially they are information processing models that are capable of constant revision in the light of emerging findings. Processing can be interrupted at any point in the information chain. Thus lesions in different locations produce variations in the disruption of the process under examination with the production of outwardly different effects or syndromes. In 1987, Kosslyn suggested the construction of a model which could be subjected to lesions: 'the effects of disrupting the model in selected ways will constitute precise predictions of behavioral deficits following brain damage. It would also be interesting to do the obverse, to start with a known deficit and see what sorts of lesions are necessary to make the simulation mimic the deficit...'. A decade later we can see that this would now be recognized as a form of 'reverse engineering' which has grown exponentially in the past decade in computer science. Such an approach could lead to the construction of constantly modifiable models of the type required by cognitive neuropsychology.

In considering DMS, an obvious major component is face recognition. At the outset a distinction should be made between face recognition deficits per se and delusional misidentification. While facial perception may form part of the disruption suffered by Capgras' patients it is only part of a complex delusional state, and it is possible to have gross facial misrecognition without accompanying delusion. Nevertheless, models accounting for facial recognition and its disruption can be helpful in understanding conditions of which it forms a part.

A fine example is offered by Ellis and Young (1990) based on the information processing model outlined earlier by Bruce and Young (1986). Their approach incorporates notions, such as that of Bauer (1984), that there are different anatomical pathways for conscious versus unconscious facial recognition. They not only put forward a model for various forms of misperception termed 'delusional misidentification', but provide a bibliography presenting a wide range of studies on normal and pathological face recognition which gives a clear appreciation of the complexity of this area (see Hay & Young 1982, Young & Ellis 1989, Young 1992).

Experimental study of DMS patients has begun in an endeavour to clarify the issues. Ellis et al (1993) employed two face processing tasks, flashing stimuli to either half visual field. When three 'non-organic' Capgras' patients were compared with matched psychiatric controls a difference was found only with the right hemisphere component. These three patients and another were later compared with psychotic controls and with the test data of the unfamiliar faces component of the Warrington Recognition Memory Test, and were found to be significantly poorer. Details and discussion of related issues are given by Ellis (1994).

ROLES FOR CLINICAL NEUROPSYCHOLOGY

As in other clinical endeavours, the two principal roles are evaluation and therapy. The first of these, outlined in Chapter 10, is relatively well developed, the second is just beginning.

Neuropsychological evaluation: an overview

The major features of evaluation relate to diagnosis and measurement of function. At the outset it should be remembered that the clinical neuropsychologist is seldom in the position of being asked to provide a definitive diagnosis. It will be argued, however, that if neuropsychologists accept the role of applied scientist rather than technician they will be in the position of offering what at times is crucial information with regard to diagnosis. The neuropsychological examination is an integral part of the neurological examination and must be seen in this context. It would be valuable if sensitive behavioural measures could be refined so as to promote the earlier diagnosis of some cerebral lesions.

There is encouraging evidence that behavioural measures may be able to detect impairment which is too subtle to be detected by many current neurological procedures, e.g. CT scan, that depend on the detection of structural alterations in the brain.

The second role lies in the assessment of cases where the diagnosis has already been verified. A systematic and comprehensive documentation of the patient's mental functions is of value in following the progress of patients suffering from cranio-cerebral trauma, cerebrovascular disorders and the numerous other neurological conditions in which mental symptoms form a prominent part. This role should not be thought of simply as a mechanical documentation but rather the examinations should be seen as providing *understanding* of the ways in which the neurological condition has affected the individual patient. This understanding forms the basis for advice on medical management and rehabilitation and for counselling the patient and relatives about the effects of the disorder. It also forms a useful basis for opinions on medico-legal matters arising from brain impairment (see below and Walsh 1991).

Other roles for assessment include the education of other professionals about the ways in which neuropsychology has developed and the ways in which it can provide useful information for patient management. This can be conveyed in well-argued written or verbal reports which should provide a reasoned argument that does not go beyond the data available. This is a well-tried method of increasing the sophistication of referral questions which, in the ideal situation, will provide the hypotheses for testing.

Neuropsychological assessment also provides an important method of evaluating various forms of medical, surgical and psychological treatment including rehabilitation.

Therapeutic intervention

The topic of treatment and rehabilitation is beyond the scope of this text but a warning note might be sounded.

The past 20 years have seen an increasing emphasis on rehabilitation and the establishment of many treatment centres. This has given rise in some instances to confident claims of the effectiveness of various procedures. However, very few well-designed outcome studies have been published. A parallel may be drawn with the long-standing division of opinion over other treatments such as psychotherapy. In 1990 Whitby pointed out that psychotherapeutic methods have remained as popular as ever with their practitioners despite the fact that, even when subjective criteria are used, only a moderate success is claimed; when objective criteria are employed, success is not even moderate. He proposed a model to account for the continuing unwarranted self-confidence: 'I propose to term the effect produced by regular, non-contingent reinforcement "assumed usefulness". In humans it produces a state of high self-esteem, directed and persistent activity, good humour and a conviction of certainty. Above all the subject assumes that what he or she is doing is really useful'. A further characteristic is to produce a 'frame of mind in which change and progress become difficult' leading to a breakdown of communication with those of opposite views.

The history of medicine is strewn with confidently upheld opinions, based on clinical appraisal, of supposedly efficacious therapeutic procedures which were eventually abandoned as ineffectual.

The evolution of a number of specialized journals such as *Cognitive Rehabilitation* may help to prevent or lessen a similar state of affairs by encouraging objectively based appraisal in this area.

Forensic neuropsychology

In recent years neuropsychologists have been called on for advice in a range of medico-legal issues. One major issue has been the residual compromise of function after moderate to severe head injury.

The neuropsychologist as expert witness

At the outset, many of the difficulties encountered by expert witnesses appear to arise from the nature of the legal process itself. In the adversarial system arguments are made eristically, i.e. more with regard to winning the argument than with establishing the truth (Trimble 1981). Neuropsychologists should familiarize themselves with the system, though they will find that it differs from their own scientific methodology.

Legal versus scientific argument. A fundamental difference between legal and psychological thinking is the mode of operation. 'Psychologists tend to describe "facts" in terms of probability estimates and confidence limits while lawyers tend to favour absolutes: true and false, yes and no' (Cooke 1990, p. 218).

Trimble (1981) has outlined other main differences between scientific and legal thinking '…the rules of science are not the rules of the courtroom… The law in taking as its starting point tradition and precedent is, of course, in direct opposition to the scientific mode of thinking, since both are highly anti-scientific… Lawyers tend to employ deductive logic, whereas doctors use inductive methods…' (pp 173–174).

Following years of research on the position of expert witnesses in English courts, Goodwin Jones (1986) commented: 'The expert witness occupies an ambivalent position at the interface between the two disciplines', i.e. 'law as a body of practice and science as a body of knowledge'. Neuropsychologists need to learn to present their evidence in ways which will minimize these differences. The ethics of expert witnessing are discussed by Sales and Shuman (1993).

The adversarial system has its critics within and outside the legal profession, particularly with regard to its most basic tenet. 'The sporting contest, which is inherent in the adversary system, seems fundamentally inappropriate to expert evidence; as the Secretary of the British Medical Association (see Havard 1983) has said 'It would be difficult to devise a system less likely to arrive at the scientific truth'. (Mason 1984). Further discussion of the system is provided by Sperlich (1985). Elsewhere, Mason (1986) has discussed modifications which might be made to the existing system. These include pre-trial consultation between experts.

Some of the difficulties posed by the adversarial system might be overcome and agreement reached more readily if courts were to set more stringent standards when it comes to qualifying the definition of an expert (see Kassin & Wrightsman 1988).

Expert evidence versus expert opinion. Expert *evidence* refers to a body of specialized knowledge related to the practice of some profession. Expert *opinion* relates to the conclusions drawn from the expert evidence.

While there may be agreement between experts about the evidence, the nature of the adversarial process means that there are almost always differences of opinion. While some of the differences are 'legitimate', very often the differences arise because of varying degrees of expertise of two or more witnesses on the particular matters under consideration. While two witnesses may appear equally expert from their qualifications, membership of learned societies and so forth, it is often the case that one individual (even one with slightly less impressive status markers in the profession) may have much greater depth of experience on the particular issues under scrutiny, in other words, possess more expertise on certain questions. It is up to counsel to bring out such features to help the court adjudge the weight to be given to individual testimony.

Inherent dangers and biases. It is clear that most lawyers in the adversarial system see the expert witness not as someone to instruct the judge or jury, but consider that the witness 'is hired to help the lawyer present "the best possible case" and as such is a tool of advocacy' (Goodwin Jones 1986), or 'made to feel a member of a team, whose object is to win' (Mason 1986). The 'reality is that experts are almost never appointed by the court, but hired by one of the parties' (Kassin & Wrightsman 1988, p. 96).

In many instances expert witnesses may be expected to assist counsel in preparation of questions for cross-examination of other experts. This instantly raises the question of 'being paid to be partisan' (Goodwin Jones 1986). If one eschews this role one is likely to be considered a less than desirable witness to be called on subsequent occasions.

In many cases of litigation over personal injury the fact that a witness has been called, and will be paid, by one side or the other already raises the possibility of preliminary bias especially where lawyers may have 'shopped around', turning down several individuals before finding one who suits their purpose. It is not without significance that those who engage in medico-legal work frequently find the same experts appearing regularly for one side, e.g. the plaintiff, and never for the other side. This immediately raises the question of bias.

Ideally, experts should express not only their opinions but also the confidence with which they hold such opinions, giving argument in favour of this degree of confidence *if called on to do so*. An eminent legal authority is quoted by Freckelton (1987): 'The one essential of all expert evidence is a frank statement by the expert of the limits of accuracy within which he is speaking, and a readiness to indicate whether asked or not, what his evidence does *not* prove or suggest as likely' (Ormrod 1972, p. 16).

Witnesses should also be aware that their opinions are often only part of the evidence on which decisions will be made, although on occasions these opinions will be the crucial evidence. Many experts, particularly in clinical matters, will already be familiar with this notion through their discussions with other experts in non-legal cases.

Biased sampling. A common complaint by experts is that they are not permitted to give a balanced account of matters since certain facts which they consider to be important and relevant are not brought out by counsel in examination. 'Not infrequently the experts are in possession of information and views that could be critical to the determination of issues by the court but which never comes before it *because of the adversary procedure*' (Freckelton 1987, p. 133, emphasis added). This means that the adversary system is directly preventing the expert from giving an unbiased presentation of the facts and favours a particular point of view. It is not surprising that, having experienced this form of constraint, many scientists are unwilling to take part in further cases.

The expert should always make clear, at least in all written submissions of expert opinion, both the factual evidence and the relative weighting to be given to the parts, separately and in combination.

When faced with biased sampling by either counsel, expert witnesses should be careful not to become personally involved and thus take up more extreme opinions than they would otherwise have done. The real expert will be able to accept possible, reasonable alternatives while still firmly maintaining the main thrust of his or her argument or opinion.

Expertise in neuropsychology

Clinical psychology, psychiatry and neuropsychology. In the recent past both clinical psychologists and psychiatrists have given expert testimony in cases of 'brain damage' and in some places continue to do so. While there has been a good deal of overlap in the medico-legal roles of the psychologist and psychiatrist, even to the extent of psychiatrists on occasion presenting the findings of the clinical psychologist as part of the basis of their own opinions, the development of clinical neuropsychology has clearly altered the situation with regard to opinion about the effects of brain impairment in civil suits. Speaking of his Australian experience, Freckelton (1989) wrote:

> The second matter concerns the interaction between *psychiatrist and psychologist*. Whilst it is probably possible for the evidence of a psychologist and a psychiatrist as to a particular subject (whether plaintiff or accused) to complement each other in a meaningful way, in practice it seems to me that this is not often done in the civil jurisdiction. Perhaps this is because of the advent of well qualified and experienced neuro-psychologists whose evidence is of particular assistance in cases involving brain damaged plaintiffs. In such cases, issues such as the capacity of the plaintiff to undertake employment or to marry and live an independent existence are the subject of neuro-psychological evidence, whilst for diagnosis and prognosis the neurologist is called. In most of such cases in my experience lawyers see little place for the psychiatrist witness. (Freckelton 1989)

Not only have clinical neuropsychologists been replacing psychiatrists in some areas, but they have also been replacing clinical psychologists who, before the advent of neuropsychology, were the experts to whom courts looked for an appraisal of the client's behavioural changes, particularly in the area of cognitive loss. Many of these clinical psychologists had developed considerable skills in the understanding of neuropsychological problems.

On the fundamental matter of expertise, Faust and Ziskin (1988) have claimed that studies of the activities of clinicians in psychology and psychiatry demonstrate that the validity and reliability of their judgments do not surpass those of the lay person. In other words they are not fit to be expert witnesses. Such an extreme position is contested by Fowler and Matarazzo (1988) who suggest that not all the evidence on classification is negative. Certainly Faust and Ziskin are correct in saying that there is substantial doubt about the reliability of diagnostic categorization in these clinical disciplines, but one should not proceed to generalize about other fields such as clinical neuropsychology, particularly that mode of operating utilized by the present authors and others which is essentially comparable to the 'medical model' long accepted by courts everywhere.

Clinical activity is about much more than diagnosis although a good deal may flow from the acceptance of a diagnostic label. Fowler and Matarazzo (1988) correctly note that courts are likely to be interested more in the expert's contribution to their 'understanding of an individual's behavior and ability to function in specific situations than on what specific diagnosis is assigned to that individual' (p. 1143).

Most of the weaknesses noted by Ziskin and Faust (1988) are related to the purely psychometric approaches which are so commonly used, particularly in the United States. They admit, for example, that the method of flexible batteries as espoused by Edith Kaplan of Boston might work well with that eminent neuropsychologist, though not with others less well trained. Just like physicians, clinical neuropsychologists must be able to demonstrate that they have received specialist training. The main point to be stressed about methods such as that of Kaplan and our own is that the psychometric data when used is only part of the total information upon which 'diagnosis' and predictive statements are made (Walsh 1995).

What is a neuropsychologist? Some lawyers are still not sufficiently conversant with specialization within psychology and may ask psychologists to testify as experts in areas such as neuropsychology where they have little or no training and experience (Haward 1981, Loftus 1983, Greene et al 1985). Psychologists should make it clear to lawyers in which areas they claim expertise. This avoids subsequent downgrading of their evidence when they are cross-examined in court on their standing.

Courts usually pay more heed to those whose credentials seem the most impressive. However, 'mere possession of generic professional credentials should not be used as justification of necessary and sufficient skill to perform in a forensic role' (Haas 1993). This means that experts with less impressive status need to be careful in their examinations of clients and as cogent as possible in their arguments, both in written and oral reports.

Opposing counsel may attempt to play down an expert's credibility by pointing to weaknesses in usually accepted criteria such as university degrees even when an overall appraisal, including lengthy experience with the particular type of problem under consideration and acceptance by other experts in the field (such as the expert's colleagues at large), provides overwhelming evidence of expertise. Occasionally such attacks backfire and make those hearing them more impressed than they were before such cross-examination.

The acceptance by courts of evidence from neuropsychologists about the relationship between injury and subsequent behavioural change has varied from complete acceptance to complete rejection, but appears to have become more generally positive in recent years. Some courts have based their rejection on the neuropsychologist's lack of medical training (Kolpan 1986). Part of the difficulty arose from the all-too-common use of the term 'brain damage' which, to most lay persons, means physical disruption of the brain substance. Some psychologists (and even some neuropsychologists) may have had very little training in medical topics such as neuroanatomy or neuropathology which would permit comment on 'brain damage', while others will have had quite extensive formal training. However, the essential expertise for the psychologist to demonstrate is that related to brain *impairment*, i.e. to explain to the court the extent to which the person wishing to be accepted as an expert is knowledgeable through training and experience in the evaluation of disorders of *function* which are known to result from brain pathology, whether from trauma, stroke, tumour, toxic substances or other causes. The psychologist is an expert in the study of behaviour. The neuropsychologist is an expert in the study of deranged functions as the result of neurological disturbances and if the claimant cannot substantiate this then he or she should not be accepted as an expert in clinical neuropsychology, no matter how well qualified and experienced in other fields of psychology. Also, a neuropsychologist with excellent academic qualifications who has published numerous research papers may have very little experience of the specific matters under debate in court, which are the province of those with extensive *clinical* experience even though the latter may be less qualified academically. The distinction between cognitive and clinical neuropsychology has become clearer as neuropsychology has developed.

Criteria for expertise in clinical neuropsychology vary a good deal from country to country. The nature of training programmes differs from place to place even in one country, and there are still many places where no formal training exists. Some of the requirements include: (i) understanding of neurologically based disorders of neuropsychological function and their distinction from non-neurological disorders – this implies training and experience with both types of cases; (ii) the effects of other medical disorders on the functioning of the brain; (iii) evaluation methods capable of being employed in appropriate cases; and (iv) assistance with rehabilitation planning on the basis of assessments.

This expertise should be integrated with a range of knowledge of the broader determinants of behaviour, test construction, measurement and application as commonly used in clinical psychology with necessary allowance for the effects of the neuropsychological disorder. For a fuller description see Meier (1987).

Keeping out of court

The pre-trial report. In a survey conducted by *The British Psychological Society* (Gudjonsson 1985) some psychologists reported having to present evidence in court on most occasions where they had submitted reports, while others had been required for court appearance for only one in a hundred reports. Some of the difference may arise from the effectiveness or otherwise of the written report. 'In reality, justice and the promotion of human welfare are probably better served when the expert's work results in a conclusion before the trial commences' (Blau 1984, p. 212).

The essence of the neuropsychologist's contribution is a well-ordered report which presents a cogent argument based on a careful examination and consideration of the history and the results of the examination and those of others. Blau (1984) recommends careful copy reading since (usually) 'the written report is the document from which the psychologist will render expert testimony at deposition or at court' (p. 168). There are numerous instances where little or no care has been given to the actual writing of the report, leaving the writer open to a harrowing cross-examination.

The report should point out not only the writer's findings and opinions but also what the expert is ready to accept in the findings and opinions presented by others, as well as a balanced consideration of apparent differences, lack of factual evidence for statements made and other major arguments which may assist in resolving differences. The neuropsychologist should note features in the documents such as deficiencies in the history, e.g. lack of information for a particular period, or conflicting statements. For example, in one of our cases, there was a major difference of opinion between a neuropsychologist and other psychologists about the degree of impairment of a man who received multiple injuries when he was struck by a motor vehicle while riding his bicycle. One psychologist, finding poor performances on a number of cognitive tests, particularly tests of memory several years after the accident, readily equated these poor performances with the severity of the injury, making use of the long period of post-traumatic amnesia (some weeks) described by the patient's wife. However, when the neuropsychologist obtained information from the hospital records several features came to light. Firstly, the patient had only a brief period of retrograde amnesia, describing an event minutes before being struck. There was little delay in getting him to hospital where he was described as being conscious and alert, speaking and complaining of pain from his limb fractures, and neurological examination was described as normal. He continued to complain of his pain for several hours until he was taken to the operating theatre for orthopaedic surgery. On another occasion the wife described him as having been unconscious for two days or more.

In this case great reliance was placed on the wife's statements since the patient was for years morose and uncommunicative. Again, the records show that she gave different statements to different individuals about her husband's cognitive disabilities. On occasions she was adamant that he had a pervasive and lasting memory defect, yet she told other examiners that her husband's memory varied depending on the day, that sometimes he would remember past events while on others he would forget easily. At times she would discuss things with him for a considerable time but he would forget within minutes, even if the matter was of some importance. On closer questioning later, she admitted that that did not always occur. She said he was unable to use public transport as he could not remember which bus to catch and at which bus stop to wait for the bus. Other inconsistencies were apparent in her declarations.

The neuropsychologist considered that her version of the man's memory disorder did not tally with the commonly seen disorder based on cerebral damage, pointing out that if the amnesic disorder were based in neural incapacity it would not fluctuate so markedly. Neither had the deficit altered with time, as documented in the extensive literature even with the most severe deficits, and examination revealed a good deal of defensiveness and 'role enactment' if not frank malingering.

Lastly, in anticipation of possible court appearance, it is well to attempt to foresee other possible interpretations of the data that are likely to be made by others and to present arguments as to why such explanations are less tenable than the opinion proposed by the present expert. In the case of injury litigation *post hoc ergo propter hoc* arguments are frequently made, and so the expert should be careful to enquire into all other possible causes such as previous injuries.

Nature of the examination

Comments on neuropsychological examination for legal purposes will be made in terms of general principles with some illustrations. Further information about the authors' methodology can be found in Walsh (1991, 1995).

The essential philosophy is centred on the concept of a syndrome or meaningful pattern of disorder. Such a notion is quite familiar in legal argument. Counsel may attempt to counter this and increase doubt in the minds of the hearers by examining test results one at a time. While it is of overwhelming value to be able to present something totally unambiguous, for example what is termed in medicine a *pathognomonic sign*, there is still strength in the notion of the collective meaning of examination data and subjective complaints together with a likely relationship to prior events based on knowledge of the literature and personal experience with similar cases.

What is a neuropsychological test? Lawyers and doctors are often uncertain about what is meant by the term 'neuropsychological test'. Is it different from other behavioural tests and, if so, in what ways? Reports from psychologists often appear to place 'neuropsychological tests' in a different category from other tests of cognition, e.g. part of a case report in Blau (1984) states that the person '…was given a series of tests of intellectual capacity, neuropsychological functioning, reading ability, skills, aptitudes, rehabilitation potential and personality' (p. 234).

In a very real sense there is *no such thing as a neuropsychological test*. All tests which involve an investigation of mental functioning can be used to gain information about the presence or otherwise of impairment of neuropsychological function. In fact, careful observation of the qualitative features and pattern of performance as well as the psychometric data derived from the Wechsler Scales alone are often quite capable of providing most of the necessary information regarding functional integrity or otherwise, since most cognitive functions are tapped in the process. It is better to specify which tests were used in the examination, for what purposes they were employed, and what conclusions are to be drawn from them singly and collectively.

Weaknesses in the examination. One of the major faults of systems which rely on fixed collections of tests is that they may not be totally relevant to the answers required by legal counsel. On the one hand, the examination may deal with matters unlikely to be of concern while, on the other, central aspects of functional capacity may be insufficiently addressed.

Part of the difficulty may arise from not placing the examination in the appropriate context. This context has several main elements, the most important being the history of events at the time of the injury and at different stages since then, the medical findings over time and the nature of the client's subjective complaints, and how, if at all, these also have changed with time. All of this must be placed against a knowledge or estimate of the individual's characteristics and known abilities before the event. Any final conclusions must be shown to be consonant with these.

Of the above factors the history of events is paramount. This may be deficient for many reasons but should be sought with assiduity '…extra time spent on the history is likely to be more profitable than extra time spent on the examination' (Hampton et al 1975, p. 489). If there are deficiencies it should be made clear that statements are made against the stated background.

With regard to the client's subjective complaints, it is usually necessary to take a separate history from the person and relatives or other close observers since the usual medical histories, though often detailed, may not address directly matters which would help to clarify the neuropsychologist's understanding of the nature of any dysfunctions, their basis in cerebral impairment or on a psychological basis or, as is so often the case, an admixture of the two. Determining this aspect of the history may be difficult in some cases depending on how the person and his or her legal advisers see the role of the individual examiner; subjects are often advised not to be too forthcoming. The reticence of some subjects may be helpful in itself.

The extent of the examination will vary from case to case, but it should be thorough enough to provide ample evidence to exemplify to counsel, and thus to the judge or judge and jury, that the expert has sufficient appropriate evidence on which to base a sound opinion: 'The ratio of fact to opinion should be high' (Cooke 1990, p. 219). This means that the medico-legal examination will often be rather more lengthy than in the common situation where a colleague refers a patient or client in the normal course of clinical consultation. In the latter case the referring agencies are already aware of the degree of expertise of their colleague and the confidence with which they can treat the proffered opinion; they will also normally have incorporated much background material from other sources, including their own examinations, which will serve as a frame of reference in interpreting the implications from the neuropsychological examination. When experts are informed that the case will feature in a legal action after they have already examined the individual they should request the opportunity to re-examine the client before the hearing. This is all the more important if some time has transpired and the client's condition may have altered, as is often the case with claims for the results of head trauma.

One fault of those who are less than expert is to believe that a very lengthy examination is necessarily better than a shorter one. One case in Blau (1984) had an examination of 14 hours (5.5 hours by an expert and 8.5 hours added examination by a technician!). One wonders just how expert the individual is who requires such a lengthy examination.

The presentation of argument from test data should be in a logical sequence, not necessarily in the order in which the tests were given. Thus the method of checking the reasons for failure on a particular test or test items by applying secondary tests might be placed with the primary findings even if it was carried out later, even at a second examination. It is important to specify what was done on each occasion. For the benefit of other experts relevant numerical data from tests should be provided in standard formats.

Weaknesses in reporting. Many reports read as though the writer has no expectation that the opinions therein will be queried, let alone taken apart with surgical precision by those adept at finding weaknesses in the reporting of facts and the sustainability or otherwise of the ensuing arguments.

With regard to the data there is often a failure to present the specific test information upon which certain, often crucial, opinions are made. On the other hand, findings may be reported which are not referred to at all or are dealt with only in passing. These may include facts which are difficult to incorporate into the general argument being made. It is well to state this at the outset. Those familiar with complex medical findings will not be surprised by the discovery of facts outside the principal diagnoses which find no ready explanation at the time of the specialist's examination but which are shown later to be of significance or whose significance is immediately apparent to others. The task of the expert is to give as complete a picture as possible, even to the extent of confessing ignorance as to the meaning of certain details. Lastly, much of the available test information may be condensed into summarizing scores such as Intelligence Quotients, Impairment Indices and the like without providing for the reader the components from which these are derived. Sometimes the provision of the component factual information might allow the parties to come closer to agreement.

Another common fault is to describe the individual's performance solely in terms of the population norms of the tests without due consideration for the relative standing of the individual should the injurious events not have occurred. The central issue for those assessing the situation from the legal point of view is an estimate of the nature and degree of any acquired deficit and its prognosis. There is also frequently a failure to provide information about the improvement or stability of deficits over time. Like other experts, neuropsychologists should resist moving outside their personal field of expertise, which in most cases does not include all aspects of their own broad subject let alone those of adjacent fields like neurology. The less-than-expert *expert* sometimes finds it difficult to say, 'I don't know'.

Courtroom performance

Communication skills. The nature of court proceedings is such that 'not only do expert witnesses need to provide evidence in their area of expertise, but also they must be expert at presenting their evidence' (Cooke 1990, p. 218). Even arguments and opinions which to the informed outsider may appear overwhelmingly in favour of a certain position may not win the day in court, '...the truth, even when we know what it is, will not always win out – the more credible witness will' (Goodwin Jones 1986, p. 14). This may happen even with the most able practitioner, but appropriate weighting is more likely to be given to evidence presented in a clear and comprehensible manner, '...one of the characteristics of the effective courtroom expert, the good forensic expert, is that he or she has acquired the skill of communicating technical matters clearly and relatively simply to a lay audience' (Freckelton 1987, p. 142). Those who have had the opportunity of prior lecturing, especially to adult education or similar 'lay' audiences, will be at a great advantage.

The need for the psychologist to develop courtroom skills was stressed by a working party of the *British Psychological Society* (Clark et al 1987). Many psychologists appear in court only infrequently, i.e. they have limited experience, which means that they are liable to be vulnerable to the rigorous cross-examination of skilled legal practitioners.

The language used should be clear and as free as possible from technical terms. It may be necessary at times to retain some technical terms but these should be explained in language that the average person can understand. The expert witness should also give some thought to expressions which may carry a different meaning in a technical sense from that employed in day-to-day usage.

The essence of good communication is to keep the audience always in mind. Outside the medico-legal setting, neuropsychological experts and others who are used to attending multidisciplinary meetings will have noticed how often some experts deliver lectures or scientific papers as though all the audience was from the same background as the speaker. In the court situation it is even more important for experts to spend time in preparation for a non-specialist audience.

Freckelton (1987) has described in detail not only the particular features in the language used by expert witnesses which may confuse jurors, but also other features which, by their very nature, may tend to alienate the hearer. These include syntactic complexity, e.g. lengthy sentences with subordinate clauses, the use of uncommon and foreign words, the use of the passive voice and of conditional terms.

A common gambit of cross-examiners is to attempt to force the witness to show loss of emotional control which may result in the hearer giving less weight to the witness's evidence. Experts should beware of being drawn into making emotionally charged, particularly hostile, statements though individuals will naturally vary in the force with which they deliver their responses, and a few clinicians are even more adept than most legal practitioners at this trial by combat.

Finally, those familiar with psychological studies of decision making may well be sceptical of all the effort put into examination and argument by numerous experts when decisions may be taken on personal grounds which have virtually nothing to do with logic and do not follow the forms of reasoning used by either legal or scientific practitioners. The way in which the expert presents the evidence, the witness's personal manner, charm, confident manner of speaking and similar factors may have much more effect than what the expert says.

Cross-examination. Cross-examination is at once the backbone of the adversarial system and the bugbear of many experts who differ enormously in their attitude to the process, many seeing its sole purpose as being to discredit the individual giving evidence, and there is a good deal of truth in this; '...(the aim is) to leave the jury with the impression that the expert witness's testimony is to be given very little weight and credibility' (Blau, 1984, p. 239). Only too often questioning in court reveals limitations of reputed experts' knowledge in the areas under question, inconsistencies in their arguments from the facts (usually centring around their examination of the cognitive or affective state of clients), and apparent inconsistencies; much of this can be attributed to incomplete preparation. Cooke (1990) points out that poor performance may not only devalue the individual expert but also influence courts about the value of psychological evidence in general. Many witnesses find the experience so traumatic that they avoid it thereafter at all costs.

Three main areas are usually the focus of cross-examination, though skilful examiners may not approach them as separate entities nor in any systematic way, at least until the latter part of the legal process. These are: (i) the adequacy of the individual as an expert; (ii) deficiencies in the factual evidence presented, usually the thoroughness of the expert's examination; and (iii) the credibility with which the opinions derived from the data can be accepted.

Careful preparation and prior discussion with counsel will help avoid inconsistencies in response to the questions likely to be posed and prevent the witness from making what appear to be contradictory statements, by which the less experienced may appear to discredit themselves.

In our own training programme for clinical neuropsychologists, the 'adversarial' system has been widely employed. During case presentations to the other trainees and supervisors the graduate is subjected to cross-examination by members of the group with regard to the adequacy of the history taking, the data elicited from the examination, and the opinions on the diagnosis or evaluation of deficits. This has proven worthwhile in getting postgraduate students to prepare material carefully and to argue cogently without going beyond the facts. In many instances, this *cross-examination* leads the professional to explore alternative hypotheses which arise as a result of questioning and it also encourages the examiners to form the habit of doing their own internal cross-examination of what they are about to give as opinion, i.e. to check how defensible is their stated position.

One of the most commonly used moves in downgrading neuropsychological opinion is for the cross-examiner to cite eminent authorities on the uncertain state of our knowledge in a particular area. In one sense, virtually any scientist can be made to agree that our knowledge of almost anything is far from complete, and such 'idealistic' statements can be heard at any interview with men of science, often accompanied by platitudes like 'the more we know the less we understand'.

Many examples of challenges on this basis are provided by Ziskin and Strauss (1988). To take one such example, they cite the authoritative work of Stuss and Benson (1984) on the functions of the frontal lobes. Our limited knowledge of the numerous and complex functions of what appear to be a number of separate functional areas in the frontal regions of the brain is stressed by these latter authorities, who say that current explanations of apparent frontal lobe function remain limited and vague. Ziskin and Faust would seem to suggest that this imperfect or restricted state of knowledge of an area should necessarily render statements about frontal lobe dysfunction valueless or virtually so.

Despite this accepted limitation of knowledge, clinicians and courts have to work in this imperfect state or world and lack of full understanding (whatever that may be) does not render useless all fact and opinion on the subject. In the case of frontal lobe damage, hundreds of papers on traumatic damage to the frontal parts of the brain in thousands of subjects attest to certain well-established consequences in the form of characteristic behavioural and personality changes which are not seen with damage to other parts of the brain, irrespective of whether we understand the mechanisms or not, and irrespective of whether scientists are able to nominate the nature of the functions served by the region or its components and connections. Moreover, it is also well established that such inimical changes, if still present after a certain lapse of time, are not likely to improve either spontaneously or with therapy. Such a state of affairs has grave implications for the injured individual's future and it is with issues such as this that courts are normally concerned. Doubt and imperfect knowledge at one level should not be taken to mean that all statements on the subject are questionable.

A different kind of ploy is to direct questions in such a way as to edge the respondent in the direction of clearly identifying with one side or the other, in other words being seen as another advocate and thereby losing the neutral position which is supposedly expected of an unbiased expert.

A variant of this tactic is to attempt to restrict the witness in some way, usually by requesting either 'yes' or 'no' to questions where the expert witness feels that further clarification is essential to an understanding of the complexity of the subject. The expert witness should become adept in serving the court's best interests, e.g. he may seek the judge's permission to expound or clarify issues within his expertise which are germane to the subject under discussion which would otherwise not be aired but which are deemed crucial to the court's understanding of the circumstances.

There may also be an attempt to argue that the claim for a certain deficit, as measured on one test, cannot be a stable deficit since the client passed a similar test for a second psychologist. Stability, it is argued, would be expected if the deficit was based on irreparable brain damage. The important thing here is to determine whether indeed the two tests measure the same function. Psychological tests are often complex in their composition: they may require the exercise of several different cognitive functions for their solution and thus they may be failed for any of a number of reasons by different individuals. Conversely, a person may be able to pass a test designed to assess and bearing the name of a certain function since, despite the fact that the person has permanently lost this function, the end result for the particular test may be reached through the use of a preserved function which is quite different from the function named. Conclusions based on tests in isolation may be quite misleading unless confirmatory checks are made. Inferences from a test about loss of a function are greatly strengthened by noting that a person fails on any test or task, whatever its name or nature, if the *particular function is necessary for its solution*.

It is not possible to cover all the specific challenges which may be encountered in cross-examination. Some appreciation of their extensive nature can be gained from studying the encyclopaedic work of Ziskin and Faust (1988), which provides an enormous storehouse of challenges for legal counsel to present to expert witnesses in psychology including neuropsychologists. The work provides lawyers and their advisers with two kinds of information: (i) the imperfect state of psychology and psychiatry in general; and (ii) details of weaknesses in arguments made from psychometric data.

Further information on forensic neuropsychology may be found in articles such as those of Farmer et al (1990) and Adams and Rankin (1996), or in textbooks, e.g. Doerr and Carlin (1991) and Valciukas (1995).

Training in neuropsychology

In 1958 Lashley, speaking of the relations between psychology and neurology, commented: 'I feel that for a synthesis of the two disciplines, individuals must be trained in both subjects. Collaboration in research or in thinking is useful after problems have been well sketched and organized, but for initiation of new thinking, I believe that it is necessary to have the material in one head. Something of value is likely to come out when you get two subjects combined in one brain…' (p. 18).

With the rapid recent evolution of neuropsychology in particular, it is highly unlikely that there will be any but a very few who would manage such a prodigious task but course designers should be encouraged to allow the possibility of trainees taking options which incorporate major conceptual features of other relevant disciplines. It is encouraging that at certain brain and behaviour conferences, it can be impossible to tell whether the speaker has received primary training in medicine or in psychology.

Finally, many years ago a psychologist coined the term 'the professional half-life' which he defined as that period of time when professionals become about half as effective as they would have been if they had kept abreast of advances in the subject. Even for the well trained and experienced there is a need for continuing education. Fortunately, this appears to be alive and well in clinical neuropsychology.

References

Abed R T, Fewtrell W D 1990 Delusional misidentification of familiar inanimate objects. British Journal of Psychiatry 157: 915–917

Adams R L, Rankin E J 1996 A practical guide to forensic neuropsychological evaluation and testimony. In: Adams R L, Parson O A, Culbertson J L et al (eds) Neuropsychology for clinical practice. American Psychological Association, New York

Anderson D N 1988 The delusion of inanimate doubles: implications for understanding the Capgras syndrome. British Journal of Psychiatry 153: 694–699

Ardila A, Rosseli M 1988 Temporal lobe involvement in Capgras syndrome. International Journal of Neuroscience 43: 219–224

Atwal S, Khan M H 1986 Coexistence of Capgras and its related syndromes. Australian and New Zealand Journal of Psychiatry 20: 496–498

Ball C, Exworthy T 1990 Capgras syndrome and town duplication. British Journal of Psychiatry 154: 889–890

Bauer R M 1984 Autonomic recognition of names and face: a neuropsychological application of the Guilty Knowledge Test. Neuropsychologia 22: 457–469

Benson D F, Gardner H, Meadows J C 1976 Reduplicative paramnesia. Neurology 26: 147–151

Berson R J 1983 Capgras' syndrome. American Journal of Psychiatry 140: 969–978

Bick P A 1984 The syndrome of intermetamorphosis. American Journal of Psychiatry 141: 588–589

Blau T H 1984 Your day in court. In: Blau T H (ed) The psychologist as expert witness. Wiley, New York

Bruce V, Young A W 1986 Understanding face recognition. British Journal of Psychology 77: 305–327

Burns A 1985 The oldest patient with Capgras syndrome. British Journal of Psychiatry 147: 719–720

Capgras J, Reboul-Lachaux J 1923 L'illusion des 'sosies' dans une délire systématise chronique. Bulletin de la Société Clinique de Médicine Mentale 2: 6–16

Caramazza A 1984 The logic of neuropsychological research and the problem of patient classification in aphasia. Brain and Language 21: 9–20
Caramazza A 1986 About drawing inferences about the structure of normal cognitive systems from the analysis of patterns of impaired performance. The case for single-patient studies. Brain and Cognition 5: 41–66
Christodoulou G N 1978 Syndrome of subjective doubles. American Journal of Psychiatry 135: 249–251
Christodoulou G N 1991 The delusional misidentification syndromes. British Journal of Psychiatry 159 (suppl 14): 65–69
Clark D F, Brittain P, Cooke D J, Hall J N, Litton R A 1987 Insurance and legal advice for psychologists. Bulletin of the British Psychological Society 40: 324–327
Coleman S M 1933 Misidentification and nonrecognition. Journal of Mental Science 79: 42–51
Colthart M, Sartori G, Job R (eds) 1987 The cognitive neuropsychology of language. Erlbaum, London
Cooke D 1990 Being an expert in court. The Psychologist 3: 216–221
Courbon P, Fail G 1927 Syndrome d'illusion de Frégoli et schizophrénie. Société Clinique de Médicine Mentale 15: 121–124
Courbon P, Tusques J 1932 Illusions d'intermetamorphoses et de charme. Annales Médico-psychologiques 90: 401–405
Crichton P, Lewis S 1990 Delusional misidentification, AIDS and the right hemisphere. British Journal of Psychiatry 157: 608–610
Cummings J L 1985 Clinical neuropsychiatry. Grune & Stratton, Orlando
Cummings J L, Trimble M R 1995 Concise guide to neuropsychiatry and behavioral neurology. American Psychiatric Press, Washington
Cutting J 1991 Delusional misidentification and the role of the right hemisphere in the appreciation of identity. British Journal of Psychiatry 159 (suppl 14): 70–75
Dally P, Gomez J 1979 Capgras: Case study and appraisal of psychopathology. British Journal of Medical Psychology 52: 556–564
Denes G, Bisiacchi P, Semenza C (eds) 1988 Perspectives in cognitive neuropsychology. Erlbaum, London
de Pauw K W, Szulecka T K 1988 Dangerous delusions: violence and the misidentification syndromes. British Journal of Psychiatry 152: 91–96
de Pauw K W, Szulecka T, Poltock T L 1987 Frégoli syndrome after cerebral infarction. Journal of Nervous and Mental Disease 175: 433–438
Diesfeldt H F, Troost D 1995 Delusional misidentification and subsequent dementia: a clinical and neuropathological study. Dementia 6: 94–98
Doerr H O, Carlin A S (eds) 1991 Forensic neuropsychology: Legal and scientific bases. Guildford, New York
Ellis H D 1994 The role of the right hemisphere in the Capgras syndrome. Psychopathology 27: 177–185
Ellis H D, Young A W 1988 Human cognitive neuropsychology. Erlbaum, Hillsdale, USA
Ellis H D, Young A W 1990 Accounting for delusional misrepresentations. British Journal of Psychiatry 157: 239–248
Ellis H D, dePauw K W, Christodoulou G N et al 1993 Responses to facial and non-facial stimuli presented tachistoscopically in either or both visual fields by patients with the Capgras delusion and paranoid schizophrenics. Journal of Neurology, Neurosurgery and Psychiatry 56: 215–219
Enoch M D, Trethowan W 1991 Uncommon psychiatric syndromes, 3rd edn. Butterworth-Heinemann, Oxford
Farmer R G et al 1990 Guidelines for the physician expert witness. Annals of Internal Medicine 113: 789
Faust D, Ziskin J 1988 The expert witness in psychology and psychiatry. Science 241: 31–35
Feinberg T E, Shapiro R M 1989 Misidentification-reduplication and the right hemisphere. Neuropsychiatry, Neuropsychology and Behavioral Neurology 2: 39–48
Fogel B S, Schiffer R B, Rao S M (eds) 1994 Neuropsychiatry. Williams & Wilkins, Baltimore
Forstl H, Almeida O P, Owens A M, Burns A, Howard R 1991a Psychiatric, neurological and medical aspects of misidentification syndromes: a review of 260 cases. Psychological Medicine 21: 905–910

Forstl H, Burns A, Jacoby R, Levy R 1991b Neuroanatomical correlates of clinical misidentification and misperception in senile dementia of the Alzheimer type. Journal of Clinical Psychiatry 52: 268–271

Forstl H, Besthorn C, Geiger-Kabisch C, Sattel H, Schreiter-Gasser U 1993 Psychotic features in the course of Alzheimer's disease: relationship to cognitive, electroencephalographic and computerized tomography findings. Acta Psychiatrica Scandinavica 87: 395–399

Forstl H, Besthorn C, Burns A, Geiger-Kabisch C, Levy R, Sattel A 1994a Delusional misidentification in Alzheimer's disease: a summary of clinical and biological aspects. Psychopathology 27: 194–199

Forstl H, Burns A, Levy R, Cairns N 1994b Neuropathological correlates of psychotic phenomena in confirmed Alzheimer's disease. British Journal of Psychiatry 165: 53–59

Fowler R D, Matarazzo J D 1988 Psychologists and psychiatrists as expert witnesses. Science 241: 1143–1144

Freckelton I R 1987 The trial of the expert: a study of expert evidence and forensic experts. Oxford University Press, Melbourne

Freckelton I R 1989 The trial of the expert. Australasian Forensic Psychiatry Bulletin (citation lost)

Fuller G N, Marshall A, Flint J, Lewis S, Wise R J 1993 Migraine madness: recurrent psychosis after migraine. Journal of Neurology, Neurosurgery and Psychiatry 56: 416–418

Goodwin Jones C 1986 Men of science v. men of law: Some comments on recent cases. Medicine, Science and the Law 26: 13–16

Greene E, Schooler J W, Loftus E F 1985 Expert psychological testimony. In: Kassin S N, Wrightsman C S (eds) The psychology of evidence and trial procedure. Sage, London

Gudjonsson G H 1985 Psychological evidence in court: Results from the BPS survey. Bulletin of the British Psychological Society 38: 327–330

Hampton J R, Harrison M J G, Mitchell J R A, Pritchard J S, Seymour C 1975 Relative contributions of history taking, physical examination, and laboratory investigation to diagnosis and management of medical out-patients. British Medical Journal ii: 486–489

Hart B 1912 The psychology of insanity. Cambridge University Press, London

Haas L J 1993 Competence and quality in the performance of forensic witnessing. Special issue, The ethics of expert witnessing. Ethics and Behavior 3: 223–229

Havard J 1983 Legislation is likely to cause more difficulties than it resolves. Journal of Medical Ethics 9: 18–20

Haward L 1981 Forensic psychology. Batsford, London

Hay D C, Young A W 1982 The human face. In: A Ellis (ed) Cognitive functions. Academic Press, New York

Hay G G 1986 Electroconvulsive therapy as a contributor to the production of delusional misidentification. British Journal of Psychiatry 148: 667–669

Hay G G, Jolley D J, Jones R G 1974 A case of the Capgras syndrome with pseudo-hypoparathyroidism. Acta Psychiatrica Scandinavica 50: 73

Hebb D O 1958 Alice in Wonderland or psychology among the biological sciences. In: Harlow H F, Woolsey C N (eds) Biological and biochemical bases of behavior. University of Wisconsin Press, Madison

Hier D B, Gorelick P B, Shindler A G 1987 Topics in behavioral neurology and neuropsychology. Butterworths, London

Hill D 1964 The bridge between neurology and psychiatry. Lancet 1: 509–514

Joseph A B 1986 Focal nervous system abnormalities in patients with misidentification syndromes. Bibliotheca Psychiatrica 164: 68–79

Joseph R 1996 Neuropsychiatry, neuropsychology and clinical neuroscience. Williams & Wilkins, Baltimore

Kapur N, Turner A, King C 1988 Reduplicative paramnesia: possible anatomical and neuropsychological mechanisms. Journal of Neurology, Neurosurgery and Psychiatry 51: 579–581

Kassin S M, Wrightsman L S 1988 The American jury on trial. Hemisphere, New York

Kertesz A (ed) 1983a Localization in neuropsychology. Academic Press, New York

Kertesz A 1983b Issues in localization In: Kertesz A (ed) Localization in neuropsychology. Academic Press, New York

Kiriakos R, Ananth J 1980 Review of 13 cases of Capgras syndrome. American Journal of Psychiatry 137: 1605–1607
Kirshner H S 1986 Behavioral neurology. A practical approach. Churchill Livingstone, New York
Kolpan K I 1986 Medicolegal issues. Journal of Head Trauma Rehabilitation 1: 79–80
Kosslyn S M 1987 Seeing and imaging in the cerebral hemispheres. Psychological Review 94: 148–175
Lashley K 1958 Cerebral organization and behavior. Research Publications, Association for Research in Nervous and Mental Disease 36: 1–18
Lees A J 1988 Editorial. Behavioural Neurology 1: 1–2
Lewis S W 1987 Brain imaging in a case of Capgras' syndrome. British Journal of Psychiatry 150: 170–171
Lipkin B 1988 Capgras syndrome heralding the development of dementia. British Journal of Psychiatry 153: 117–118
Lishman W A 1987 Organic psychiatry: the psychological consequences of cerebral disorder, 2nd edn. Blackwell Scientific, Oxford
Lishman W A 1992 Neuropsychiatry. A delicate balance. Psychosomatics 33: 4–9
Lishman W A 1995 Psychiatry and neuropathology: the maturing of a relationship. Journal of Neurology, Neuropsychology and Psychiatry 58: 284–292
Loftus E F 1983 Silence is not golden. American Psychologist 38: 564–572
McCarthy R A, Warrington E K 1987 The double dissociation of short-term memory for lists and sentences. Brain 110: 1545–1563
McCarthy R A, Warrington E K 1990 Cognitive neuropsychology: a clinical introduction. Academic Press, San Diego
McShane J, Dockrell J, Wells A 1992 Psychology and cognitive neuroscience. The Psychologist 6: 252–255
Malloy P, Cimino C, Westlake R 1992 Differential diagnosis of primary and secondary Capgras delusions. Neuropsychiatry, Neuropsychology and Behavioral Neurology 5: 83–96
Margolin D I (ed) 1992 Cognitive neuropsychology in clinical practice. Oxford University Press, New York
Mason J K 1984 New hope for expert evidence. Bulletin of the Royal College of Pathologists 43: 3–4
Mason J K 1986 Expert evidence in the adversarial system of criminal justice. Medicine, Science and the Law 26: 8–12
Meier M J 1987 Continuing education: An alternative to respecialization in clinical neuropsychology. The Clinical Neuropsychologist 1: 9–20
Mendez M F 1992 Delusional misidentification of persons in dementia. British Journal of Psychiatry 160: 414–416
Mendez M F, Martin R J, Smyth K A, Whitehouse P J 1992 Disturbances of person identification in Alzheimer's disease. A retrospective study. Journal of Nervous and Mental Disease 180: 94–96
Merrin E L, Silberfarb P M 1976 The Capgras phenomenon. Archives of General Psychiatry 33: 965–968
Mesulam M-M 1981 A cortical network for directed attention and unilateral neglect. Annals of Neurology 10: 309–325
Mesulam M-M 1985 Principles of behavioral neurology. Davis, Philadelphia
Miller L 1986 'Narrow localizationalism' in psychiatric neuropsychology. Psychological Medicine 16: 729–734
Mojtabai R 1994 Frégoli syndrome. Australian and New Zealand Journal of Psychiatry 6: 94–98
Molchan S E, Martinez R A, Lawlor B A, Grafman J H, Sunderland T 1990 Reflections of the self: atypical misidentification and delusional syndromes in two patients with Alzheimer's disease. British Journal of Psychiatry 157: 605–608
Murray J R 1936 A case of Capgras's syndrome in the male. Journal of Mental Science 82: 63–66
Ormrod R F 1972 Evidence and proof: scientific and legal. Medicine, Science and the Law 12: 9–20

Pick A 1903 Reduplicative paramnesia. Brain 26: 260–267
Rapcsak S Z, Polster M R, Comer J F, Rubens A B 1994 False recognition and misidentification of faces following right hemisphere damage. Cortex 30: 565–583
Rastogi F C 1990 A variant of Capgras syndrome with substitution of inanimate objects. British Journal of Psychiatry 156: 883–884
Reynolds E H, Trimble M R (eds) 1989 The bridge between neurology and psychiatry. Churchill Livingstone, London
Riddoch M J, Humphreys G W 1994 Cognitive neuropsychology and cognitive rehabilitation. Erlbaum, Hove, England
Sales B D, Shuman D W 1993 Reclaiming the integrity of science in expert witnessing. Special issue, The ethics of expert witnessing. Ethics and Behavior 3: 223–229
Sartori G 1988 From neuropsychological data to theory and vice versa. In: Denes G, Bisiacchi P, Semenza C (eds) Perspectives in cognitive neuropsychology. Erlbaum, London, ch 3
Semenza C, Bisiacchi P, Rosental V 1988 A function for cognitive neuropsychology. In: Denes G, Bisiacchi P, Semenza C (eds) Perspectives in cognitive neuropsychology. Erlbaum, London, ch 1
Shallice T 1979 Case-study approach in neuropsychology. Journal of Clinical Neuropsychology 1: 183–211
Shallice T 1988 From neuropsychology to mental structure. Cambridge University Press, Cambridge
Shapiro M B 1966 The single case in clinical-psychological research. Journal of General Psychology 74: 3–23
Shapiro M B 1973 Intensive assessment of the single case. In: Mettler P E (ed) The psychological assessment of mental and physical handicaps. Tavistock Publications, London
Shapiro M B, Litman G K, Nias D K B, Hendry E R 1973 A clinician's approach to experimental research. Journal of Clinical Psychology 29: 165–169
Signer S F 1987 Capgras syndrome: the delusion of substitution. Journal of Clinical Psychiatry 48: 147–150
Signer S F 1994 Localization and lateralization in the delusion of substitution. Capgras symptom and its variants. Psychopathology 27: 168–176
Silva J A, Leong G B 1992 The Capgras syndrome in paranoid schizophrenia. Psychopathology 25: 147–153
Silva J A, Leong G B, Shaner A L 1991 Syndrome of intermetamorphosis. Psychopathology 24: 158–165
Silva J A, Leong G B, Wine D B, Saab S 1992 Evolving misidentification syndromes and facial recognition deficits. Canadian Journal of Psychiatry 37: 574–576
Silva J A, Leong G B, Weinstock R, Wine D B 1993a Delusional misidentification and dangerousness: a neurobiologic hypothesis. Journal of Forensic Science 38: 904–913
Silva J A, Leong G B, Wine D B 1993b Misidentification delusions, facial misrecognition, and right brain injury. Canadian Journal of Psychiatry 38: 239–241
Silva J A, Leong G B, Garza-Trevino E S et al 1994a A cognitive model of dangerous delusional misidentification syndromes. Journal of Forensic Science 39: 1455–1467
Silva J A, Leong G B, Weinstock R, Sharma K K, Klein R L 1994b Delusional misidentification syndromes and dangerousness. Psychopathology 27: 215–219
Silva J A, Leong G B, Weinstock R, Klein R L 1995 Psychiatric factors associated with dangerous misidentification delusions. Bulletin of the American Academy of Psychiatry 23: 53–61
Silver J M, Yudovsky S C, Hales R E (eds) 1994 Neuropsychiatry of traumatic brain injury. American Psychiatric Press, Washington
Sims A (ed) 1991 Delusions and awareness of reality. The 4th Leeds psychopathology symposium. British Journal of Psychiatry 159 (suppl 14): 5–112
Sperlich P W 1985 The evidence on evidence. Science and law in conflict and cooperation. In: Kassin S N, Wrightsman L S (eds) The psychology of evidence and trial procedure. Sage, London, pp 325–361
Staton R D, Brumback R A, Wilson H 1982 Reduplicative paramnesia: a disconnection syndrome. Cortex 18: 23–36
Stuss D T, Benson D F 1984 The frontal lobes. Raven, New York

Taylor M A 1988 An introductory statement. Neuropsychiatry, Neuropsychology and Behavioral Neurology 1: 1–2
Thomson M I, Silk K R, Hover G L 1980 Misidentification of a city: delimiting criteria for Capgras syndrome. American Journal of Psychiatry 137: 1270–1272
Todd J 1957 The syndrome of Capgras. Psychiatric Quarterly 31: 250–265
Trimble M R 1981 Post-traumatic syndrome. Journal of the Royal Society of Medicine 74: 940–941
Tzavaras A, Luauté J-P, Bidault E 1986 Face recognition dysfunction and delusional misidentification syndromes. In: Ellis H D, Jeeves M A, Young A (eds) Aspects of face processing. Martinus Nijhoff, Dordrecht
Valciukas J A 1995 Forensic neuropsychology: Conceptual foundations and clinical practice. Haworth, New York
Van Lancker D 1991 Personal relevance and the right hemisphere. Brain and Cognition 17: 64–92
Vié J 1930 Un trouble de l'identification des personnes. Annales Medico-Psychologiques 88: 214–237
Vié J 1944 Les Méconnaissances systématiques. Annales Médico-psychologiques 102: 229–252
Walsh K W 1991 Understanding brain damage. A primer of neuro-psychological evaluation, 2nd edn. Churchill Livingstone, Edinburgh
Walsh K W 1992 Some gnomes worth knowing. The Clinical Neuropsychologist 6: 119–133
Walsh K W 1995 A hypothesis-testing approach to assessment. In: Mapou R L, Spector J (eds) Neuropsychological assessment of cognitive function. Plenum, New York
Warrington E K 1984 The Recognition Memory Test NFER. Nelson, Windsor
Weinstein E A, Kahn R L, Sugarman L A 1952 Phenomenon of reduplication. Archives of Neurology and Psychiatry 67: 808–814
Weston M J, Whitlock F A 1971 The Capgras syndrome following head injury. British Journal of Psychiatry 119: 25–31
Whitby P 1990 Assumed usefulness. The Psychologist 3: 308–310
Wright S, Young A W, Hellewell D J 1993 Frégoli delusion and erotomania. Journal of Neurology, Neurosurgery and Psychiatry 56: 322–323
Young A W 1992 Face recognition impairments. Philosophical Transactions of the Royal Society of London. B Biological Sciences 335: 47–54
Young A W, Ellis H D 1989 Handbook of research on face processing. Amsterdam, North Holland
Young A W, Ellis H D, Szulecka T K et al 1990 Face processing impairments and delusional misidentification. Behavioral Neurology 3: 153–168
Young A W, Reid I, Wright S, Hellawell D J 1993 Face processing impairments and the Capgras delusion. British Journal of Psychiatry 162: 695–698
Yudovsky S C, Hales R E 1992 (eds) American Psychiatric Press Textbook of neuropsychiatry. American Psychiatric Press, Washington
Yudovsky S C, Hales R E (eds) 1994 Synopsis of neuropsychiatry. American Psychiatric Press, Washington
Ziskin J, Faust D 1988 Coping with psychiatric and psychological testimony. Law and Psychology Press, Venice, California, vols 1–3
Zurif E B, Gardner H, Brownell H H 1989 The case against group studies. Brain and Cognition 10: 237–255

Index